Textbook of
URORADIOLOGY
Second Edition

Textbook of
URORADIOLOGY

Second Edition

N. Reed Dunnick, M.D.
Professor and Chair
Department Radiology
University of Michigan
Ann Arbor, Michigan

Carl M. Sandler, M.D.
Professor of Radiology and Surgery (Urology)
Vice Chair, Department of Radiology
University of Texas Medical School at Houston
Chief, Radiology Service
Lyndon B. Johnson General Hospital
Adjunct Professor of Radiology
Baylor College of Medicine
Houston, Texas

E. Stephen Amis, Jr., M.D.
Professor and Chairman
Department of Radiology
Albert Einstein College of Medicine
Montefiore Medical Center
The Bronx, New York

Jeffrey H. Newhouse, M.D.
Professor of Radiology
Director of Abdominal Imaging
Department of Radiology
Columbia-Presbyterian Medical Center
New York, New York

With contributions from the First Edition by
Ronald W. McCallum, M.B., FRCP (C), FACR
Professor Emeritus of Radiology
University of Toronto
St. Michael's Hospital
Toronto, Ontario, Canada

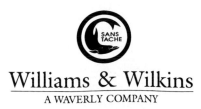

Williams & Wilkins
A WAVERLY COMPANY

BALTIMORE • PHILADELPHIA • LONDON • PARIS • BANGKOK
BUENOS AIRES • HONG KONG • MUNICH • SYDNEY • TOKYO • WROCLAW

Editor: *Charles W. Mitchell*
Managing Editor: *Marjorie Kidd Keating*
Production Coordinator: *Marette Magargle-Smith*
Typesetter: *Peirce Graphic Services, Inc.*
Printer & Binder: *RR Donnelley & Sons Company*

ISBN 0-683-02697-6

90000

9 780683 026979

351 West Camden Street
Baltimore, Maryland 21201-2436 USA

Rose Tree Corporate Center
1400 North Providence Road
Building II, Suite 5025
Media, Pennsylvania 19063-2043 USA

Accurate indications, adverse reactions and dosage schedules for drugs are provided in this book, but it is possible that they may change. The reader is urged to review the package information data of the manufacturers of the medications mentioned.

Printed in the United States of America

First Edition,

Library of Congress Cataloging-in-Publication Data

Textbook of uroradiology / N. Reed Dunnick . . . [et al.]. — 2nd ed.
   p.   cm.
  Prev. ed. cataloged under Dunnick.
  Includes bibliographical references and index.
  ISBN 0-683-02697-6
  1. Genitourinary organs—Radiography. 2. Genitourinary organs—Diseases—Diagnosis. I. Dunnick, N. Reed.
   [DNLM: 1. Urologic Diseases—radiography. 2. Genital Diseases, Male—radiography. 3. Urography. WJ 141 T355
1997]
RC874.D86 1997
616.6'0757—dc20
DNLM/DLC
for Library of Congress
                                                   96-14722
                                                      CIP

The publishers have made every effort to trace the copyright holders for borrowed material. If they have inadvertently overlooked any, they will be pleased to make the necessary arrangements at the first opportunity.

To purchase additional copies of this book, call our customer service department at **(800) 638-0672** or fax orders to **(800) 447-8438.** For other book services, including chapter reprints and large quantity sales, ask for the Special Sales department.

Canadian customers should call **(800) 268-4178,** or fax **(905) 470-6780.** For all other calls originating outside of the United States, please call **(410) 528-4223** or fax us at **(410) 528-8550.**

Visit Williams & Wilkins on the Internet: http://www.wwilkins.com or contact our customer service department at **custserv@wwilkins.com.** Williams & Wilkins customer service representatives are available from 8:30 am to 6:00 pm, EST, Monday through Friday, for telephone access.

97 98 99
1 2 3 4 5 6 7 8 9 10

This book is dedicated to our residents who

inspired us to present this material in an easily readable text,

and to our families whose patience and understanding made it possible.

Preface to the *Second Edition*

In the fall of 1990, two new books on radiology of the urinary tract were published. *Essentials of Uroradiology* by E. Stephen Amis, Jr. and Jeffrey H. Newhouse was aimed primarily at radiology residents; it attempted to impart the scope of adult uroradiology that needed to be mastered prior to completion of training. *Textbook of Uroradiology* had very similar goals; it was intended to be read in its entirety and thus to be attractive to both radiology and urology residents. It was also hoped that physicians in practice would find the book sufficiently comprehensive for daily practice yet not be overwhelmed with the encyclopedic information found in reference texts. The authors sought to keep *Textbook of Uroradiology* to a manageable size by applying the standard "what one ought to know, rather than what there is to know" when deciding how much material to include. Both books met their goals and were well accepted by readers and book reviewers alike.

Dr. Ronald McCallum decided to retire after the publication of *Textbook of Uroradiology,* so the initial planning of a revision for *Textbook of Uroradiology* was undertaken by Drs. Dunnick and Sandler while Drs. Amis and Newhouse considered a revision of *Essentials of Uroradiology.* It became apparent that separate revisions would create considerable overlap since our original goals had been similar; an amalgamation of both books would allow the best elements of the first editions of each of the works to be retained. The four of us quickly agreed to undertake this project as a joint effort and that the new edition would retain the title, organization, and design elements of *Textbook of Uroradiology.* Dr. Newhouse was instrumental in gaining permission from Little, Brown & Co. so that material previously published in *Essentials of Uroradiology* could be used in the revised *Textbook of Uroradiology.*

We hope that the resultant text achieves our goal of combining the best features of both works. The authors are all members of the Society of Uroradiology, are intimately involved in residency training programs and are actively practicing uroradiologists. We have made a conscious decision to expand those elements of the book that facilitate learning by trainees but have retained a level of comprehensiveness such that practicing radiologists will find *Textbook of Uroradiology* useful as a reference in daily practice. We have added illustrations, line drawings, and tables. We have retained the basic chapter organization of the first edition but have moved the chapters on medical renal disease and renal transplantation forward. The chapter on interventional techniques has been incorporated into Chapter 3, and all of the material on the urinary bladder has been consolidated into one chapter.

We hope that the revised *Textbook of Uroradiology* will achieve a level of acceptance similar to our first effort.

N. Reed Dunnick
Carl M. Sandler
E. Stephen Amis, Jr.
Jeffrey H. Newhouse

Preface to the First Edition

Our goal in producing *Textbook of Uroradiology* was to provide both the practicing radiologist and the radiology resident with a comprehensive, single-volume text that integrates all aspects of adult uroradiology. In order that the book be kept to a manageable size, the standard, "what one ought to know" rather than "what there is to know," was applied.

In any work of this type, there are many arbitrary decisions as to the material to be included and as to the placement of that material. We have presented the material on the anatomy, embryology, and congenital anomalies of the urinary tract as one unit because these topics are so interrelated that to disseminate this material in several different chapters would diminish the readers' ability to understand these important relationships. Chapter 3 provides an overview of the diagnostic imaging techniques that are discussed throughout the remainder of the book. Contrast material, which is fundamental to the practice of uroradiology, is included as Chapter 4. The remainder of the chapters have been divided into those dealing with various types of renal pathology (i.e., vascular disease, inflammatory disease, etc.), those dealing with anatomic regions of the urinary tract (i.e., adrenal gland, bladder, etc.), and topics that seemed best treated as a whole (i.e., trauma and transplantation).

The placement of material related to interventional uroradiology was especially problematic. For the most part, interventional topics have been placed adjacent to the material dealing with the underlying pathologic conditions for which the procedure is indicated. Thus, abscess drainage is discussed along with renal inflammatory disease, ureteral stenting with the ureter, and percutaneous stone extraction with stone disease. A separate interventional chapter has been included to provide a discussion of percutaneous nephrostomy and percutaneous biopsy as well as a general overview of these procedures.

This work represents the equal efforts of three practicing uroradiologists. Each of us reviewed and critiqued all of the material, and thus we decided not to assign authorship to any of the individual chapters.

Although *Textbook of Uroradiology* is intended to serve as a source of information about uroradiology for practicing radiologists and radiology residents, we believe that urologists, general surgeons, and nephrologists will also find the book useful. We hope it has been written in such a clear and succinct manner that it will not only be used as a reference source, but that it will also be read in its entirety.

N. Reed Dunnick
Ronald W. McCallum
Carl M. Sandler

Acknowledgments

We gratefully acknowledge the many contributions of individuals at our respective institutions as well as the highly skilled professionals at Williams & Wilkins who made this book possible.

At the University of Michigan, Bob Combs provided many high quality prints for reproduction. Anita Demario flawlessly converted pages of scribbled handwriting to readable text and painstakingly reformatted the entire manuscript into the publisher's format.

Case material was provided by Drs. Ted Dubinsky, Akira Kawashima, H. R. Parvey, Bharat Raval, Nabil Maklad, and Stanford Goldman at the University of Texas Medical School at Houston. Jay Johnson and Dan Klepac provided photographic support while Miriam Ullmann provided valuable research assistance. Katie Isch helped to coordinate all of these activities as well as supply secretarial support.

At the Albert Einstein College of Medicine, Renata Gobbo provided secretarial assistance and manuscript preparation while Eleanor Murphy was responsible for coordinating the photographic work.

Additional images were provided by Drs. Judith Fayter and Rashid Fawwaz from Columbia-Presbyterian Medical Center. Karen Hackney cheerfully typed more revisions than any decisive author would have generated.

Ronald W. McCallum, M.B., F.R.C.P.(C), F.A.C.R., has been an inspiration to all of us. This project had its origin in discussions between Dr. McCallum and Williams and Wilkins. In the preparation of the second edition, we missed his knowledge, experience, wisdom, and pithy comments as we wrestled with controversial topics and struggled to present detailed information in a readable text.

Finally, we would like to thank our wives, Marilyn, Susan, Anne, and Nancy, and our families, for tolerating the nights and weekends we worked on this manuscript.

N.R.D.
C.M.S.
E.S.A.
J.H.N.

Contents

1

Anatomy and Embryology

ANATOMY

Kidney

The kidneys are paired, retroperitoneal structures that parallel the psoas muscle on either side of the lumbar spine. The left kidney is usually slightly higher than the right and is slightly more medially located. The vertical axis of the kidneys is approximately 20°, with the top of the kidneys closer to the spine. There is often considerable motility of each kidney, which varies with respiration and with body position; several centimeters of excursion may be demonstrated on deep inspiration or in the upright position.

The kidney is composed of a variable number of structural units known as the renal pyramids. Each pyramid consists of a minor calyx and its associated papillary ducts. The base of the pyramid is formed by its overlying renal cortex, and its apex is formed by the renal papilla, which projects into the renal sinus. The papillae are cone-shaped structures that contain the openings of the distal collecting ducts (the ducts of Bellini), which empty into the minor calyces. The peripheral portion of the minor calyx is called the fornix and projects slightly above the central papillary portion; this appearance is responsible for the cup-like configuration of a normal minor calyx. The minor calyces are arranged into three groups: an upper group, a middle or interpolar group, and a lower group. Each group contains anterior and posterior calyces. On urography, anterior calyces are generally projected en face, whereas the posteriorly located calyces are seen in profile. Four to six minor calyces come together to form a major ca-

lyx or infundibulum; these join together to form the renal pelvis.

On cut surface, the kidney may be divided into two discrete regions: the outer cortex and the inner medulla. The arcuate artery at the base of each pyramid marks the junction between the cortex and the medulla. The cortex overlying each pyramid is sometimes known as the *centrilobar cortex*. Columns of cortical tissue, however, may be found between each pyramid. These columns have been termed the septal cortex, but they are more commonly referred to as the columns of Bertin or Bertini. The minor calyces, the infundibulae, and the renal pelvis are jointly referred to as the *renal collecting system*. The renal sinus surrounds the collecting system and is filled with a variable amount of fat.

The kidneys and their surrounding fascial covering, Gerota's fascia, define the boundaries of the retroperitoneum (Fig. 1.1). The retroperitoneum is divided into three discrete compartments: the anterior pararenal space, the perirenal space, and the posterior pararenal space.

The anterior pararenal space extends from the posterior portion of the peritoneal cavity to the anterior layer of Gerota's fascia. The anterior pararenal space contains the pancreas, the second through fourth portions of the duodenum, the ascending and descending colon, and the hepatic and splenic arteries. Laterally, the posterior layer of peritoneum and the anterior layer of Gerota's fascia merge into the lateroconal fascia.

The perirenal space is defined by the anterior and posterior layers of the perirenal fascia. The two layers of perirenal fascia are usually fused in the midline, then open to surround the kidney, the adrenal gland, and the proximal ureter, and finally fuse again to merge into the lateroconal fascia laterally. The perinephric space, as defined by the perirenal fascia, is cone shaped and filled with perinephric fat. The perinephric space is open at its top where it extends to the diaphragm and becomes progressively smaller inferiorly where it communicates through its open end with the pelvic extraperitoneal space. The ureter passes into the pelvic extraperitoneal space through this open end. Recent evidence from cadaver dissections suggests that the renal fasciae fuse to create an anatomic barrier to disease extension between the perinephric space and the extraperitoneal pelvis.

The posterior pararenal space is defined anteriorly by the posterior layer of the perirenal fascia (Zuckerkandl's

1

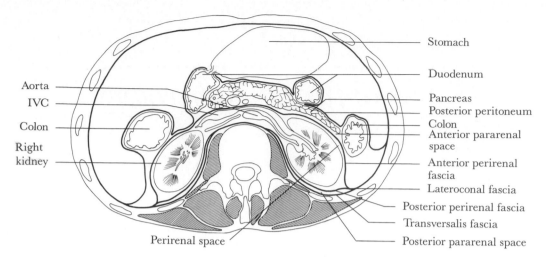

Aorta
IVC
Colon
Right kidney

Stomach
Duodenum
Pancreas
Posterior peritoneum
Colon
Anterior pararenal space
Anterior perirenal fascia
Lateroconal fascia
Posterior perirenal fascia
Transversalis fascia
Posterior pararenal space

Perirenal space

Figure 1.1.   Retroperitoneal anatomy. Note the potential for communication between the right and left perirenal spaces across the midline. IVC = inferior vena cava. (From Amis ES Jr, Newhouse JH: *Essentials of Uroradiology.* Boston, Little, Brown & Co, 1991.)

layer) and posteriorly by the fascia that covers the psoas and quadratus lumborum muscles. The posterior pararenal space contains no organs. Laterally, it merges into the transversalis fascia; thus, the fat in the posterior pararenal space communicates with the properitoneal fat of the anterior abdominal wall. The fat between the lateroconal fascia and the transversalis fascia is continuous with the fat in the posterior pararenal space; laterally, it is known as the "flank stripe." The posterior space is quite small at the level of the kidneys as the posterior layer of Gerota's fascia inserts on the quadratus lumborum at this level; inferiorly, it extends more medially to insert on the psoas muscle itself.

Unlike the retroperitoneum, the pelvic extraperitoneal space is not truly anatomically divided; however, it often is classified into four potential spaces for descriptive purposes: (*a*) the space of Retzius (the anterior extraperitoneal space) between the symphysis pubis and the bladder; (*b*) the retrovesicle space between the rectum and the bladder; (*c*) the presacral space between the rectum and the sacrum; and (*d*) the perirectal space that surrounds the rectum. The functional anatomy of the kidney is discussed in Chapter 4 and the vascular anatomy is described in Chapter 8.

Ureter

The ureter is a muscular conduit that transports urine from the renal pelvis to the bladder. It begins at the ureteropelvic junction, which is usually a gentle tapering of the pelvis to join the ureter. The ureter remains retroperitoneal throughout its course, extending from lateral to medial across the psoas muscle. At its most anterior portion, the ureter crosses anterior to the common or external iliac artery. The ureter then passes posteroinferiorly to enter the pelvis and courses laterally before entering the posterolateral aspect of the bladder wall.

The ureters enter the bladder obliquely, tunneling for approximately 2 cm in the muscular wall before emptying into the bladder lumen at the trigone. The ureterovesical junction is the narrowest portion of the ureter.

The ureter is composed of mucosal, muscular, and adventitial layers. The mucosa is covered by transitional epithelium that is continuous with that of the renal pelvis proximally and the bladder distally. When the ureter is empty, the mucosa collapses into longitudinal folds.

The muscular layer has both circular and longitudinal muscle fibers separated by fibroareolar connective tissue. In the distal ureter, longitudinal muscle fibers continue in the intravesical portion of the ureter and decussate with muscles of the trigone.

The distal ureter has both a superficial and a deep periureteral sheath that is derived from the bladder. A plane of cleavage containing loose connective tissue provides mobility for the intravesical ureter. The outer or adventitial layer is composed of fibrous tissue that blends with this outer sheath of the ureter.

The normal resting pressure of 8 to 15 mm Hg within the bladder compresses and closes the ureter. During peristalsis, pressures of 20 to 35 mm Hg are sufficient to propel a bolus of urine from the ureter into the bladder. The length of the intramural ureter and the configuration of the longitudinal muscle that inserts into the trigone are critical to the prevention of reflux.

The ureter receives arterial supply from many sources. The renal arteries provide branches to the renal pelvis and proximal ureter. The aorta, lumbar, gonadal, and iliac arteries supply the midportion of the ureter. The predominant vessel supplying the distal ureter is the inferior vesical artery. The uterine artery often sends branches to the ureter in females.

Urine is moved from the kidney to the bladder primarily by peristalsis, although gravity does play a small role as well. Contractions begin in the calyces and propel urine toward the renal pelvis. These contractions are propagated in the renal pelvis, although they contribute relatively little to urine flow. Most of the urine enters the ureter during the resting phase, when the renal pelvis and ureter are in open communication.

Ureteral peristalsis results from the continuation of peristaltic waves initiated in the intrarenal collecting system and propagated into the renal pelvis. Stretching of the renal pelvis or ureteropelvic junction also contributes to the initiation of peristaltic activity. Increases in urine flow and ureteral distention increase the frequency of peristaltic contractions.

Bladder

The bladder is a hollow pelvic viscera consisting of smooth muscle, lamina propria, submucosa, and mucosa. The muscle is the detrusor muscle and consists of three layers: an inner longitudinal, a middle circular, and an outer longitudinal layer. Each layer is closely applied to the other without separating laminae or fascia. The detrusor body is expandable and rises higher in the pelvis as it fills with urine. The three muscle layers condense inferiorly to form the trigone or bladder base plate. The ureters enter the bladder at the posterior aspect of the trigone. Between the ureteric orifices is a muscular ridge, the interureteric ridge, at the posterior aspect of the trigone. Outer longitudinal muscle fibers extend inferiorly to the undersurface of the base plate and may contribute to the opening of the bladder neck when the detrusor muscle contracts during voiding. There is, however, a separate circular smooth muscle sphincter at the bladder neck, the internal sphincter.

The adult bladder lies deep in the pelvis when empty, but flexibility of the detrusor muscle fibers allows the bladder walls and dome to rise high in the pelvis when the bladder is full. The flexibility of the bladder is, however, limited because it is firmly fixed in position. The allantois obliterates to become the middle umbilical ligament. Obliterated umbilical arteries form lateral umbilical ligaments that attach the bladder to the anterior abdominal wall. The puboprostatic ligament extends from the pubic bone to the prostate gland and contributes fibers to the anteroinferior aspects of the bladder. Posteriorly, the rectovesical ligaments represent condensations of Denonvilliers' fascia, which is a double-layered fascia separating the bladder and urethra from the rectum and anus. The external longitudinal smooth muscle fibers of the detrusor muscle contribute muscle fiber insertions into the puboprostatic and rectovesical ligaments. The trigone is triangular in shape, with the base at the interureteric ridge and the apex anteriorly, extending around the urethral orifice or bladder neck to form the bundle of His.

The bladder dome and proximal one third of the lateral walls are loosely covered by the peritoneum. When the bladder is empty, the peritoneum extends deep to the pelvis; when the bladder is full, the peritoneum is elevated. The male bladder is adjacent to the rectum posteriorly, the ampulla of the vas deferens and seminal vesicles posteroinferiorly, and the prostate base inferiorly. In the female, the uterus and vagina lie inferiorly and posteriorly to the bladder, and the fallopian tubes, fimbria, and ovaries lie laterally and superiorly to the empty bladder. Anteriorly, the space of Retzius lies between the anterior bladder wall and the posterior aspect of the symphysis pubis.

The blood supply of the bladder originates from the hypogastric arteries with branches that supply the bladder dome; the superior, posterior, and anterior parts of the walls (superior vesical artery); the middle parts of the lateral, posterior, and anterior walls (middle vesical artery); and the inferior, posterior, and lateral bladder walls and the trigone (inferior vesical artery). Additional arterial blood may come from branches of the obturator artery, the vas deferens artery, and the inferior gluteal artery. In the female, additional branches from the uterine and vaginal arteries may supply the lateral and inferior bladder walls. Capillaries from these supply arteries form a rich arterial network around the bladder. Consequently, there is a rich vesical venous plexus that surrounds the bladder and flows directly into the hypogastric (internal iliac) veins. Auxiliary veins connect the vesical venous plexus to the hemorrhoidal veins that drain into the intervertebral venous plexus. This is the route of vesical venous drainage when the inferior vena cava is blocked. In addition, a rich network of vesical lymphatics drain into the internal and external iliac nodes, with continued drainage into the common iliac and paraaortic nodes.

The nerve supply to the bladder is from the autonomic system. The parasympathetic nerves (the pelvic nerves) are motor to bladder function and are responsible for the micturition reflex arc (S2–S4) and for the emptying of the bladder. The sympathetic (hypogastric) nerves also supply the bladder and internal and intrinsic urethral sphincters. Sympathetic stimulation initiates α- and β-receptors within smooth muscle. Sympathetic stimulation of β-receptors causes smooth muscle relaxation, whereas stimulation of α-receptors stimulates smooth muscle contraction.

The bladder body is rich in β-receptors. During bladder filling, receptor sympathetic stimulation causes detrusor relaxation. The internal sphincter at the bladder neck is rich in α-receptors, and causes contraction of the bladder neck sphincter. Consequently, bladder filling and retention of urine in the bladder is the result of sympathetic activity. When the bladder is fully stretched, receptors in the detrusor muscle stimulate the parasympathetic and micturition reflex arc to activity, causing motor activity in the parasympathetic pelvic nerves, resulting in reciprocal reduction of sympathetic activity and relaxation of the smooth muscle sphincters to allow voiding. Voluntary relaxation of the striated external sphincter and pelvic floor muscles under the voluntary and reflex activity of the pudendal nerves (S2–S4) also allows normal voiding. Any abnormal activity of the parasympathetic, sympathetic, or pudendal nerve results in an abnormal voiding pattern such as that found in patients with a neurogenic bladder.

The bladder mucosa is composed of transitional cells and contains pain receptors. The mucosa is more sensitive to extreme temperature changes than to pain. The instillation of ice-cold water into the bladder stimulates detrusor contraction. Afferent pain and temperature impulses are conveyed via the parasympathetic (pelvic) and sympathetic (hypogastric) nerves. Consequently, pain and temperature stimulation result in detrusor contraction, which produces more frequent voiding.

Prostate

The normal prostate gland weighs up to 20 g and has a wider base (approximately 4.5 cm) than length (approximately 3.5 cm). Five prostatic lobes are present in the early fetus. By birth, the anterior lobe has atrophied and the lateral lobes have extended anteriorly to surround the urethra. Thus, there are four recognized lobes in the adult. The median lobe lies posterior and above the ejaculatory duct (Fig. 1.2), while the posterior lobe lies below the ejaculatory duct. The posterior lobe is

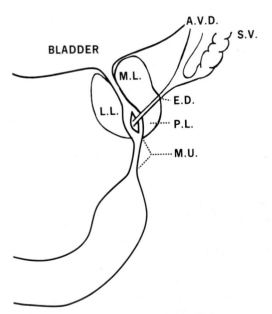

Figure 1.2. Diagram of normal prostate lobes in relation to bladder base, ejaculatory duct (ED), and membranous urethra (MU). AVD = ampulla of vas deferens; LL = lateral lobe; ML = medial lobe; PL = posterior lobe; SV = seminal vesicle. (From McCallum R: The adult male urethra. *Radiol Clin North Am* 27:227–244, 1979.)

fan-shaped and is palpated on rectal examination. The lateral lobes extend laterally and anteriorly. Through the posterior prostate pass the ejaculatory ducts that divide the median and posterior lobes. Microscopic studies of the prostate reveal an extensive fibrous tissue stroma more prominent in the transitional and central zone.

The prostate is fixed in position by two main attachments. The puboprostatic ligament extends from the posterior aspect of the pubis to the prostatic capsule and the bladder anteroinferiorly. The prostate often is represented diagrammatically as an upside-down pear, with the apex resting on the superior fascia of the urogenital diaphragm and the base resting against the bladder trigone. Multiple microscopic studies of this region have not revealed any superior fascia of the urogenital diaphragm. The studies do reveal that the apex of the prostate is embedded in the striated muscle fibers of the external sphincter. True prostatic glands intermingle with these striated muscle fibers. Posteriorly, the prostate is separated from the rectum by Denonvilliers' fascia, which supplies posterior ligamentous fibers to the posterior bladder base. Thus, the prostate is held firmly in position by the puboprostatic ligament, bladder trigone, and external sphincter fibers at the urogenital diaphragm (which is not a true diaphragm).

In 1954, Franks described two separate types of glands and named them the inner and outer periurethral glands. The inner periurethral glands are mucosal and submucosal, and are only present above the verumontanum. He attributed prostatic hypertrophy and hyperplasia to these glands. The outer periurethral glands are the true prostatic lobes and never undergo hypertrophy, but are subject to carcinoma and infection.

In 1972, McNeal's anatomic dissections and microscopic studies emphasized the different types and sites of glandular tissue within the prostate. Rather than designating lobes, McNeal described three separate zones within the prostate. Corresponding to the inner periurethral glands of Franks, McNeal described a transitional zone that undergoes hypertrophy and hyperplasia to produce fibroadenomata. This zone represents only 5% of prostatic volume and is only seen above the verumontanum. McNeal's central zone is said to be true prostatic tissue centrally and above the verumontanum, the glands of which also undergo hypertrophy. The peripheral zone is true prostatic tissue, comprises the bulk of the prostate gland, and is subject to the development of carcinoma and infection. Hypertrophy of transitional zone glands centrally and posteriorly may result in an apparent intravesical filling defect, the so-called "lobe of Albarran."

Vas Deferens and Seminal Vesicles

Vas Deferens

The vas deferens arises from the tail of the epididymis, passes along the spermatic cord, and enters the pelvis through the internal spermatic ring. In the pelvis the vas deferens follows the lateral pelvic wall, curving infero-posteriorly and medially. It crosses superficial to the external iliac vessels, the vesical arteries, the obturator nerve and vein, and the ureter. As the vas deferens crosses the ureter it becomes convoluted and dilated, increasing in diameter from 1 mm up to 1 cm. This is the ampulla of the vas deferens (Fig. 1.3). The diameter of the ampulla of the vas deferens varies from approximately 3 mm to 1 cm. The total length of the vas deferens including the ampulla is 35 to 45 cm.

The beginning of the ampulla as it crosses the ureter is within 1.5 cm of the fundus of the seminal vesicle. The inferomedial course brings the vas deferens medial and adjacent to the seminal vesicle. As the ampulla courses to the midline it meets the excretory duct of the seminal vesicle. The distal ampulla and excretory duct join to form the ejaculatory duct. The ejaculatory duct is almost midline, coursing through the prostate posteriorly to empty into the verumontanum 1 mm lateral to midline. The ejaculatory duct is a continuation of the excretory duct, with the ampulla contributing as a tributary in approximately 50% of males. In the other 50% of males, the ejaculatory duct is a confluence of the excretory duct and the ampulla with equal contribution. The duct is approximately 1.5 cm in length and 1.5 mm in width.

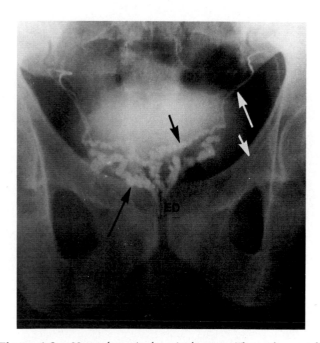

Figure 1.3. Normal seminal vesiculogram. Through scrotal incisions contrast medium is injected into the vas deferens and outlines the vas deferens (*white arrows*), the ampulla of the vas deferens (*black arrow*) the ejaculatory duct (ED), and reflux of contrast medium into the seminal vesicles (*long black arrow*). (From Putman C, Ravin C: *Textbook of Diagnostic Imaging,* vol. 2. Philadelphia, WB Saunders, p. 1358, 1988.)

The ejaculatory ducts are straight, parallel, and symmetric. Rarely, they are slightly curved or hooked. In anatomically normal males, the opening of the ejaculatory ducts into the verumontanum is 2 to 2.5 cm below the bladder neck. The vas deferens consists of three layers: an areolar layer externally, a smooth muscle layer, and a mucosal layer.

The muscle layer at the origin of the duct consists of three layers: an outer longitudinal, a middle circular, and an inner longitudinal layer. Shortly after the commencement of the duct, the inner longitudinal layer disappears, leaving most of the length of the vas deferens with outer longitudinal and inner circular layers of smooth muscle. Most of the epithelial layer consists of one layer of columnar epithelium, which is not ciliated. Near the origin of the vas deferens at the testicular end there is a double layer of columnar epithelium, the superficial layer of which is ciliated. The dilated convoluted ampulla of the vas deferens consists of the same structure as most of the length of the vas deferens. The ampullae of the vas deferens are generally symmetric in size and angulation.

Seminal Vesicles

Like the vas deferens, the seminal vesicles are paired structures that are usually symmetric. Each seminal vesicle is approximately 4.5 to 5 cm in length and 2 cm in width when measured in its normal state. The seminal vesicle is a blind-ending tube, coiled on itself and convoluted, giving the appearance of numerous diverticula. The seminal vesicle is pyramidal in shape with the broader end directed laterally and posterosuperiorly. The lower end is funneled to form the excretory duct that joins with the distal end of the ampulla of the vas deferens to form the ejaculatory duct. The anterior surface of the seminal vesicle is in close contact with the posterior bladder wall and reaches to the fundus of the empty bladder. When the bladder is distended with fluid, the seminal vesicle reaches almost halfway up the posterior bladder wall. The posterior surface of the seminal vesicle lies on Denonvilliers' fascia, separating it from the rectum. The distal posterior surface is closely adjacent to the base of the prostate. The seminal vesicle is adjacent to the ampulla of the vas deferens. Laterally and posteriorly it reaches to the level of the pelvic ureter.

Like the vas deferens, the microscopic structure of the seminal vesicles consists of three layers enveloped in a dense fibromuscular sheath. The outer layer consists of fibroareolar tissue. The middle layer consists of two smooth muscle layers: an outer longitudinal and an inner circular layer. An internal mucosa consists of columnar epithelium. Within the pseudodiverticulae are numerous goblet cells that contribute to the seminal fluid. Arterial supply and venous drainage originate from the middle and inferior vesicle arteries and from the middle hemorrhoidal artery and vein. The nerve supply is autonomic, arising from the pelvic parasympathetic plexus.

Urethra

Anterior Urethra

The urethra consists of anterior and posterior portions, each of which is subdivided into two parts (Fig. 1.4). The anterior urethra extends from the external meatus to the inferior edge of the urogenital diaphragm. The penile (or pendulous) urethra extends from the external meatus to the penoscrotal junction inferiorly, and to the suspensory ligament superiorly. This is a relatively fixed point, although the suspensory ligament has some elasticity, allowing approximately 1 cm of inferior motion. The penile urethra has a slightly dilated segment approximately 1.5 to 2 cm proximal to the external meatus, which is known as the fossa navicularis and is approximately 1 to 1.5 cm in length.

The bulbous urethra extends from the penoscrotal junction to the inferior fascia of the urogenital diaphragm. There is a dilatation in the proximal half of the bulbous urethra, termed the bulbous urethral sump, where the diameter of the anterior urethra is greatest. The bulbous sump is approximately 2 to 3 cm long and is the most inferior part of the urethra.

The anterior urethra is lined by stratified columnar epithelium except at the external meatus, where it changes to stratified squamous epithelium, which covers the glans penis. Along the length of the anterior urethra are small mucus-secreting submucosal glands, termed the glands of Littre, which are more numerous in the bulbous sump and in the superior aspect of the penile urethra. These glands secrete mucus into the urethra during sexual stimulation. Two ducts empty into the sump of the bulbous urethra. These are the long ducts of the pea-sized glands of Cowper, which lie on either side of the membranous urethra, within the urogenital diaphragm. Cowper's glands also secrete mucus during sexual stimulation.

A small striated musculotendinous sling of the bulbocavernous muscle extends from the anterior and lateral surfaces of the proximal bulbous urethra. This structure is known as the musculus compressor nuda (Fig. 1.5) and may indent the proximal bulbous urethra on dynamic retrograde urethrography or, rarely, on voiding urethrography. It should not be mistaken for stricture formation. The bulbocavernous muscle is involved in emptying the anterior urethra at the end of micturition. The levator ani muscles, the ischiocavernous muscles, and the superficial and deep transverse perineii are pelvic floor muscles involved in the active inhibition or interruption of micturition. Both anatomic dissections and dynamic retrograde urethrographic studies have shown a convex symmetric cone shape to the proximal bulbous urethra (Fig. 1.5). The tip of the cone shape is the point at which the bulbous urethra enters the urogenital diaphragm to continue as the membranous urethra.

Posterior Urethra

The posterior urethra extends from the bladder neck to the inferior aspect of the urogenital diaphragm and is divided into the prostatic and membranous portions.

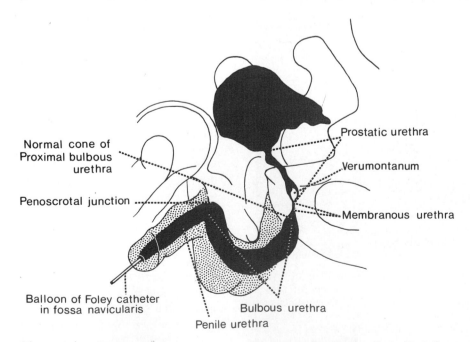

Figure 1.4. Diagram of urethra with normal anatomic landmarks. (From McCallum R: The adult male urethra. *Radiol Clin North Am* 27:227–244, 1979.)

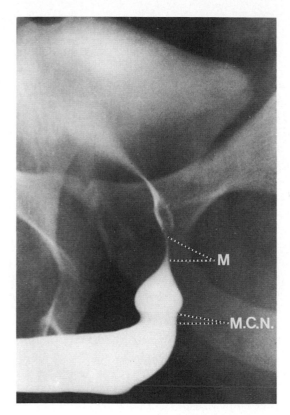

Figure 1.5. Dynamic retrograde urethrogram. M = membranous urethra; MCN = musculus compressor nuda. (From McCallum R: The adult male urethra. *Radiol Clin North Am* 27:227–244, 1979.)

The prostatic urethra is approximately 3.5 cm in length and passes through the prostate gland slightly anterior to midline. It continues as the membranous urethra, which is approximately 1 to 1.5 cm in length and ends at the inferior aspect of the urogenital diaphragm. A longitudinal ridge of smooth muscle extends from the bladder neck to the membranous urethra on the posterior wall of the posterior urethra. This longitudinal smooth muscle bundle swells just proximal to the membranous urethra to form an ovoid mound, the verumontanum (colliculus). The bulk of the verumontanum is posterior, is approximately 1 cm in length, and tapers distally in the prostatic urethra to continue as the urethral crest, which flattens in the membranous urethra.

The prostatic urethral mucosa is continuous with the bladder mucosa and is composed of transitional cells, but changes to stratified columnar epithelium at the membranous urethra. The supracollicular prostatic urethra is the widest part of the prostatic urethra. During voiding, the normal diameter of the bladder orifice and supracollicular prostatic urethra is approximately 1 to 1.5 cm. The submucosa in the supracollicular prostatic urethra differs from the submucosa at the verumontanum and inferiorly. Above the verumontanum, small mucosal and submucosal glands known as the inner periurethral glands that correspond to McNeal's transitional zone are present. These periurethral glands are only present above the verumontanum and undergo hypertrophy and hyperplasia. Consequently, the supracollicular prostatic urethra may be compressed by prostatic adenomata that may enlarge to obstruct the bladder neck or indent the bladder base. Occasionally adenomata are so numerous and large that they may push the verumontanum inferiorly. Rarely do prostatic adenomata extend below the verumontanum. The inner periurethral glands or glands of the transitional zone empty into the supracollicular prostatic urethra and into the prostatic sulcus on both sides of the verumontanum.

There are three distinct orifices in the verumontanum. The most proximal orifice is central and represents the prostatic utricle, a vestigial remnant of the müllerian duct. On either side of the midline below the prostatic utricle are two openings of the ejaculatory ducts formed at the junction of the ampulla of the vas deferens and the short duct of the seminal vesicles. The verumontanum tapers inferiorly to continue as the urethral crest, which is longitudinal smooth muscle and continues to the membranous urethra. Within the submucosa of the posterior urethra is a network of blood vessels that predominate over the verumontanum and urethral crest. The verumontanum and urethral crest form a smooth muscle organ involved in lengthening the posterior urethra during voiding and shortening the urethra at the end of voiding. This muscular organ also is likely involved in contracting the posterior urethra during emission and ejaculation, directing the emission through the membranous urethra and into the bulbous urethra for ejaculation by contraction of the bulbocavernous muscle.

Urethral Sphincters

The internal urethral sphincter lies in the trigourethral area and is the primary muscle of passive continence (Fig. 1.6). There are two schools of thought regarding this complex area. Tanagho, Lapides, and Hutch believe that a true circular sphincter does not exist, and that the outer longitudinal muscle fibers from the detrusor muscle are inserted below the trigone. These investigators claim that detrusor contraction when the bladder is full pulls the base plate open from below, allowing the internal urethral orifice to open. This opinion is in direct contrast to the microscopic studies of McCallum and Colapinto as well as those of McNeal, Uhlenhuth, Woodburne, and Gil-Vernet, which found that compact circular smooth muscle fibers at the bladder neck (unlike detrusor muscle fibers) represent a true internal sphincter. In addition, physiologic studies by Kleeman have shown that the bladder neck sphincter can be made to contract under the action of sympathomimetic drugs, even while the detrusor muscle is contracting. There is

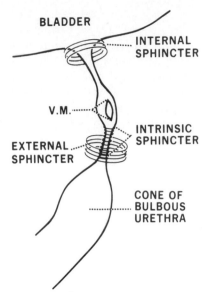

BLADDER

INTERNAL
SPHINCTER

V.M.

EXTERNAL
SPHINCTER

INTRINSIC
SPHINCTER

CONE OF
BULBOUS
URETHRA

Figure 1.6. Diagram of the three urinary sphincters. The internal and intrinsic sphincters are smooth muscle, while the external sphincter is striated voluntary muscle. VM = verumontanum. (From McCallum R: The adult male urethra. *Radiol Clin North Am* 27:227–244, 1979.)

sufficient evidence to state that there is a true circular internal sphincter at the bladder neck that acts as the primary muscle of passive continence. Detrusor external longitudinal smooth muscle fibers inserting into the inferior surface of the trigone are present and undoubtedly contribute to the opening of the bladder neck during voiding.

Below the mound of the verumontanum in the distal one third of the prostatic urethra and surrounding the membranous urethra is a second smooth muscle sphincter, the intrinsic sphincter (Fig. 1.6). Microscopic cross-sections through the distal prostatic urethra show a longitudinal smooth muscle elevation in the posterior wall of the cross-section that is the urethral crest. Surrounding the distal prostatic urethra is a thick band of circular smooth muscle that continues inferiorly to surround the membranous urethra. The urethral crest flattens in the membranous urethra. Adjacent to the membranous urethra submucosa is a thick band of circular smooth muscle that constitutes the intrinsic sphincter surrounding the membranous urethra and distal prostatic urethra up to the inferior edge of the mound of the verumontanum. Only sparse circular or arcuate striated and smooth muscle fibers lie between the internal sphincter at the bladder neck and the intrinsic sphincter. Consequently, there appear to be two separate smooth muscle sphincters in the posterior urethra. Both of these sphincters function as muscles maintaining passive continence. If the internal sphincter at the bladder neck is ablated, as it is in any kind of prostatectomy, or as a result of trigourethral injury in pelvic fracture (rare), the intrinsic

sphincter becomes the primary smooth muscle of passive continence. If both internal and intrinsic sphincters are damaged, the patient will be passively incontinent. The degree to which this condition is present usually depends on the extent of damage to the intrinsic sphincter.

The external sphincter is a striated voluntary muscle and is involved in active continence or the interruption of micturition. There also is reflex activity of the external sphincter, which contracts reflexly (along with the pelvic floor muscles) on increased intraabdominal pressure and inhibits stress incontinence. The external sphincter surrounds the membranous urethra peripheral to the intrinsic sphincter and, in addition, sends arcuate fibers proximally beneath the prostatic capsule almost to the bladder base. The external striated sphincter plays no part in maintaining passive continence. Although the striated muscle fibers maintain tone, the resting tone of the striated muscle fibers is insufficient to maintain passive continence.

Microscopic studies through the membranous urethra and urogenital diaphragm clearly show that the external striated muscle fibers lie in close apposition to the smooth muscle fibers of the intrinsic sphincter and, in fact, intermingle with peripheral smooth muscle fibers. It is postulated that, when micturition is physiologically necessary but socially unsuitable, voluntary contraction of the pelvic floor muscles including the external sphincter actively inhibits micturition by the transference of electrical impulses from the intermingling striated fibers of the external sphincter to the smooth muscle fibers of the intrinsic sphincter. Thus, active continence becomes passive continence within a few minutes.

Contraction of voluntary muscles including the external sphincter can only be maintained for a few minutes, after which striated muscle fibers tire. Consequently, when it is inconvenient to micturate but the urge to micturate is strong, micturition can be controlled by initiating active continence, maintained for a few minutes, after which continence becomes passive and the immediate necessity to void passes.

The smooth muscle sphincters of the posterior urethra are rich in α-receptors that cause contraction with sympathetic stimulation. Consequently, passive continence is controlled by sympathetic (T11–L2) stimulation with reciprocal relaxation of the parasympathetic nerves to allow the bladder to fill. The filled bladder stimulates the parasympathetic (S2–S4) nerves to cause motor activity in the detrusor muscle and bladder contraction. Reciprocal sympathetic relaxation causes the smooth muscle sphincters to relax, allowing micturition to take place. The external striated sphincter and pelvic floor muscles also relax reflexly by reduced activity of the pudendal nerves (S2–S4), allowing good urinary flow.

The intrinsic sphincter has a second function that involves a milk-back action at the end of micturition. The milk-back action empties the posterior urethra at the end of micturition, projecting the 1 to 2 cm of urine in the posterior urethra back into the bladder. This function is likely the result of both the striated external sphincter and intrinsic sphincter. The bulbocavernous muscle empties the anterior urethra at the end of micturition; therefore, the whole urethra is empty of urine at the end of micturition.

The urethra is fixed at two points: the penoscrotal junction and the urogenital diaphragm. Consequently, the urethra normally maintains a reverse horizontal S-shape. Thus, passage into the urethra of any straight metallic instrument that is maintained in position for a significant time may cause pressure necrosis at the fixed points, leading to scarring and stricture formation.

Penis

The penis is suspended superiorly from the pubic bone by the suspensory ligament. Inferiorly, the bulbous penis is longer and extends proximally between the testicles, where the bulbocavernosus muscle covers the bulbous urethra. The penis consists of two separate bodies of cavernous tissue. The corpus spongiosum, through which the urethra passes, lies inferior to two parallel cavernous bodies, the corpora cavernosa (Fig. 1.7). The corpus spongiosum is longer than the corpora cavernosa and is bulbous at both ends. The distal end of the corpus spongiosum is formed by the glans penis, which fits like a cap on the blunt ends of the corpora cavernosa. The proximal end of the corpus spongiosum dilates as the bulbous penis, which is bound to the pu-

bic arch by the inferior fascia of the urogenital diaphragm (i.e., the perineal membrane).

The corpora cavernosa are symmetric cavernous bodies capped distally by the glans penis. Proximally at the root of the penis, they become pointed and separated, and each is firmly connected to the rami of the pubic arch. Each corpus cavernosa is separated by a perforated septum, the septum pectiniform. Both corpora cavernosa and corpus spongiosum are bound together by a fibrous envelope, the deep (Buck's) fascia that is surrounded by the tunica albuginea. Within this fibrous tunica albuginea lies the deep dorsal vein, dorsal artery, and dorsal nerve of the penis. The tunica albuginea is surrounded by a loose areolar layer below the skin. The superficial dorsal vein of the penis lies within the areolar layer and drains the prepuce and skin of the penis.

The arterial supply to the penis is from the internal pudendal artery, which is a branch of the anterior division of the internal iliac artery. The four branches of the internal pudendal artery are the pelvic, gluteal, ischiorectal, and perineal. The dorsal penile artery usually arises from the perineal branch. Rarely, the dorsal penile artery arises from branches of the external pudendal artery, or from the inferior vesical artery. The deep dorsal artery extends to the glans penis and sends circumflex branches to the sinusoids of the spongy tissue of the three corpora. An increase in arterial blood flow to these sinusoids, as in sexual stimulation, results in erection.

The venous drainage of the penis is via the superficial and deep dorsal veins. The superficial vein drains the penile skin and prepuce, and drains into the external

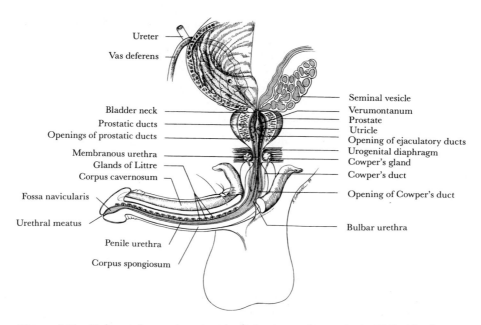

Figure 1.7. Male urethra and periurethral structures. (From Amis ES Jr, Newhouse JH, Cronan JJ: Radiology of male periurethral structures. *AJR* 151:321–324, 1988.)

pudendal vein and saphenous vein. Circumflex veins interconnecting the superficial and deep dorsal veins are present and function when the penis is in the flaccid state. These circumflex veins are compressed during erection between tunica albuginea and the deep (Buck's) fascia and are temporarily obliterated, thus reducing venous drainage. The deep dorsal vein and circumflex veins of the penis have been shown to contain valves. These valves are closed during erection, further reducing venous drainage. The deep dorsal vein drains into the vesicoprostatic plexus. In the flaccid penis, cavernosography shows symmetric corpora cavernosa and shows the deep dorsal vein draining into the vesicoprostatic plexus. During erection, the valves in the deep dorsal vein are closed and may not be visualized during cavernosography in normal erection. The vesicoprostatic plexus and the superficial venous system should not be visualized. Because communications are temporarily obliterated during erection, these anatomic conditions are the basis for cavernosography in the assessment of impotence that may be due to venous leakage.

The dorsal nerve that lies within the deep fascia is a branch of the pudendal nerve and provides sensory input to the glans penis, penile skin, and urethra. Accompanying the dorsal nerve of the penis are branches of the parasympathetic nerves, which are the autonomic nerve supply that produces erection. Both the parasympathetic and the pudendal nerves arise from the sacral segments S2–S4. The sympathetic nerve supply (i.e., hypogastric nerve) is responsible for emission of semen into the posterior urethra. The pudendal nerve supplying the bulbocavernous and pelvic floor muscles is responsible for ejaculation. Emission of semen and ejaculation are not yet fully understood, because the bladder neck must remain closed to avoid retrograde ejaculation into the bladder, and the external and intrinsic sphincter (supplied by the pudendal nerve and sympathetic, respectively) must relax to allow the seminal emission to pass into the proximal bulbous urethra for ejaculation by the bulbocavernosus, which is supplied by the pudendal nerve. Emission and ejaculation are believed to be a matter of precise timing, and the bladder neck is thought to be closed by contraction of the arcuate fibers of the external sphincter that pull the verumontanum up to the bladder neck to mechanically close the orifice. The emission then goes the route of least resistance and passes into the bulbous urethra.

Scrotum and Contents

The scrotum and contents are best considered as evaginations of the anterior abdominal wall produced by testicular descent through the inguinal canal and superficial inguinal ring. Consequently, the scrotal contents have eight different layers of tissue. By the time the testes and epididymis are ready for descent through the

inguinal canal, they are already invested by the tunica albuginea, which is closely applied to the seminiferous tubules. The tunica albuginea extends septa between the seminiferous tubules that converge on the rete testis and divide the testis into seminiferous lobules. About the same time, a peritoneal fold on the anterior abdominal wall termed the saccus vaginalis evaginates into the inguinal canal. Consequently, as the testicle descends through the inguinal canal and superficial inguinal ring, it becomes invested by three tunica: (*a*) the tunica albuginea, which is closest to the seminiferous tubules; (*b*) the tunica vasculosa, which consists of a plexus of blood vessels lining the tunica albuginea and interlobular septa, thereby allowing adequate blood supply to the testis; and (*c*) the tunica vaginalis, a peritoneal layer that is continuous with the saccus vaginalis and that surrounds both inner tunica. The tunica vaginalis is double layered, consisting of visceral and parietal layers with a cavity between them. The saccus vaginalis proximal to the testis obliterates, leaving no connection between the testis and peritoneal cavity.

As the testis descends through the inguinal canal, it carries the layers of the anterior abdominal wall including tunica vaginalis, subperitoneal fat, transversalis fascia, transversus, internal oblique and external oblique aponeurosis, subcutaneous fat, and skin. Within the subcutaneous fat layer extending to the scrotum is a layer of Colles fascia and the Dartos muscle.

The normal testis is 4 to 5 cm in length, 3 cm in width, and 2.5 cm in breadth. Testicular weight varies from 10 to 14 g. The epididymis lies along the lateral posterior border of the testis. The testicular appendix, a minute oval sessile body, lies at the upper end of the testis adjacent to the head of the epididymis. This is the hydatid of Morgagni, a vestigial remnant of the müllerian duct. The head of the epididymis has a small appendix that is thought to be the result of detached efferent ducts. The internal structure of the testis consists of 250 to 400 lobules. Each lobule consists of several (one to five) convoluted tubules, supported by interstitial cells. From these convoluted tubules spermatogonia, spermatids, and spermatozoon develop. Cells of Sertoli are also present in the tubules and appear to be necessary for the progress of the spermatozoa along the tubules. Toward the hilum, the tubules become straight and coalesce to form 20 to 30 straight ducts that enter the fibrous tissue of the mediastinum testis. Here the tubules lose their walls and simply become channels through the fibrous tissue of the mediastinum, producing a fine network of channels called the rete testes. The channels of the rete testes progress to the proximal end of the mediastinum where a number of ducts develop for perforation of the tunica albuginea. These efferent ducts pass through the tunica albuginea in the head epididymis.

EMBRYOLOGY

Upper Urinary Tract

The human kidney develops in three discrete stages (Fig. 1.8). The first such stage, the *pronephros,* appears during the end of the third week of gestation and is so named because of its relatively cephalic position. The tubules of the pronephros drain into an excretory duct that terminates in the cloaca. After the third week of gestation, the pronephros involutes and is replaced by the *mesonephros,* which develops immediately caudal to the pronephros. The mesonephros consists of a series of uriniferous tubules, each of which is associated with a group of blood vessels to form primitive glomeruli. The uriniferous tubules develop from a pair of laterally placed mesodermal structures known as the nephrogenic cord. The tubules on each side drain into a medially located structure called the mesonephric or wolffian duct. The mesonephric duct in turn drains into the same excretory duct that had its origins in the pronephros stage. The mesonephric duct then begins to involute; however, remnants of this duct persist in both sexes into adulthood. In males, the mesonephric duct serves as the precursor of the vas deferens, the seminal vesicles, and the ejaculatory ducts. In females, remnants of the mesonephric duct are vestigial.

Late in the fifth week of gestation, the final stage of development of the human kidney, the *metanephros,* begins. At the level of the 28th somite (the future site of the first sacral vertebra) a diverticulum forms from the mesonephric duct. This outpocketing is known as the ureteral bud. The tissue that surrounds the ureteral bud is known as the metanephric blastema and is derived from the caudal end of the nephrogenic cord. The metanephric blastema is induced to develop into nephrons under the influence of the ureteral bud, beginning at about the seventh week of gestation. The metanephric blastema will not develop nephrons unless the ureteral bud is present. The ureteral bud itself elongates and undergoes multiple divisions to form the renal tubules, the major and minor calyces (Fig. 1.9), the renal pelvis (Fig. 1.10), and the ureter. The divisions of the ureteral bud are dichotomous; however, more divisions occur in the polar regions of the kidney than in its midportion. For this reason, the renal parenchyma contains more nephrons and is thicker in its poles. This division process results in the formation of the renal pyramids. A pyramid together with its overlying cloak of renal cortex is known as a primitive renal lobe. The number of renal lobes formed thus depends on the number of calyces present. Also, between the fourth and eighth weeks, the developing kidneys migrate in a cephalic direction out of the pelvis to assume their adult position opposite the second lumbar vertebra. During the course of this migration, the kidneys rotate 90° about their longitudinal axis, so that the renal pelvis lies in a medial position.

At the fourth month of gestation, there are classically 14 discrete renal lobes, seven anterior and seven posterior, separated by a fibrous longitudinal groove. Following the 28th week of gestation, assimilation of the boundary between these lobes occurs. Persistence of these grooves into adulthood results in a grooved appearance to the surface of the kidney known as persistent fetal lobulation. In addition, some of the calyces become fused so that the one-to-one relationship between the calyces and the papillae in the fetal kidney is lost in the adult kidney. This process also is more pronounced in the polar region of the kidney and results in the development of compound calyces, each of which drains two to four papillae.

During this same period, there is assimilation of the septal cortex, which also is more pronounced in the

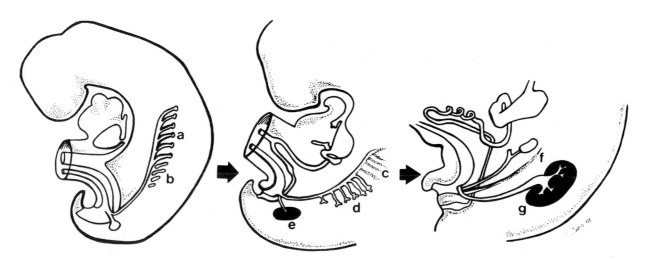

Figure 1.8.   Embryogenesis of the kidney. **a,** pronephros; **b,** early mesonephros; **c,** degenerating pronephros; **d,** mesonephric duct; **e,** ureteral bud; **f,** degenerating mesonephros; **g,** metanephros.

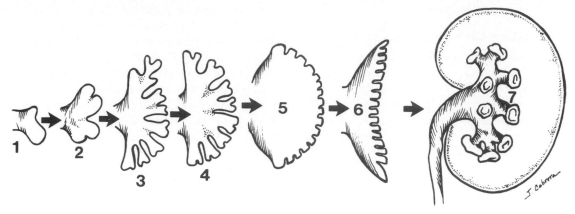

Figure 1.9. Development of calyx. New generations of branches are formed from the ureteral bud (**1–3**); early configuration of calyx (**4**); progressive distention of the cavity (**5**); invagination of the cavity (**6**); cup-like structure of calyx is formed (**7**). (Modified from Potter EL: *Normal and Abnormal Development of the Kidney,* Chicago, Year Book Medical Publishers, 1972.)

polar regions of the kidney. When such fusion is complete, the medulla between adjacent lobes directly abut one another; where relatively little fusion is present, characteristically in the interpolar regions of the kidney, columns of cortical tissue may be found between adjacent medullary lobes. When these columns have a slightly bulbous appearance, an indentation on one of the major calyces or the renal pelvis may be produced, which simulates an intrarenal mass; such a renal "pseudotumor" is known as a hypertrophied column of Bertin.

Lower Urogenital Tract

The embryology of the lower urogenital tract is best considered as consisting of four separate developmental stages: (*a*) development of the cloaca; (*b*) separation of the cloaca into dorsal and ventral portions; (*c*) development of these into the bladder, allantois, and uro-

genital sinus; and (*d*) development of the ventral and vesicourethral portions of the bladder, and division of the urogenital sinus into pelvic and phallic portions.

The cloaca is a dilatation of the entodermal hindgut formed after fetal flexion and anterior movement of the allantois into the body stalk. Solid rods of cells form in the mesoderm of the lateral cell masses. These rods of cells move caudally to reach the ventral portion of the cloaca and become canalized to form the wolffian ducts. This process occurs at 4 to 5 weeks of gestation. Shortly after the formation of the wolffian ducts, a second pair of ducts develop lateral to the wolffian ducts. These are the müllerian ducts that develop from coelomic evaginations. The cloaca is closed inferiorly from the exterior by the cloacal membrane, which consists of a thin entodermal layer and a thick ectodermal layer.

After the development and insertion of the wolffian

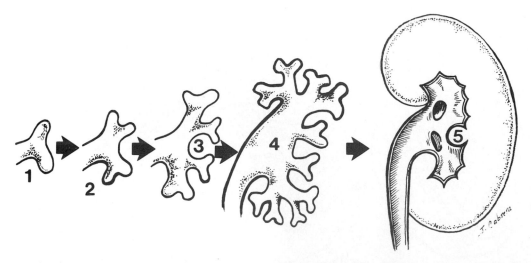

Figure 1.10. Development of renal pelvis. Divisions of ureteral bud (**1**), polar divisions (**2**), interpolar divisions (**3**), dilatation of individual branches (**4**), developed renal pelvis (**5**). (Modified from Potter EL: *Normal and Abnormal Development of the Kidney,* Chicago, Year Book Medical Publishers, 1972.)

and müllerian ducts into the ventral aspect of the cloaca, the cloaca is divided into dorsal and ventral portions by the cloacal septum (urorectal septum). The cloacal septum arises from the ridge separating the communication of the allantois with the intestine and the communication of the cloaca with the intestine. The dorsal portion of the cloaca becomes the rectum, and the ventral portion becomes the allantois, bladder, and urogenital sinus. The urogenital sinus divides into pelvic and phallic portions, and the allantois finally atrophies as the umbilical ligament.

The ventral bladder produces the bladder dome, the ventral bladder wall, and the urachus. The vesicourethral portion of the ventral bladder is the site of insertion of the wolffian and müllerian ducts. The lateral and posterior bladder walls, the bladder trigone, internal sphincter, and proximal urethra are formed from the vesicourethral portion of the ventral bladder. The two wolffian and two müllerian ducts develop into distinctive features that separate the sexes. In the male, the wolffian duct develops into the epididymis, the vas deferens, the seminal vesicles, the ejaculatory ducts, and the verumontanum. The proximal prostatic urethra and the proximal part of the prostate also are developed from the vesicourethral portion of the ventral bladder. The müllerian ducts atrophy but persist as a vestigial remnant as the prostatic utricle in the verumontanum and by appendices of the testes (the hydatid of Morgagni).

In the female, the müllerian ducts develop into the fallopian tubes and by fusing together produce the uterus, cervix, vagina, and proximal urethra while the distal wolffian ducts atrophy. The proximal wolffian ducts develop into long ducts, the ducts of Gartner.

The pelvic portion of the urogenital sinus also develops into the features differentiating the sexes. In the male, the pelvic portion produces the distal prostatic urethra, the membranous urethra, the distal prostate gland, and the urogenital diaphragm. In the female, the pelvic portion produces the distal urethra, the vestibule, and the greater vestibular gland.

In the male, the phallic portion of the urogenital sinus produces the bulbous and penile urethra, the glands and ducts of Cowper, the glands of Littre, the corpora cavernosa, and the corpus spongiosum. In the female, the phallic portion produces the clitoris, the labia major and minor, and the hymen.

Initially the development of the testes and ovaries is essentially the same in both sexes. Initial development consists of coelomic cavity epithelial thickening, which forms the genital ridge. Both ovaries and testes develop from this genital ridge. By the end of the seventh week, sex distinction is apparent anatomically and microscopically.

The ovary develops from the genital ridge as a central mass of cells with a layer of surface epithelium, while ova develop from the central cell mass. Within the central cell mass is a connective tissue stroma. Each ova develops a covering of connective tissue resulting in rudimentary follicles, and these form an aggregate that becomes covered by a tunica albuginea. Caudal movement of the ovary to the uterus is effected by uterine adhesions that become the ovarian ligament.

The testis develops in a similar fashion to the ovary, arising as a central mass of cells. Within the central mass a series of epithelial cords arise from the surface epithelium, and aggregation of these epithelial cords covered by surface epithelium forms the rudimentary testes. The testis develops a tunica albuginea that separates the surface epithelium from these epithelial cords. The epithelial cords converge toward a hilum that becomes the rete testes, and the epithelial cords also develop peripherally into the seminiferous tubules. Residual mesonephros cells become the efferent ducts of the testis. The seminiferous tubules connect with these efferent ducts to form the functioning testis. At this stage the testis is attached to the posterior abdominal cavity by peritoneum. Peritoneal folds form the inguinal fold and inguinal crest. The gubernaculum testis develops within the inguinal crest and guides the testis and testicular vessels through the inguinal canal into the scrotum.

SUGGESTED READINGS

Anatomy

Bors ET, Commarr AE: *Neurological Urology.* Baltimore, University Park Press, 1971.

Chesbrough RM, Burkhard TK, Martinez AJ, Burks DD: Gerota versus Zuckerkandl: the renal fascia revisited. *Radiology* 173: 845, 1989.

Franks LM: Benign nodular hyperplasia of the prostate: review. *Am R Coll Surg* 14:92, 1954.

Gil-Vernet S: *Morphology and Function of Vesico-prostato-urethral Musculature.* Canora, Treviso, p. 172, 1968.

Hunter DW: A new concept of urinary bladder musculature. *J Urol* 71:645, 1985.

Hutch JA, Rambo ON: A study of the anatomy of the prostate, prostatic urethra and the urinary sphincter system. *J Urol* 104:443, 1970.

Kaye KW, Reinke DB: Detailed caliceal anatomy for endourology. *J Urol* 132:1085, 1984.

Kleeman FJ: The physiology of the internal urinary sphincter. *J Urol* 104:549, 1970.

Lafortune M, Constantine A, Greton G, et al.: Sonography of the hypertrophied column of Bertin. *AJR* 146:53, 1986.

Lapides J, Ajemian EP, Stewart BH, Breakey BA, Lichtwardt JR: Further observations on the kinetics of the urethrovesical sphincter. *J Urol* 84:86, 1960.

McCallum RW: The radiologic assessment of the lower urinary tract in paraplegics: a new method. *J Can Assoc Radiol* 25:34, 1974.

McCallum RW: The adult male urethra: normal anatomy, pathology and method of urethrography. *Radiol Clin North Am* 17:227, 1979.

McCallum RW, Colapinto V: *Urological Radiology of the Adult Male Lower Urinary Tract.* Springfield, IL, Charles C Thomas, 1975.

McCallum RW, Colapinto V: The role of urethrography in urethral disease: part I. accurate radiological localization of the membranous urethra and distal sphincters in normal male subjects. *J Urol* 122:607, 1979.

McNeal JE: The prostate and prostatic urethra: a morphological synthesis. *J Urol* 107:1008, 1972.

Mindell HJ, Mastromatteo JF, Dickey KW, et al.: Anatomic communications between the three retroperitoneal spaces: determination by CT-guided injections of contrast material in cadavers. *AJR* 164:1173, 1995.

Mitty HA: Embryology, anatomy and anomalies of the adrenal gland. *Semin Roentgenol* 23(4):271, 1988.

Raptopoulos V, Kleinman PK, Marks S, Jr., et al.: Renal fascial pathway: posterior extension of pancreatic effusions within the anterior pararenal space. *Radiology* 158:367, 1986.

Raptopoulos V, Lei QF, Touliopoulos P, Vrachliotis TG, Marks SC Jr: Why perirenal disease does not extend into the pelvis: the importance of closure of the cone of the renal fasciae. *AJR* 164:1179, 1995.

Rifkin MD: *Diagnostic Imaging of the Lower Genitourinary Tract.* New York, Raven Press, p. 7, 1985.

Sampaio FJB, Aragao AHM: Anatomical relationship between the intrarenal arteries and the kidney collecting system. *J Urol* 143:679, 1990.

Tanagho EA, Smith DR: The anatomy and function of the bladder neck. *Br J Urol* 38:54, 1966.

Uhlenhuth E, Hunter DW, Loechel W: *Problems in the Anatomy of the Pelvis.* Philadelphia, JB Lippincott, 1953.

Woodburne RT: The structure and function of the urinary bladder. *J Urol* 84:79, 1960.

Embryology

Arey LB (ed): *Developmental Anatomy,* ed 7. Philadelphia, WB Saunders, 1966.

Potter EL: *Normal and Abnormal Development of the Kidney.* Chicago, Year Book Medical Publishers, 1972.

Sadler TW (ed): *Langman's Medical Embryology,* ed 5. Baltimore, Williams & Wilkins, 1985.

2

Congenital Anomalies

UPPER URINARY TRACT ANOMALIES

Kidney

Anomalies of Position

MALROTATION. Malrotation of a normally positioned kidney most commonly occurs as a result of failure of rotation of the kidney about its vertical axis. This results in an anterior position of the renal pelvis. In many cases, a partial malrotation is present with the renal pelvis located in an anteromedial position. The abnormality may be bilateral or unilateral. Under rare circumstances, overrotation of the kidney may result in a laterally facing renal pelvis.

On urography, malrotation can be diagnosed when calyces are projected medial to the renal pelvis (Fig. 2.1). Rarely the appearance of malrotated kidney may be mistaken for a more significant renal abnormality, such as the presence of a medially located renal mass. Occasionally malrotation about the vertical axis of the kidney will be present. This is most commonly associated with a deformity of the spine and results in a foreshortened appearance of the affected kidney.

RENAL ECTOPY. As the fetal kidneys ascend from their pelvic position to meet the adrenal glands, each kidney acquires blood supply from the neighboring vessels. The initial supply from the external and internal iliac vessels is lost during this process, and blood supply directly from the aorta is acquired around the eighth week of development. Any abnormality in acquiring such blood supply or an associated abnormality of the spine may prevent cephalic migration from occurring. This will result in a condition known as renal ectopy or an abnormal position of the kidney. The most common form of simple renal ectopy is a *pelvic* kidney in which the kidney is located in the true pelvis or adjacent to the sacrum (sacral kidney). Occasionally the kidney may lie at the level of the iliac crest; such a position is termed abdominal ectopy. The reported incidence of renal ectopy varies between 1:500 and 1:1200. The exact incidence is difficult to determine, because in many cases the condition is clinically silent. With any congenital anomaly, the likelihood of finding other anomalies in the same or other organ systems is increased. Therefore, it is not unusual to find pelvic kidneys associated with a pathologic process such as hydronephrosis or vesicoureteral reflux. Clinical symptoms related to the presence of a pelvic kidney are usually due to one of its associated conditions, such as pain from obstruction or infection related to reflux; because of the location of the kidney, these conditions may mimic gastrointestinal disease.

The findings on urography depend on the degree of renal function in the pelvic kidney and the presence of associated abnormalities. When the ectopic kidney is small and no hydronephrosis is present, the kidney may be obscured by the bony pelvis. Tomography over the pelvis or an oblique view is frequently helpful (Fig. 2.2). On rare occasions, both kidneys may be ectopic in the pelvis (Fig. 2.3). Computed tomography (CT) or ultrasound may be used to demonstrate a small ectopic kidney that has not been demonstrated on urography. On ultrasound, the reniform mass will be found in the pelvis with a characteristic pattern of renal sinus echoes. On CT, a functioning mass of renal parenchyma can usually be identified. Angiography is customarily employed before any contemplated surgical procedure on a pelvic kidney because of the highly variable nature of its blood supply.

INTRATHORACIC KIDNEY. This rare anomaly occurs when the kidney ascends to a position higher than the second lumbar vertebra. The kidney may reach an intrathoracic location through a posterior diaphragmatic aperture that may be congenital or acquired. The anomaly is more common in males and is more commonly found on the left side. The blood supply to an intrathoracic kidney

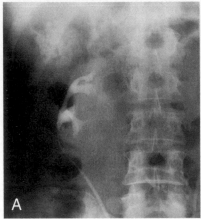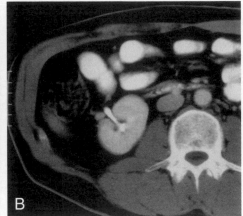

Figure 2.1. Malrotated kidney. **A,** Excretory urography shows the calyces of the right kidney projecting medial to the laterally displaced renal pelvis and proximal ureter. **B,** Com- puted tomography confirms the anterolateral position of the small intrarenal pelvis.

generally arises from the abdominal aorta in its normal location. Congenital intrathoracic kidney occurs in 1:15,000 births and often is diagnosed by the finding of a posterior thoracic mass, which appears to arise from the diaphragm on a chest radiograph (Fig. 2.4).

Anomalies of Number

RENAL AGENESIS.   True renal agenesis is defined as the complete congenital absence of renal tissue. This con- dition is to be distinguished from acquired forms of age- nesis, in which renal tissue develops but atrophies dur- ing development or during childhood because of an associated malfunction. Renal agenesis occurs in ap- proximately one in 1000 births. It is thought to occur as the result of failure of formation of the ureteral bud or because of an inherent deficiency of the metanephric blastema. In the latter case, partial development of the ureter may be present. In true agenesis, an ipsilateral ab- sence of the trigone and ureteral orifice will be found in the bladder on cystoscopy. No renal artery is present. The colon occupies the renal fossa on the affected side, which may suggest the diagnosis on plain film exami- nation or contrast studies of the colon; this is especially true on the left. The ipsilateral adrenal gland is absent in 8 to 10% of the cases.

Compensatory hypertrophy of the contralateral kidney almost always accompanies renal agenesis. This begins in utero and also can be found when the other kidney is compromised by any other process. Compensatory hy- pertrophy may occur whenever the contralateral kidney is removed or is functionally compromised. However, the older the patient at the time of renal damage, the less compensatory hypertrophy will occur.

Genital abnormalities also may be associated with unilateral renal agenesis and, when present, suggest an etiology that also affects the mesonephric duct. In

males, such abnormalities include cysts of the ipsilateral seminal vesicle (Fig. 2.5), absence of the ipsilateral vas deferens, hypoplasia or agenesis of the testicle, and hy- pospadias. In females, renal agenesis may be associated with a unicornuate or bicornuate uterus, absence or hy- poplasia of the uterus, and absence or aplasia of the vagina (Rokitansky-Kuster-Hauser syndrome).

Bilateral renal agenesis is extremely rare and incom- patible with life. Males are affected in three fourths of the cases. Infants with this abnormality exhibit the char- acteristic features of Potter's facies, which include low- set ears and a prominent palpebral fold.

RENAL HYPOPLASIA AND DYSPLASIA.   Renal hypoplasia is a distinctly unusual renal anomaly in which the kidney is 50% or more smaller than normal and typically contains

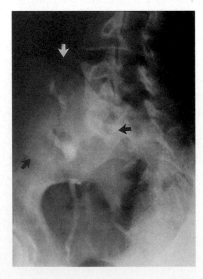

Figure 2.2. Pelvic kidney. A right posterior oblique view shows the collecting system projected over the right iliac crest. *Arrows* outline the renal parenchyma.

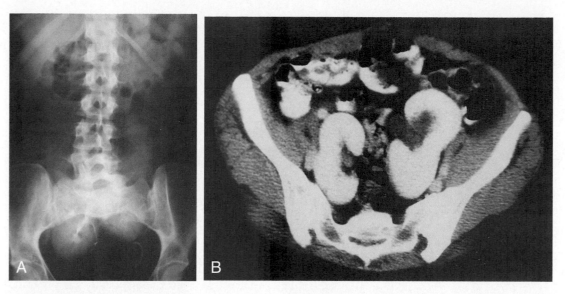

Figure 2.3. Bilateral pelvic kidneys. **A,** Excretory urography and **B,** computed tomography reveal both kidneys in the pelvis. (From Amis ES Jr, Newhouse JH: *Essentials of Uroradiology,* Boston, Little Brown & Co, 1991).

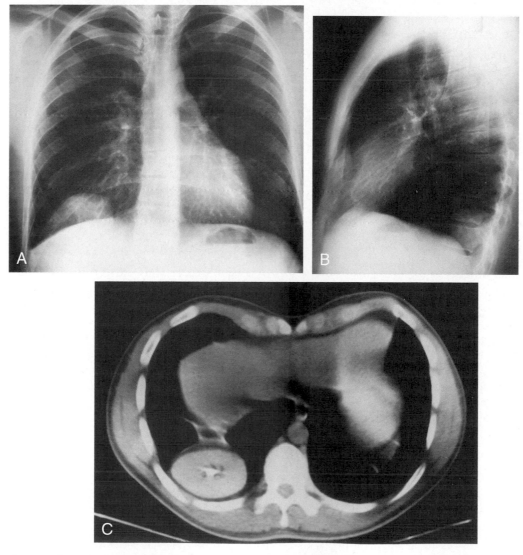

Figure 2.4. Intrathoracic kidney. **A,** A posterior thoracic mass is seen on posteroanterior and **B,** lateral chest radiograph. **C,** A thoracic kidney is confirmed on computed tomography.

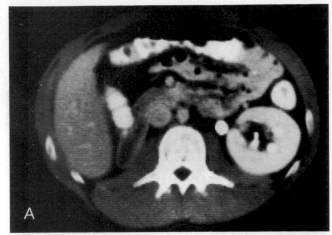

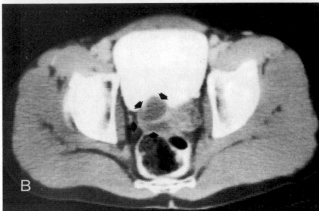

Figure 2.5. Agenesis of the right kidney. **A,** Computed tomography shows bowel loops occupying the right renal fossa and hypertrophy of the left kidney. **B,** Pelvic computed tomography demonstrates a cyst of the right seminal vesicle (*arrows*). (From Sandler CM, Raval B, David C: Computed tomography of the kidney. *Urol Clin North Am* 12(4):657, 1985.)

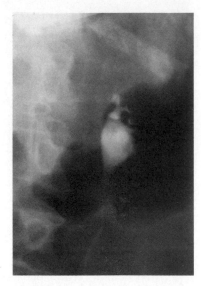

Figure 2.6. Hypoplastic kidney. Retrograde pyelography reveals a diminutive kidney with fewer than the normal number of calyces. The calyces are normally cupped. (From Amis ES Jr, Newhouse JH: *Essentials of Uroradiology*, Boston, Little Brown & Co, 1991.)

fewer than the normal number of calices (Fig. 2.6). The condition is usually unilateral, and the kidney functions normally for its size. Most unilaterally small kidneys are acquired because of chronic ischemia, reflux (chronic atrophic pyelonephritis), or long-standing obstruction (hydronephrotic atrophy). However, these conditions can be differentiated from hypoplasia by the normal number of calices and the fact, that in reflux or obstruction, the calices are not normally cupped.

The Ask-Upmark kidney (*see* Chapter 9) was thought by some to be a variant of renal hypoplasia. The kidney is small, predominantly because of cortical loss in the upper pole associated with cortical indentations. However, most patients also have associated reflux and infection. The Ask-Upmark kidney is currently thought to be caused by scarring due to chronic pyelonephritis rather than a true congenital lesion.

Renal dysplasia also results in a small kidney, but there is usually no function and the collecting system is grossly distorted. This condition typically results from an

ectopic insertion of the ureter far from its normal location on the trigone.

SUPERNUMERARY KIDNEY. A supernumerary kidney is extremely rare. Cleavage of the metanephric blastema has been suggested as the cause for this abnormality. Most supernumerary kidneys are caudally placed and are hypoplastic; they may be connected to the ipsilateral dominant kidney either completely or by loose areolar connective tissue. A separate collecting system in the supernumerary kidney is generally present.

Anomalies of Form

CROSSED ECTOPY. Crossed ectopy is defined as a kidney located on the opposite side of the midline from its ureter. The crossed kidney usually lies below the normally situated kidney. In 90% of the cases, at least partial fusion between the kidneys is present (crossed fused ectopy). In the remainder, two discrete kidneys on the same side are present (crossed unfused ectopy). Other variations of crossed ectopy, including solitary crossed ectopy and bilateral crossed ectopy, have been described (Fig. 2.7). The anomaly is more common in males (2:1) and left-to-right ectopy is three times more common than right-to-left ectopy. Crossed fused ectopy has been estimated to occur in approximately 1:1000 births.

The anomaly is thought to result because of an abnormally situated umbilical artery that prevents normal cephalic migration from occurring; in such cases, the developing kidney takes the path of least resistance and crosses to the opposite side, where cephalic migration resumes. Others have postulated that the abnormality occurs when the ureteral bud crosses to the opposite

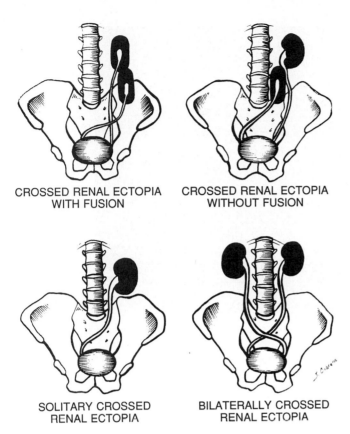

CROSSED RENAL ECTOPIA
WITH FUSION

CROSSED RENAL ECTOPIA
WITHOUT FUSION

SOLITARY CROSSED
RENAL ECTOPIA

BILATERALLY CROSSED
RENAL ECTOPIA

Figure 2.7. Schematic drawing showing the variations of crossed-renal ectopy.

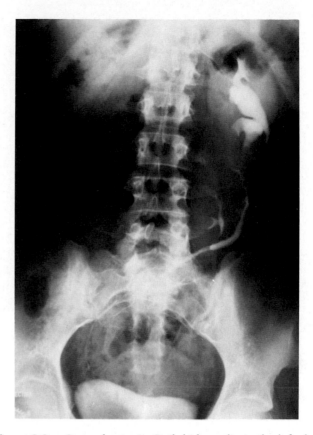

Figure 2.8. Crossed ectopia. Both kidneys lie in the left abdomen and are malrotated.

side, where it induces nephron formation in the contralateral metanephric blastema.

In most cases of crossed renal ectopy, the ureters are not ectopic and cystoscopy reveals a normal trigone. The incidence of associated congenital anomalies is low. Symptoms of crossed renal ectopy are rare; however, these patients may present in adulthood with abdominal pain, pyuria, or urinary tract infection. A slightly higher incidence of urinary tract calculi associated with crossed renal ectopy is thought to be related to stasis. On urography, the abnormality is readily detected (Fig. 2.8), although differentiation of the fused from the unfused variety may require additional imaging studies such as ultrasound or CT. On ultrasound, crossed-fused ectopy can be identified by a characteristic anterior or posterior "notch" between the two kidneys (Fig. 2.9). The blood supply to the crossed renal unit is generally anomalous; as with pelvic kidney, angiography is usually recommended before surgical procedures.

HORSESHOE KIDNEY. Horseshoe kidney is the most common anomaly of renal form, occurring in approximately 1:400 births. There is a 2:1 male predominance. The abnormality occurs when the two kidneys on either side of the midline are connected by an isthmus. The anomaly is thought to occur because an abnormal position of the umbilical artery results in disturbance of the

normal pattern of cephalic migration. As a result, there is contact between the developing metanephric blastema on each side that leads to partial fusion.

The isthmus of a horseshoe kidney usually consists of a band of parenchymal tissue that has its own blood supply. In some cases, the band consists merely of fibrous

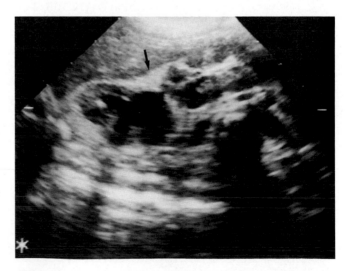

Figure 2.9. Cross-fused ectopy. Sonogram showing the notch (*arrow*) between the two kidneys. Mild dilatation of the collecting system of the upper kidney is present.

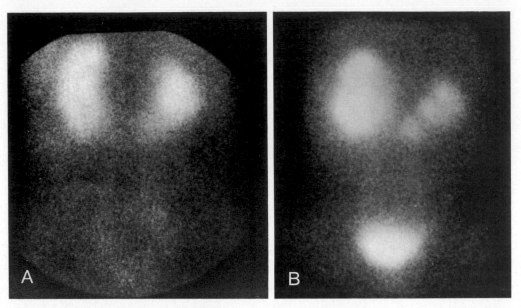

Figure 2.10.   Horseshoe kidney. **A,** Radionuclide examination using technetium-99m diethylenetriaminepentaacetic acid (^{99m}Tc-DTPA) showing that the isthmus of the kidney is not composed of functioning renal tissue. **B,** Delayed image shows an accumulation of tracer within the pelvis of the left kidney consistent with an associated ureteropelvic junction obstruction.

tissue (Fig. 2.10**A**). Usually, the band joins the lower poles of the kidney and prevents normal rotation from occurring, so that on each side the renal pelvis is in an anterior position. Rarely, the band connects the upper poles rather than the lower poles. The band is usually located anterior to the aorta and inferior vena cava (IVC), but posterior to the inferior mesenteric artery, which is thought to prevent further cephalad migration from occurring. Alterations in this arrangement, however, are common so that the position of the kidneys, their blood supply, their relation to the major vessels, and even the size of the kidney on either side is variable. Horseshoe kidney commonly has an associated ureteropelvic junction (UPJ) obstruction (Fig. 2.10**B**, 2.11).

Many patients with horseshoe kidney remain asymptomatic throughout their lifetimes; in the remainder of patients, symptoms of obstruction, infection, or a renal calculus bring the abnormality to medical attention. In some patients, symptoms may be thought to be referable to the gastrointestinal tract. An increased incidence of renal malignancies is reported in patients with a horseshoe kidney. Carcinoma of the renal pelvis is more common in patients with a horseshoe kidney, and Wilms' tumor has a predilection to originate in the isthmus.

Several investigators report that a horseshoe kidney is more prone to suffer injury in patients suffering blunt

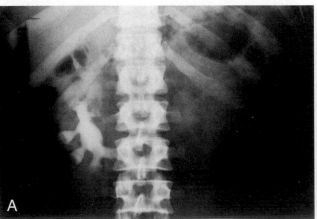
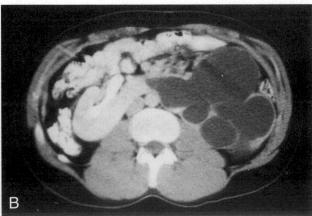

Figure 2.11.   Horseshoe kidney with left ureteropelvic junction obstruction. **A,** Excretory urography reveals function only on the right. The axis of the right kidney is reversed suggesting a horseshoe kidney. **B,** Computed tomography reveals severe hydronephrosis of the left portion of the horseshoe kidney with only a thin rim of functioning parenchyma remaining.

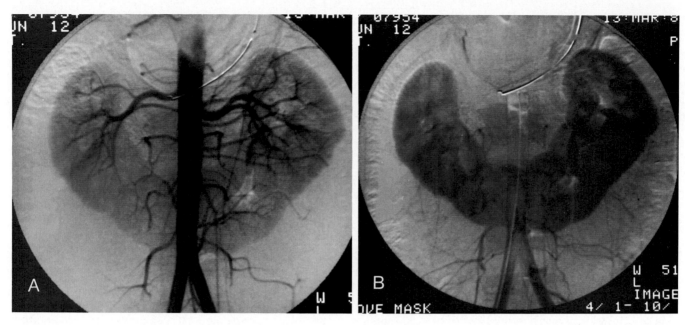

Figure 2.12.   Horseshoe kidney. **A,** Intraarterial digital subtraction angiogram demonstrates that multiple renal arteries supply the kidney, all of which arise from the abdominal aorta.

B, Nephrogram phase showing persistent fetal lobulation in the kidney.

abdominal trauma, presumably because of its relatively less protected, more anterior position.

The blood supply to a horseshoe kidney is quite variable, the majority of patients having multiple bilateral renal arteries (Fig. 2.12). The isthmus may be supplied by branches of the renal arteries or directly from the abdominal aorta, the inferior mesenteric artery, or the iliac arteries.

Urographic findings (Fig. 2.13) in patients with horseshoe kidneys include: (*a*) an abnormal axis for each kidney with their lower poles more medially located than their upper poles; (*b*) the kidneys are found in a somewhat more caudad position; and (*c*) there is bilateral

malrotation with the renal pelves in an anterior position so that the lower calyces are projected in a more medial position than the proximal ureter. The isthmus may be visualized if it is composed of functioning renal tissue.

On CT (Fig. 2.14), the isthmus of a horseshoe kidney is usually easily identified. Computed tomography also is helpful in defining the relationship of the kidney to the major vessels.

OTHER FUSION ANOMALIES.   A variety of other fusion abnormalities may occur much less commonly than crossed renal ectopy. These include the *donut* kidney, a kidney

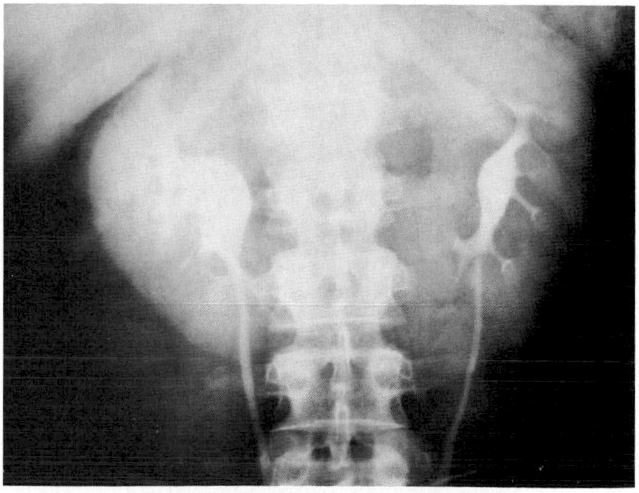

Figure 2.13.   Horseshoe kidney. Typical urographic finding in a horseshoe kidney where isthmus is composed of functioning renal tissue.

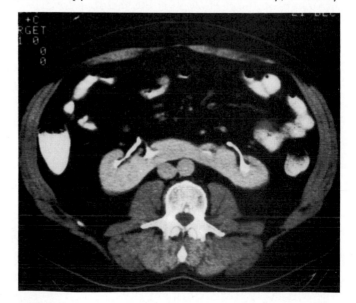

Figure 2.14.   Horseshoe kidney. Computed tomography clearly demonstrates the isthmus.

that is joined medially at its poles to form a ring-like renal mass. The *lump* or *pancake* kidney is a rare abnormality marked by extensive fusion between the two renal masses. The kidney is found in the midline or slightly to one side, generally no higher than the sacral promontory. The renal pelves are anterior and drain separate portions of the kidney. The ureters generally do not cross.

Renal Pelvis and Ureter

Unipapillary Kidney and Polycalicosis

The normal human intrarenal collecting system typically has 10 to 14 calyces. The kidneys in many mammals, including the dog, cat, sheep, rabbit, monkey, and rat, contain only a single papilla. On rare occasions, a unipapillary kidney (as this condition is called) can be found in humans, usually associated with other significant anomalies, such as ipsilateral hypoplasia and frequent abnormalities of the contralateral kidney. Conversely, polycalicosis (also known as a multiplicity of calices) signifies an increased number of calyces; this is usually an isolated finding in an otherwise normal kidney.

Congenital Megacalyces

Many investigators believe that congenital megacalyces, also known as megacalicosis, is an acquired condition. The calyces are all symmetrically enlarged, although the renal pelvis and ureter are of normal size. Furthermore, there is no history to suggest previous obstruction or reflux. Involvement is almost always unilateral, and the kidney is typically normal in size and functions well. While megacalyces may be congenital, clinically silent obstruction or reflux in the distant past, perhaps even during fetal life, may be the cause. Another factor that favors an acquired etiology is the fact that congenital megacalyces are typically seen in adults.

Abortive Calyx

An abortive calyx is small and may arise from a renal pelvis or infundibulum; however, it is also abnormally formed. Instead of the delicately cupped calyx seen in either the normal or microcalyx, an abortive calyx has a blunt termination and may be broader than it is tall. It is most often found near the base of the upper pole infundibulum, and only one abortive calyx is seen in a kidney.

Microcalyx

A microcalyx resembles a normal calyx in every way but size. It may arise from the renal pelvis or an infundibulum, and ends at a papillary tip. The microcalyx is formed normally with a fornix and tubules draining into it.

ABERRANT (ECTOPIC) PAPILLA.   Most renal papilla empty into a minor calyx. In the renal polar regions, where compound calyces are common, several papillae may empty side by side into a major calyx. Rarely, a papilla may have an aberrant insertion into the collecting system and may present as a filling defect that must be differentiated from stones, tumors, or other pathologic processes. The aberrant papilla can protrude into virtually any part of the collecting system surrounded by renal parenchyma, including an infundibulum or the intrarenal portion of the renal pelvis. The resultant finding on excretory or retrograde pyelography is a smooth round or ovoid lucent defect in the contrast-filled collecting system (Fig. 2.15). The smooth border and fixed location on a margin of the collecting system tend to differentiate the finding from a tumor or stone. Oblique views may show the extrinsic origin of the papilla.

Ureteropelvic Junction Obstruction and Congenital Megaureter

Although occurring at either end of the ureter, UPJ obstruction and congenital megaureter are discussed together because of their histologic and physiologic similarities. Both conditions are caused by deficiency and derangement of the ureteric smooth muscle fibers with associated fibrosis, resulting in a failure of normal peristalsis in the affected segment and subsequent functional obstruction. Congenital obstruction of the UPJ is a common anomaly of the urinary tract. The disorder produces caliectasis and marked pelviectasis as a result of a functional narrowing of the UPJ. Secondary UPJ obstruction due to an acquired disorder of the renal pelvis or vesicoureteral reflux will not be considered in this section.

In approximately 5% of cases, extrinsic compression of the UPJ by an aberrant renal artery can result in a similar radiographic pattern (Fig. 2.16).

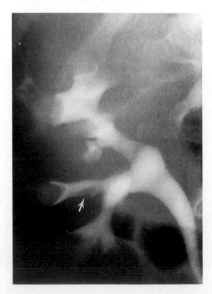

Figure 2.15.   Ectopic papilla. A smooth ovoid filling defect (*arrow*) in an infundibulum is seen on an excretory urogram.

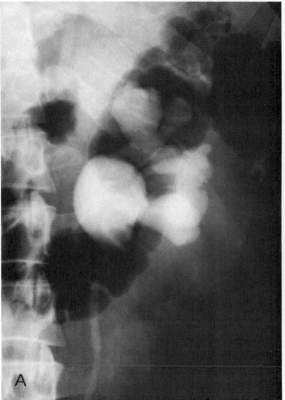

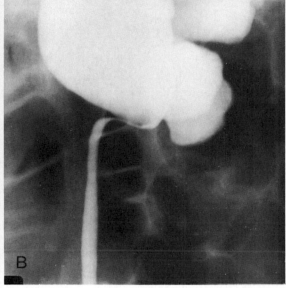

Figure 2.16. Ureteropelvic junction obstruction. **A,** Radiograph from an excretory urogram demonstrates a dilated renal pelvis and caliectasis. **B,** On retrograde pyelography, a "kink" in the proximal ureter is clearly demonstrated. At surgery, an aberrant lower pole renal artery was found.

Congenital UPJ obstruction is the most common cause of an abdominal mass in a neonate. The disorder is being discovered increasingly in the antenatal period because of the almost routine use of obstetric ultrasound. In a significant number of cases, however, the abnormality is clinically silent until adulthood, when hematuria, flank pain, fever, or, rarely, hypertension cause the patient to seek medical attention. Cases in which presentation has been delayed well into the sixth or seventh decade have been reported. In some patients, the finding is coincidental on studies performed for other disease. Males are affected more often than females by a 2:1 ratio, and the left side is more commonly affected than the right for unknown reasons. A familial tendency toward the disorder also has been reported.

In some cases, symptoms may only be present in the setting of a sustained diuresis, a condition that has become known as "beer-drinker's hydronephrosis." Such cases have been attributed to a very mild form of UPJ obstruction such that under conditions of normal urine volumes the UPJ is compensated. Urograms made while such a patient is asymptomatic may show only an extrarenal pelvis; the use of a diuretic renogram or a urographic study during acute symptoms has been advocated to demonstrate the underlying abnormality.

On urography, a dilated renal pelvis and calyces will be demonstrated. Because of the dilatation, slow opacification of the affected side is the rule and delayed radiographs are usually necessary to demonstrate that the UPJ is, in fact, the point of obstruction (Fig. 2.17). With longstanding or very high-grade obstruction, a virtually nonfunctioning kidney may be present. The renal pelvis may be markedly dilated; in fact, when the dilated renal pelvis has a capacity over 1 L, the term "giant hydronephrosis" applies. In rare instances, giant hydronephrosis can occupy almost the entire abdomen, extending well across the midline.

The UPJ itself may be difficult to visualize; in some cases, it appears to join the renal pelvis in a higher or more medial position. Care must be taken to differentiate a true UPJ obstruction from a large extrarenal pelvis (Fig. 2.18). In the latter case, the renal pelvis may appear quite dilated; however, in the absence of caliectasis, the diagnosis of UPJ obstruction should not be entertained. Variable filling of the ureter may occur distal to the UPJ. When there is significant kinking of the UPJ, the possibility that the obstruction is secondary to an aberrant vessel should be considered.

When there is insufficient contrast excretion on urography or when the ureter itself is not visualized, the

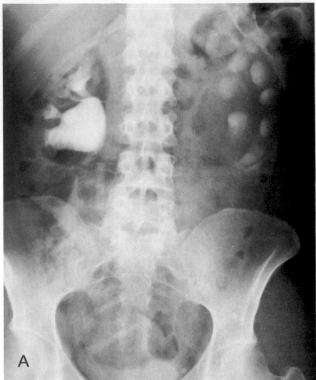

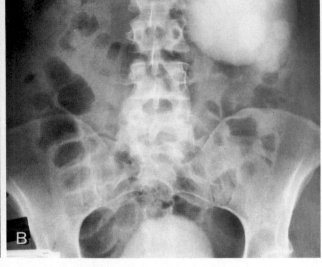

Figure 2.17. Ureteropelvic junction obstruction. **A,** Ten-minute film from an excretory urogram demonstrating dilated calyces with delayed opacification of the remainder of the col-lecting system. **B,** Twenty-four-hour delayed radiograph shows a markedly dilated renal pelvis.

diagnosis may be established by antegrade or retrograde pyelography. The former is preferred as a predecessor to percutaneous nephrostomy; the latter may be performed to confirm the diagnosis immediately before a contemplated surgical procedure, because a retrograde injection into an obstructed system may introduce infection. Some authorities advocate voiding cystourethrography in all patients with suspected UPJ obstruction to exclude vesicoureteral reflux as a cause of the renal pelvic dilatation, especially if there is any dilation of the ureter below the UPJ.

On ultrasound (Fig. 2.19), hydronephrosis associated with a very dilated renal pelvis may be readily identified. This finding in association with the inability to demonstrate a dilated ureter suggests the diagnosis of UPJ obstruction with a high degree of certainty. The diagnosis also may be suggested by CT; however, such studies are rarely indicated or necessary in uncomplicated UPJ obstruction.

In patients with equivocal UPJ obstruction, or in cases where there is a discrepancy between the patient's clinical symptoms and the radiologic findings, diuresis renography or the Whitaker procedure may be employed to assess whether functionally significant obstruction is present (*see* Chapter 16).

Pyeloplasty has been considered the treatment of choice for UPJ obstruction. Recently, however, the use of percutaneous nephrostomy followed by balloon pyeloplasty (Fig. 2.20) or by endoscopic endopyelotomy has been reported as a primary procedure and as a secondary procedure in patients in whom surgical therapy has failed. While success rates of up to 85% have been reported with endopyelotomy, pyeloplasty consistently corrects the defect in 85 to 90% of patients. Endopyelotomy probably should not be used in small infants and has a higher failure rate in patients with extremely redundant renal pelves or long UPJ strictures.

Congenital megaureter, as noted above, is a functional obstruction of the distal ureter. Typically, approximately 2 cm of the ureter just above the ureteral orifice is involved and this abnormal segment is usually of normal caliber. However, the ureter proximal to this improperly functioning segment is variably dilated. It is not unusual to see this dilation involving only the distal one third of the ureter, although if the obstruction is severe enough, significant hydronephrosis may occur. As with UPJ obstruction, a normal sized ureteral catheter can be easily passed through the abnormal ureteral segment. Thus, this narrowing is not an anatomic stricture, but rather is a failure of the abnormal ureteral segment to undergo normal peristalsis. Treatment for severe cases includes excision of the abnormal distal segment, surgi-

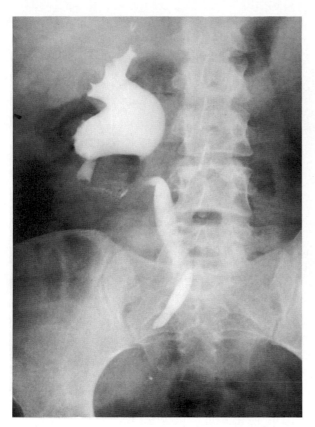

Figure 2.18. Dilated extrarenal pelvis. Retrograde pyelogram showing a dilated extrarenal pelvis. Note that the calyces are not dilated, which helps to differentiate this condition from true ureteropelvic junction obstruction. Mild fullness of the ureter secondary to pregnancy dilatation also is present.

cal tapering of the dilated "normal" ureter, and re-implantation of the tapered ureter into the bladder using antirefluxing techniques (*see* Chapter 16).

Circumcaval Ureter

While most deviations of the ureter are caused by pathologic processes in the retroperitoneum, one congenital anomaly, circumcaval ureter, results in a pathognomonic ureteral course. The IVC develops embryologically from persisting portions of the posterior cardinal, subcardinal, and supracardinal veins. Normally, the suprarenal IVC derives from the right subcardinal vein, and the infrarenal IVC derives from the right supracardinal vein. Circumcaval ureter results from formation of the infrarenal IVC from the persistent right posterior cardinal vein rather than from the right supracardinal vein. The right ureter is carried medially by the migration of the posterior cardinal vein toward the developing IVC. Symptoms of circumcaval ureter, if any, relate to the degree of ureteral obstruction.

The typical pattern on urography is a tortuous, dilated proximal right ureter and associated hydronephrosis. The course of the proximal ureter is described as having a "reverse J" configuration before it crosses behind and around the IVC and then descends medial to the ipsilateral lumbar pedicle (Fig. 2.21**A**). This severe medial deviation is the hallmark of circumcaval ureter. Confirmation of the diagnosis can be made with CT, which shows the ureter passing posterior and medial to the IVC (Fig. 2.21**B,C**).

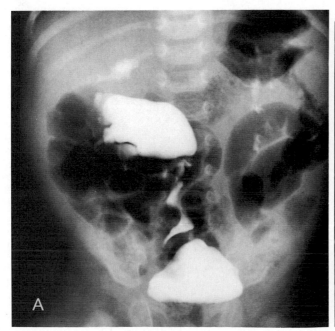

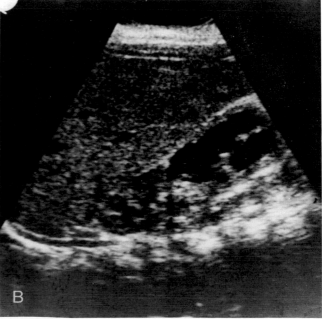

Figure 2.19. Ureteropelvic junction obstruction. **A,** Excretory urogram and **B,** sonogram demonstrate a ureteropelvic obstruction in the lower pole moiety of a duplicated renal collecting system.

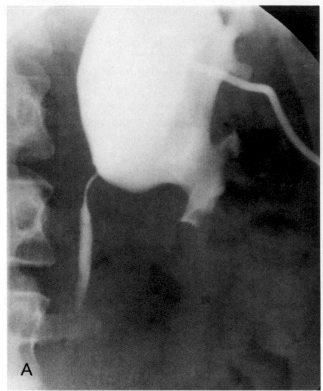

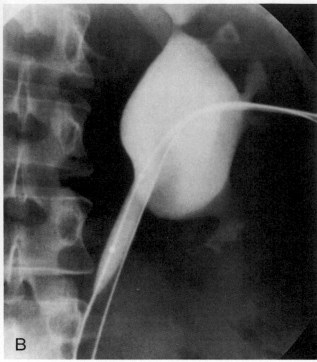

Figure 2.20. Balloon pyeloplasty. **A,** Nephrostogram demonstrates typical appearance of ureteropelvic junction (UPJ) obstruction. **B,** Balloon catheter has been inflated in the UPJ to perform pyeloplasty.

Duplex Collecting Systems

Duplication of the collecting system may be partial or complete. Partial duplication is the most frequently occurring congenital anomaly in the urinary tract. The duplex collecting system and its related abnormalities can result in some of the most complicated patterns detected on imaging studies in both children and adults.

The autopsy incidence of partial duplication is approximately 1 in 150 cases, while complete duplication is found approximately once in every 500 cases. However, the incidence in clinical series for this anomaly is up to 6 times higher, probably reflecting the likelihood for this anomaly to produce symptoms. Complete duplications are bilateral in up to 20% of cases.

Embryology

The ureter forms as a bud from the mesonephric duct (Fig. 2.22). The normal kidney is formed when this bud invaginates the metanephric blastema and, through multiple branchings, forms the collecting system and distal collecting ducts. Partial duplication results from the branching of the ureteral bud before it connects with the metanephric blastema. The point at which the ureteral bud branches will determine the level at which the two ureters join; this bifurcation may occur anywhere from the bladder wall to the renal pelvis. The latter will result in a bifid renal pelvis. On rare occasions, the single ureteral bud may trifurcate or may even branch into 4 or 5 segments before meeting the metanephric blastema, resulting in multiplication of the renal pelvis. Another variation occurs when one branch of a partially duplicated system fails to reach the kidney and becomes a blind-ending stump connected to the functional ureter (Fig. 2.23). This branch is sometimes short and is referred to as a ureteral diverticulum. However, because all layers of the ureteral wall are present, this branch is not a diverticulum and is more properly termed a blind-ending ureteral bud.

Complete duplication of the ureter occurs when two separate buds arise from the mesonephric duct. These buds invaginate the metanephric blastema separately, resulting in formation of separate upper and lower intrarenal collecting systems. Each of these systems is known as a moiety, and each is drained by a separate ureter. As the mesonephric duct migrates caudally during embryonic life, the ureter from the lower moiety is deposited near its expected normal location in the bladder, and its ureterovesical junction is therefore usually close to its normal position on the trigone. The ureter from the upper moiety remains attached to the mesonephric duct longer during its caudal migration, and eventually con-

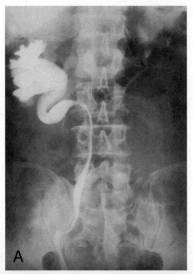

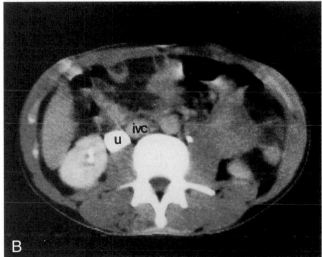

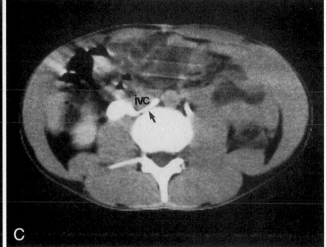

Figure 2.21.   Retrocaval ureter. **A,** Retrograde pyelography shows moderate right hydronephrosis with the characteristic "reversed J" appearance of the proximal ureter. The midportion of the ureter is medial to one lumbar pedicle. (From Amis ES Jr, Newhouse JH: *Essentials of Uroradiology.* Boston, Little

Brown & Co, 1991.) **B,** Computed tomography at the level of the lower pole of the right kidney shows the dilated proximal right ureter (u) lateral to the inferior vena cava (ivc). **C,** A section slightly lower reveals the ureter sweeping medially behind the inferior vena cava (*arrow*).

nects with the bladder inferiorly and medially. The Meyer-Weigert law states that the ureter from the upper moiety will enter the bladder inferiorly and medially (the ectopic ureter) in relation to the ureter draining the lower moiety (the orthotopic ureter).

The majority of complete and incomplete duplications are associated with normal function, and thus, are incidental findings on urography. Typically, the upper moiety is the smaller of the two, containing only two or three calices on average. This moiety drains approximately 25% of the upper portion of the kidney. On rare occasions, this configuration can be reversed. In cases of incomplete duplication the point at which the two proximal ureters join can actually occur in the bladder wall. In these cases, it may be impossible to differenti-

ate partial from complete duplication without cystoscopic evaluation to determine whether there are one or two orifices on the side in question. In uncomplicated complete duplications, the two orifices usually enter the bladder adjacent to each other in a relatively normal position on the trigone.

On ultrasound, a duplication may be demonstrated on longitudinal scans as two distinct groups of renal sinus echoes. Some investigators have reported, however, that this finding may be absent in a significant number of cases. Uncomplicated duplication may be difficult to demonstrate on CT because of the cross-sectional nature of the technique. Often, the two ureters may be demonstrated on caudal sections, but no one section will demonstrate both renal pelves. Scans obtained through

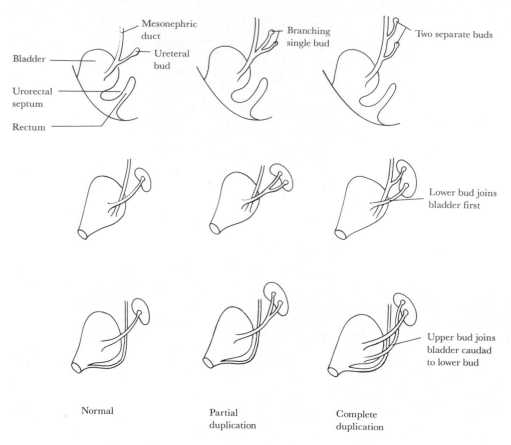

Figure 2.22. Embryology of duplex collecting systems. (From Amis ES Jr, Newhouse JH: *Essentials of Uroradiology.* Boston, Little Brown & Co, 1991.)

the junction of the upper and lower pole moieties (Fig. 2.24), however, will demonstrate an absence of collecting system elements or renal sinus fat. This feature has been termed the "faceless kidney" and may help identify duplication even in the absence of contrast enhancement.

Four distinct abnormalities of the termination of the ureters in complete duplications can result in significant pathologic changes in the duplicated kidney: (*a*) stenosis of the orifice of the upper pole ureter (resulting in hydronephrosis of the upper collecting system); (*b*) maldevelopment of the valve mechanism at the ureterovesical junction of the lower pole ureter (resulting in reflux); (*c*) ectopic insertion of the upper pole ureter outside the bladder; and (*d*) ectopic ureterocele also involving the ureter draining the upper moiety.

Stenosis of the Upper Pole Ureter

Because the orifice of the ureter draining the upper pole moiety enters the bladder in an ectopic location, its orifice may be stenotic leading to obstruction. Obstruction of the upper pole moiety may be present without reflux into the lower segment, reflux into the lower segment may be present without upper pole obstruction, or both abnormalities may be present concomitantly.

Maldevelopment of the Valve Mechanism of the Lower Pole Ureter

Improper development of the valve mechanism at the ureterovesical junction involves the orifice of the ureter draining the lower pole moiety. This orifice may be slightly above and lateral to its normal position on the trigone. Because of this abnormal location, there is shortening of the submucosal tunnel for the distal ureter, and thus, a more direct course through the bladder wall, a condition that facilitates reflux. The incidence of reflux into the lower moiety in complete duplications is significantly higher than for a single collecting system. Reflux into the lower moiety is the most common abnormality associated with complete duplications.

Radiographically, reflux can be demonstrated by voiding cystourethrography. The spectrum of radiographic appearances ranges from reflux into a nondilated normal-appearing lower pole collecting system to massive dilation of the lower moiety with complete loss of function. In addition, one usually finds reflux nephropathy, including focal or diffuse lower pole renal scarring with clubbing of the underlying calyces (Fig. 2.25).

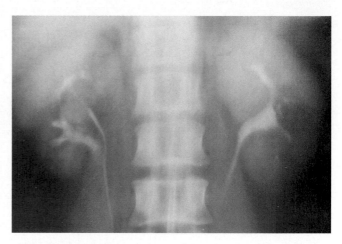

Figure 2.25. Reflux nephropathy in lower pole of a completely duplicated system. A nephrotomogram obtained during excretory urography reveals duplication on the right. The lower pole calyces are clubbed and there is loss of parenchyma in the right lower pole. Note the normal appearance of the right upper pole.

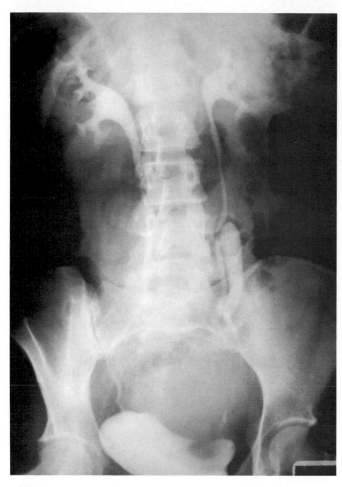

Figure 2.23. Ureteral diverticulum. Oblique film demonstrates origin of a ureteral diverticulum from the junction of the middle and distal thirds of the left ureter.

Ectopic Insertion of the Ureter

Another major abnormality associated with complete duplication is ectopic insertion of the ureter draining the upper pole. Typically, the insertion is extravesical in lo-

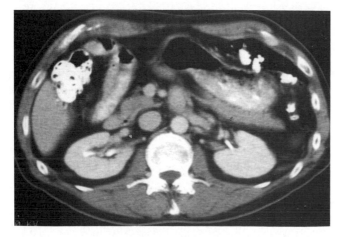

Figure 2.24. Duplicated collecting system. A computed tomography scan between the two renal pelves has been described as a "faceless kidney."

cation, resulting in obstruction and possible dysplasia of the upper moiety. More than two thirds of all extravesical ectopic ureteral insertions are associated with complete duplication. Figure 2.26 illustrates the sites of extravesical ectopic ureteral insertion. Remnants of the embryonic mesonephric duct can be found in the walls of the vagina, uterus, and broad ligaments in approximately one fourth of all adult females. These vestigial structures explain the ectopic insertion of the ureter into these female reproductive organs. In the male, ectopic insertion of the ureter into the vas deferens and seminal vesicles is easily explained by the fact that these organs are derived from the mesonephric duct, which also gives rise to the ureter. Ectopic ureters terminating outside the urinary tract tend to obstruct the upper pole moiety. Generally speaking, the more distal the ectopic orifice, the more dysplastic the upper moiety it drains will be.

Clinically, extravesical ectopic ureters in girls are commonly beyond sphincter control, resulting in continual dribbling incontinence of urine. This is not the case in males, because all ectopic orifices occur above the level of the external urethral sphincter. In males, a typical clinical presentation is chronic or recurrent epididymitis due to ectopic insertion of the ureter into the ipsilateral vas deferens or seminal vesicle.

Urographic findings range from an easily visualized dilated upper pole collecting system to complete nonvisualization of the upper moiety (Fig. 2.27). The presence of a nonfunctioning upper pole collecting system often can be inferred from the appearance of the visualized lower moiety. In these cases, the lower collecting system will usually exhibit reversal of its normal axis, fewer than the normal number of calyces expected for a

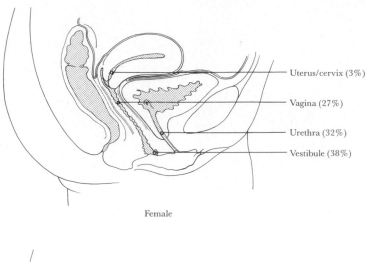

Female

Uterus/cervix (3%)

Vagina (27%)

Urethra (32%)

Vestibule (38%)

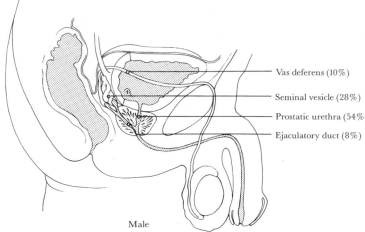

Male

Vas deferens (10%)

Seminal vesicle (28%)

Prostatic urethra (54%)

Ejaculatory duct (8%)

Figure 2.26. Sites of extravesical insertions of the upper moiety ureter in completely duplicated collecting systems.

(From Amis ES Jr, Newhouse JH: *Essentials of Uroradiology.* Boston, Little Brown & Co, 1991.)

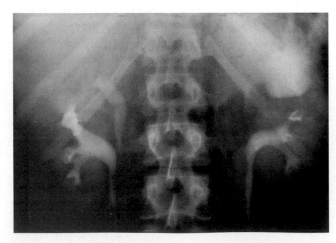

Figure 2.27. Bilateral duplication. There is mild blunting of calyces in upper pole of right kidney. The left upper pole moiety is hydronephrotic, creating a "drooping lily" appearance of the lower pole moiety.

nonduplicated kidney, and lateral deviation of the proximal ureter due to the medial location of the dilated ureter from the nonfunctioning upper pole. The appearance of the lower collecting system has been termed the "drooping lily" sign.

In patients in whom a nonfunctioning obstructed upper moiety is suspected, ultrasound typically shows an echo-free cystic area in the medial upper pole of the kidney (Fig. 2.28**A**). This represents the dilated upper collecting system, and its dilated ureter often can be traced distally to its insertion (Fig. 2.28**B**). Computed tomography also can demonstrate the hydronephrotic upper moiety and its dilated ureter. If necessary, antegrade pyelography usually delineates the anatomy of the ectopic insertion. In some cases, the ectopic orifice can be identified and catheterized, and retrograde studies can be performed. Voiding cystourethrography should be performed in all cases of duplication in which pathology is suspected, because it may demonstrate reflux into either moiety.

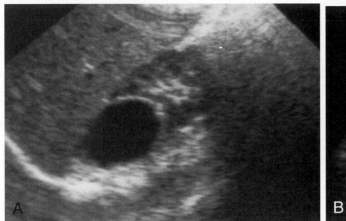

Figure 2.28. Ectopic ureteral insertion in a completely duplicated system. **A,** Sonography shows an echo-free mass in the
upper pole of the right kidney. **B,** The dilated ureter can be
seen coursing behind the bladder on the right in this transverse
sonogram through the pelvis. (From Amis ES Jr, Newhouse JH:
Essentials of Uroradiology. Boston, Little Brown & Co, 1991.)

Ectopic Ureterocele

A ureterocele is a focal dilatation of the submucosal
portion of the distal ureter. Ureteroceles may be orthotopic (simple) or ectopic. An orthotopic ureterocele is
associated with a single collecting system and is discussed in the next section (see Anomalous Termination
of the Ureter). Virtually all *ectopic ureteroceles* are associated with ipsilateral complete duplication. The ureterocele is always associated with the ureter from the upper moiety. This dilatation may extend to the bladder
neck or even into the posterior urethra (Fig. 2.29). Approximately one half of all ectopic ureteroceles terminate within the bladder, where they may be associated
with vesicoureteral reflux into the lower pole moiety.
The majority, however, have stenotic orifices that do not

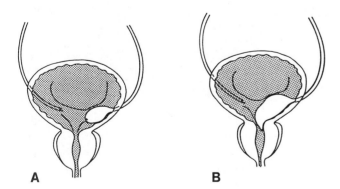

Figure 2.29. Diagram of types of ectopic ureteroceles. **A,**
Approximately one half of ectopic ureteroceles terminate in
the bladder. **B,** The remainder extend through the bladder
neck and terminate in the proximal urethra. (From Amis ES Jr,
Newhouse JH: *Essentials of Uroradiology.* Boston, Little Brown
& Co, 1991.)

reflux, but are associated with hydronephrosis of the
upper pole. Ectopic ureteroceles also may course submucosally through the bladder neck and may terminate
in the posterior urethra, where a widely patent orifice is
the rule rather than the exception.

This latter ureterocele often refluxes during voiding,
but is obstructed when the patient is not voiding because it empties into the normally closed urethra.
Overall, almost one half of ureteroceles may demonstrate reflux during cystourethrography, at least during
voiding.

As with ectopic ureteral insertions, ectopic ureteroceles may be associated with little or no function of their
associated ipsilateral upper pole collecting systems, or
obstruction by the ureterocele may be mild, allowing
good visualization of the upper moiety. Because of their
size and location, large ectopic ureteroceles may distort
the ipsilateral lower pole ureteral orifice, and thereby
may increase the incidence of reflux into the lower moiety. Conversely, large ectopic ureteroceles may directly
compress and obstruct the ipsilateral lower pole orifice.
In fact, an ectopic ureterocele may be large enough to
extend across the midline and obstruct the contralateral
ureteral orifice or prolapse into the bladder neck with
subsequent bladder outlet obstruction.

An ectopic ureterocele typically presents during urography or cystography as a smooth rounded or ovoid filling defect in the bladder base (Fig. 2.30). While they
tend to be laterally oriented, if large enough, they can
be midline. Ectopic ureteroceles may range in size from
1 cm to several centimeters in diameter.

Urographic upper tract findings in completely duplicated systems complicated by either ectopic ureteral insertion or an ectopic ureterocele tend to be identical, as

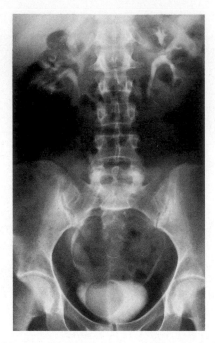

Figure 2.30. Ectopic ureterocele with minimal obstruction. An excretory urogram reveals complete duplication on the right with minimal dilation of the upper pole moiety. The dilated ureter from the right upper pole can be seen terminating in a round ectopic ureterocele clearly defined within the bladder.

both abnormalities affect the upper moiety, often resulting in dilation and nonfunction (Fig. 2.31). Therefore, ultrasonographic findings will be similar to those described in earlier paragraphs for ectopic ureteral insertion. If it is difficult to determine the pathologic change

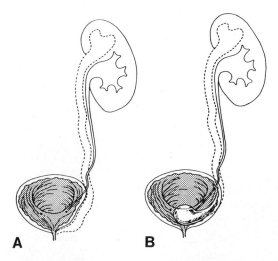

Figure 2.31. Similar upper urinary tract changes caused by ectopic insertion and ectopic ureterocele in completely duplicated systems. **A,** Ectopic insertion into the urethra results in upper moiety hydronephrosis with an associated dilated ureter. **B,** An ectopic ureterocele can result in identical upper urinary tract changes. (From Amis ES Jr, Newhouse JH: *Essentials of Uroradiology*. Boston, Little Brown & Co, 1991.)

involving the distal ureter, antegrade pyelography via the nonfunctioning dilated upper pole system will allow opacification of the entire pathologic drainage. Unlike ectopic insertion of the ureter, in which the dilated distal ureter is seen coursing posteriorly or laterally to the bladder, pelvic sonography for ectopic ureterocele will demonstrate a thin septation in the bladder representing the distended ureterocele.

Anomalous Termination of the Ureter

The anomalies involving the termination of the ureter have been discussed to large degree in the above sections on primary megaureter and ureteral duplications. However, orthotopic ureterocele, ectopic ureteral orifice, and reflux can occur in nonduplicated systems and deserves further brief discussion.

Ureterocele

Orthotopic ureteroceles occur in normal position on the trigone and also are known as simple or adult-type ureteroceles. The etiology of both types of ureteroceles is probably the same, although there is no well-defined theory regarding how they are formed. The remainder of this discussion deals with orthotopic ureteroceles.

During excretory urography, the orthotopic ureterocele is seen as "cobra head" or "spring onion" deformity of the distal ureter protruding into the bladder lumen in the region of the trigone (Fig. 2.32). If the ureter is opacified with contrast, the central portion of the ureterocele also is opacified in continuity with the remainder of the ureter, but is surrounded by a lucent rim, representing the bladder mucosa around the ureterocele (Fig. 2.33). There is typically no or very little obstruction, although on rare occasions the ureterocele may cause rather severe upper tract dilation.

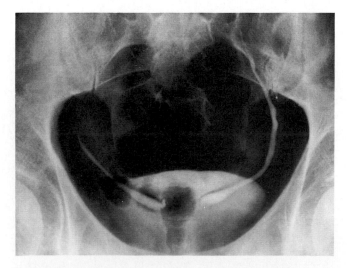

Figure 2.32. Excretory urogram showing bilateral simple ureteroceles with classic "cobra head" appearance.

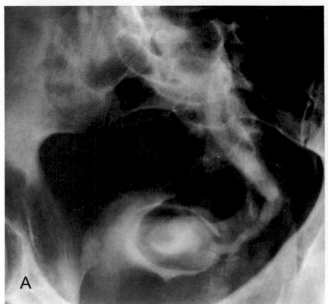

Figure 2.33.   A, Oblique supine view of excretory urogram showing large simple ureterocele containing contrast medium. The distal one third of the left ureter is slightly dilated. **B,** Same patient. Upright prevoid film showing ureterocele has filled with contrast medium. The double layer of mucosa compressing the wall of the ureterocele is radiolucent.

Ectopic Ureteral Insertion

An ectopic ureter is defined as a ureter that does not terminate in the normal location on the trigone of the bladder. By convention, the term is used to define a ureter that opens outside the urinary bladder. Eighty percent of ectopic ureters are found in association with complete duplication of the ureter. The anomaly is more common in female patients by a 6:1 ratio. In male patients, however, the majority of ectopic ureters drain single systems (Fig. 2.34). With ectopic insertion of a nonduplicated ureter, an absent hemitrigone will be found in the bladder on the side of ectopic insertion. The possible sites of ectopic insertion have been previously discussed in the section on ureteral duplication. The more distal the insertion (e.g., into the vas deferens in the male), the more dysplastic will be the ipsilateral kidney. In such cases, there will be minimal, if any, kidney function. For more proximal extravesical insertions, such as into the posterior urethra, obstruction and reduced function of the involved kidney will be the predominant finding.

Vesicoureteral Reflux

The normal ureterovesical junction acts as a one-way valve that allows urine to flow freely from the ureter into the bladder, but prevents reverse flow. The ureter traverses the bladder wall at a slightly oblique angle and then courses submucosally for approximately 2 cm to the ureteral orifice. As the bladder fills, the intravesical pressure is exerted on the wall of the bladder equally in all directions; this results in pressure on the bladder epithe-

lium overlying the submucosal ureter and subsequent flattening of this portion of the ureter against its muscular backing, preventing reflux. This flattening, however, does not prevent normal ureteral peristalsis from propelling a bolus of urine from the ureter into the bladder as long as bladder pressure remains within normal limits.

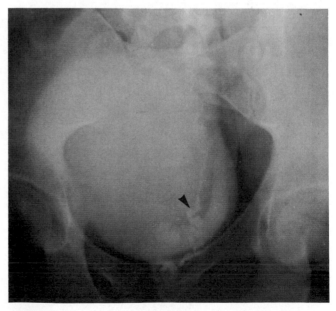

Figure 2.34.   Excretory urogram in a patient with lower abdominal and perineal pain. Ectopic insertion of the left ureter into the left seminal vesicle is seen. The ejaculatory duct and refluxing contrast medium into the ampulla of the vas deferens (*arrowhead*) is seen.

If the course of the ureter through the bladder wall is more direct, and if the submucosal course is shortened, this valve mechanism fails to function properly, and vesicoureteral reflux occurs. The hydrostatic effect of reflux alone can result in reflux atrophy of the kidney. However, intrarenal reflux of urine can occur, resulting in reflux nephropathy, a combination of clubbed calyces and overlying parenchymal scarring. This is also known as chronic atrophic pyelonephritis. These findings tend to occur in the renal polar regions. The presence of compound calyces in these areas is believed to facilitate reflux into the collecting ducts. Normally, duct orifices on the papillae have an antirefluxing configuration; but in compound calyces, this configuration is distorted, allowing the intrarenal reflux to occur.

PRUNE BELLY SYNDROME

Prune belly syndrome (Eagle-Barrett syndrome) is a rare congenital syndrome characterized by the classical triad of absent abdominal musculature, undescended testicles, and urinary tract abnormalities initially described in the late 19th century. Although absence of abdominal musculature has been described in female patients, the full syndrome including the urinary tract abnormalities only develops in males.

Clinically, the syndrome is recognizable at birth because of the characteristic features produced by the absent abdominal musculature (Fig. 2.35). The deficiency typically affects the lower abdominal wall; the upper abdomen has a normal appearance. In some cases, the

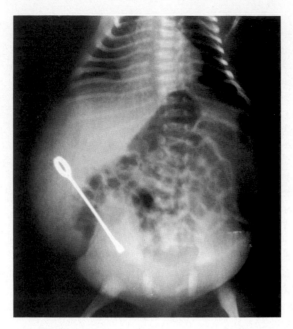

Figure 2.35. Prune belly syndrome. An abdominal radiograph of a newborn with prune belly syndrome shows bulging of the flanks as a result of the absence of abdominal musculature.

muscular defect is partial or asymmetric. The overlying skin has a wrinkled appearance reminiscent of a prune; in older children, the wrinkling tends to disappear and is replaced by a "potbelly" appearance. The precise cause of the syndrome has been a matter of dispute; some authorities believe that the distended urinary tract sec-

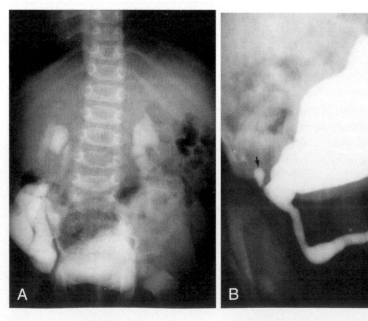

Figure 2.36. Prune belly syndrome. **A,** Excretory urography reveals bilaterally dilated and extremely tortuous ureters. By contrast, the kidneys reveal only minimal hydronephrosis. **B,** Voiding cystourethrography reveals wide dilation of the prostatic urethra. The utricle (*arrow*) is mildly dilated. (From Amis ES Jr, Newhouse JH: *Essentials of Uroradiology*. Boston, Little Brown & Co, 1991).

ondary to outlet obstruction prevents abdominal muscle development. Others have postulated that prostatic dysgenesis and transient neonatal ascites are responsible; still others believe that the urinary tract abnormalities and the abdominal wall defect are secondary to a mesodermal deficiency.

The urinary tract abnormalities affect the kidneys, the ureters, the bladder, and the urethra. Although the kidneys may be normal, renal dysplasia or hydronephrosis often is described. The findings in the kidneys may be asymmetric, with a normal renal unit on one side while the opposite kidney is dysplastic. The ureters tend to be tortuous and dilated (Fig. 2.36**A**), most often in a segmental distribution. Vesicoureteral reflux is common. The ureteral abnormalities have been attributed to a deficiency of smooth muscle. The bladder is typically very large and may be associated with a patent urachus. The prostatic urethra is characteristically dilated and tapers rapidly at the membranous urethra (Fig. 2.36**B**), occasionally resembling posterior urethral valves. The dilated posterior urethra is believed to be secondary to prostatic hypoplasia. The anterior urethra is usually normal, although an association with megalourethra has been described. The testes are cryptorchid, usually in an abdominal location.

Extraurinary abnormalities that may be present include intestinal malrotation, congenital heart defects, and musculoskeletal deformities.

Patients with urinary tract abnormalities characteristic of the prune belly syndrome, but who have normal abdominal musculature, have been described. Such cases are thought to represent an incomplete or variant manifestation of the syndrome.

LOWER URINARY TRACT ANOMALIES

Bladder

Exstrophy

The most common congenital bladder lesion is exstrophy. It is the result of a deficiency in development of the lower abdominal wall musculature, so that the bladder is open and the mucosa of the bladder is continuous with the skin. There is associated epispadias in which the urethra is open dorsally and urethral mucosa covers the dorsum of a short penis. The condition occurs in approximately 1 in 50,000 births and has a male/female ratio of 2:1.

Skeletal and gastrointestinal anomalies are commonly associated with exstrophy. Separation of the symphysis pubis correlates directly with the severity of the exstrophy-epispadias complex. In full-blown exstrophy, the pubic bones are widely separated (Fig. 2.37). The exstrophy-epispadic anomaly may be associated with ureteric obstruction and unilateral or bilateral pelvicaliectasis due to fibrosis at the ureterovesical junction. However, in

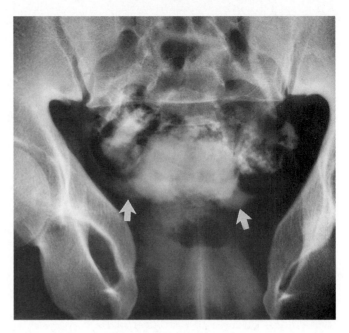

Figure 2.37. Exstrophy of the bladder. Excretory urogram in this patient who has not had bladder repair reveals the typical "Hurley stick" deformity of the distal ureters just proximal to the ureterovesical junctions (*arrows*). The bladder is ill-defined because it has failed to close in the midline. Note the widely separated pubic symphysis.

most cases the upper tracts are normal, but there may be widening of the distal ureters. This widening has been likened to a "Hurley," the stick used in the traditional Irish game of hurling. Umbilical and inguinal hernias are frequently present. In the past, management typically consisted of excision of the bladder and urinary diversion by ureterosigmoidostomy. Radiologic assessment in such patients is required at periodic intervals to exclude the adenocarcinoma of the colon that may develop at the ureterosigmoid anastomosis. More recently, most children with exstrophy are treated with a primary closure of the bladder and subsequent bladder augmentation.

Bladder Duplication

Bladder duplication is extremely rare and may be complete or incomplete. Variations include bladder septum, which may be multiple and which divides the bladder into two or more compartments. The embryogenesis of bladder duplication is not clearly understood. Complete duplication may result from a bifurcation of the cloacal septum, resulting in two ventral bladders and urogenital sinuses. In complete duplication, both bladders lie side by side, separated by a peritoneal fold. Each bladder has normal musculature and mucosa, and the ipsilateral ureter drains into each bladder. Each bladder has a separate urethral orifice that may drain into a common urethra with a single penis, or there may be complete duplication of the urethra and penis. Lower gastrointestinal anomalies are commonly associated.

Partial duplication occurs when a coronal or sagittal septum completely or incompletely divides the bladder and there is a single urethra for drainage. In cases of complete division, one of the ureters may drain into a segment of the bladder not drained by the urethra, resulting in nonfunctional dysplasia of the associated kidney.

Agenesis of the bladder is usually incompatible with life, death resulting from obstruction and renal failure. A few cases of bladder agenesis have been reported in children who lived long enough for a diagnosis to be made. Most of these patients were females.

Congenital Bladder Diverticulum

A congenital diverticulum occurs in close relationship to the ureteral orifice, typically opening just above and lateral to it. Such a finding often is called a Hutch diverticulum. Because of distortion of the valve mechanism at the ureterovesical junction by the diverticulum, vesicoureteral reflux may result.

Bladder Ears

Bladder ears are seen in infants or very young children during urography or cystography as inferolateral protrusions of the bladder, usually bilaterally, into the regions of the inguinal canals. These become less apparent as the bladder fills to capacity, and disappear as the child grows. They are probably due to a close relationship of the bladder to the inguinal rings in infants, and are not considered true herniations of the bladder.

Urachus

The allantois is the attachment of the bladder dome to the umbilicus. Initially the bladder is an abdominal organ, but it then descends into the pelvis. As this happens, the bladder dome narrows to form the urachus, which elongates with bladder descent. Normally this umbilical attachment of the bladder becomes a completely obliterated fibrous cord (umbilical ligament). Failure of this fibrous closure results in a patent urachus through which urine can flow from the bladder to the umbilicus. The male:female ratio of patent urachus is 3:1. Segmental failure of closure of the urachus at the bladder attachment results in a urachocele, or diverticulum in the dome of the bladder. Failure of closure at the umbilical attachment results in a draining umbilical sinus. Failure of closure in any other part of the duct results in a urachal cyst. Urachal cyst (Fig. 2.38, 2.39) is usually clinically silent unless infection supervenes. Calculi have been reported within urachal cysts and may be seen on plain film as small punctate calcifications above the bladder outline.

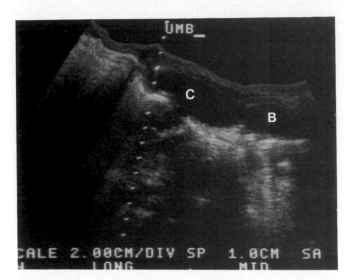

Figure 2.38. Transabdominal ultrasound longitudinal scan in a 3-year-old boy with a palpable abdominal mass. The study shows a urachal cyst (C) with clear definition of space between the cyst and the bladder (B). (Courtesy of A. Daneman, M.D.)

Müllerian Duct Cyst and Dilated Prostatic Utricle

Normal müllerian duct atrophy occurs in about the sixth week in the fetus. The vestigial remnants of this ductal obliteration are the prostatic utricle and the appendix of the testis. Nonatrophy of the müllerian duct may produce cystic dilatations along the route of the vas deferens from the scrotum to the ejaculatory ducts. Müllerian duct cysts are rare, but most commonly occur in the midline just above the prostate. They may occasionally become large enough to cause an impression on the posterior bladder wall or to obstruct the bladder outlet.

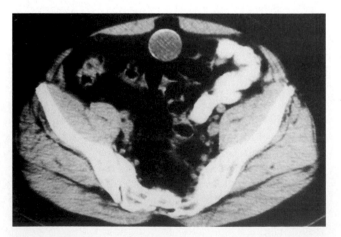

Figure 2.39. Urachal cyst. Computed tomography reveals a midline cystic structure with thin peripheral calcification behind the anterior abdominal wall. There is no soft tissue component to suggest tumor or infiltration of the surrounding fat to indicate infection.

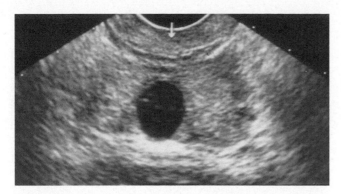

Figure 2.40.   Müllerian duct cyst. A cystic mass is well defined in this transrectal ultrasound examination.

If infection supervenes, suprapubic and rectal pain occur. Fluid aspirated from a müllerian duct cyst may be serous, mucoid, purulent, or hemorrhagic, but it contains no spermatozoa. These cysts can be imaged with ultrasound (Fig. 2.40), CT, or magnetic resonance imaging (MRI).

Another müllerian remnant problem is a dilated utricle, which is commonly associated with hypospadias and incomplete testicular descent, a complex of findings suggesting intersex. The normal prostatic utricle is 8 to 10 mm in length, narrow at its orifice (2 mm) in the verumontanum, and bulbous at its blind end. Because the dilated utricle communicates with the urethra, it can be imaged during antegrade or retrograde urethrography (Fig. 2.41).

Seminal Vesicles

Congenital seminal vesicle anomalies result from interruption or failure of the normal development of the mesonephric duct. The mesonephric duct develops ureteric buds dorsomedially after 5 weeks of gestation. The ureteric buds grow cranially and dorsally to meet the nephrogenic ridge and form the metanephros, which becomes the normal kidney. As fetal growth continues, the ureters derive separate openings into the bladder, and the mesonephric duct moves caudally and ends as the ejaculatory duct. Small buds develop in the distal mesonephric duct that become the seminal vesicles.

Any deviation in the development of the ureteric bud or the seminal vesicle bud results in a congenital anomaly. When both buds fail to develop, the ipsilateral kidney, ureter, hemitrigone, and seminal vesicle are lost. Failure to develop the normal ureteric bud results in renal agenesis and a normal seminal vesicle. Failure to develop a normal seminal vesicle bud results in a normal kidney, ureter, and hemitrigone and absent seminal vesicle. Abnormal development of the distal mesonephric bud may result in atresia of the seminal vesicle duct, resulting in seminal vesicle obstruction producing a seminal vesicle cyst (Fig. 2.42). Seminal vesicle cyst is commonly associated with ipsilateral absence of the kidney and ureter (Fig. 2.5). Rarely, the anomaly involves delay in the origin of the ureteric bud such that the seminal vesicle bud gives rise to the ureteric bud, resulting in ectopic insertion of the ureter into the seminal vesicle. Seminal vesicle cysts rarely enlarge enough to be of clinical significance. They most commonly present in the third decade but have been reported in patients up to

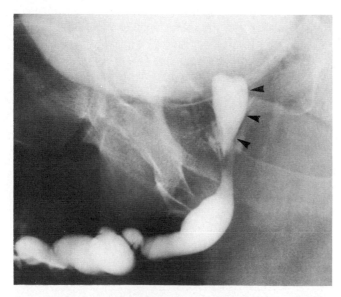

Figure 2.41.   Dynamic retrograde urethrogram in a patient with hypospadias and multiple postoperative anterior urethral strictures. Congenital cystic dilatation of the prostatic utricle (*arrowheads*) is demonstrated. (From McCallum RW, Colapinto V. *Urologic Radiology of the Adult Male Lower Urinary Tract*. Springfield, IL, Charles C Thomas, p. 55, 1976.)

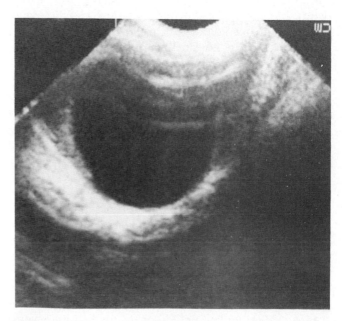

Figure 2.42.   Transrectal ultrasound in a 50-year-old man with lower abdominal pain. A 4-cm cyst is seen arising from the left seminal vesicle.

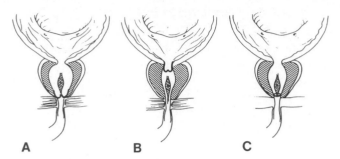

A   **B**   **C**

Figure 2.43. Classification of posterior urethral valves. **A,** Type 1 valves are leaflets extending from the distal verumontanum to the walls of the urethra. **B,** Type 2 valves are seen in the proximal prostatic urethra and probably represent redundant mucosal folds. **C,** Type 3 valve is a diaphragm extending across the distal prostatic urethra. The size of the opening in this diaphragm determines the degree of obstruction. (From Amis ES Jr, Newhouse JH: *Essentials of Uroradiology.* Boston, Little Brown & Co, 1991.)

60 years of age. When such cysts are large, patients present clinically with urgency, frequency, and dysuria. Pelvic and perineal pain are common.

Urethra

Many of the congenital urethral lesions discussed in the following paragraphs are obstructive and consequently produce vesical and ureteric dilatation. Severe obstruction results in gross hydronephrosis with renal obstructive atrophy. Because the lower urinary tract has completely formed by the end of the fourth month of gestation and because fetal micturition also occurs at this time, complete obstruction may lead to intrauterine death. Incomplete obstruction may be compatible with a live birth, but failure to thrive and vomiting in the neonate or early life are symptoms of renal failure, which raises the possibility of outlet obstruction from a urethral anomaly.

Posterior Urethral Valves

The continuation of the inferior aspect of the verumontanum is the urethral crest, which is a mucosal fold that is originally midline but divides into two to four fins (plicae colliculi) that take a spiral course to end inferiorly in the membranous urethra, anteriorly and midline. These plicae colliculi are vestigial remnants of the migrating wolffian duct orifices. When the origin of the wolffian duct orifice is too far anterior, normal migration is altered, leading to abnormal fusion and insertion of the plicae colliculi and resulting in thick valve cusps.

In 1919, Young classified urethral valves into three types (Fig. 2.43). Type 1 is the most common and consists of valve leaflets extending from the distal verumontanum to the urethral walls. These valves act as sails, ballooning out during voiding and resulting in out-

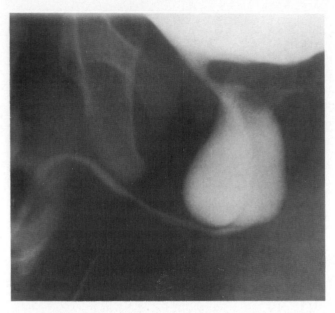

Figure 2.44. Voiding cystourethrogram in a 2-year-old boy. The posterior urethra is dilated down to the membranous urethra. The valves are visible. (Courtesy of A. Daneman, M.D.)

let obstruction (Fig. 2.44). Type 2 posterior urethral valves are mucosal folds extending proximally from the verumontanum to the bladder neck. These are rare and are probably caused by mucosal redundancy secondary to current or prior, more distal urethral obstruction. Thus, many authorities no longer consider type 2 valves to be true valves because they are acquired rather than congenital. A type 3 posterior urethral valve also is rare and is unrelated to the verumontanum. It occurs in the distal prostatic urethra as an iris-like membrane with a central pinhole orifice (Fig. 2.45).

Posterior urethral valves are the most common cause of obstructive symptoms in infants and very young

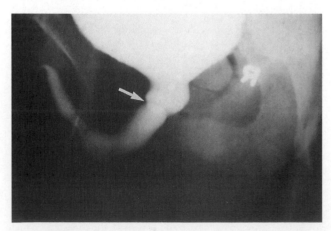

Figure 2.45. Type 3 posterior urethral valve. Voiding cystourethrogram reveals an iris diaphragm type of valve (*arrow*) extending across the prostatic urethra causing proximal dilation.

boys; they occur only in males. The condition may cause complete obstruction leading to renal failure, oligohydramnios, and intrauterine death. Vesicoureteral reflux (occurring in approximately 50% of patients) or high intravesical pressure can result in massive hydrostatic pressure in the kidney, leading to calyceal rupture and resultant subcapsular or perirenal urinomas. Fetal and/or neonatal urine ascites also may occur. Neonatal clinical diagnosis therefore includes palpable kidneys and bladder, abdominal distention, ascites, straining to void, and an absent or dribbling urinary stream. Blood urea nitrogen and creatinine levels are usually elevated, indicating renal impairment. Renal function may return to normal after the obstruction is relieved, depending on the degree of renal damage. Occasionally, chronic renal failure may occur in spite of surgical intervention to relieve obstruction.

Young children may present with symptoms of urinary tract infection; fever, vomiting, and hematuria should lead to an investigation of the urinary tract. This also may occur in older children and young adults when the degree of obstruction due to posterior urethral valves may be so mild that investigation is delayed until superimposed infection occurs. The variability of the degree of obstruction may lead to dilemmas of diagnosis and management, whereby some cases are mistakenly diagnosed as neurogenic bladder. It is therefore mandatory to include posterior urethral valves in the differential diagnosis of urinary tract infection or outlet obstruction in male infants, children, and young adults.

Posterior urethral valves are best demonstrated in children and young adults by voiding cystourethrography. There is no difficulty with the insertion of a catheter into the bladder in type 1 valves, but catheter insertion may be difficult in type 3 valves. Bladder filling demonstrates a large-capacity bladder, bladder trabeculation with diverticula, or vesicoureteral reflux in approximately one half of the cases, and a somewhat narrowed bladder neck due to hypertrophy of the bladder detrusor. The voiding study demonstrates a dilated posterior urethra with poor distention of the membranous and anterior urethra. The valves occasionally may be seen as lucent bands bulging distally across the prostatic urethra and impeding the flow of urine.

Fibroepithelial Polyp

Fibroepithelial polyp in the urethra is rare and is of embryonic origin, usually originating in the prostate and projecting into the urethra. This condition presents at birth with difficulty in micturition or intermittent stream that may progress to retention. The polyp is connected to the verumontanum via a stalk, which allows it to rest in the prostatic urethra or even extend through the bladder neck into the bladder; during the voiding phase of cystourethrography it is typically seen as a smooth filling defect extending into the midportion of the bulbar urethra.

Atresia Ani-Urethralis

Anal atresia in the male may be associated with a fistulous tract between the bowel and posterior urethra, resulting in difficulty catheterizing the bladder. If the fistulous tract goes untreated, recurrent urinary tract infection may eventually result in renal failure. Treatment of the anal atresia by colostomy is insufficient, because urine passes along the fistulous tract into the bowel forming "bowel calculi," the result of urinary crystalloids combining with colonic mucous.

Meatal Stenosis

Congenital meatal stenosis can account for severe outlet obstruction in the male and can produce the same degree of hydronephrosis, bladder dilatation, and trabeculation as urethral valves. Meatal stenosis of this degree is a much less common cause of hydronephrosis than is posterior urethral valves. Catheter insertion through the external meatus is difficult or impossible. The stenosis is easily treated by a meatotomy. An associated wide-necked diverticulum may arise from the dorsal urethra within the glans penis; this is referred to as a lacuna magna and also can be an isolated occurrence. Diagnosis of meatal stenosis is clinical.

Hypospadias

In hypospadias, the external urethral meatus is found on the ventral surface of the penis, anywhere from just proximal to its normal location to the perineum. Although clinically obvious on physical examination, hypospadias is usually asymptomatic until bladder training has been completed, after which the urinary stream is found to be difficult to direct and may require, depending on the severity of the anomaly, sitting to void. Urethroplasty to construct a new distal urethra is required.

Epispadias

Epispadias is less common than hypospadias. The external urethral orifice opens onto the dorsum of the penis, and as for hypospadias, urethroplasty is required for correction. In patients with exstrophy, epispadias is complete with the entire urethra lying open along the dorsum of a foreshortened penis.

Anterior Urethral Diverticulum

Congenital urethral diverticulum occurs only in males and arises from the ventral surface of the anterior urethra. Urethral diverticulum in the adult female is thought to be acquired. In the male, anterior urethral diverticulum is the result of failure of closure of urethral folds or an abortive attempt at urethral duplication. The diverticulum has a somewhat narrow neck and fills during voiding. As the diverticulum fills, it increases in size and compresses the true urethra. This may result in significant obstructive voiding symptoms. At the end of micturition, the diverticulum empties, causing postvoid dribbling. Diagnosis is best accomplished by voiding cystourethrography. Removal of the diverticulum requires urethroplasty to repair the defect in the urethral floor.

Anterior urethral valves also have been described, and result in a clinical and radiographic pattern difficult to distinguish from an anterior urethral diverticulum (Fig. 2.46). Currently it is unclear whether such a valve is a true entity or is simply the anterior lip of a diverticulum.

As mentioned in association with meatal stenosis, a dorsal urethral diverticulum can occur in the region of the fossa navicularis. These diverticula are typically round and are known as lacuna magna. Their opening is obscured during retrograde urethrography but, if suspected, can usually be demonstrated by voiding studies.

Urethral Duplication

No satisfactory embryologic explanation has been suggested to explain urethral duplication, which may be complete or incomplete.

In complete duplication in the male patient, there may be accompanying bladder or penile duplication or both. The two urethras lie one above the other in males, and the ventral channel usually proves to be the more functional and normal appearing. In female patients, duplicated urethrae lie side by side. When the anomalous urethra lies outside the control of the internal and distal sphincter mechanism, urinary incontinence is the presenting symptom. The anomalous urethra has an epispadiac or hypospadiac external meatus and is subject to recurrent infection. Indications for removal of the anomalous urethra are urinary incontinence and urethritis in the anomalous urethra.

In incomplete duplication, two external meati may be found with two urethras joining near the bladder neck or two urethrae may originate from the bladder neck and may join at some point distally to form a single urethra (Fig. 2.47). Both retrograde and voiding urethrography may be necessary to completely define the extent of this anomaly.

Congenital Urethral Stricture

Congenital urethral stricture has been reported in children, but not in neonates or infants. It is questionable whether urethral stricture is ever congenital. More likely such strictures result from some form of trauma.

Retention Cyst of Cowper's Duct

Cowper's glands are two pea-sized glands lying within or at the inferior fascia of the urogenital diaphragm. The ducts of these glands are approximately 2 cm in length, extend from the urogenital diaphragm inferiorly, and pass through the corpus spongiosum to enter the mid-bulbous urethra on both sides of midline. Rarely the ducts join before entering the urethra as a single opening. Cowper's glands secrete mucin that is a lubricator for semen and prevents coagulation of spermatozoa during ejaculation. Cowper's duct cysts have been reported in newborn infants and are thought to be the result of a congenital malformation of the ostia producing ductal obstruction resulting in retention cyst swelling. The retention cyst projects into the bulbous urethra and may cause minor urinary symptoms such as frequency or

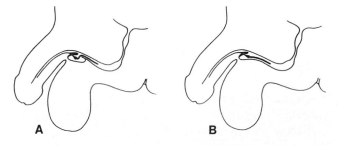

Figure 2.46. Diagram of anterior urethral diverticulum and anterior urethral valve. **A,** Note that the proximal portion of the diverticulum forms an acute angle with the urethra. Elevation of the distal lip of the diverticulum against the roof of the urethra acts as an obstruction as the diverticulum fills. **B,** An anterior urethral valve, if such an entity truly exists, has the same obstructive mechanism as a diverticulum. Note that there is no proximal angulation such as that seen with the diverticulum. (From Amis ES Jr, Newhouse JH: *Essentials of Uroradiology.* Boston, Little Brown & Co, 1991.)

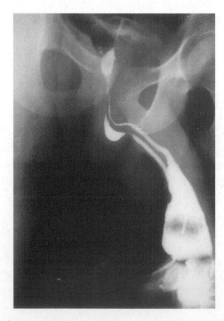

Figure 2.47. Urethral duplication. Retrograde urethrography is performed with the balloon inflated in the common distal channel. Note that the ventral urethra is more normal appearing.

strangury; large retention cysts may cause obstructive symptoms. Retention cysts of Cowper's ducts may burst spontaneously into the urethra without causing symptoms and may be more common than appreciated. Retention cysts in adults are generally the result of an inflammatory process such as infection or trauma.

On urethrography, a Cowper's duct cyst is seen as an indentation on the floor of the mid- or proximal bulbar urethra (Fig. 2.48).

Undescended Testicle

Undescended testicle, also known as cryptorchism or cryptorchidism, commonly occurs as an isolated phenomenon or may be associated with other urogenital anomalies, such as renal agenesis or ectopia, prune belly syndrome, and epispadias. Up to 20% of premature males are born with undescended testes. In most of these infants, normal descent into the scrotum occurs within the first few weeks to months of life. In term infants, the incidence is significantly lower, and further decreases to approximately 1% by 1 year of age because of spontaneous descent.

The undescended testicle often is smaller than the normal descended testis. In a small number of these patients, testicular agenesis occurs. The most common ectopic position for the undescended testicle is in the inguinal canal. However, arrested descent of the testes may occur in the abdomen, pelvis, or high in the scrotum after passage through the inguinal canal. Failure of normal testicular descent into the scrotum is caused by hormonal dysfunction or mechanical obstruction. The hormonal stimulus for testicular descent is testosterone, the production of which by the fetus is dependent on adenohypophyseal gonadotrophin. Abnormality in the secretion of either hormone may result in arrested descent of the testes. Gonadotrophin secretion is commonly normal, but the normal response of the gubernaculum in guiding the testes into the scrotum is lacking.

The testis itself may be abnormally formed, resulting in a lack of testosterone production. When secretion of gonadotrophin and testosterone are normal, arrested descent is caused by mechanical obstruction. Because the most common site for an undescended testicle is the inguinal canal, one can assume that hormonal secretion has been normal to get the testes so far descended, and that the lack of further descent is mechanical, due to obstruction of the process vaginalis or to the formation of a septum at the scrotal neck. Complications of the undescended testicle include malignant change, sterility, and testicular torsion. A testis arrested in the inguinal canal also is subject to accidental injury. The incidence of malignant change in the undescended testicle is high. In the normal male population, the incidence of testis tumor is approximately 2:100,000. This increases to 10:100,000 in inguinally placed undescended testis, and the rate is even higher in arrested descent in the pelvis or abdomen.

Imaging modalities used in the detection of undescended testicle include ultrasound, CT, MRI, and spermatic venography. Ultrasound is useful in the detection of the undescended testicle when the arrest is in the inguinal canal. However, ultrasound is of little value in detecting arrested descent in the abdomen or pelvis unless malignant change has occurred producing a mass. High-frequency transducers can successfully define the undescended inguinal testis in most cases. Both sides should be examined for symmetry. An asymmetric mass in the inguinal region with the echogenic characteristics of the normal testes is the most common finding. However, the mediastinum testes must be identified. Rarely, the pars infravaginales gubernaculi can present a similar echogenic appearance to the testis and may be distant from the undescended testis that may be in the pelvis. The pars infravaginales gubernaculi does not show the characteristic mediastinum testes. The undescended testis that is atrophic is more difficult to identify because its echogenicity may be variable and, unlike the normal testis, the epididymis may not be seen. Malignant change in the undescended testis is seen on ultrasound as a mass of indefinable echogenicity in the inguinal canal.

Computed tomography accurately identifies the undescended testicle in and adjacent to the inguinal canal (Fig. 2.49). Contiguous 5-mm collimation from the scrotum up to the iliac crest is recommended. Normally structures in this region are symmetric. In undescended testes, asymmetry occurs with the presence of a small mass on the affected side corresponding to the undescended testicle. An asymmetric mass larger than the expected testicular size raises the possibility of malignant change. Because an undescended testicle may be as small as 1 cm, it is necessary to opacify bowel with oral contrast material. Magnetic resonance imaging has similar spatial resolution to CT

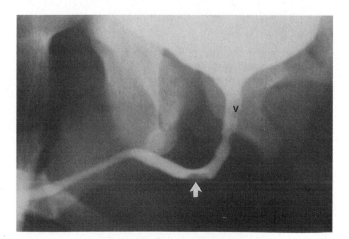

Figure 2.48.   Cowper's duct cyst. Voiding cystourethrogram reveals a well-defined indentation on the floor of the midbulbar urethra (*arrow*). There is no urethral obstruction in this case. The verumontanum is clearly seen (v).

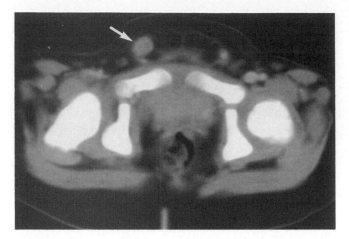

Figure 2.49. Undescended testicle. A computed tomography scan through the level of the symphysis pubis demonstrates the right testis (*arrow*) in the inguinal canal.

(Fig. 2.50). The undescended testis is seen as a medium-signal mass on T1-weighted images and as a high-signal mass on T2-weighted images.

The normal spermatic cord may be identified low in the inguinal canal medial and anterior to the femoral vessels. The cord usually contains fat and is slightly larger than the femoral vessels. If the undescended testis lies in the inguinal canal, the spermatic cord of the undescended testicle is not seen at the level of the normal spermatic cord. As sequential cephalad images are obtained, a mass representing the undescended testicle may be demonstrated. In such a case, the spermatic cord may be seen in the inguinal canal owing to the normal evolution of the vas deferens.

Spermatic venography is useful in identifying the nonpalpable undescended testicle. Localization of the abdominal or pelvic undescended testicle is demonstrated by visualization of the pampiniform plexus,

which is seen as a collection of linear coalescing vessels. Agenesis of the testis is presumed when no pampiniform plexus is seen and the spermatic vein exhibits a blind end. In film interpretation, care should be taken not to mistake the epididymal veins for the pampiniform plexus. The epididymal veins are commonly much lower in the abdomen or pelvis than the pampiniform plexus, because the vas deferens and epididymis descend ahead of the testes. Successful demonstration of the pampiniform plexus is approximately 80% on the left. Because of more difficult catheterization of the right spermatic vein and since valves are more common in the right spermatic vein, successful demonstration of the right pampiniform plexus is reduced to 60%. Although the imaging findings may be helpful, in most cases, preoperative imaging is not necessary.

IN UTERO ANOMALIES

Using state-of-the-art ultrasound equipment, it is widely accepted practice to evaluate the fetus in utero for anomalies. The urinary tract lends itself well to such evaluation, because the fetal kidneys are discernible at 13 to 14 weeks of fetal age using high-quality transabdominal techniques or a vaginal probe. The fetal bladder can be imaged as early as 11 weeks of gestation. Care must be taken not to overcall hydronephrosis, since it is not uncommon for the renal pelvis to be distended to 1 cm when measured in anteroposterior diameter in the normal fetus. Many anomalies can, however, be diagnosed with some degree of certainty; although to date there has been no significant success in treating these conditions in utero (Table 2.1). The ultrasonographic findings in these anomalies are generally the same as those described in the term infant after delivery and are discussed previously in this chapter or elsewhere in this book.

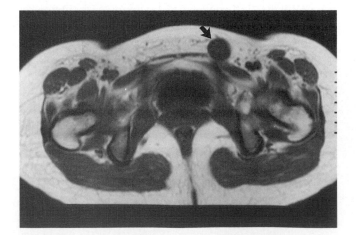

Figure 2.50. Magnetic resonance imaging (MRI) of undescended testicle. A T1-weighted MR image clearly shows the medium signal intensity testicle (*arrow*) in the left inguinal area.

Table 2.1.
Genitourinary Anomalies Detectable by In Utero Sonography

Renal agenesis
Renal ectopy
Multicystic dysplastic kidney
Polycystic renal disease
   Autosomal recessive
   Autosomal dominant
Ureteropelvic junction obstruction
Hydronephrosis with ureterectasis
   Reflux
   Primary megaureter
   Ureterocele
   Posterior urethral valve
Patent urachus
Bladder exstrophy
Scrotal hydrocele
Mesoblastic nephroma

SUGGESTED READINGS

Upper Urinary Tract Anomalies and Duplex Collecting Systems

Amis ES Jr, Cronan JJ, Pfister RC: Lower moiety hydronephrosis in duplicated kidneys. *Urology* 26:82, 1985.

Blair D, Rigsby C, Rosenfield AT: The nubbin sign on computed tomography and sonography. *Urol Radiol* 9:149, 1987.

Cronan JJ, Amis ES Jr, Zeman RK, et al.: Obstruction of the upper pole moiety in renal duplication in adults: CT evaluation. *Radiology* 161:17, 1986.

Curtis JA, Sadhu V, Steiner RM: Malposition of the colon in right renal agenesis ectopia, and anterior nephrectomy. *AJR* 129:845, 1977.

Daneman A, Alton DJ: Radiographic manifestations of renal anomalies. *Radiol Clin North Am* 29:351, 1991.

Friedland GW, Cunningham J: The elusive ectopic ureteroceles. *AJR* 116:792, 1972.

Gay BB, Jr, Dawes RK, Atkinson GE, et al.: Wilms' tumor in horseshoe kidneys: radiologic diagnosis. *Radiology* 146:693, 1983.

Gerber GS, Lyon ES: Endopyelotomy: patient selection, results, and complications. *Urology* 43:2, 1994.

Goodman JD, Norton KI, Carr L, et al.: Crossed fused renal ectopia: Sonographic diagnosis. *Urol Radiol* 8:13, 1986.

Hartman GW, Hodson CJ: The duplex kidney and related abnormalities. *Clin Radiol* 20:387, 1969.

Hohenfellner M, Schultz-Lampel D, Lampel A, et al.: Tumor in the horseshoe kidney: clinical implications and review of embryogenesis. *J Urol* 147:1098, 1992.

Hulnick DH, Bosniak MA: "Faceless Kidney": CT sign of renal duplicity. *J Comput Assist Tomogr* 10:771, 1986.

Kunin M: The abortive calix: variations in appearance and differential diagnosis. *AJR* 139:931, 1982.

Lee WJ, Badlani GH, Karlin GS, et al.: Treatment of ureteropelvic strictures with percutaneous pyelotomy: experience in 62 patients. *AJR* 151:515, 1988.

Macpherson RI: Supernumerary kidney: typical and atypical features. *J Can Assoc Radiol* 38:116, 1987.

Mascatello VJ, Smith EH, Carrera GE, et al.: Ultrasonic evaluation of the obstructed duplex kidney. *AJR* 129:113, 1977.

Share JC, Lebowitz RL: Ectopic ureterocele without ureteral and calyceal dilatation (ureterocele disproportion): findings on urography and sonography. *AJR* 152:567, 1989.

Yeh HC, Halton KP, Shapiro RS, et al.: Junctional parenchyma: revised definition of hypertrophic column of Bertin. *Radiology* 185:725, 1992.

Prune Belly Syndrome

Berdon WE, Baker DH, Wigger JH, et al.: The radiologic and pathologic spectrum of the prune belly syndrome. *Radiol Clin North Am* 15(1):83, 1977.

Fallat ME, Skoog SJ, Belman AB, et al.: The prune belly syndrome: a comprehensive approach to management. *J Urol* 142:802, 1989.

Greskovich FJ, Nyberg LM: The prune belly syndrome: a review of its etiology, defects, treatment and prognosis. *J Urol* 140:707, 1988.

Lower Urinary Tract Anomalies and Undescended Testicle

Amins M, Wheeler CS: Selective venography in abdominal cryptorchidism. *J Urol* 115:760, 1976.

Herman TE, McAlister WH: Radiographic manifestations of congenital anomalies of the lower urinary tract. *Radiol Clin North Am* 29:365, 1991.

Hollowell JG, Hill PD, Duffy PG, Ransley PG: Lower urinary tract function after exstrophy closure. *Pediatr Nephrol* 6:428, 1992.

Hrebinko RL, Bellinger MF: The limited role of imaging techniques in managing children with undescended testes. *J Urol* 150:458, 1993.

Lee JKT, McClennan BL, Stanley RJ, et al.: Utility of computed tomography in localization of the undescended testicle. *Radiology* 135:121, 1980.

Miyano T, Kobayashi H, Shimomura H, et al.: Magnetic resonance imaging for localizing the nonpalpable undescended testis. *J Pediatr Surg* 26:607, 1991.

Weiser WJ, Montanera W: Ultrasonographic demonstration of a ureterocele in an adult: a case report. *Medical Ultrasound* 8:160, 1984.

Young HH, Frontz WA, Baldwin JC: Congenital obstruction of the posterior urethra. *J Urol* 2:298, 1919.

In Utero Detection of Genitourinary Anomalies

Glazebrook KN, McGrath FP, Steele BT: Prenatal compensatory renal growth: documentation with US. Radiology 189:733, 1993.

Hill MC, Lande IM, Larsen JW Jr: Prenatal diagnosis of fetal anomalies using ultrasound and MRI. *Radiol Clin North Am* 26:287, 1988.

Sanders RC: In utero sonography of genitourinary anomalies. *Urol Radiol* 14:29, 1992.

3

Diagnostic and Interventional Techniques

DIAGNOSTIC TECHNIQUES
Excretory Urography

Despite recent declines in its popularity, excretory urography remains the cornerstone of radiologic diagnosis of the urinary tract. The strength of urography lies in its ability to provide an overall survey of the urinary tract; anatomic definition of the kidney, collecting system, and lower urinary tract; as well as information about renal function. Thus, a disease process that is primarily manifested by an acute impairment of renal excretion (e.g., unilateral ureteral obstruction), without much change in renal anatomy, may be readily diagnosed using urography. The strength of urography also is its greatest limitation; when the ability of the kidneys to excrete the contrast is impaired, the information obtained from the study is markedly reduced.

The use of urography has declined as a result of the increased availability of other imaging studies of the urinary tract, the need for cost containment, a hesitancy to expose certain patients to contrast material, and the elimination of urography as a screening study for patients with nonspecific complaints. However, for most patients with specific complaints related to the urinary tract (i.e., flank pain, hematuria, urinary retention), urography remains a highly efficacious and cost-effective examination. Routine urography in patients with recurrent urinary tract infection, however, has been shown to yield little information that directly affects the patient's therapy. The value of urography in selected patients with urinary tract infection, however, remains unquestioned (*see* Chapter 7). Both Donker and Bauer demonstrated that routine urography before prostatectomy did not significantly alter the therapy in the group of patients they studied. The value of routine urography also has been questioned in patients with stress urinary incontinence, in patients undergoing hysterectomy, and as a screening study to exclude a renovascular cause for hypertension.

Routine Urographic Technique

The radiologist should monitor closely the technical factors employed during urography to optimize the diagnostic information obtained from the study. A film–screen combination with a relatively long gray scale should be employed. Close attention should be paid to positioning and collimation, and the films should be free from artifacts and should not be degraded by respiratory motion. To optimize the subject contrast, a peak kilovoltage (KvP) level no higher than 60 to 75 with the milliampere seconds (MAS) varying with the patient's size should be employed.

The advisability of routine bowel preparation with laxatives before urography remains unsettled. Many radiologists believe that if routine tomography is employed, there is no necessity to "cleanse" the bowel prior to urography. Others believe that this procedure, although uncomfortable for the patient, may improve the quality of the study and should be employed when urography is performed on an elective basis. This is particularly true when renal calculi are suspected, because fecal material in the colon may obscure their presence.

When bowel preparation is desired, the use of an oral laxative administered 12 to 18 hours before the examination, supplemented by a rectal suppository on the morning of the examination is suggested. Although uncommon, care should be taken that the patient does not become inadvertently dehydrated as a result of the bowel preparation.

When symptoms are acute, there is little justification to deny urography merely because the patient has not received bowel preparation. It is not advisable to employ cleansing enemas in this situation, because a large quantity of air inadvertently introduced during the enema may obscure detail further. Solid food should be withheld for several hours before the examination to reduce the risk from vomiting should it occur after injection of the contrast material; however, clear liquids are permitted.

There is no universally accepted filming sequence for an excretory urogram. Perhaps in no other radiologic study is there such variability in the number and sequence of films that are made as part of a "routine" urogram. "Optimal" urography is most likely to be obtained if the study is monitored by the radiologist and modified to answer the clinical question posed. Certain essential features include the following.

THE SCOUT FILM.   The preliminary or scout radiograph is an indispensable part of every excretory urogram. This is usually performed as a single radiograph that includes the upper abdomen and pelvis. If the patient is too large to fit on a single film, a second collimated radiograph of the kidneys or the pelvis to include the symphysis pubis should be obtained. A preliminary tomogram also should be made to evaluate the technique and the level of tomographic cuts to be obtained after the contrast material is injected. The scout should be obtained after the patient has voided and immediately prior to the injection of the contrast material. This will ensure that the excreted contrast will not be diluted by a large amount of unopacified urine in the bladder and that the position of calculi subsequently identified on the urogram will be accurately portrayed.

Scout films may reveal errors in positioning or radiographic technique that must be corrected before the injection of contrast material. Calcifications within the urinary tract also must be detected prior to contrast injection, because they often are obscured after the contrast administration. Oblique scout films or tomograms of the kidneys may be obtained to help distinguish renal from extrarenal calcifications that overlie the kidneys in the anteroposterior projection. However, oblique films to determine whether a calcification lies in the urinary tract but outside the kidney are of no value, because the precise course of the ureter cannot be determined until after contrast material is injected.

Many common extraurinary calcifications are visible on scout radiographs (Fig. 3.1); only a small number, however, have pathologic significance. Gallstones or pancreatic calcifications might aid in elucidating the etiology of upper abdominal pain. Vascular calcifications in the aorta, splenic, renal, or iliac arteries may be incidental findings; however, when both walls are calcified and widely separated, aneurysmal dilatation can be diagnosed. Arterial calcifications can occasionally extend throughout the intrarenal arterial tree (Fig. 3.2). Incidental calcifications include those in the costochondral cartilage, splenic and hepatic granulomas, calcified mesenteric nodes, and old hemorrhage or granulomatous disease in otherwise normal-sized adrenal glands. Phleboliths are seen as small rounded calcifications in the pelvis, usually with lucent centers. These are thought to result from thrombosis in the deep pelvic veins. Phleboliths may lie over the course of the distal ureters and may be confused with distal ureteral calculi. Prostatic calcifications are seen as an aggregate of multiple small calcific densities usually protruding above the pubic symphysis. These may be idiopathic or secondary to infection. Calcification of the vasa deferentia is of clinical significance, because approximately 90% of men with this diagnosis have diabetes mellitus (Fig. 3.3).

The detection of calcification in the lower urinary tract (i.e., the bladder or ureter) is equally important. Faintly opaque bladder stones may be easily overlooked, and their subsequent discovery may be a source of embarrassment to the responsible radiologist.

Another use of the scout radiograph is to detect ab-

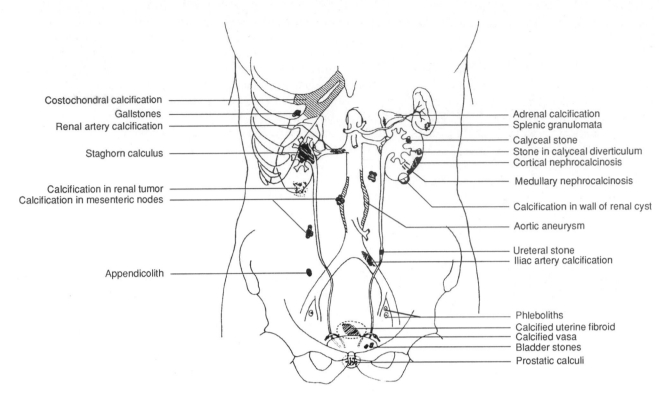

Costochondral calcification
Gallstones
Renal artery calcification

Staghorn calculus

Calcification in renal tumor
Calcification in mesenteric nodes

Appendicolith

Adrenal calcification
Splenic granulomata
Calyceal stone
Stone in calyceal diverticulum
Cortical nephrocalcinosis
Medullary nephrocalcinosis
Calcification in wall of renal cyst
Aortic aneurysm
Ureteral stone
Iliac artery calcification
Phleboliths
Calcified uterine fibroid
Calcified vasa
Bladder stones
Prostatic calculi

Figure 3.1. Abdominal calcification. Schematic representation of a number of pathologic and physiologic calcifications that may be found on abdominal radiology. (Modified with permission from Amis ES Jr, Newhouse JH: *Essentials of Uroradiology*. Boston, Little Brown & Co, 1991.)

normal soft tissue densities. The presence of unilateral or even bilateral small kidneys may be a clue to the nature of the underlying pathology. Enlargement or displacement of an organ often can be detected; loss of the psoas silhouette may represent underlying pathology in the retroperitoneum. However, the psoas margin may not be clearly seen on one side or the other in as many as 50% of patients. A bulge in the psoas shadow or displacement of the flank stripe is more clearly an indication of a soft tissue mass in the retroperitoneum.

Detection of abnormal gas collections also is an important role of the scout radiograph. The presence of free intraperitoneal air or gas within the biliary tree or gall bladder may be important evidence that the gastrointestinal tract rather than the urinary tract is the source of the patient's complaints. Detection of air within the urinary tract almost always signals important underlying pathology, including the presence of infection or a fistulous communication between the urinary tract and the gastrointestinal tract. The presence of a small amount of air in the urinary bladder in a patient with a Foley catheter, however, may be normal as air can be introduced during placement of the catheter.

Bone abnormalities also may indicate underlying urinary tract pathology. Characteristic osteoblastic metastases from carcinoma of the prostate may be the first indicator of this disease. The presence of an abnormal

spinal column may be the clue to urinary tract dysfunction on the basis of an occult neurogenic bladder.

EARLY NEPHROGRAM FILMS.   The rate of excretion of the contrast material is directly related to the level of the plasma concentration of the contrast material (*see* Chapter 4). Therefore, the nephrogram is at its peak intensity with maximum concentrations in the nephron 30 sec-

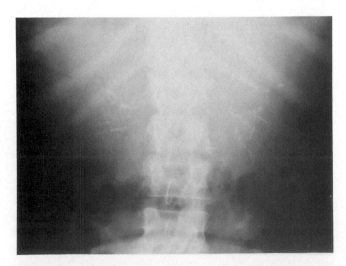

Figure 3.2. Extensive intrarenal vascular calcifications are present. (Reprinted with permission from Amis ES Jr, Newhouse JH: *Essentials of Uroradiology*. Boston, Little Brown & Co, 1991.)

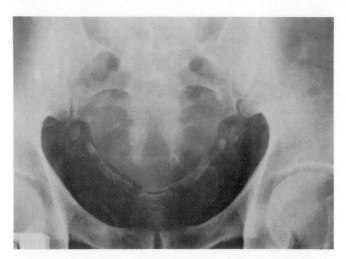

Figure 3.3. Calcified vas deferentia. (Reprinted with permission from Amis ES Jr, Newhouse JH: *Essentials of Uroradiology*. Boston, Little Brown & Co, 1991.)

onds to 1 minute after the injection of contrast material (Fig. 3.4). An immediate postinjection coned view of the kidneys or a tomogram of the kidneys will allow the best visualization of the renal parenchyma. For this reason, masses that distort the renal parenchyma are most readily evaluated on early films.

TOMOGRAPHY. The routine use of tomography increases the detection of renal masses and thereby increases the sensitivity of the urogram. This is obtained at a relatively small cost (i.e., the increased radiation exposure to the patient and increased film costs). In a prospective study, Lloyd determined that only 29% of renal masses observed would have been detected without the routine use of tomography. In a study from the

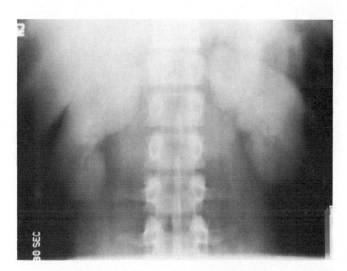

Figure 3.4. Early nephrogram film. A 30-sec tomogram shows the renal margins to be sharply demarcated with intense enhancement of the renal parenchyma. Faint early opacification of the calyces is evident.

Mayo Clinic, only one third of renal masses less than 2.5 cm in diameter would have been detected without the aid of tomographic sections. Routine tomograms also are used in evaluating abnormalities of the collecting system, particularly subtle changes in calyceal anatomy and filling defects within the collecting system.

Almost all available tomographic-urographic tables employ linear tomographic motion. An arc of 25° provides adequate blurring, yet covers the thickness of an average kidney with three exposures. Therefore, this angle is recommended for screening tomography. A tomographic angle of 40° will increase the amount of blurring and decrease the thickness of each slice, but to cover the entire thickness of the kidneys, multiple slices must be obtained. A tomographic cut of 5° provides insufficient blurring for routine use.

The optimal level for the tomographic cuts of the kidneys is most highly correlated with the anteroposterior thickness of the patient (Table 3.1). The midcoronal plane of the kidney often can be determined in the scout tomogram when the pedicles of the L2 vertebral body are in sharpest focus. Sections 1 cm above and 1 cm below this level are usually sufficient (Fig. 3.5).

The optimal timing for the tomographic sections is a matter of preference. Many authorities argue that because the major value of the tomogram lies in the detection of renal masses, the tomograms should be carried out immediately after injection when the nephrogram is at its peak. However, if tomographic evaluation of the collecting system also is desired, it is necessary to delay the timing of the tomograms until approximately 5 minutes after the initial injection (Fig. 3.6); at this time, both the parenchyma and the collecting system will be opacified.

ABDOMINAL COMPRESSION. The purpose of the compression device is to assure that the pelvocalyceal system and ureters are adequately filled. In the uncompressed patient, normal peristaltic activity, as well as layering of the contrast material in the dependent portions of the collecting system, frequently result in underfilling of one or more portions of the collecting system. This may be a special problem with the use of

Table 3.1.
Tomographic Levels for Nephrotomography

Anteroposterior diameter (cm) Including Table Pad	Tomographic Levels
14–17	6, 7, 8
18–22	7, 8, 9
23–26	8, 9, 10
27–29	9, 10, 11
>30	10, 11, 12

From Newberg AH, Mindell HJ: Predicting tomographic levels for urography. *Radiololgy* 118:460, 1976.

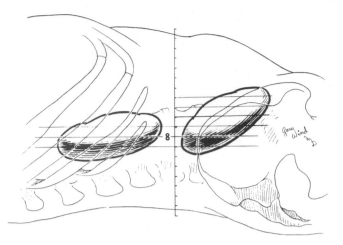

Figure 3.5. Approximate levels for tomographic sections. (From Amis ES Jr: Excretory urography. In Tavaras JM and Ferrucci JT [eds], *Radiology: Diagnosing-Imaging-Intervention,* Philadelphia, JB Lippincott, 1988.)

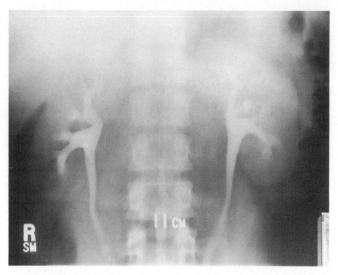

Figure 3.6. A tomographic section 11 cm above the tabletop made approximately 5 minutes after contrast material injection demonstrates the midcoronal plane of the kidney. The minor calyces are sharply focused in the right kidney. Both renal outlines are well demonstrated.

low-osmolar or nonionic contrast materials that produce a smaller diuresis than do the older ionic contrast agents. To be effective, the abdominal compression device must be placed so that it will compress the ureters where they cross the pelvic brim (Fig. 3.7). The use of a device placed around the patient rather than a device that attaches to the x-ray table is preferred. The device must be placed tightly enough that the patient is not able to tense the abdominal musculature and overcome

the pressure exerted by the compression. In addition, if the device is improperly positioned (i.e., too high or too low), effective compression will not be achieved.

Contraindications to the use of abdominal compression include a known abdominal aortic aneurysm, ureteral obstruction, recent abdominal surgery, and the

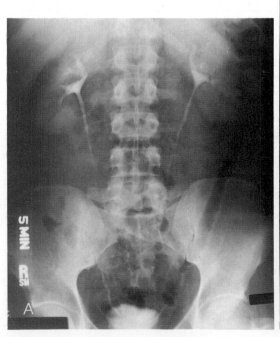

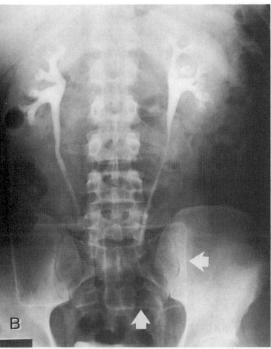

Figure 3.7. Effect of abdominal compression. **A,** In the uncompressed patient, the calyces and proximal ureters are poorly distended. **B,** After application of the compression device (*arrows*), the calyces and proximal ureter are much better demonstrated.

presence of an ostomy. As with the routine use of to-mography, the use of abdominal compression improves the diagnostic utility of the urogram without appreciable cost to the patient.

EXCRETION FILMS.   A series of two or three films should be made between 5 and 15 minutes after the injection of the contrast agent for an overall evaluation of the urinary tract. Some radiologists prefer one of these films to be collimated to the kidneys, particularly if tomograms are not made. The exact choice and timing of the radiographs is a matter of preference.

ADDITIONAL VIEWS.   In addition to the standard views obtained routinely during the urogram, many additional views should be used to evaluate specific clinical problems. Some of these views may, by preference, be incorporated into the "routine" urogram. *Oblique plain films* or *oblique tomograms* more precisely localize a suspected defect within the collecting system and are useful to define the presence of a mass in the renal parenchyma. These are preferably performed on films collimated to the kidney. Both oblique views are frequently necessary to completely evaluate a filling defect or to differentiate an impression due to a crossing vessel from an intraluminal defect. The *prone radiograph* is useful to evaluate the ureters when supine films do not adequately demonstrate their course. The prone radiograph is particularly helpful in a patient in whom acute

ureteral obstruction is present, but the exact point of obstruction has not been demonstrated. Because contrast material is heavier than unopacified urine, in the prone position, the contrast and nonopacified urine will exchange; thus, the point of obstruction may be demonstrated without resorting to further delayed radiographs. A film made with the patient in the *upright* position after release of abdominal compression is very useful in assessing the effect of gravity on the "drainage" of the upper urinary tract. This is especially helpful when there is equivocal dilatation of one or both of the ureters (Fig. 3.8); drainage of the contrast material from the collecting system on the upright radiograph indicates that the dilatation is not due to obstruction. The upright radiograph also allows the contrast material to optimally demonstrate the base of the bladder. The routine use of such a radiograph will indicate the presence of such bladder abnormalities as cystocele, pelvic floor relaxation, and bladder hernia that might not be appreciated on routine supine views (Fig. 3.9). The upright radiograph also may be useful in patients with ureteral obstruction in that the most distal extent of the contrast column can more readily be identified.

Traditionally, the *postvoid film* has been used to evaluate the patient's ability to empty the bladder. This is a frequent concern, especially in older men with suspected bladder outlet obstruction. However, a postvoid

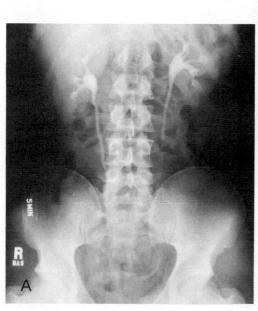
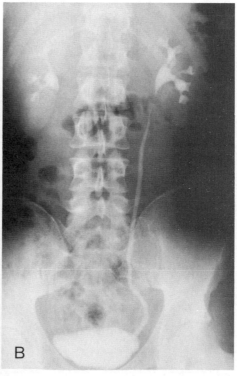

Figure 3.8.   Value of the upright film. **A,** A 5-minute radiograph demonstrates equivocal dilatation of the distal left ureter. **B,** The upright film made a few moments later shows poor drainage of the left collecting system as a consequence of a partially obstructing distal left ureteral calculus.

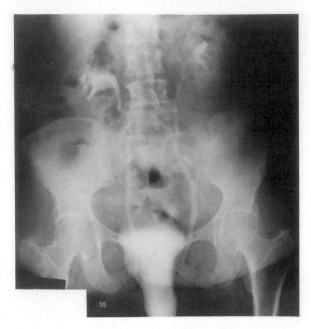

Figure 3.9.   Large cystocele is demonstrated on an upright radiograph from an excretory urogram.

radiograph that shows residual contrast opacified urine does not mean that the patient *could* not empty his bladder, but only indicates that he *did not* do so. Conversely, a nearly empty bladder may be demonstrated, but only after considerable effort on the part of the patient. An important use of the postvoid radiograph, however, is to evaluate the distal ureters that are frequently hidden behind the distended bladder on the prevoiding radiographs. This is especially important in patients with suspected distal ureteral calculi (Fig. 3.10). *Oblique postvoid radiographs* also may be very useful in

this regard. The postvoid radiograph allows evaluation of the bladder mucosa (Fig. 3.11) and may be the only radiograph on which small filling defects or other urothelial lesions of the bladder are demonstrated.

DELAYED RADIOGRAPHS.   In patients with acute ureteral obstruction, delayed filling of the collecting system and ureter is the rule. The amount of delay is highly variable and depends on the acuity and the degree of obstruction. In this situation, delayed radiographs are frequently necessary to demonstrate the precise point of obstruction, and these should be obtained until this point is demonstrated. The precise timing for these delayed films varies from department to department, but a reasonable schedule would include films at 1, 3, 6, 12, and 24 hours after injection or until the point of obstruction is demonstrated. Rarely, films obtained as long as 48 hours after the initial injection may be necessary to demonstrate the point of obstruction.

The Normal Excretory Urogram

Analysis of the excretory phase of the urogram begins with the kidneys.

SIZE.   There is a wide variation in the size of "normal" kidneys. As determined radiographically, renal size varies according to a number of factors unrelated to intrinsic renal pathology. Such factors include the degree of magnification, the amount of diuresis induced by the contrast material, and the patient's state of hydration. Ordinarily, the left kidney is approximately 0.5 cm larger than the right kidney. Thus, there should be no discrepancy in the length of the two kidneys greater than 1.5 cm if the right kidney is larger than the left, or no more than 2 cm if the left kidney is larger than the right.

Because the size of the kidneys varies with the size

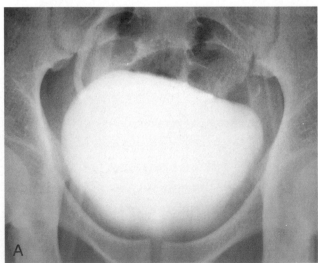

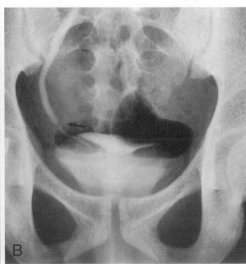

Figure 3.10.   **A,** The exact point of ureteral obstruction secondary to an impacted stone is hidden behind the contrast-filled bladder, but is well demonstrated on **B,** the postvoid radiograph (*arrow*).

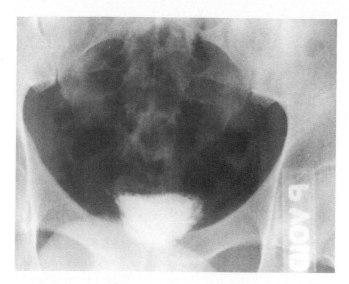

Figure 3.11. Postvoid film. The normal mucosal pattern of the bladder is demonstrated.

and sex of the patient, an average renal length of three to four vertebral bodies is normal. Simon evaluated 100 kidneys that were normal on autopsy and found a range of 9.4 to 13.7 cm, with a mean length of 11.7 cm on standard abdominal radiographs. He found that two standard deviations of normal would yield a measurement of 2.6 to 3.6 times the height of the L2 vertebral body and its interspace. As a practical matter, experienced radiologists can usually visually inspect the kidneys and determine whether or not the renal size falls within the range of normal.

POSITION. The kidneys lie in the retroperitoneum with their long axes parallel to the outer border of the psoas muscle. In heavier patients, the kidneys may assume a more vertical configuration. The renal hilus usu-

ally sits at the level of the L2-L3 vertebral body. Abnormal position of the kidneys may be related to a variety of processes, including patient habitus; the presence of spinal abnormalities, such as rotoscoliosis; developmental failures, such as a failure of ascent and/or rotation; and/or displacement of the kidney by a variety of pathologic processes in the kidney or adjacent to it.

ABNORMALITIES OF CONTOUR. The normal kidney should be sharply marginated and smooth in contour. The normal shape of the kidney is usually referred to as "reniform." Occasionally, in very asthenic individuals with little perinephric fat, the superior margins of the kidneys may be in contact with other intraabdominal organs. For example, the superior border of the right kidney may contact the liver, and its margins may be difficult to appreciate even on tomographic sections. With this aside, failure to completely visualize the renal outlines segmentally should be considered to represent an abnormality until proven otherwise (Fig. 3.12).

Indentations on the contour of the kidney are frequently seen. A lobulated contour of the renal margin, either in its entirety or segmentally representing fetal lobulation (Fig. 3.13), may be present. These indentations represent incomplete fusion of the embryologic renal lobules. They are usually differentiated from pathologic scarring by their smooth contour and regular spacing. A pyelonephritic scar, for example, is usually deeper than a renal lobulation and is always located adjacent to an underlying abnormal calyx (Fig. 3.14). Renal infarcts tend to occur randomly without the regular spacing associated with renal lobation (Fig. 3.15). Especially prominent grooves may sometimes be seen in the superior or inferior margins of the kidneys. These grooves also represent a residua of the fetal renal anatomy and are sometimes termed the sulcus interpartialis superior or inferior, respectively.

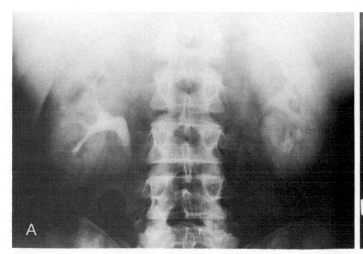

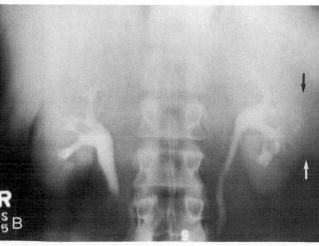

Figure 3.12. **A,** The left renal margin is incompletely visualized along its lateral margin. **B,** Tomogram demonstrates typical findings of a simple cortical cyst (*arrows*).

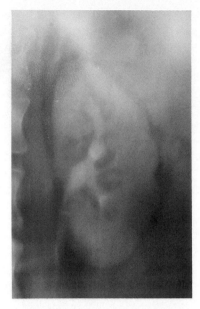

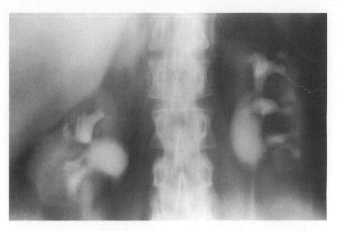

Figure 3.15. Multiple cortical infarcts. Multiple irregular scars, most pronounced in the right kidney, are now present as a result of multiple cortical infarcts.

Figure 3.13. Fetal lobation. Regularly spaced indentions along the renal margin are typical of fetal lobation (lobulation).

A prominent bulge on the lateral border of the left kidney is sometimes appreciated. This has been called a dromedary hump (Fig. 3.16) and represents a normal variation caused by molding by the spleen. Occasionally, enlargement of the liver or the spleen may compress the kidney anteriorly, producing the appearance of the unilaterally enlarged kidney. A soft tissue density caused by fluid in the fundus of the stomach is frequently seen overlying the upper pole of the left kidney, especially on tomograms. This shadow often is confused with a renal or adrenal mass (Fig. 3.17); the true nature of the "mass"

can be appreciated by shallow oblique tomograms or with a prone radiograph in which the "mass" will be seen to fill with air.

THE PELVOCALYCEAL SYSTEM. The average human kidney contains 10 to 15 calyces; however, this number may vary considerably and may still fall within the normal range. The calyceal systems are roughly divided into upper, middle, and lower calyceal groups. Calyces in the polar regions, in particular, the right upper pole, may be compound (i.e., two or more calyces may share a common infundibulum). The calyces should be deeply cupped and delicate in appearance without blunting or distortion. The infundibulae should be straight with no bowing or displacement. Occasionally, a small blush of contrast may be noted in the renal papilla just outside the calyx, which is related to a relatively high concentration of contrast material in the distal collecting ducts as they enter the minor calyces. This appearance is quite normal and should not be confused with the dilatation

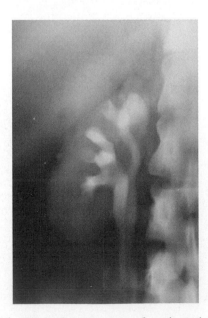

Figure 3.14. Typical appearance of pyelonephric scarring of the upper pole is demonstrated.

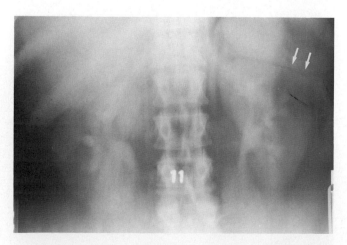

Figure 3.16. Dromedary hump. A prominent bulge (*arrows*) is present on the superior border of the left kidney produced by compression of the renal margin by the spleen.

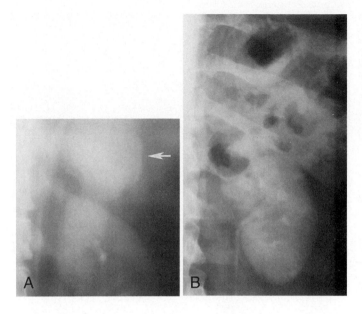

Figure 3.17. Renal pseudotumor. **A,** Nephrotomogram demonstrates a soft tissue mass above the left kidney (*arrow*). **B,** Prone plain film demonstrates air in the region of the "mass," indicating that it represents the fundus of the stomach. (Reprinted with permission from Amis ES Jr, Newhouse JH: *Essentials of Uroradiology.* Boston, Little Brown & Co, 1991.)

of the distal collecting ducts seen in medullary sponge kidney (see Chapter 13). In older patients, especially, the calyces and renal pelvis may be compressed by an accumulation of fat in the renal sinus. This condition, termed *renal sinus lipomatosis* (Fig 3.18) , may produce a spidery and attenuated appearance of the collecting system and may prevent adequate calyceal distention, but otherwise carries no pathologic significance. Frequently, impressions are present on the infundibula of the major or minor calyces produced by segmental arteries or by veins (Fig. 3.19). The defects are sharply marginated, and when produced by a crossing vein, may occasionally be eliminated with tight abdominal compression. An extrinsic impression on the infundibulae or

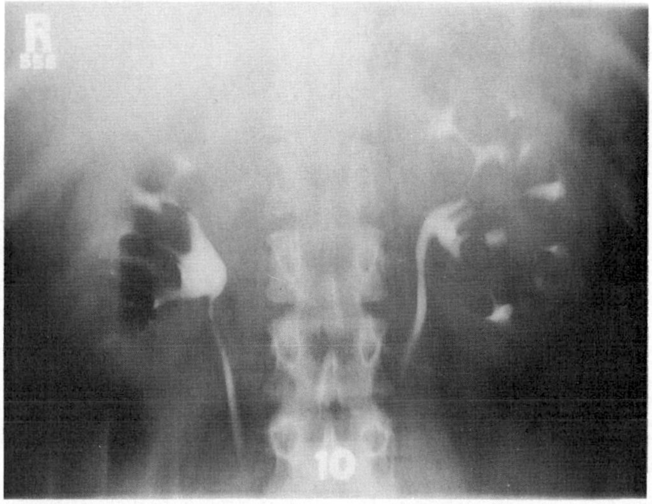

renal pelvis may be produced by a hypertrophied column of Bertin. This is most common at the junction of the upper and middle thirds of the kidney (Fig. 3.20).

The major calyces come together to form the renal pelvis, which can be extremely variable in appearance. In some patients, the renal pelvis is entirely intrarenal in location (i.e., surrounded by renal sinus fat), whereas in others it appears to be outside the confines of the kidneys and has a ballooned appearance (the extrarenal pelvis). If the calyces are normal in appearance, significant obstruction is not present, even though the renal pelvis may appear to be quite large in relation to the calyces. There is usually a smooth transition between the renal pelvis and the proximal ureter.

Although there is a tendency toward symmetry of the collecting systems in the two kidneys, there may be considerable variation in any patient. A lack of symmetry

Figure 3.18. Renal sinus lipomatosis. The calyces have a compressed appearance because of an accumulation of fat in the renal sinus. This fat appears relatively radiolucent on the tomographic section.

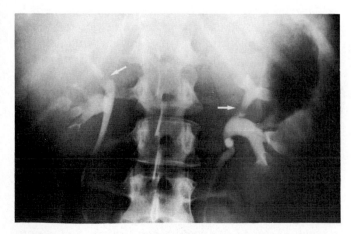

Figure 3.19. Crossing vessel defects. Extrinsic compression (*arrows*) on the upper pole infundibulae bilaterally produced by crossing segmental arteries.

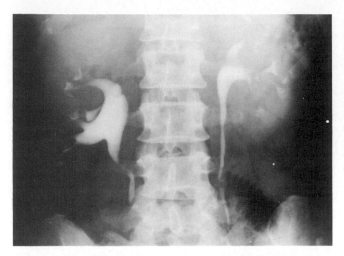

Figure 3.20. Hypertrophied column of Bertin. There is bowing of the upper pole infundibulum and an impression on the renal pelvis of the right kidney secondary to hypertrophy of a column of Bertin.

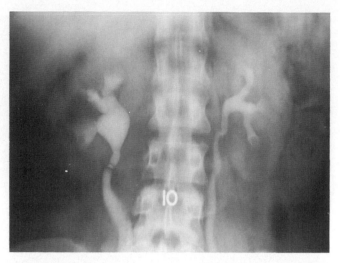

Figure 3.21. Transverse ureteral folds. Several band-like constrictions are present in the right proximal ureter that have no physiologic or pathologic consequence.

should not be considered abnormal, because it has been said that renal morphology may be as distinctive as a person's fingerprints.

THE URETER.   The ureters generally exit from the renal pelvis at the level of the second lumbar vertebra and descend through the cone of renal fascia just lateral to the transverse processes of the upper lumbar vertebra. The middle third of the ureter usually overlaps the transverse processes of the lower lumbar vertebra to the level of the pelvic brim. The ureter is at its most anterior location where it crosses the iliac vessels; it then descends into the pelvis, taking a more lateral course before finally entering the bladder at the trigone. Because of active peristalsis, the degree to which the ureters are normally filled on any single radiograph is highly variable; lack of filling of a particular segment of the ureter is not necessarily pathologic. An attempt should be made to visualize as much of the course of the ureter as possible by using the additional views described above. One or more slight constrictions of the ureter sometimes may be visualized at the level of the ureteropelvic junction (Fig. 3.21). These constrictions are transverse folds that represent physiologic indentations of the ureter rather than true anatomic sphincters. They are frequently more prominent in infants and young children. Normal indentations on the course of the ureter that may be present include an impression at the level of the L3-L4 interspace caused by hypertrophy of the ovarian vessels in women, and tortuosity of the ureter as it crosses the iliac vessels, particularly in older patients. In younger male patients, the ureters may appear to have a more medial course in their middle and distal third due to large psoas muscles (Fig. 3.22).

BLADDER.   The size and contour of the bladder vary with the degree of filling. In its usual state of distention, the bladder has a roughly spherical or oblong shape with the superior portion indented by the overlying viscera. The normal bladder is smooth in contour with rounded borders. Any straightening or deformity of one of the contours of the bladder should be considered a

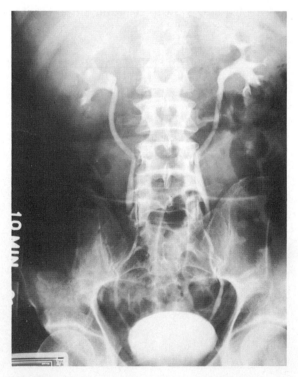

Figure 3.22. The ureters have a more medial course secondary to large psoas muscles in this young male patient. This condition is sometimes referred to a psoas "hypertrophy."

sign of bladder pathology until proven otherwise. On the postvoid radiograph, the mucosal pattern of the bladder should be identified.

Retrograde Pyelography

Retrograde injection of contrast material directly into the ureter or ureteral orifice allows visualization of the collecting system and ureter without relying on the ability of the kidneys to excrete contrast media. In addition, the degree of opacification and the degree of distention of the collecting system can be controlled by varying the amount and concentration of the contrast material that is injected. To perform retrograde pyelography, the ureteral orifice in the bladder is cannulated cystoscopically. The catheter may be advanced to the renal pelvis, or the contrast material may be injected into the lower ureter and filling of the ureter and the collecting system may be monitored fluoroscopically. In other instances, a bulb-shaped catheter is wedged into the ureteral orifice and the contrast material is injected from this location. This technique is sometimes referred to as a bulb pyelogram. If the room is so equipped, spot filming and positioning may be done directly in the cystoscopy suite, or the catheter may be placed in the cystoscopy suite and the patient brought to the radiology department, where the injection of contrast and the filming is performed. When a urothelial lesion is suspected on the basis of the film studies, brushing of the lesion for cytologic evaluation may be accomplished at the same time.

The advisability of performing bilateral retrograde pyelograms has been debated by urologists for many years. Edema at the ureteral orifice may rarely produce transient bilateral ureteral obstruction. Another danger is the introduction of infection into a previously uninfected renal unit. With modern urography, however, bilateral retrograde pyelograms are rarely necessary.

Care must be exercised in filling the collecting system, because inadvertent overdistention of the calyces can occur easily. This overdistention may result in pyelovenous extravasation, in which contrast material escapes from the collecting system into the veins; pyelosinus extravasation, which results from rupture of a fornix and extravasation of the contrast material into the renal sinus; pyelolymphatic extravasation, which results in filling of the perirenal lymphatics; and pyelotubular back flow, in which there is retrograde filling of the distal collecting ducts at the level of the renal papilla (Fig. 3.23 and Fig. 14.1–14.4). In addition, the contrast material should be diluted so that small urothelial lesions will not be obscured by dense contrast material.

The primary use of retrograde pyelography is to evaluate suspected ureteral obstruction in the patient in whom the ability of the kidney to excrete contrast material is significantly impaired, or to evaluate possible filling defects in the collecting system or the ureter where urography has failed to adequately demonstrate a suspected lesion. In addition, on rare occasions, retrograde pyelography may be useful in localizing a suspected calculus or in evaluating a duplicated collecting system.

Retrograde pyelography should not be used as a primary diagnostic procedure, because it offers no evaluation of the renal parenchyma and because it is relatively invasive since cystoscopy is required for placement of

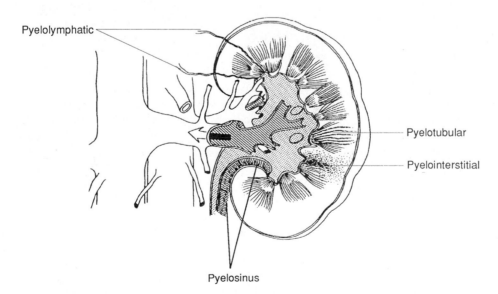

Figure 3.23. Diagrammatic representation of the routes for extravasation that may be found on retrograde pyelography. (Modified with permission from Amis ES Jr, Newhouse JH: *Essentials of Uroradiology.* Boston, Little Brown & Co, 1991.)

the catheters. Retrograde pyelography should be used as an adjunctive technique when conventional imaging studies fail to adequately demonstrate the suspected pathology.

A variation of retrograde pyelography termed air pyelography is occasionally useful. In such instances, air rather than opaque contrast material is injected in the collecting system. This technique can be used when the suspected filling defect, such as a stone, is obscured with the injection of conventional contrast media.

Antegrade Pyelography

Antegrade pyelography is a study of the collecting system of the kidney and ureter made through the direct injection of contrast material into the collecting system. As a diagnostic study, antegrade pyelography is usually performed when urography fails to demonstrate the desired information regarding the collecting system, or when retrograde pyelography is either hazardous or cannot be performed.

Antegrade pyelography is usually performed using a direct puncture of one of the calyces or the renal pelvis using a 20- or 22-gauge needle. Direct needle puncture is generally easily accomplished when the collecting system is dilated; in a nondilated system, direct puncture is much more difficult to perform. The collecting system may be localized using fluoroscopy, ultrasonography or, rarely, computed tomography (CT). Fluoroscopic guidance is usually preferred, because it permits filming after the collecting system is opacified. If ultrasonic or CT guidance is used, the patient is generally transferred to a fluoroscopy room after placement of the needle or catheter.

Indications

The indications for antegrade pyelography are listed in Table 3.2. The antegrade approach to opacification of the urinary tract for the study of suspected urinary tract obstruction may be preferable in patients with ileal conduits and in patients in whom ureteroneocystostomy has been performed. In both instances, the ureteral orifice may be very difficult to catheterize from a retrograde approach. In addition, the antegrade study is preferred in boys, in whom cystoscopy and the introduction of a catheter often is technically very difficult and hazardous because of their small urethras and because of the small instruments that must be used.

Ureteral perfusion studies to assess the functional integrity of the collecting system and ureter have been proven to be a useful adjunct in the evaluation of anatomic abnormalities of the upper urinary tract (*see* Chapter 14). Antegrade pyelography also is commonly performed as a prelude to percutaneous nephrostomy and other percutaneous interventional procedures in the urinary tract.

Table 3.2.
Indications for Antegrade Pyelography

Morphologic (pathologic anatomy)
    Confirmation and evaluation of hydronephrosis
    Determination of resting pressure
    Urinalysis: cystologic study, culture, biochemical analysis
    Site and etiology of obstruction
Urodynamic (perfusion, pressure-flow)
    Assessment of ureteral resistance
        Congenital and acquired dilatation
        Following corrective treatment
        Effect of bladder distention
Prior to percutaneous nephrostomy and other interventional procedures
    Drainage
    Dilatation of stenosis
    Stenting
    Balloon occlusion
    Stone removal
    Biopsy

From Pfister RC, Papanicoulaou N, Yoder IC: Diagnostic morphologic and urodynamic antegrade pyelography. *Radiol Clin North Am* 24(4):561–571, 1986.

Technique

To perform antegrade pyelography, the patient is placed prone on the fluoroscopy table, and the soft tissues of the back and flank are prepared and draped as for any sterile procedure. It is prudent to evaluate bleeding parameters and to discontinue anticoagulation therapy before the procedure. If infection in the upper urinary tract is suspected and is the prime indication for the procedure, prophylactic broad-spectrum antibiotics should be considered, because the distention that may accompany antegrade pyelography in a patient with a distal obstruction may place the patient at risk for the development of sepsis.

After the appropriate site is selected for the puncture, the skin and soft tissues of the flank are anesthetized with 1 or 2% lidocaine, and the needle puncture is accomplished during suspended respiration. When urine is aspirated from the kidney, the correct needle placement is confirmed via the injection of contrast material. The calyces and ureter are filled to the point of obstruction. A tilting table is helpful so that gravity may be used to carry the contrast material to the most dependent portion of the urinary tract. If this is not available, contrast may be instilled directly into the collecting system, the needle can be removed, and filming then can be accomplished in supine, prone, and upright positions. If there is any suspicion of infection, urine should be aspirated and sent for bacteriologic studies.

Complications

In general, antegrade pyelography is safe and easily performed. Complications of the procedure include bleeding, sepsis, and inadvertent puncture of an adjacent organ. Pneumothorax may occur if the pleural space is traversed during the introduction of the needle. This complication can be minimized when a direct posterior approach is used, because the costophrenic sulcus is generally shallower in the direct posterior position than in an approach from the posterior axillary line. Virtually all patients in whom antegrade pyelography is performed will develop at least microscopic hematuria, which is usually transient and is not considered a complication.

Cystography

Static cystography is performed to assess bladder rupture, low-pressure vesicoureteral reflux or to demonstrate vesical fistula. Three hundred to four hundred ml of contrast material (20–30% weight/volume) is instilled into the bladder using a Foley catheter, and radiographs in the anteroposterior, oblique and lateral positions are obtained. A postdrainage view also is obtained and is considered a mandatory part of a trauma cystogram, so that small amounts of contrast material extravasation that can be hidden behind a distended bladder will not be overlooked. Occasionally, static cystography using more diluted contrast material is useful in assessing suspected intravesical filling defects, bladder diverticula, or congenital anomalies of the lower urinary tract.

Voiding cystourethrography is used to diagnose high-pressure vesicoureteral reflux and to evaluate the urethra. The bladder is filled with contrast material infused using a Foley catheter as for a static cystogram. The bladder should be filled until the patient is certain he or she can void when the catheter is removed, and voiding cystography is performed with fluoroscopy. A video recording of bladder emptying may be obtained, and the procedure may be recorded using spot films, 100-mm cut film, or continuous 105-mm film. High-pressure reflux, bladder extravasation, or a small-necked diverticulum may not be apparent until the voiding study is obtained. In female patients, anteroposterior radiographs of the urethra are adequate. In male patients, however, the voiding films should be obtained in a 45° oblique position, so that the entire length of the urethra is demonstrated. Some films should be centered on the bladder, particularly when vesicoureteral reflux is suspected. If reflux is present, the highest level of that reflux should be documented on spot radiographs.

Ileal Conduit Studies

After cystectomy, an ileal conduit is commonly constructed for supravesical urinary diversion. One end of an isolated segment of ileum is brought to the skin as an ileocutaneous stoma. The ureters are implanted in the opposite end of the loop, which is closed off and placed retroperitoneally, if possible. As the ureters are anasto-

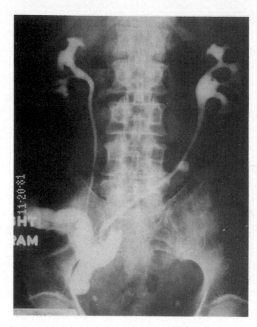

Figure 3.24.   Loopogram. Contrast material is instilled via a Foley catheter into the ileal conduit and refluxes up both ureters, thereby demonstrating the renal collecting system.

mosed to the loop in an end-to-side fashion, there is generally ready reflux from the conduit into the ureters. Therefore, contrast material instilled into the ileal loop may be used to demonstrate the ureters and the renal collecting systems. Such a study is called an ileal conduit study or a "loopogram" (Fig. 3.24).

To perform a loopogram, an appropriate Foley catheter (generally between 20 and 26 French) is inserted into the stoma and the balloon is inflated to a volume of 5 to 8 ml within the stoma. Contrast material is then instilled into the Foley catheter by gravity infusion or by hand injection. Gravity infusion is generally preferred, as the pressure is limited by the height of the bottle of contrast material. Under fluoroscopic observation, contrast material fills the loop and will usually reflux into the ureters. The study is especially useful in patients with impaired renal function and serves in lieu of retrograde pyelography to exclude ureteral obstruction.

Urethrography

The male urethra may be visualized in a retrograde or antegrade fashion. Retrograde urethrography and voiding cystourethrography may be performed separately, but the best method for assessing urethral disease is dynamic retrograde urethrography immediately followed by a voiding study.

Dynamic retrograde urethrography is the method of choice for the study of the urethra. The study is termed "dynamic," because it implies that the exposure is obtained during the active injection of contrast material into the urethra. In this fashion, optimal distension of the anterior urethra is obtained, and visualization of the deep bulbous and posterior urethra is achieved. Static retrograde urethrography in which contrast material is merely injected into the urethra results in inadequate distention of the urethra and should not be performed. Two main methods of dynamic retrograde urethrography are in use.

1. The Foley catheter method. A 12- or 14-French Foley catheter is inserted 2 to 3 cm into the penis, and the balloon of the catheter is inflated with 1 to 1.5 ml of saline in the fossa navicularis, enough to keep the balloon fixed in position, but insufficient to tear the urethral mucosa. The catheter is connected to a 50-ml syringe filled with water-soluble contrast medium. Injection of contrast medium outlines the whole urethra, and films are exposed during retrograde injection. Some investigators have found that by having the patient himself actually inject the contrast material (autourethrography), more consistent filling of the prostatic urethra can be obtained.
2. The Brodny clamp method. The Brodny clamp consists of a clamp apparatus containing an external meatal plug through which contrast medium can be injected from a syringe attached to the apparatus. The plug is held in position by a clamp fitted over the glans penis. Injection of contrast medium outlines the whole urethra if films are exposed during retrograde injection.

Either method is successful in obtaining dynamic retrograde urethrography. The Foley catheter method has some advantages: (*a*) the operator's hands are farther away from the x-ray beam; and (*b*) it provides more control of the injection, and penile and patient positioning. Both methods require gentle traction on the penis to straighten the urethra at the penoscrotal junction. Traction on the Brodny clamp may be painful and may injure the mucosa of the glans penis.

Both methods are best performed with fluoroscopic control, but may be done using an overhead tube; the technologist is instructed to expose the film while the operator is injecting. After obtaining two or three dynamic retrograde films, the same Foley catheter can be advanced into the bladder to obtain a voiding cystourethrogram. During the retrograde and voiding studies, the patient should remain positioned 40° oblique to the right. The retrograde study is usually obtained with the patient supine; the voiding study is usually obtained with the patient in the semierect or erect position. In both dynamic retrograde and voiding studies, the patient's thighs should be separated as far as possible to minimize the reduction in urethral visibility caused by the soft tissue shadow of the thigh. The dynamic retrograde and voiding cystourethrogram can be completed in 15 to 20 minutes.

Excretory voiding cystourethrography is a voiding cystourethrogram obtained at the end of an excretory urogram. After the urogram is completed, but before voiding, the patient is given water to drink to fill the bladder and spot films of voiding are obtained. There are several flaws in this method:

1. It is commonly time consuming, and patients must occupy a room intermittently when they think they are ready to void and do not;
2. It usually involves extended time in the radiology department, which is not always convenient for the patient;
3. No information about possible vesicoureteral reflux can be obtained;
4. Most importantly, voiding cystourethrography alone may provide misleading information on the extent of urethral disease and does not demonstrate anterior urethral pathology as well as does retrograde urethrography.

Cavernosography

Corpus cavernosography has been traditionally performed for the evaluation of Peyronie's disease, penile fracture, or priapism. The technique of the examination is straightforward. The skin on the dorsal lateral shaft of the penis just proximal to the glans is optionally infiltrated with 1% lidocaine for local anesthesia. A 21-gauge scalp vein needle is then inserted into one of the corporal bodies with a sharp thrusting motion that facilitates puncture of the tunica albuginea. Test injection of diluted contrast material will confirm the intracorporeal location of the needle tip. Under fluoroscopic guidance, additional diluted contrast material is injected until the body of the corpora is filled with contrast material. Injection of one of the corpora fills both, because there are multiple anastomoses between the two corporeal bodies. Anteroposterior and oblique film studies are generally obtained.

Recently, there has been increased interest in corpus cavernosography for the evaluation of organic impotence. Current thinking suggests that approximately 50% of the cases of organic impotence are vasculogenic in origin. Vasculogenic impotence is, in turn, subdivided into arterial impotence (i.e., an inadequate in-flow of blood to the corpora) and venous impotence (due to a defect in the venoocclusive mechanism of the corpora cavernosa, such that rapid blood flow out of the corpora prevents an erection from occurring or being maintained despite adequate inflow). Failure of this venoocclusive mechanism of the corpora is commonly referred to as venous leakage. Cavernosography in such cases is usually combined with corpus cavernosometry so that correlation of the images with intracorporeal pressure measurements can be obtained.

The technique of cavernosometry/cavernosography

for the assessment of impotence is similar to that used for standard cavernosography, except that two needles are placed, one in each corpora. The first needle is used to infuse diluted contrast material or saline at standard infusion rates, while the second needle is used to monitor intracorporeal pressure during these infusions. Most authorities now believe that the use of supraphysiologic infusion rates (up to 400 ml/min) in an attempt to produce an artificial erection is not valid, and therefore, that cavernosometry should only be performed after injection of pharmacologic agents designed to activate the corporal venoocclusive mechanism. A variety of pharmacologic regimens have been used, however, a mixture of papaverine, (a smooth muscle dilator), phentolamine, and prostaglandin E-1 is most commonly recommended. Infusion of normal saline is then performed at an initial rate of 30 to 40 ml/min and, if necessary, to a maximum of 120 ml/min. If infusion at these rates does not produce an artificial erection, the study is terminated and no conclusion about the relative contribution of venous leakage to the patient's impotence can be drawn. If, however, a rigid erection occurs, the infusion is terminated and the decrease in corporeal pressure monitored. If there is a precipitous decrease in intracorporeal pressure, the presence of a venous leak is inferred. In addition, some authorities recommend the measurement of the pharmacologic maintenance erectile flow (PMEF), which is the rate of infusion necessary to maintain the erection. This measurement is used to quantitate the degree of venous leakage that is present. Normal males demonstrate a PMEF of between 2 and 12 ml/min; a higher rate indicates a venous leak.

If a leak is demonstrated by cavernosometry, cavernosography is performed by repeating the infusion using diluted contrast material to demonstrate the sites of leakage. Film studies are generally performed in the anteroposterior and both oblique projections. Common sites of venous leakage include the deep crural veins, the glans penis, and the deep and superficial dorsal veins of the penis. If no leak is indicated by cavernosometry, cavernosography is unnecessary.

Vasography

A seminal vesiculogram is an operative procedure in which the vas deferens is cannulated after making a small incision in the scrotum. Injection of contrast medium into the vas outlines the course of the vas and the ampulla. The ejaculatory duct is visualized and reflux of contrast medium into the seminal vesicle occurs. Contrast medium passing into the prostatic urethra is normally propelled retrogradely into the bladder.

In patients who have had transurethral prostatectomy or in patients who have had severe urethral and prostatic infection, dynamic retrograde urethrography and voiding urethrography occasionally show the ejacula-

tory ducts, the seminal vesicles, and the vas deferens. This results from reflux of contrast medium into the ejaculatory ducts due to patency of these ducts from infection or operation.

Cross-Sectional Imaging

Ultrasonography

The physical principles of ultrasonography are beyond the scope of this book. Sonography offers a painless and noninvasive method of visualizing soft tissue structures within the urinary tract that does not require the use of contrast agents or ionizing radiation. Real-time sonography has essentially replaced the older static gray-scale images for the evaluation of the urinary tract. Real-time equipment allows the physician to closely monitor the examination, and its resolution now surpasses that of the older static units.

RENAL SONOGRAPHY. The forte of sonography is its ability to differentiate fluid-filled structures from solid tissue. For this reason, one of the earliest applications of ultrasonography in the urinary tract was its use in differentiating solid renal mass lesions from renal cysts. Ultrasound is still used for this purpose and at an accuracy rate reported as high as 98% in the hands of an experienced sonographer.

The uses of sonography in the urinary tract have expanded to include the evaluation of a wide variety of morphologic diseases of the kidney, including renal cystic disease, medical renal disease, perirenal fluid collections, renal transplants, and nonfunctioning kidneys. In patients in whom urography demonstrates a poorly visualized kidney or shows a questionable abnormality, sonography often is the next imaging study. Sonography has become the imaging method of choice for the initial evaluation of the azotemic patient. It also may be used as a primary imaging method in patients with severe contrast allergies, for the evaluation of the urinary tract in infants, and in children with palpable abdominal masses.

Ultrasonography has been particularly useful in the evaluation of hydronephrosis, especially when it is of long-standing duration. Opaque and nonopaque renal calculi may be detected by ultrasound because of their highly echogenic nature and characteristic acoustic shadow caused by the attenuation of the sound beam behind the stone. Intraoperative sonography may facilitate complete stone removal in patients undergoing operative pyelolithotomy. Sonography also is used as a guidance technique for a variety of invasive procedures, including antegrade pyelography, percutaneous nephrostomy, percutaneous renal biopsy, and percutaneous abscess drainage. Ultrasound also may be used in the evaluation of pregnant patients because, to date, no adverse biologic effects of the technique have been demonstrated.

As with any diagnostic technique, the limitations and

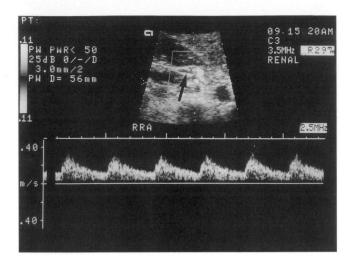

Figure 3.25. Pulsed duplex ultrasound. The Doppler gate is positioned over the renal artery (*arrow*). The resulting waveform is displayed below the gray-scale image.

disadvantages of sonography should be recognized. The technique offers a purely anatomic demonstration of the morphology in a single plane. The technique is much more operator-dependent than virtually any other method of diagnostic imaging, and therefore, the results often depend on the experience of the operator, as well as the quality of the equipment. The right kidney is generally better imaged than the left kidney because the liver can be used as a sonographic window. Sound waves are completely reflected by gas and are completely absorbed by bone. For this reason, the bony pelvis and intestinal gas often pose significant limitations within the abdomen. The lower pole of the left kidney, in particular, can be difficult to image because of overlying intestinal gas. The technique is difficult to use to evaluate the ureter because it is impossible to distinguish a nondistended ureter from its surrounding retroperitoneal fat. In addition, since the transducer must be directly applied to the patient's skin, recent surgery, bandages, or ostomies may pose significant limitations. With obese patients, greater absorption of the sound waves is apparent, which significantly decreases the resolution of the images.

DOPPLER SONOGRAPHY. The Doppler effect is a well-known physical phenomenon that states that the apparent shift in frequency of a wave reflecting from a moving object is proportional to the speed of that object relative to the observer. The principle is named for the Austrian physicist, Christian Doppler, who first described it in 1842. Thus, in theory, the Doppler effect may be used to determine the velocity of a moving object, such as flowing blood, using an ultrasound wave. While a number of factors in practice may limit the accuracy of quantitative blood flow measurements using the Doppler effect, modern ultrasound equipment can be used to accurately as-

sess relative flow. Three types of Doppler ultrasound instruments are available: 1) continuous wave, 2) pulsed duplex, and 3) color flow instruments.

Continuous wave instruments are small, relatively inexpensive devices used to assess flow in superficial vessels by subjectively listening for the Doppler signal as the transducer is placed in proximity to the vessel. No image is produced. Pulsed duplex devices allow the operator to display the flow in an area on a corresponding gray-scale image as a continuous time-velocity waveform (Fig. 3.25). With a color flow device, a color-encoded Doppler signal is superimposed on a gray-scale image; red is used to indicate flow (Fig. 3.26) toward the transducer (i.e., arterial flow) whereas blue is used to indicate flow away from the transducer (i.e., venous flow). A paler color is used to indicate a large Doppler shift (high flow), while a deeper hue is used to indicate slower flow. In comparison to a pulsed duplex device, a color flow device is capable of displaying the flow over a large area of an image simultaneously. A modification of standard color Doppler ultrasound, called "power Doppler" offers extended dynamic range, and therefore can demonstrate the perfusion of a small tissue sample.

Applications of Doppler imaging in uroradiology are extensive and include the evaluation of renal transplants; the detection of arteriovenous fistulae; the assessment of renal artery stenosis and occlusion; renal vein thrombosis; the evaluation of suspected testicular torsion, varicoceles, and vasculogenic impotence; and the relative assessment of urine flow from the ureteral orifices (ureteral jet phenomena) (Fig. 3.27).

BLADDER SONOGRAPHY. The full bladder is well visualized using the transabdominal or transurethral approach.

The *transabdominal approach* is most commonly used, but requires a full bladder. This is best done by

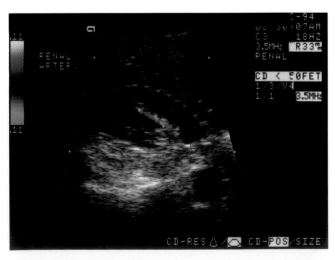

Figure 3.26. Color Doppler image showing arterial flow (*red*) in the renal artery.

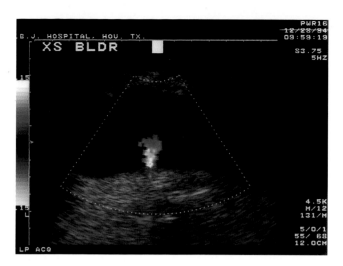

Figure 3.27. Ureteral jet. A transverse image of the bladder showing a jet of urine (*red*) from the ureteral orifice.

waiting until the patient's bladder naturally fills with urine, or if there is renal impairment, the bladder may be filled with normal saline using a urethral catheter. Transverse and longitudinal views are essential. The transducer is placed in the suprapubic area adjacent to the pubic bone and is angled inferiorly toward the bladder trigone. For visualization of structures on the right side of the bladder, the transducer should be placed to the left of midline and angled obliquely toward the right; the opposite should be done for visualization of structures on the left side of the bladder. Gain control adjustment may be necessary to make the bladder content echo free at the beginning of the procedure. The filled bladder was initially used to provide an acoustic window for the visualization of the uterus and ovaries in female patients and for visualization of the prostate in male patients. However, intrinsic bladder lesions are relatively well seen. Bladder stones that move with alteration of patient position are seen as hyperechoic areas with acoustic shadowing. Isoechoic lesions without acoustic shadowing generally represent bladder tumors that remain fixed in position. Bladder foreign bodies may be hyperechoic if calcified or isoechoic if not calcified, but usually move with the patient. Bladder diverticula are well seen on transabdominal ultrasound. Extravesical fluid collections are demonstrated as hypoechoic areas adjacent to the bladder. These can represent urine, urachal cystic fluid, or lymph. Old hemorrhage is mixed echogenicity and usually contains numerous bright echoes without acoustic shadowing. Bladder residual volumes can be estimated by transabdominal ultrasound. Measurements in the transverse and longitudinal planes give width, length, and depth measurements. Using the empirical formula, bladder volume may be calculated as follows:

$$\textit{Bladder volume } Vc = 0.7(W \times H \times D) \quad \text{(Eq. 3.1)}$$

Such estimation of bladder residual volume is accurate within approximately 20%, which is considered acceptable.

Specialized *transurethral* probes have been recently developed and provide excellent assessment of the bladder. Unlike transabdominal ultrasound, transurethral ultrasound usually requires heavy sedation or anesthesia, particularly in male patients. The transurethral ultrasound transducer is large enough to require a 24-French cystoscope for passage into the bladder and the examination performed at the time of cystoscopy. The bladder must be fluid-filled after removal of the cystoscope light. As the transducer is passed through the cystoscope into the bladder, its progress toward the bladder dome is monitored. Half-centimeter-spaced transverse images are obtained from the bladder dome to the bladder trigone. This method provides excellent detail of the bladder wall.

PROSTATE SONOGRAPHY. Initially, a 3-MHz transducer was able to use the full bladder as an acoustic window for visualization of the prostate. The size and shape of the prostate size, as well as the effect of the prostate on the bladder base could be assessed. However, transrectal ultrasound has become the method of choice for prostate assessment. A transducer with a radial head is used to obtain transverse images of the prostate, and a linear array transducer with a varying number of transducers (between 64 and 120) is used to visualize the prostate in longitudinal fashion.

Transrectal sonography is used to assess carcinoma of the prostate. While the efficacy of this method has never been shown, the method has proven useful to localize suspicious nodules for biopsy.

Proper positioning and assessment of echogenicity is time-consuming and difficult, and requires considerable experience. Sonographers disagree about the appearance of prostate carcinoma as seen by transrectal ultrasound. Generally sonographers agree that hypoechoic areas within the prostate should be biopsied and that operable prostatic carcinoma is more commonly hypoechoic. However, transrectal ultrasound usually clearly delineates the central zone from the peripheral zone. Prostatic carcinoma arises in the peripheral zone. Any hypoechoic or hyperechoic area in the peripheral zone requires biopsy, since some hyperechoic areas in the peripheral zone also have been shown to be carcinoma by biopsy.

Biopsy of hypoechoic and hyperechoic areas is guided by transrectal ultrasound. Attached to the handle of the transrectal transducer is a fitting which takes the biopsy needle for transrectal or perineal biopsy and this can be guided to the appropriate area. Prostatic carcinomas which have gone through the capsule or are locally invasive are not so readily distinguished by echogenicity from prostatic hypertrophy.

SEMINAL VESICLE SONOGRAPHY. On transabdominal sonography, the seminal vesicles are visualized, using the filled bladder as an acoustic window, as hypoechoic linear or crescentic areas. They are not quite as hypoechoic as the bladder. On longitudinal views, the nechogenicity of the seminal vesicles approaches that of the prostate, and they appear as proximal extensions of the prostate.

The seminal vesicles are well seen on transrectal ultrasound, which is usually performed as a method of assessing the prostate gland. Following a Fleet enema (C.B. Fleet Co., Lynchburg, Va.), the transrectal probe is gently passed into the rectum. If the probe is inserted up to the base of the prostate and bladder trigone, the seminal vesicles are well seen. The transverse views show the seminal vesicles as hypoechoic with a bow tie or crescentic shape. Longitudinal views show the seminal vesicles as linear hypoechoic areas adjacent to the base of the prostate, where they present as beak-shaped areas in most patients. Absence of the beak appearance on longitudinal transrectal scan raises the possibility of invasion from prostatic carcinoma.

SCROTAL SONOGRAPHY. Over the past several years, the development of high-resolution, short-focused 7.5–12 MHz real-time transducers has allowed detailed resolution of the scrotal contents. The normal testis has a homogeneous echo texture and can easily be differentiated from the epididymis, which is located superior and posterior to the testicle itself.

The most common indication for scrotal ultrasonography is for scrotal enlargement and to differentiate such benign conditions of the testis as hydroceles from solid tumors of the testis. The accuracy of scrotal sonography in differentiating solid lesions of the testis from cystic lesions and in differentiating intratesticular disease from extratesticular disease has been reported to approach 100% in some series.

Scrotal sonography also may be of value in finding the cause of male infertility in that varicoceles may readily be detected. Cryptorchid testes below the inguinal ligament may be evaluated by sonography.

Computed Tomography

Computed tomography uses the same ionizing radiation as conventional radiography. With CT, the data from multiple planar projections are mathematically recombined to produce a cross-sectional image. Images can be reformatted into coronal, sagittal, or oblique projections, but these are seldom needed. Although the spatial resolution of CT is less than conventional film–screen radiography, the contrast resolution is far superior. Thus, fat is easily distinguished from other soft tissues of muscle or organ density, and contrast enhancement is an important diagnostic feature.

There have been several generations of CT equipment, but the basic process of image generation remains the same. A series of exposures from different projections is made. The image is formed by back-projecting the relative densities into a matrix that assigns a value to each element. These back-projections are then filtered to eliminate star artifact. The result is a matrix of numbers corresponding to the attenuation of volume elements (voxels) of the patient. A water phantom is used to calibrate the scanner and to allow conversion of the relative tissue densities to Hounsfield units (HU) which range from −1000 to +1000. Air measures −1000 HU, water is 0 HU, and bone approaches +1000 HU.

The CT image consists of a matrix, usually 512 × 512 picture elements (pixels), of numbers ranging from −1000 to +1000. Although the computer image contains 2000 levels, the human eye can perceive only 16 to 20 gray levels. Thus, the computer data are combined into 16 displayable levels.

The display can be varied in both width and level. A wide window allows visualization of the greatest amount of tissue, but minimizes the differences of density. A narrow window accentuates subtle differences and is useful for carefully examining a relatively homogeneous organ such as the liver. Wider windows are used when tissues with a broad range of densities are examined.

The optimal window level depends on the tissue density. Pulmonary parenchyma, for instance, must be viewed at a low level such as −700 HU, but the mediastinum will be completely white at this level. The mediastinum is better imaged near 0, whereas bony structures often are best imaged at +100 to +200 HU. Current CT scanners are either third or fourth generation. Third-generation scanners use a system of parallel detectors in which the x-ray tube and detectors rotate in unison. Fourth-generation scanners have a complete ring of stationary detectors such that only the x-ray tube moves. Resolution is a function of the number, size, and efficiency of the detectors and their distance from the x-ray source.

In addition to these conventional CT scanners, an electron beam sweep with fixed detector array has been designed to provide ultrafast scans and to eliminate motion artifact. Scans as fast as 50 msec can be used to image dynamic structures such as the heart. It also may prove useful in examining uncooperative patients such as children or trauma victims, because the rapid scan speed prevents motion artifact.

The many advantages of CT scanning have made a dramatic impact on genitourinary radiology. Computed tomography is essential in the examination of the adrenal glands and is an important modality for imaging the kidney and retroperitoneum. Although CT is seldom used to directly image the bladder, prostate, or testes, it is commonly employed to stage tumors arising in those organs.

There are, however, some disadvantages to CT scanning. It is expensive. CT table incrementation may not be accurate when large patients (over 300 lbs) are scanned; very large patients may even have to be pushed, because the table may not move automatically. Biopsy procedures also may be limited by the size of the patient opening in the gantry.

HELICAL CT. A recent technical advance in CT has been the development of spiral or helical CT. Helical CT allows the acquisition of volumetric image data on a continuous basis such that the entire abdomen can be scanned in one or two breath holds. Three technical refinements in CT hardware have been crucial to the development of spiral CT: 1) the invention of the slip-ring gantry, 2) improved detector efficiency, and 3) improved x-ray-tube cooling capacity. Slip-ring technology allows the gantry of the scanner to rotate in one continuous motion without the use of electrical cables which, in a conventional gantry, prevent this continuous rotation from occurring. Thus, the x-ray tube is energized and data are transferred from the detectors through the slip-rings while the patient is transported through the gantry in one continuous motion. Because the data are acquired volumetrically, high-quality three-dimensional reconstruction of the data is possible without the necessity of acquiring the data in overlapping scans, as would be necessary with conventional CT. The number of scans, and consequently, the radiation dose received by the patient is reduced. Three-dimensional software packages that can be used to produce a CT angiogram (i.e., a surface rendering of the major blood vessels) are available. Such displays have been shown to be capable of demonstrating the extrarenal portions of the renal arteries and veins and their relationship to the great vessels. Such studies may obviate the need for conventional angiography in selected patients.

Non-contrast helical CT has recently been shown to be a cost-effective and efficent alternative to urography for the assessment of patients with acute flank pain secondary to ureteral calculi. Advantages of this technique include its speed (the entire examination may be completed in a few minutes and delayed radiographs as required with urography are not necessary), the absence of a requirement for the adminstration of contrast media, and the ability to detect extraurinary pathology which may be responsible for the patient's symptom. (See Chapter 12)

Magnetic Resonance Imaging

The physics of image production from magnetic resonance (MR) is complicated and beyond the scope of this text, but a simplified model can explain the phenomena of imaging. Protons within the patient can be thought of as small spinning bar magnets. Hydrogen molecules have a single proton. When a patient is placed in a large magnetic field, the hydrogen protons within the body align, and this alignment leads to the formation of a net magnetic vector within the patient. By applying radiofrequency (RF) pulses to the patient, this vector can be made to spin. A wire (the antenna) lying outside the patient will have a current induced within it by the spinning bar magnet. This current originates from the tissues and its magnitude is related to the intensity of the pixel in the MR image.

The intensity of the signal from the tissues is related to both tissue and system parameters. The tissue parameters are the number of protons that have aligned within the voxel (initial magnetization, MO), the T1 relaxation time, the T2 relaxation time, the affects of flow and motion in the tissues, and local changes to the magnetic field. T1 and T2 are time constants that describe delay mechanisms of the spinning bar magnet. System parameters that affect the intensity of the signal from the tissue include the manner in which the RF pulses are applied to the patient and the time between the application of these RF pulses.

Images can be created with contrast between tissues dependent primarily on the T1 values of tissues (T1-weighted images), or the T2 values of the tissues (T2-weighted images). One of the most common ways to do this is to use a sequence of RF pulses known as the spin-echo pulse sequence. Timing parameters in the spin-echo pulse sequence are repetition time (TR) and echo time (TE). An image of which the contrast is primarily due to the differences of T1 values in the tissues is produced by a relatively short TR (approximately 250–600 msec), and a relatively short TE (approximately 12–25 msec). T2-weighted images have a long TR (TR = 2000–4000 msec) and a relatively long TE (TE = 40–120 msec). Values of TR and TE between these ranges produce images with a mix of T1 and T2 contrast. Other pulse techniques are available that will allow adjustment of contrast between the soft tissues depending on their MO, T1, or T2 values, or on techniques that will accentuate blood flow within vessels.

Although conventional spin echo technique remains the mainstay of MR imaging, they take the longest amount of time to perform. A variety of faster pulse sequences including gradient echo, fast spin echo, and echo planar techniques have been described which decrease image acquisition times to as little as 20 milliseconds.

Three basic magnet types are currently used for imaging. Resistive magnets operate up to the field strength of 0.15 Tesla (T). They are the least expensive to build and do not require cryogens. However, there is a significant cost in electrical energy and only lower field strengths are available.

Permanent magnets allow field strengths up to approximately 0.35 T. These units do not require cryogens and use only a moderate electric current. However, they are permanent magnets, are very heavy, and cannot be disabled.

Clinically used superconductive magnets operate with a field strength up to 2.0 T. This higher field strength results in improved contrast resolution and is essential for spectroscopy. Although the electrical requirements are not high, the basic unit is quite expensive and the use of cryogens adds to the continuing operating expense. Furthermore, shielding requirements may add significantly to the cost and space needed for installation.

KIDNEY.   There is no single scanning technique that is universally used for MR imaging of the kidney. The profusion of techniques in the literature probably has to do with the ongoing rapid advancement of the field, differing capabilities of available machines, and the continued predominance of CT as the most definitive imaging modality for the kidneys. Magnetic resonance imaging is thus used as a problem-solving technique, rather than as a primary diagnostic modality.

A few principles always apply, however. The examination should be individually tailored and monitored to address the specific clinical question. Body coils should be used for native kidneys; surface coil use is largely restricted to transplanted kidneys that are near the skin surface. The field of view should be sufficiently large to include both the kidneys and the perirenal regions. Very thin slices are generally not necessary; slices of 7 to 10 mm in thickness with gaps ranging from 0 to 3 mm are appropriate. Slice orientation is determined by the clinical question; coronal and transverse slices are commonly used, sagittal sections occasionally yield additional information. Specific slice orientation is most important when neoplastic invasion across perirenal tissue planes is in question; in such cases, slices should be perpendicular to the plane of possible invasion. The number of slices also should be tailored. When masses or morphologic abnormalities are to be investigated, there should be a sufficient number of slices to cover both the kidneys and the perirenal regions. When functional studies, such as those intended to display any asymmetry in renal perfusion are performed, one or two planes imaged dynamically and containing representative portions of the central parts of the kidneys (i.e., midtransverse or midcoronal views) are generally sufficient. Fat saturation techniques may be useful when the kidneys are bright (i.e., when T2-weighted or gadolinium-enhanced T1-weighted images) are used. Frequency-selective fat-saturation techniques should be used; short T1 inversion recovery techniques for nulling fat has not been found to be frequently useful. The optimal matrix size is largely determined by a trade-off among imaging time, signal-to-noise ratio, and in-plane spatial resolution; matrix sizes ranging from 128×256 to 256×256 are most often used.

The selection of pulse sequences and paramagnetic enhancement protocols also are important. T1-weighted spin-echo images (Fig. 3.28) are a good way to assess renal morphology and may initially be performed in the transverse or coronal plane. Often these images will reveal flow voids in the renal vein and inferior vena cava,

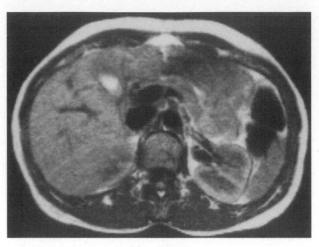

Figure 3.28.   T1-weighted spin-echo image of normal left kidney. Corticomedullary differentiation is well seen.

a phenomenon that may permit an evaluation of the extent of any intravascular thrombi. Repetition times ranging from 300 to 600 ms are generally used (higher TR values, especially in high-field devices, may make corticomedullary distinction hard to see); the TE should be the shortest the machine can perform. Even though these images require sufficient time that true dynamic imaging is not possible, the addition of gadolinium enhancement (0.1 mmol/kg) may be useful to demonstrate the renal parenchyma and the perfused regions of renal pathology (Fig. 3.29).

T2-weighted spin-echo images (Fig. 3.30) are less frequently useful, but may permit visualization of certain focal tumors and cysts. T2-weighted images also are useful to demonstrate corticomedullary abnormalities reflecting intrarenal iron deposition. The TR should be relatively long (at least 2000 ms for high-field machines) and the TE should be long (80–130 ms) as well. Fast T-2 weighted spin-echo images can be used instead of standard T-2 weighted spin echo images. The increased speed of data acquisition permitted by fast spin-echo technique can be used either to improve signal to noise ratios or to shorten scanning times. TR and effective TE values should be in the same range as the TR and TE values for standard T2 weighted spin-echo sequences.

Gradient-echo images are useful for several reasons; they can be performed sufficiently fast to use breath-holding as a motion-reducing technique, to permit dynamic imaging after a bolus of gadolinium and to make venous blood bright to assess the presence and extent of thrombi. The parameters of these sequences are usually designed to provide T1 weighting to exploit the enhancement effects of gadolinium; TRs between 30 and 40 ms, short TEs (16 ms or less), and flip angles between 45 and 90° have been reported. If the renal parenchyma is to be evaluated, images obtained before and after

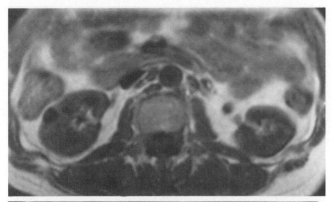

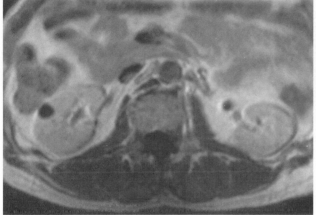

Figure 3.29.   Top, T1-weighted spin-echo image; small right renal cyst. **Bottom,** T1-weighted spin-echo imaging after administration of gadolinium-DTPA 0.1 mmol/kg. The renal parenchyma is enhanced, but the cyst is not.

gadolinium administration (images may be obtained immediately after, approximately 1 minute after, and several minutes after the bolus) are useful (Fig. 3.31). If the parenchyma need not be evaluated, but many closely spaced delay times are needed, one or two slices may be imaged every few seconds before and for several minutes after a bolus of gadolinium.

For all imaging techniques, from 1 to 4 excitations

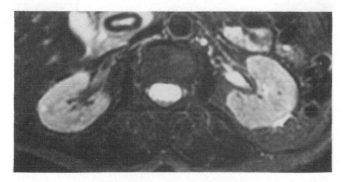

Figure 3.30. T2-weighted spin-echo image of normal kidneys. The parenchyma is bright, and no corticomedullary distinction is visual. The patient has a large gallstone (*dark oval*).

may be used; as always, there is a trade-off between rapid imaging and improved signal-to-noise ratio, which can be tailored to the specific clinical question.

ADRENAL.   Most adrenal imaging can be done in the transverse plane; this may be augmented by coronal or sagittal views, if these are needed to establish the organ of origin of a mass that appears in the adrenal region. Standard body coils suffice for most imaging. Although some reports describe the use of surface coils, the adrenal glands are not close to the skin, and adrenal imaging relies to a great degree on uniform sensitivity throughout the imaged volume. Therefore, surface coils are not commonly used.

When trying to detect small (less than 1 cm) adrenal masses, it is important not to use very thick slices or very large gaps. However, multislice imaging eliminates the possibility of respiratory misregistration even with standard breathing, so that most investigators are satisfied with slices of 7 to 10 mm in thickness using no gap or gaps up to 3 mm in width.

The initial pulse sequence should be a transverse T1-

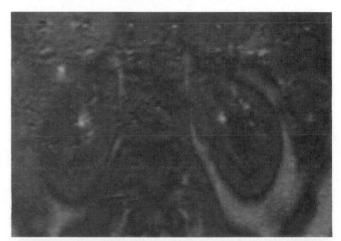

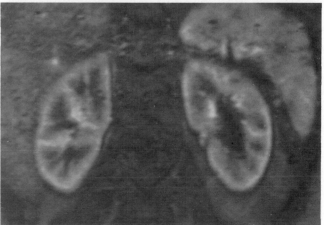

Figure 3.31.   Top, T2-weighted gradient-recalled-echo image of normal kidneys. **Bottom,** Image obtained during cortical enhancement phase after gadolinium bolus. The paramagnetic agent has not yet reached the medullary pyramids.

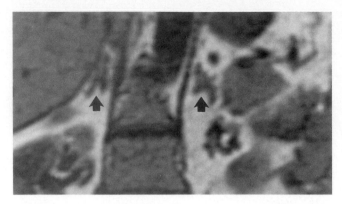

Figure 3.32. Coronal T1-weighted images through normal adrenals (*arrows*). The adrenal limbs are well outlined by bright retroperitoneal fat.

weighted spin-echo series. The TE should be as low as the scanner permits; TR is less crucial, but should be within the range of approximately 300 to 700 ms. Fat saturation pulses are recommended by some authors, but retroperitoneal fat provides such striking contrast against which both normal and abnormal adrenals can be seen that it is not generally necessary.

If good-quality T1-weighted spin-echo images (Fig. 3.32) reveal the adrenal anatomy to be normal, the examination can be terminated (unless the clinical situation warrants a search for extraadrenal pheochromocytomas). If a mass is seen, a T2-weighted spin-echo or fast spin-echo series should be performed (Fig. 3.33). Standard spin-echo imaging should employ a TR of at least 2000 ms and a TE within the range of 75 to 110 ms. Because a dual-echo study can be conducted without incurring extra scan time, a short-TE spin-density series can be done simultaneously. If a fast spin-echo program is available, a TR of approximately 4000 ms or more and an effective TE of 70 to 110 ms are suitable.

If a mass is encountered that might be an adenoma, in-phase and out-of-phase gradient-recalled-echo images should be performed (Fig. 3.34). For these masses, the TE is crucial. The out-of-phase TE should be one, three, or five times the interval required for lipid and water spins to be maximally out of phase (2.24 ms at 1.5 T) and the in-phase images should be two, four or six times this value. Flip angles ranging from 15 to 90° have been described, as have TRs from 30 to 60 ms.

Some authors have suggested using dynamic fast imaging after administration of a bolus of gadolinium to distinguish between adenomas and other masses, including medullary and malignant neoplasms. A single-slice dynamic sequence may be performed before, during, and at 1-minute intervals for 5 minutes or so after the administration of gadolinium; the imaging sequence should be continued at several-minute intervals for at least 15 minutes as well.

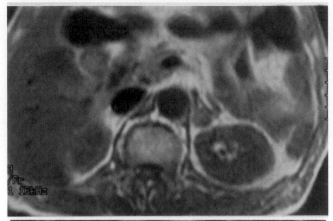
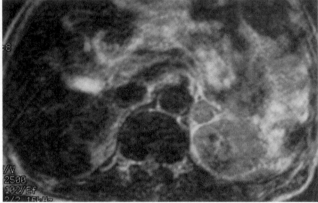

Figure 3.33. Top, T1-weighted spin-echo image of metastasis to left adrenal. **Bottom,** T2-weighted fast spin-echo image. The adrenal mass is brighter than the liver and is approximately isointense with the kidney.

PROSTATE. The primary use for prostate MR imaging is the staging of prostate cancer. Body coil images alone have an insufficient signal-to-noise ratio to provide the necessary spatial resolution, so that images performed using an intrarectal surface coil are now considered necessary for definitive evaluation.

The examination should, nonetheless, include body-coil transverse spin-echo images of the pelvis and lower abdomen to assess lymphadenopathy. For these images, the TE should be as short as the machine will permit, the TR may be anywhere from 800 ms to considerably lower values, the slice thickness should be from 7 to 10 mm, and slice gaps should be 0 to 3 mm. The field of view should be sufficient to include the retroperitoneal lymph nodes, and respiratory compensation should be used. A saturation band may be placed superior to the imaged volume to reduce pulsation artifacts and anterior to the retroperitoneum to reduce respiration artifacts from anterior subcutaneous fat. Since lymphadenopathy is the major finding, fat saturation is probably not necessary, nor is there reason to use routine T2-weighted images or gadolinium enhancement.

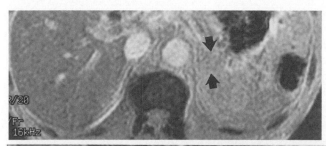

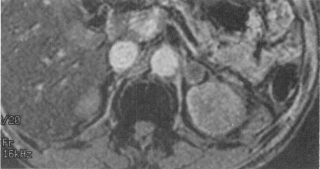

Figure 3.34. **Top,** In-phase gradient-recalled-echo image of left adrenal adenoma (*arrows*). The lesion is nearly isointense with its surroundings and is very difficult to discern. **Bottom,** Out-of-phase gradient-recalled-echo image. The adrenal adenoma is now less intense and is easily seen.

These parameters also will be useful when the retroperitoneum needs to be imaged for other diseases that may involve the urinary tract (Fig. 3.35). If retroperitoneal fibrosis or neoplasms are encountered, T2-weighted images (fast spin-echo images using TR values of several thousand and effective TEs approaching 100 ms) may be useful to determine tissue intensity and distinguish stable fibrosis from neoplasms, inflammatory lesions, and rapidly progressive desmoplastic reactions.

Placement of the intrarectal coil for high-resolution imaging of the prostate and periprostatic structures should be performed carefully and should proceed only after the examiner is satisfied that there is no rectal stricture or neoplasm that may be injured by the coil. The details of the procedure should be explained to the patient after which the balloon of the coil should be tested, lubricated, and then inserted into the rectum; 60 to 90 ml of air is an appropriate volume range. Correct placement of the coil is essential: the wire loop should be in the coronal plane, and the coil should be prevented from migrating proximal to the prostate by an external perineal stop placed on the handle.

T1-weighted spin-echo images of the prostate should be acquired. A field of view of approximately 10 cm is appropriate (the periprostatic tissues, bladder base, pubic symphysis, and seminal vesicles should be included), in addition to the entire prostate gland. Interleaved images of 3 to 4 mm in thickness should be acquired, using a TR of approximately 500 to 800 ms with the short-

est TE the machine will permit. Using the same field of view, slice thickness, and orientation, fast T2-weighted images should be acquired, using a TR of 4 to 5 seconds and an effective TE of 100 ms or slightly more. Some investigators repeat the transverse T2-weighted images using fat-saturation. T2-weighted images in the sagittal plane and in the coronal (or angled coronal, to be aligned with the long axis of the prostate) should also be acquired. To keep any motion artifact from the coil away from the main portions of the prostate, a side-to-side, rather than anterior-to-posterior, direction should be chosen for the phase-encoding gradients.

BLADDER. The most important application of MR imaging of the bladder is the staging of bladder carcinoma. A number of pulse sequences and paramagnetic contrast agent protocols have been tested, but no one sequence is universally accepted. Certain principles, however, seem to be emerging. Magnetic resonance imaging should be used to stage rather than to detect the tumor. It cannot improve on clinical diagnosis (including cystoscopy and biopsy) for very superficial tumors; T1-weighted spin-echo images are best for detecting lymphadenopathy, and techniques that display the tumor itself as relatively intense are best for staging the primary lesion. The bladder should be filled prior to imaging; this is usually accomplished by instructing the patient to drink water without voiding for a couple of hours before the examination. Either a body coil or sandwich-type pelvic surface coil may be used.

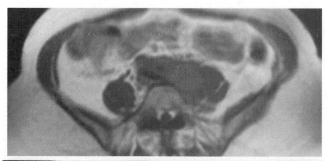

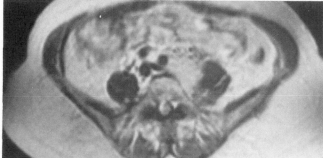

Figure 3.35. **Top,** T1-weighted spin-echo image; patients with confluent lymphadenopathy from non-Hodgkin's lymphoma. The tumor is of relatively low intensity. **Bottom,** T2-weighted spin-echo image. The tumor now appears relatively bright. Stable fibrosis would appear darker.

Standard T1-weighted multiplanar MR images may be used to begin; the TR may range from 400 to 800 ms and the TE should be as short as the scanner will permit. The field of view should include the bladder and region of pelvic lymph nodes; slice thickness should ideally be less than 1 cm, and gaps should be narrow or nonexistent. This sequence is good for demonstrating gross extension of tumor into perivesical fat, and may be acquired in whatever orientation is perpendicular to the bladder wall at the site of the tumor.

T2-weighted spin-echo sequences are good to display intrinsic contrast between the margin of the tumor and muscular layer of the bladder wall. Fast spin-echo sequences have largely supplanted standard spin-echo sequences for this purpose; a TR of at least 2000 ms and a TE of 80 to 120 ms are acceptable ranges.

Gadolinium may sufficiently enhance tumor tissue so that it appears to be of different intensity from bladder wall on T1-dependant images. The maximum contrast is achieved just a few seconds after intravenous injection has yielded the highest systemic arterial concentration of the paramagnetic agent, so that fast scanning is essential. A fast T1-weighted spin-echo sequence, using a TR of approximately 100 and a TE of 14 ms has been suggested; data acquisition should begin almost immediately after intravenous injection. Faster dynamic gradient-echo variations also have been described; very short TE values should be used, as should relatively short TR values and flip angles of at least 45° to produce T1 weighting.

SCROTUM.   Magnetic resonance imaging of the scrotum can produce highly accurate images of both anatomy and pathology, but scrotal ultrasound provides similar information more cheaply; scrotal MR imaging has therefore not become a primary imaging technique.

Imaging of the scrotum and its contents should be done with a surface coil. Frequently, evaluation of patients with scrotal pathology requires imaging of the pelvis and retroperitoneum as well; if this is performed by MR imaging, the techniques are not significantly different from those described above for pelvic and retroperitoneal applications.

Patients may be examined in the prone or supine positions; the former may reduce motion artifact, because the scrotum and surface coil are held motionless against the table. A 12- or 13-cm circular surface coil is most frequently used; this should be placed around the scrotum and oriented in a plane parallel to the main magnetic field. T1-weighted images are acquired and usually involve a spin-echo technique using a TR of 400 to 600 ms and the shortest TE the machine can perform. T2-weighted images also should be acquired; the TR should be at least 2000 ms and the TE should be in the range of 80 to 110 ms; although most reports in the literature describe standard spin-echo imaging, fast spin-echo imaging can be used routinely in their place. The field

of view should be sufficiently large to include the entire scrotum and distal portions of the spermatic cord; sizes ranging from 16 to 24 cm have been described. Slice thickness of 3 to 5 mm are appropriate and may be contiguous or involve gaps up to several millimeters. As usual, the increased signal-to-noise ratio provided by increasing scanning time needs to be balanced against patient throughput and the likelihood of motion; two excitations are frequently used.

No single slice orientation has emerged as the best one. Because the orientation of the scrotal contents is variable, all three of the standard planes have been found to be useful. A good routine would be to use a transverse or coronal plane for T1-weighted images, followed by T2-weighted images in the transverse and coronal planes, with sagittal images added only if needed.

Invasive Techniques
Angiography

Despite advances in noninvasive imaging modalities, arteriography and venography remain important techniques in genitourinary radiology.

ARTERIOGRAPHY.   Diagnostic arteriography may be used to define either the renal arteries or mass lesions. The renal arteries are most commonly studied for suspected renovascular hypertension in which the stenosis is usually in the main renal artery, and often at the origin from the aorta. Smaller renal arteries may be studied in patients with vasculitis, such as polyarteritis nodosa, in which the renal arteries are commonly affected. However, renal arteriography also may be used to identify an embolus or renal infarction.

Arteriography may be needed to define the organ of origin of an abdominal mass or to delineate the vessels in a variety of clinical situations. When a mass becomes large, it compresses adjacent structures and obliterates fat planes. When other organs are distorted, it may not be possible to determine the tissue of origin of the mass. This is especially true in the upper abdomen, where an adrenal mass may be indistinguishable from an exophytic renal mass, liver mass, or even primary retroperitoneal tumor. By defining the vessels supplying these large tumors, it may be possible to predict the tissue type.

Arterial access is usually gained through the right femoral artery, but the left femoral, the left brachial, or even the right brachial arteries may be used if necessary. Most angiographers prefer working with 5-French catheters. Thin-walled catheters allow high flow rates while preserving the small outer diameter. Larger catheters may be required for some interventional procedures, and smaller catheters (3 or 4 French) may be used with digital techniques.

If evaluation of the main renal arteries is desired, a flush aortogram should be performed as the initial run.

This allows visualization of the origin of the renal arteries, although oblique views are occasionally needed to see the renal origin in profile. The flush aortogram also provides visualization of the renal arteries before a catheter or guidewire is introduced into the renal artery, because this manipulation may cause vascular spasm.

Abdominal aortography may be performed with pigtail or straight end and side hole catheters. The straight end catheter has a slight advantage, because it avoids the potential problem of uncoiling and unwanted selective vessel catheterization that can occur with a pigtail catheter. However, this is a rare complication, and most angiographers believe that the tighter bolus obtained with the pigtail configuration more than compensates for this potential problem.

The ideal position of the catheter tip in the abdominal aorta depends on the specific indication for the arteriogram, however, it is usually placed just above or just below the renal arteries. If the pigtail is placed just below the renal arteries, contrast injection will reflux 2 or 3 cm cephalad and will provide opacification of the renal arteries. This avoids reflux into the celiac and superior mesenteric arteries, which may obscure portions of the renal arteries by opacifying overlying vessels.

A variety of catheters is available for selective catheterization of the renal arteries. A simple J hook is all that is required; but a specific renal curve, the Mikaelson curve, and the visceral cobra curve are popular catheter shapes. The choice of catheter depends on personal preference and what other maneuvers may be needed during the arteriogram.

Selective adrenal arteriography is much more demanding because the adrenal arteries are small. Flush aortography may be useful, but the adrenal arteries often are difficult to identify because of the many overlying vessels. The easiest adrenal artery to opacify is the superior adrenal artery, which arises from the inferior phrenic artery. Selective injection of the ipsilateral inferior phrenic artery usually provides adequate opacification of the superior adrenal artery. The inferior adrenal artery arises from the renal artery, and injection of the renal artery usually results in sufficient visualization of the inferior aspects of the adrenal gland. The smallest of the adrenal arteries is the middle adrenal artery, which arises directly from the aorta. Unless this artery is enlarged, it is difficult to catheterize and is seldom worth the time required and possible damage to the vessel.

Diagnostic arteriography of the other genitourinary structures is seldom required, although there has been increased interest in the arterial supply and venous drainage of the penis for problems of impotence. Selective injection of the internal iliac arteries with an oblique projection will demonstrate medium-sized vessels supplying the dorsal penile artery. A flush aortogram also may be useful to see if a common iliac artery stenosis

might be amenable to percutaneous transluminal angioplasty.

DIGITAL SUBTRACTION ANGIOGRAPHY.   Digital subtraction techniques may be used to image arteries or veins, but are most often applied to procedures to screen for abnormalities of the renal arteries and to guide interventional procedures. In digital subtraction angiography (DSA), the analog information obtained with fluoroscopy is digitized. Similar digital information from a mask obtained before contrast injection is subtracted from the frames obtained during contrast injection. Digital computers capable of making these subtractions at very high speed allow visualization of the subtracted images during the procedure. The technique has very high contrast sensitivity, but does not have the spatial resolution of conventional film–screen angiography.

Because contrast sensitivity is high, less contrast material is needed to adequately image the vessel. Thus, DSA may be used to image arteries after an intravenous injection. This may be done to screen patients for renovascular hypertension or to look for anomalies of the renal arteries in potential renal transplantation donors. With a peripheral injection of 40 ml of 60% iodinated contrast material at 10 ml/sec, the renal arteries can be imaged. An alternative approach, injecting contrast into the inferior vena cava or right atrium, requires a caval catheter. However, both of these are intravenous injections and avoid the potential complications of arterial catheterization.

If the contrast material is injected directly into the artery studied, adequate images can be obtained with much less contrast material than with conventional arteriography. This may be desired in a patient with renal failure in whom the contrast load should be minimized to decrease the risk of contrast nephropathy. It is important to dilute the contrast material to 30 to 50% of the conventional concentration rather than decrease the volume, because a small volume will not replace blood flow and will produce artifacts.

During lengthy interventional procedures such as embolization or angioplasty, DSA may save time. The digital image is available for immediate viewing, since film loading and processing is not required.

VENOGRAPHY.   Access to the venous system is usually gained through the right femoral vein, although the left femoral vein or a vein in the antecubital fossa may be used if needed. The most common use of venography in uroradiology is collection of blood samples from the renal veins for renin assay in patients suspected of having renovascular hypertension.

When blood samples are obtained from a large vein, such as the renal vein, a side hole near the catheter tip often is helpful, as the end hole of a downward-directed catheter tip may be occluded by the wall of the vein. It is important to be aware of the location of veins such as the inferior phrenic vein or left gonadal vein that drain into the renal vein, as inadvertent catheterization of these vessels will result in a spurious result. The use of a small amount of contrast material to confirm location of the catheter tip does not affect the blood sample if the catheter is flushed and blood is re-aspirated to avoid dilution. If there is suspicion of a branch artery stenosis, narrowing of an accessory renal artery or a renin-producing tumor, samples should be taken from smaller renal vein branches to reflect the upper and lower poles, as well as the central portion of the kidney.

Adrenal venography is occasionally needed to identify an autonomous hyperfunctioning adrenal tumor. Selective catheterization of the left adrenal vein may be accomplished through the femoral and left renal veins. The left adrenal vein joins the inferior phrenic vein, which enters the superior aspect of the left renal vein just to the left of the vertebral body. This vein can usually be catheterized with a variety of catheters, but a double-curved catheter specifically designed for this purpose is available.

The right adrenal vein is more difficult to catheterize because of its small size and variable entrance directly into the inferior vena cava. A down-pointing tip with a secondary curve which reaches the opposite wall of the inferior vena cava is needed. This can be accomplished by forming a catheter to fit the expected shape or using a preformed catheter such as a Mikaelson or sidewinder configuration. In either case, heparin irrigation is useful to prevent clot formation in the small adrenal veins partially occluded by the catheter or in the catheter itself. Adrenal venous sampling can be a slow and tedious process and should be performed by experienced angiographers.

Gonadal venography is used to prepare for occlusion therapy for a varicocele or to identify the pampiniform plexus of an undescended testis. Catheterization of the left gonadal vein is accomplished with a variety of catheters, but a visceral cobra often is used. Because the left gonadal vein enters the inferior surface of the left renal vein, it is usually easy to find. The right gonadal vein enters the inferior vena cava below the level of the renal veins, usually at L2 or L3. Because a variety of catheters can be used, the choice of the specific catheter should be determined by the other goals of the procedure.

Lymphography

Lymphography was introduced for human use in 1952 and subsequently gained widespread acceptance to evaluate the retroperitoneal lymph nodes. Although it has largely been replaced by CT, lymphography can identify smaller metastatic foci by detecting alterations in internal architecture. The injected contrast material remains within lymph nodes 1 to 2 years, providing visualization of opacified nodes on surveillance abdominal radiographs.

Superficial lymphatic vessels, usually in the dorsum of the foot, are cannulated and an iodinated oily contrast material is infused. Much of this contrast is retained in the draining lymph nodes, resulting in prolonged opacification. Contrast that is not taken up by the lymph nodes is trapped by pulmonary capillaries. This creates multiple small pulmonary emboli that result in a predictable impairment of pulmonary function. The diffusion capacity is most severely affected, although a decrease in vital capacity also has been shown. The maximum impairment is seen approximately 36 hours after contrast infusion, and recovery is usually complete in 3 to 5 days. Thus, significant impairment of pulmonary function is a contraindication to lymphangiography. If any doubt exists, pulmonary function tests should be obtained.

The presence of normal lymphaticovenous shunts will increase the pulmonary embolic load if they are present before the lymph nodes, as the shunts decrease the extent of lymph node uptake of contrast. These lymphaticovenous communications are undesirable, but still keep the oily contrast material on the right side of the heart. However, the presence of a right-to-left shunt is an absolute contraindication to lymphography, as the contrast will bypass the lung and become a systemic embolus, possibly leading to stroke or other neurologic dysfunction.

Although technically more challenging, lymphography may be performed in children as well as in adults. In a review of 1079 cases from three institutions, Castellino and associates reported successful bilateral studies in 90% of children 15 years of age or younger. An additional 8.7% had successful unilateral lymphograms so that the bilateral failure rate was only 1.3%. Ketamine hydrochloride anesthesia is recommended in younger children, and care should be taken to limit proportionately the amount of contrast infused.

The interpretation of lymphograms in patients with solid tumors differs from the interpretation of patients with malignant lymphomas. Metastases to lymph nodes from solid tumors tend to produce peripheral filling defects. As criteria for metastases, these defects are most reliable if they are greater than 1 cm in diameter and multiple. It is important to check the 2-hour channel films to be sure that lymphatic channels do not traverse these filling defects, as channels will not pass through a metastatic deposit. Small filling defects are much less reliable even if they are multiple, as they may be caused by a variety of etiologies, such as fat, fibrosis, or an irregularly shaped lymph node. If the metastasis becomes large, it may totally obstruct the lymphatic channel and prevent opacification of a lymph node or group of nodes. Although this is a reliable criteria, it often is difficult to be sure that lymphatic obstruction is present. Persistent filling of lymphatic channels at 24 hours or evidence of an unopacified mass seen on other studies such as CT help to confirm this impression.

In each case, the lymphogram should be interpreted with knowledge of the pertinent clinical information. The type, location, and extent of the tumor are important, because lymphatic metastases follow the normal lymphatic drainage routes. Testicular neoplasms metastasize to the high paraaortic regions, whereas prostatic tumors are usually first seen in the iliac chains. If, however, the tumor has locally invaded beyond the fascial confines of the gland, it may take alternate pathways, and the usual drainage patterns are no longer reliable. Finally, the presence of an unopacified mass recognized by other means, such as CT or ultrasound, may indicate a lymph node or group of nodes that are not filled on the lymphogram.

Percutaneous Biopsy

Although exquisite images can be provided by a variety of radiographic modalities, the precise nature of the abnormal tissue is seldom certain. Pathologic proof, in the form of histology or cytology, often is required. Percutaneous needle biopsy guided precisely into the area of abnormality by an imaging modality has achieved a high level of success. Pathologic diagnoses can be made without subjecting the patient to the morbidity, mortality, or long recovery time associated with open surgery. These techniques are now commonly used for masses in the adrenal glands, kidney, and prostate gland, as well as other sites that may represent metastatic disease.

Cutting needles provide tissue for histologic evaluation. Aspirating needles provide material for cytopathology and may be used to diagnose the primary tumor, but they are more commonly used to confirm the presence of malignant tissue, especially metastases when the primary tumor has been diagnosed previously.

NEEDLE SELECTION. Needles ranging from 23 to 14 gauge are frequently used for radiologically guided percutaneous aspiration biopsy. In general, the smaller needles offer greater safety than the larger needles. However, smaller needles less consistently obtain an adequate sample for diagnosis. The specific needle choice should be individualized for each patient, biopsy target, and clinical setting. Furthermore, the experience of the radiologist and the pathologist, as well as the guiding modality also must be considered.

Fine 22- or 23-gauge needles achieved popularity in the early experience of radiologically guided percutaneous biopsy. They were used for fluoroscopically guided lung biopsies and then were applied to abdominal lesions where CT or ultrasound was used as the guiding modality. Using 22-gauge needles, Wittenberg and colleagues reported an overall accuracy of 85% in percutaneous biopsy of 150 patients with suspected abdominal tumors.

However, these thin needles are frequently difficult to direct into a small, deep lesion. The 22- and 23-gauge needles take the path of least resistance and often "bow" out of the line of direction during insertion. Thus, greater skill may be required to direct these needles into the target or more passes may have to be made. This can be expected to decrease patient comfort and increase the complication rate.

Medium-size needles, 18 to 20 gauge, provide larger samples than the 22- or 23-gauge needles. Andriole and associates reported the average weight of the liver biopsy specimen using a variety of needles (Table 3.3). They demonstrated a progressive increase in sample weights as larger needles were used. They also demonstrated that, for any given needle size, the more acute angle of the bevel (usually 30°), provided more tissue than needles with a flat 90° bevel.

These medium-size needles are easier to direct into the target, which enables the biopsy procedure to be performed more quickly. The larger diameter of the needle makes it more apparent under fluoroscopy or ultrasound guidance. When CT is used, these needles are easier to keep within the axial scan plane, and this requires fewer images to track the course of the needle.

Cutting needles often are employed when the diagnosis of the primary tumor has not yet been made. The target mass should be large enough that the entire specimen can be obtained from the suspected tumor. Adjacent structures, especially arteries, must be avoided. The most commonly used cutting needles are those with a "slot" or cutting gap into which the sample falls before it is cut off by a sheath. Cutting needles used for percutaneous biopsy are usually 20 to 16 gauge.

To improve the consistency of biopsy samples, a spring-loaded biopsy gun was developed by Lindgren. One model (Biopty gun, Bard (CR Bard Inc., Covington, GA)) achieved popularity for ultrasound-directed prostate biopsies. Although designed for use in prostate biopsies, it has been applied to a variety of organs.

Parker and colleagues recently reported their results using a biopsy gun for 182 percutaneous biopsies from a variety of anatomic sites. They obtained high-quality

Table 3.3.
Size of Biopsy Specimen

Needle (gauge)	Sample Weight (mg)
22	4.0
20	7.6
19	12.5
18	16.2
16	37.3

From Andriole JG, Haaga JR, Adams RB, *et al.*: Biopsy needle characteristics assessed in the laboratory. *Radiology* 148:659–662, 1983.

histopathologic specimens in 177 (97%) of their biopsies. "Crush" artifact and obscuring blood were eliminated, and patient discomfort was decreased.

The biopsy gun is designed for an 18- or 20-gauge slotted cutting needle. The spring-loaded gun is cocked, and the hub of the needle is placed into the gun. The covering panel of the gun is closed, and the needle tip is advanced into the patient. When released, the spring of the gun moves the needle 2.3 cm further into the patient and then advances the sheath, which cuts off the core specimen. Thus, the needle tip must be positioned in front of the target to be sampled. A 1×17 mm core of tissue is consistently obtained. The speed of the needle movement seems to lessen patient discomfort.

While the biopsy gun is ideal for ultrasound-guided biopsies, it also can be readily applied to procedures guided by fluoroscopy. For biopsies requiring CT guidance, modified biopsy devices, in which the gun is retrofitted onto the needle after it has been placed into the target, have been developed.

Renal Biopsy

Renal Mass

There are many indications for biopsy of a renal mass, but relatively few are actually performed. A renal mass suspicious for primary renal adenocarcinoma is usually staged radiographically, and the patient is taken to surgery on the assumption that the mass is malignant. Percutaneous aspiration is performed if metastases are suspected and if tissue confirmation is needed to avoid surgery. However, even when metastatic disease is present, nephrectomy may be performed to treat or prevent complications of the tumor, such as pain, hematuria, or a paraneoplastic syndrome.

Because a negative aspiration does not necessarily exclude malignancy, few urologists are willing to forego possible curative surgery on the assumption that a suspicious renal mass is not malignant. Similarly, aspiration of indeterminate or cystic renal masses can only provide further support for a benign etiology, but cannot exclude cancer.

The needle size and route are seldom a problem when performing a biopsy of a renal mass. Aspirating needles, usually 20- or 22-gauge, are routinely used. The approach is dictated by the location of the mass in the kidney. If possible, normal renal parenchyma and hilar structures should be avoided. Larger cutting needles can be employed, but because renal carcinomas are usually hypervascular, bleeding complications are more likely.

Serious complications are uncommon, but include local bleeding, hematuria, arteriovenous fistula, or false aneurysm formation and, rarely, tumor seeding along the needle tract.

Medical Renal Disease. Biopsy of the kidney used for diagnosis of medical renal disease is commonly performed under ultrasound guidance. Most operators prefer to perform a biopsy of the right kidney to minimize the risk of splenic injury. Traditionally, a 14-gauge Vim Silverman needle has been used to provide sufficient material for both light and electron microscopy. Some interventional radiologists prefer to perform the procedure using CT guidance, because this modality allows more precise needle placement in the peripheral renal cortex, and thereby lessens the risk of major vessel injury. Others have advocated the use of smaller biopsy needles and/or the use of a spring-loaded device to accomplish this same purpose.

PROSTATE.   Prostate biopsy is an integral part of the endorectal ultrasound examination of the prostate gland (*see* Chapter 18). Since sonography is used to guide the needle into the most abnormal portion of the gland, the approach depends on the equipment available. If a rectal biopsy probe is used, an 18-gauge needle can fit into a biopsy guide and can be advanced into the suspicious area. Since the rectal mucosa is not sterile, antibiotics often are given to the patient before the biopsy study to prevent or minimize bacterial seeding.

Radionuclide Evaluation

The biodistribution of a small amount of radiotracer injected intravenously and detected with an external scintillation counter forms the basis for radionuclide evaluation of the urinary tract. The evaluation of the kidney is one of the oldest techniques in nuclear medicine. Initially, because of limitations in radiopharmaceuticals and radiation dose considerations, only functional information about the distribution of the tracer was available from such studies. With the development of newer radiopharmaceuticals, functional and limited anatomic information regarding the urinary tract can now be obtained. Modern radiopharmaceuticals often provide information about the urinary tract at a radiation dose well below a number of common radiologic procedures. Because the information is quantifiable and can be acquired by computer, the information can be stored, manipulated, and analyzed in detail. The most common scintillation detector used today is the gamma camera fitted with a crystal that is large enough that both kidneys may be analyzed simultaneously.

Radiopharmaceuticals

A number of radiopharmaceuticals have proven useful in evaluation of the urinary tract (Table 3.4). Unlike contrast materials used for conventional radiologic studies, radiopharmaceuticals are remarkably free of adverse reactions.

Eighty percent of an injected dose of iodine-131-labeled orthoiodohippurate (OIH) is excreted by tubular secretion. Because of its relatively high extraction efficiency (the percentage of radiopharmaceutical extracted

Table 3.4.
Radiopharmaceuticals for Urinary Tract Imaging

Radiopharmaceutical	Principle Gamma Energy (keV)	Physical Half-life	Usual Dose
^{131}I Orthoiodohippurate (OIH)	364	8 days	300 μCi
^{99M}Technetium	140	6 hr	
Diethylenetrianine pentacetic acid (DTPA)			10–20 mCi
Dimercaptosuccinic acid (DMSA)			1–5 mCi
Glucoheptonate			10–20 mCi
Mercaptoacetyltriglycine (MAG$_3$)			5–10 mCi

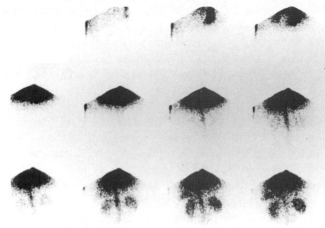

Figure 3.36. Radionuclide angiogram. A bolus of ^{99m}Tc-DTPA has been injected. The activity can be seen circulating through the heart (*top row*), the lungs (*middle row*), and into the abdominal aorta and kidneys (*bottom row*).

on each pass through the kidney), this agent is particularly useful in the evaluation of patients with diminished renal function. However, given the relatively long half-life of I 131 and its associated radiation dose, only relatively small amounts of this isotope (microcuries) can be used. Therefore, this agent is unsuitable for an evaluation of renal perfusion. Since such a high percentage of OIH is excreted by tubular secretion, the isotope may be used to calculate effective renal plasma flow. Iodine-123-labeled OIH has the same chemical and physiologic properties as the I-131-labeled variety, but has a much shorter half-life and as a consequence, a lower radiation dose. In addition, its gamma emission is much better suited to imaging than is the energy of I 131. Unfortunately, it is expensive to produce and has a very short shelf-life, which limits utility, and is, therefore, no longer commercially available in the United States.

Technetium-99m–diethylenetrianine pentacetic acid (^{99m}Tc-DTPA) is useful for evaluation of renal perfusion as well as for imaging the kidneys and the urinary tract. A small percent of this radiopharmaceutical is protein bound, but the majority is excreted by glomerular filtration without significant tubular resorption or secretion. Approximately 90% of an injected dose of DTPA is excreted within 4 hours. Because it can be administered in relatively large (millicurie) amounts, the arrival of the tracer can be documented on camera images made every 2 or 3 seconds. In this fashion, a "radionuclide angiogram" can be obtained (Fig. 3.36). Since DTPA is cleared so rapidly from the kidneys, it is not suitable as a cortical imaging agent. In addition, DTPA is considered to be a relatively poor agent for the evaluation of renal function, because it has an extraction efficiency of only 20%, even in patients with normal renal function.

Technetium-99m–glucoheptonate is a labeled carbohydrate that, in contrast to DTPA, is excreted very slowly by the kidney. Approximately 50% of this agent is pro-

tein-bound, and while about 40% is excreted within the first hour, approximately 15% of the injected agent is retained within the renal cortex. The primary use of glucoheptonate, therefore, is as a cortical imaging agent when anatomic information about the kidney is desired in addition to information about perfusion and excretion.

Technetium 99m dimercaptosuccinic acid (^{99m}Tc-DMSA) is cleared from the kidney even more slowly than is glucoheptonate. Approximately 50% of the injected dose remains in the renal cortex 6 hours after the injection. DMSA is of particular value when high-resolution images of the renal cortex are needed and when little information about the excretion of the material is desired. Only about 15% of the dose of DMSA is excreted in the urine, and there is significant excretion of this agent by the liver as well. Because there is so much binding of this agent to the renal cortex, the radiation dose is higher than with other technetium-labeled isotopes. Thus, unlike the other technetium agents, DMSA is not suitable for perfusion studies.

Technetium-99m–mercaptoacetyltriglycine (^{99m}Tc-MAG$_3$) has functional properties similar to those of Hippuran, but as a technetium-labeled compound, has physical properties which make it an excellent agent for both perfusion and imaging studies. Thus, MAG$_3$ as a single agent can yield anatomic and functional information that heretofore required two different radiopharmaceuticals (i.e., Hippuran and DTPA). The biological properties of MAG$_3$, however, are not identical to those of OIH; in fact, MAG$_3$ has been shown to have a 50 to 60% lower clearance than OIH. However, because of its increased protein binding, the agent stays in the vascular compartment for a longer period. Glomerular filtration accounts for 11% of the clearance of MAG$_3$ compared with 27% for OIH; tubular secretion is responsible for the remainder. The extraction efficiency of MAG$_3$ is approximately 40 to 50%. Effective renal plasma flow (ERPF) measurements made with MAG$_3$ are consistently lower than those obtained with OIH, but an excellent correlation between the two agents over a wide range of renal function has been reported. Because of its high rate of plasma clearance compared with DTPA, MAG$_3$ is suitable for imaging patients with impaired renal function.

Since its introduction into clinical use in the early 1990s, MAG$_3$ has become the standard renal imaging agent in the United States for a wide range of clinical applications, including renal transplant evaluation, diuretic renography, and the assessment of renal perfusion. One potential disadvantage for MAG$_3$ in the evaluation of transplants is in the detection of postoperative urinary leaks. In some formulations of MAG$_3$, as much as 10% of the agent is excreted through the gastrointestinal tract; thus, differentiating bowel activity from extraurinary activity caused by urinary extravasation may be difficult.

The Radioisotope Renogram

The major radionuclide tool for evaluation of renal function is the radioisotope renogram, a curve demonstrating the radioactivity within the kidney plotted against the time after injection of the radiopharmaceutical. The renogram curve also is referred to as a time-activity curve. Renogram curves may be constructed for studies performed with DTPA, MAG$_3$, (Fig. 3.37) or Hippuran. Analysis of the shape of the renogram curve can be used to suggest the diagnosis of many pathologic

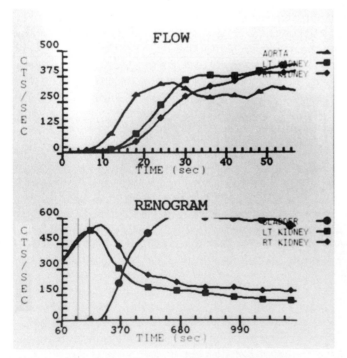

Figure 3.37. Radioisotope renogram performed using ^{99m}Tc-MAG$_3$. The upper set of curves shows the flow of the radioisotope in the aorta and to both kidneys. The renogram curves demonstrate the excretion of the isotope by each kidney and the corresponding increase in bladder activity.

conditions of the kidney, including acute tubular necrosis, suspected urinary tract obstruction, and renal transplant rejection. A modification of the standard radioisotope renogram, called the *diuretic renogram,* is useful in differentiating functionally insignificant urinary tract dilatation from that caused by urinary tract obstruction. With this technique, a diuretic, commonly furosemide, is injected shortly after the radiopharmaceutical appears in the collecting system, and the effect of the diuretic on the shape of the renogram curve is analyzed. In patients with functionally insignificant urinary tract dilatation, the diuretic will cause a prompt reduction in the amount of activity in the renal collecting system, whereas, in those with true urinary tract obstruction, the amount of activity in the collecting system will increase after the diuretic is administered (*see* Chapter 16).

Radionuclide Renal Imaging Studies

RENAL PERFUSION.   A renal perfusion study may be obtained after the intravenous administration of 10 to 20 mCi of ^{99m}Tc-DTPA or glucoheptonate, or 5 to 7 mCi of MAG$_3$ (Fig. 3.37) given as a compact bolus. Images are obtained on the gamma camera every 2 to 5 seconds for the first 1 minute after the injection and demonstrate the arrival of the bolus of activity in the abdominal aorta and the iliac vessels, as well as the arrival of the tracer in the kidneys. On the early images, the circulation of the radiopharmaceutical in the liver and spleen also is visualized. The camera should be positioned posterior to the patient when native kidneys are being evaluated and anterior to the iliac fossa for the evaluation of a transplanted kidney. Data from the perfusion study (first minute after injection) may be acquired in a computer and a time-activity curve can be generated for each kidney. Such a curve will demonstrate the relative perfusion of each kidney. Data acquired between 1 and 3 minutes after injection also may be used to generate a time-activity curve that can be used to calculate the relative contribution of each kidney to total renal function (also known as split renal function studies) (Fig. 3.38). Static images are normally obtained 3 to 5 minutes after the injection as well. A modification of the standard renogram obtained following administration of a dose of captopril, an angiotensin-converting enzyme (ACE) inhibitor, has proven to be useful as a screening study for renovascular hypertension (*see* Chapter 9).

RENAL CORTICAL IMAGING.   Renal cortical imaging may be performed after intravenous administration of 10 to 20 mCi ^{99m}Tc-glucoheptonate or 1 to 5 mCi of ^{99m}Tc-DMSA. One of the more common uses of these agents is in the evaluation of renal pseudotumors, normally functioning renal tissue that simulates a renal mass lesion. The uptake of the radiopharmaceutical by such pseudotumors differentiates them from pathologic renal masses, which will not accumulate any activity. This

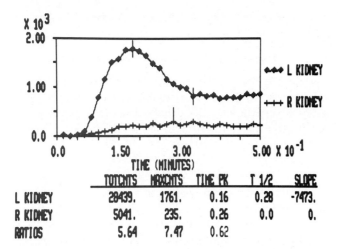

Figure 3.38. Split renal function studies performed using ^{99m}Tc-DTPA. Computer-generated curves of activity (*x-axis*) plotted against time after injection (*y-axis*) for each kidney. The activity in the right kidney is demonstrated to represent 15% of the total renal function (activity left kidney plus activity right kidney divided into activity right kidney).

technique is frequently used to evaluate such conditions as a "hilar lip," a hypertrophied column of renal tissue medially that may impress the renal pelvis; a "dromedary hump" or splenic impression on the lateral portion of the left kidney; or a hypertrophied column of Bertin, an invagination of the cortex into the medullary portion of the kidney that may simulate an intrarenal mass.

RENAL FUNCTIONAL IMAGING. Renal functional imaging may be carried out following intravenous administration of 300 µCi of Hippuran OIH I 131, or 5 to 7 mCi of MAG$_3$. Sequential images are frequently obtained every 2 to 3 minutes for a period of 20 to 30 minutes. Such studies will demonstrate the excretion of the radionuclide by the kidney into the bladder. Because relatively small amounts of activity are used, no radionuclide angiogram is possible and unless obstructed, the collecting system and the ureter are not visualized when OIH is used. A renogram curve is frequently obtained simultaneously when imaging with Hippuran is performed.

RENAL TRANSPLANT EVALUATION. A major use of radionuclides in the urinary tract is the evaluation of the status of a renal transplant. Many different radiopharmaceuticals have been used for this purpose. Most typically, renal perfusion using ^{99m}Tc-DTPA (Fig. 3.39) and delayed images of the kidney were obtained. In some institutions, a combination of ^{99m}Tc-DTPA perfusion and OIH I 131 images were generally obtained. The combination of these two studies frequently was believed to be helpful in evaluating such complications of transplantation as obstruction of the renal artery, acute tubular necrosis, rejection, perirenal fluid collections, cyclosporine nephrotoxicity, and various mechanical complications, such as ureteral obstruction and urinary

extravasation. In most institutions that use radionuclide studies to evaluate transplants, however, a single study using MAG$_3$ is now performed and yields similar information to that formerly obtained with the two agents. As indicated earlier, some confusion between bowel activity and urinary extravasation has, however, been reported.

Radionuclide Renal Function Studies

GLOMERULAR FILTRATION RATE. A radionuclide estimation of glomerular filtration, while not as accurate as an inulin clearance performed under strict laboratory conditions, provides a reasonable estimate of the glomerular filtration rate (GFR). ^{99m}Tc-DTPA is normally used for radionuclide calculation of the GFR. Three to five blood samples drawn over a 2- to 4-hour period after the injection of a known dose of the radiopharmaceutical are obtained, and a plasma disappearance curve for the DTPA is calculated.

EFFECTIVE RENAL PLASMA FLOW. Effective renal plasma flow can be calculated using ^{131}I-labeled OIH. Many methods for this determination, which is qualitatively similar to that used for determination of GFR, have been described. Both blood and urine samples are usually required. Modification of the technique, which requires only a single blood sample, also has been described.

Nonrenal Imaging Studies

RADIONUCLIDE CYSTOGRAPHY. Radionuclide cystography can be performed in children to follow the course of vesicoureteral reflux. A dose of 0.5–1 mCi of technetium pertechnetate is instilled via a Foley catheter into the bladder and is diluted with an appropriate amount of saline. While the method offers considerably less spatial resolution than conventional voiding cystourethrography made with fluoroscopic spot films, it has the significant advantage of offering a lower radiation dose. Although it has a lower spatial resolution than the radi-

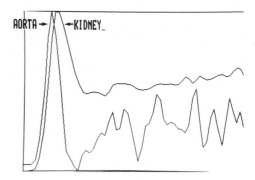

Figure 3.39. Renal perfusion curve of a transplant obtained with ^{99m}Tc-DTPA. The arrival of the bolus activity into the kidney as compared with the aorta is demonstrated in the first 1 minute after injection. Relative activity is plotted on the x-axis and time is plotted on the y-axis.

ologic techniques, the sensitivity of a scintigraphic voiding cystourethrogram is said to be the same or greater than the radiologic study for the detection of vesicoureteral reflux greater than grade 1. When an initial radiographic study shows that reflux is present, this technique provides a relatively sensitive method for following the course of the reflux in children with minimal radiation exposure. If the radionuclide study suggests that an increased amount of reflux is present, repeat radiographic studies should then be obtained.

The amount of reflux that is present on the radionuclide study can be quantitated by evaluating specific regions of interest over the distal ureters.

SCROTAL IMAGING.   Radionuclide techniques have been used extensively to evaluate patients who present with acute, painful scrotal swelling. The primary purpose of these techniques is to differentiate patients with epididymoorchitis from those with testicular torsion or a testicular abscess. Scrotal imaging is performed as a perfusion study centered over the pelvis after intravenous administration of 10 to 20 mCi of technetium pertechnetate. Dynamic scintiphotos made at 2- to 3-second intervals followed by static images are used for this purpose.

ADRENAL IMAGING.   A resurgence in interest in radionuclide imaging of the adrenal gland has occurred as the result of the introduction of ^{131}I-labeled metaiodobenzylguanidine (MIBG). This compound is taken up by the adrenal medulla and is capable of demonstrating adrenal medullary hyperplasia and pheochromocytomas.

Adrenal cortical imaging with [131]I- or I-123–19-iodocholesterol has never achieved great clinical popularity because of relatively low uptake of the precursor by the adrenal gland and because delayed imaging for up to 15 days is required. I-131-iodomethyl 19-norcholesterol (NP 59) has been somewhat more successful in its evaluation of patients with Cushing's or Conn's syndrome in differentiating patients with adrenal hyperplasia from those with functioning adenomas and contralateral adrenal suppression.

INTERVENTIONAL TECHNIQUES

The development of interventional uroradiology has allowed the diagnostic radiologist to participate in the therapy of disease processes. During the past 15 years, interventional techniques in uroradiology have become among the best accepted and most widely practiced procedures in interventional radiology. Information concerning procedures relating to a specific disease process are included adjacent to the discussion of the diagnostic aspects of that disease (i.e., abscess drainage in Chapter 7, "Renal Inflammatory Disease," and stone management in Chapter 12, "Nephrocalcinosis and Nephrolithiasis"). Percutaneous nephrostomy is applicable to multiple disorders and is the prelude to many of the other interventional techniques used in the urinary tract; it is therefore discussed in the following section.

Percutaneous Nephrostomy

Percutaneous nephrostomy (PCN) is the single most valuable interventional technique in uroradiology. It relieves obstruction of the urinary tract and provides access to the collecting system for a variety of diagnostic and therapeutic procedures.

Indications

Percutaneous nephrostomy is indicated in a large variety of clinical situations (Table 3.5). Each patient must be considered individually, and some may have both indications and contraindications to the procedure. The decision whether or not to undertake PCN must depend on other available options.

Obstruction

The most common indication for PCN is relief of obstruction, but there are several subcategories. Infection in an obstructed collecting system requires urgent decompression. If the patient is toxic, PCN may be an emergency procedure.

Acute obstruction often causes ureteral colic as the ureter attempts to overcome the obstruction with active peristalsis. Analgesics are usually employed to control pain until the obstruction can be relieved. Occasionally, decompression with a PCN may be elected until the obstruction can be relieved.

Chronic obstruction results in dilation of the collecting system, tubular damage, parenchymal loss, and deterioration of renal function. Percutaneous nephrostomy may be used to prevent renal damage if the cause of obstruction cannot be adequately treated (Fig. 3.40). If

Table 3.5.
Percutaneous Nephrostomy Indications

Relief of obstruction
  Preserve renal function
  Treatment of infection
  Relieve pain
Urinary diversion
  Heal leak or fistula
Diagnostic study
  Antegrade pyelogram
  Whitaker test
  Biopsy or brushing for cytology
Removal of solid material
  Stone
  Foreign body
Access for ureteral intervention
  Stricture dilation
  Stenting
  Ureteral occlusion
Infusion of chemolytic agents
Access for nephroscopy

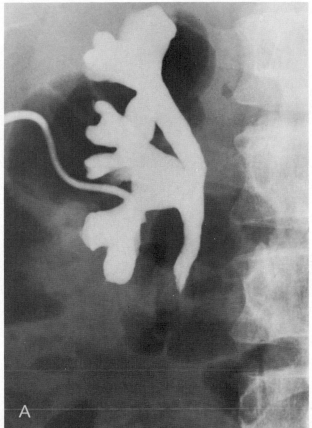

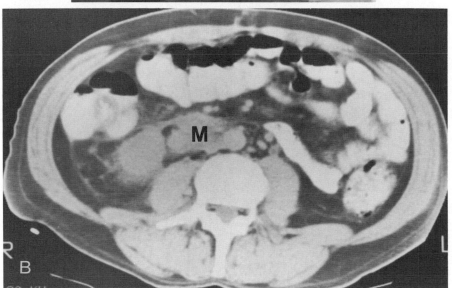

Figure 3.40.   Percutaneous nephrostomy. **A,** Antegrade pyelogram after percutaneous nephrostomy demonstrates proximal ureteral obstruction. **B,** Computed tomography demonstrates a tumor mass (*M*) causing the ureteral obstruction.

there is bilateral obstruction, impaired renal function may result in electrolyte abnormalities (Fig. 3.41).

Most urinary tract infections respond to appropriate antibiotics. If there is obstruction, however, even sensitive bacteria may not be eradicated, because the kidney may be unable to excrete a sufficient quantity of the anti-

biotic to reach an effective therapeutic concentration. Drainage of the closed infection can be readily performed with PCN to alleviate this concern.

A nephrostomy performed for an elective indication should be delayed until the urinary tract infection is eradicated. However, obstruction must be relieved before the

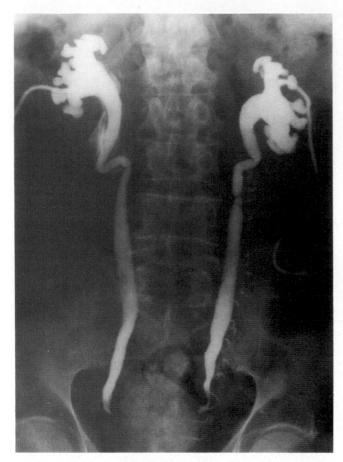

Figure 3.41. Bilateral percutaneous nephrostomy. Obstruction of both distal ureters by prostate cancer necessitated bilateral nephrostomy.

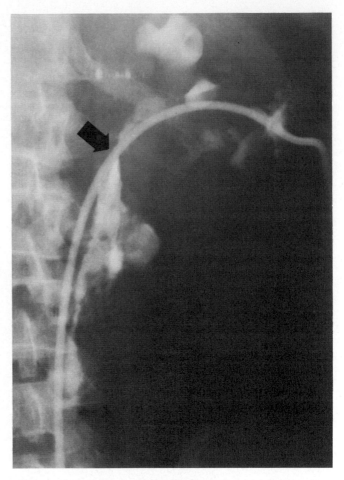

Figure 3.42. Diverting nephrostomy. Traumatic injury to the ureter has resulted in persistent leak (*arrow*) with urinoma formation. Percutaneous nephrostomy with urinary diversion and ureteral stenting.

infection can be cleared. Thus, PCN must be performed as an urgent procedure despite the contraindications.

Urinary Diversion

Traumatic extravasation from the urinary tract usually heals spontaneously. If there is continued urine flow through the leak, however, healing will be delayed and a chronic fistula may develop. Even those cases that heal spontaneously may have a large urinoma that is fed by extravasated urine until the perforation seals. These patients are usually helped by a diverting nephrostomy.

When a nephrostomy catheter is placed in the renal pelvis, urine takes the path of least resistance and flows out the catheter. The amount of urine flowing out the site of extravasation is markedly reduced, promoting healing (Fig. 3.42).

In patients who are incontinent, a variety of methods, including catheter drainage of the bladder, may be used to prevent continued urine leak and soiling of the patient. Occasionally a nephrostomy may be needed to divert the urine before it reaches the bladder.

Removal of Stones or Foreign Bodies

Percutaneous nephrostomy is the first step in extracting solid material from the collecting system. The most common use is nephrostolithotomy, which is discussed in Chapter 12. However, other materials, such as broken catheters or ureteral stents, also may be removed (Fig. 3.43). Simple guidewire snares are used most frequently, because they require the least dilation of the nephrostomy track; however, any number of other instruments, including grasping forceps, may be used for this purpose.

Access for Ureteral Intervention

Percutaneous nephrostomy also is used to gain access to the ureter for interventional techniques. Stricture dilation and ureteral stenting are discussed in Chapter 16. Rarely there may be a desire to occlude the ureter. Temporary occlusion is readily accomplished with a balloon catheter. However, the pressure of the balloon against the ureteral mucosa may create sufficient ischemia to in-

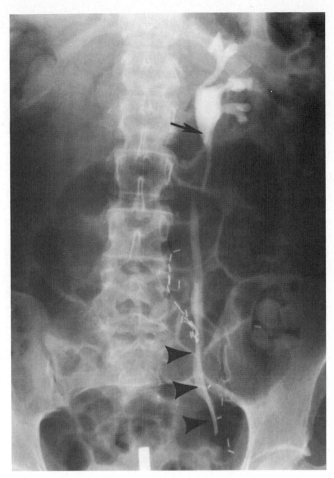

Figure 3.43.   Broken ureteral stent. A double-J ureteral stent catheter has broken into three pieces. Percutaneous nephrostomy was used for access to remove the portions from the renal pelvis (*arrow*) and distal ureter (*arrowheads*).

duce necrosis or stricture formation. Deposition of embolic materials, such as cyanoacrylate and vascular coils, also has been used to accomplish ureteral occlusion.

Infusion of Chemolytic Agents

Chemical stone dissolution is discussed in Chapter 10. Two catheters often are required, one for infusion and a second for drainage. They should be placed on either side of the stone to obtain maximal bathing of the calculus.

Other therapeutic agents also can be instilled through a PCN. This technique allows a high concentration of the drug in the collecting system with a minimal systemic level.

Access for Nephroscopy

In the past several years, there has been a dramatic increase in endourologic procedures. Most of these require access to the collecting system through a PCN. Earlier instruments were rigid and a straight track was

needed. Furthermore, the position of the nephrostomy limited access to only one portion of the collecting system. Flexible nephroscopes alleviate this problem to a large degree, but still may not provide access to the entire collecting system and limit the types of instruments that can be inserted through an operating port. Thus, the exact position of the PCN contributes significantly to the success or failure of the procedure.

Anatomy

The kidneys are retroperitoneal organs surrounded by perinephric fat and enclosed by Gerota's fascia. The pleura extends down to the 12th vertebral body, posteriorly, then extends laterally crossing the 12th, 11th, and 10th ribs as they angle caudally. Although there is great normal variation, approximately one half of the right kidney and one third of the left kidney lie above this posterior reflection of the pleural surface.

The liver is anterolateral to the upper pole of the right kidney. In occasional patients, however, a portion of the right lobe of the liver may extend posterolateral to the upper pole of the kidney.

The position of the spleen is more variable. It classically lies superolateral to the kidney, but often is adjacent to the lateral margin and may frequently be posterolateral to the upper pole.

The colon also may lie along the proposed route of the nephrostomy (Fig. 3.44). The descending colon lies in the anterior pararenal space and its position depends on the position of the lateroconal fascia. In approximately 10% of patients, the descending colon lies behind a horizontal line at the posterior edge of the left kidney. In 1% of patients, the descending colon actually extends behind the left kidney. Thus, in 1% of patients, the descending colon would be punctured if the stan-

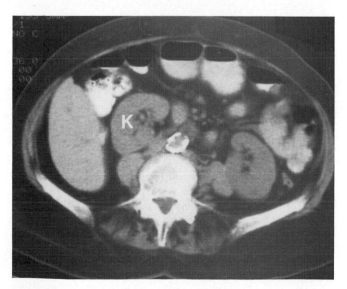

Figure 3.44.   Anterior position of right kidney (*K*) places liver and colon along proposed percutaneous nephrostomy tract.

dard nephrostomy approach is used. Occasionally, the ascending colon is seen posterolateral to the right kidney, medial to the liver.

The calyces are generally arranged in two rows, anterior and posterior. At either pole, fusion results in compound calyces. In the interpolar region posterior calyces often are seen "end on" during urography, while anterior calyces are seen extending laterally. This appearance reflects the classic description by Brodel. However, there is significant normal variation. The significant normal variation in this anatomy requires that the urogram include anteroposterior and both oblique views that can be carefully examined before the nephrostomy route is chosen.

The main renal artery and vein lie anterior to the renal pelvis. There is, however, a posterior branch of the renal artery which courses behind the renal pelvis to supply the dorsal segments. The segmental arteries divide into interlobar and the arcuate arteries which enter the renal parenchyma, usually at the corticomedullary junction. The closer to the calyx, the smaller the artery has become. Thus, a puncture into the calyx traverses a much smaller artery than a needle passing into an infundibulum.

Technique

Percutaneous nephrostomy is performed by visualizing the target, identifying the tract for the PCN, and placing the catheter. The procedure may be guided with fluoroscopy, ultrasound, or even CT. Fluoroscopy is the most convenient method of guidance and is used for the vast majority of these procedures. Visualization of the collecting system requires its opacification by contrast material. This may be accomplished by renal excretion after intravenous injection or by blind percutaneous puncture of the renal pelvis.

Ultrasound may be used in conjunction with fluoroscopy to eliminate the need for contrast material to opacify the collecting system. This is most conveniently done by moving an ultrasound unit to the fluoroscopy table. Ultrasound can not only identify the targeted collecting system, but also can assure that adjacent organs do not lie along the proposed nephrostomy tract. However, it is only successful if the collecting system is dilated. In rare instances, CT may be the preferred method of guidance for PCN, particularly in patients whose anatomy is distorted or whose body habitus precludes conventional positioning. Computed tomography also is sometimes used for placement of a PCN in a kidney in an anomalous position.

Many variations on the basic PCN technique may be used, depending on the clinical setting and specific patient anatomy. The two basic procedures are the trocar technique and the needle-guidewire-catheter exchange system described by Seldinger for arterial catheterization.

The trocar technique consists of passing a draining catheter and trocar needle together into the collecting system. The trocar is removed, and the catheter is se-

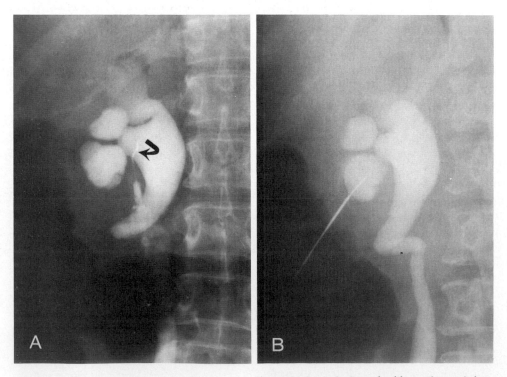

Figure 3.45.   Percutaneous nephrostomy technique. **A,** A 3- French dilator (*arrow*) has been passed over a 0.018-inch guidewire and is used to opacify the collecting system. **B,** With good opacification, the desired calyx can be punctured.

cured in position. Because this involves an initial puncture with a large needle, it is used primarily for large, superficial targets.

This trocar method also can be adapted to a two-puncture technique. An initial puncture with a small (22- or 23-gauge) needle is made through which contrast media can be injected to opacify the collecting system. The trocar can then be placed more confidently in the desired location.

As experience with interventional techniques increases, however, most radiologists prefer variations on the Seldinger technique. With this method, a smaller needle, usually 20- to 22-gauge, is used for the initial puncture. Thus, if needle placement is undesirable, it can be withdrawn and repositioned after having created only a small perforation.

If the collecting system is not well seen because of poor renal function, a direct puncture of the renal pelvis with a 22-gauge needle may be performed. Contrast can then be introduced to opacify the collecting system (Fig. 3.45). This technique also is used when there is no dilation of the intrarenal collecting system. A 0.018-inch guidewire is passed through the 22-gauge needle. After removal of the needle, a 3-French multiside-hole catheter is passed over the guidewire into the renal pelvis. Injection of contrast material not only opacifies but also dilates the collecting system.

Percutaneous nephrostomy may be performed in the prone, prone-oblique, or supine-oblique positions. The prone position is the most stable for the patient, but requires an angled needle approach. This is facilitated if C- or U-arm fluoroscopy is available. The prone-oblique position elevates the ipsilateral side 30 to 45° so that a vertical puncture can be made. Thus, patient positioning compensates for a fixed fluoroscope. The supine-oblique position consists of elevation of the ipsilateral side and a horizontal needle entry. It is used for very sick or immobile patients.

The collecting system should be punctured through the kidney. Direct access to the renal pelvis has a higher incidence of vascular complications. The needle should pass through the least vascular plane of the kidney (Brodel's line). A needle traversing this route into a calyx avoids all but the smallest intrarenal arteries. This long route through the renal parenchyma increases catheter purchase and minimizes urine leakage or catheter dislodgment. This posterolateral track results in catheter exit near the posterior axillary line, which allows the patient to lie supine without kinking the catheter or causing undue discomfort.

Results

The results of PCN procedures are excellent. In 1978, Stables and colleagues reported a technical success rate greater than 90% and major complications of only 4%.

With increased experience and improvements in equipment and technique, even better results can be expected. A successful PCN placement should be accomplished in almost every obstructed system if there is dilation of the collecting system. Failure is more likely in the rare case of nondilated obstruction or in patients with urinary leaks or fistulas that keep the collecting system decompressed.

Similar excellent success rates can be achieved in infants and children by modifying the equipment and by paying close attention to the special needs of these very young patients. Stanley and associates were successful in each of 28 PCNs performed in children ranging in age from 1 day to 18 years, whereas Ball and colleagues reported a 98% success rate in 61 interventional uroradiologic procedures.

Complications

The most common complications of PCN are related to bleeding, urine extravasation (Fig. 3.46), and infection. The kidney is a highly vascular organ, and puncture of at least small intrarenal arteries cannot be avoided (Fig. 3.47). However, the PCN catheter usually provides

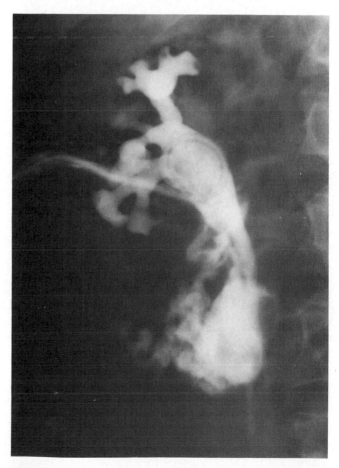

Figure 3.46. Extravasation. Inadvertent puncture of the renal pelvis has resulted in contrast extravasation. This condition usually heals within 2 days with nephrostomy drainage.

sufficient tamponade to prevent significant blood loss. Retroperitoneal hemorrhage will be an even greater problem in patients with clotting deficiencies. However, these patients may not be surgical candidates, and PCN is still appropriate if the collecting system is dilated and if no technical difficulties are anticipated in catheter placement.

In addition to hematoma formation (Fig. 3.48), an arteriovenous fistula or a pseudoaneurysm may be created. Either of these may result in delayed bleeding or bleeding when the PCN catheter is removed. Arteriography with selective renal artery injection is indicated in these patients to better define the source of bleeding. In many patients, selective occlusion of a branch renal artery can be performed and surgery can be avoided.

Infection is the other common complication of PCN. Sepsis is more likely to occur in patients with preexisting pyonephrosis, which is exacerbated by the procedure. Catheter manipulation or injection of contrast material into an infected closed space may force bacteria into the circulation and may cause septicemia or septic

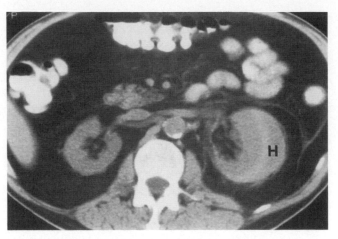

Figure 3.48. Subcapsular hematoma. A left subcapsular hematoma (*H*) is seen on this unenhanced computed tomography scan.

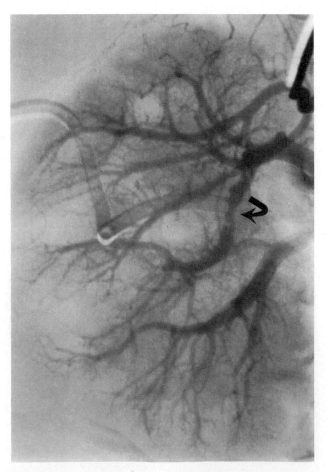

Figure 3.47. Arterial injury. Persistent hematuria after percutaneous nephrostomy (PCN) prompted this selective renal arteriogram. Note the arterial damage (*arrow*) adjacent to the PCN catheter.

shock. Thus, a urinary tract infection is a contraindication to PCN placement. However, infection of an obstructed collecting system often is a medical emergency requiring percutaneous relief. In these patients, antibiotics often are administered before beginning the procedure. If the sensitivity of the infecting organism is unknown, a broad-spectrum antibiotic should be used. The PCN should be placed with as little manipulation as possible, and only small amounts of contrast, if any, should be used to confirm catheter position. Larger contrast injections for diagnostic purposes (antegrade pyelogram) should be delayed at least 1 day until the infection is under control.

An indwelling nephrostomy catheter will become colonized with bacteria. However, as long as there is adequate drainage of the collecting system, through the ureter or the PCN, infection will not be a problem.

Cronan and colleagues studied a series of patients with indwelling percutaneous nephrostomy catheters and urinary tract infections to see how often bacteremia occurred during catheter manipulation and whether or not antibiotics affected the incidence of bacteremia. Asymptomatic bacteremia was documented in 11 of 104 (11%) nephrostomy tube exchanges, but there was no difference in incidence between the group receiving prophylactic antibiotics and those patients who did not have antibiotic coverage.

Failure to respond to percutaneous drainage may indicate a perinephric abscess. Perinephric abscesses require ultrasound or CT for detection, and are usually amenable to percutaneous catheter drainage.

Occasionally, adjacent organs are traversed during nephrostomy placement. This is more likely to occur if a specific portion of the collecting system must be entered, such as for percutaneous nephrostolithotomy or in patients with variations of normal anatomy.

Pneumothorax is more likely to occur if the upper pole collecting system must be entered. In many patients, an entry site above the 11th or 12th rib is selected, and the pleural space is traversed. An expiratory chest film should be obtained to look for pneumothorax when a high puncture is used. Most small pneumothoraces resolve spontaneously and only observation is required. Large or symptomatic pneumothoraces can be treated by the radiologist with a small chest tube.

Variations of normal anatomy may result in liver, spleen or colon lying in the path of the nephrostomy tract. In many patients, the position of the kidneys or the identification of bowel gas may suggest this interposition. An ultrasound or CT examination may be very helpful in confirming the position of the interposed organ and in identifying a path through which the nephrostomy can be safely placed (*see* Fig. 3.43).

Ureteral Intervention

With the nephrostomy catheter providing access to the collecting system, interventional procedures can be performed in the ureter. This direct antegrade approach avoids problems associated with traversing the urethra, bladder, and ureterovesical junction. Ureteral stents may be placed to bypass obstruction, to heal a ureteral leak, or to prevent stricture formation. In patients in whom a stricture has already occurred, angioplasty balloon catheters may be used to dilate the stricture (*see* Chapter 16). Stone removal has been discussed in Chapter 12, but other solid materials, such as broken ureteral catheters, often may be removed more easily using this antegrade approach than using retrograde catheterization of the ureter.

SUGGESTED READINGS

Excretory Urography

Banner, MP, Pollack HM: Evaluation of renal function by excretory urography. *J Urol* 124:443, 1980.

Bauer DL, Garrison RW, McRoberts JW: The health and cost implications of routine excretory urography before transurethral prostatectomy. *J Urol* 123:386, 1980.

Choyke PL: The urogram: are rumors of its death premature? *Radiology* 184(1):33, 1992.

Collie DA, Paul AB, Wild SR: The diagnostic yield of intravenous urography: a demographic study. *Br J Urol* 73(6):603,1994

Daughtridge TG: Ureteral compression device for excretory urography. *AJR* 95(2):431, 1965.

Dawson P: Intravenous urography revisited. *Br J Urol* 66(6):561, 1990.

Donker PJ, Kakisilatu F: Preoperative evaluation of patients with bladder outlet obstruction with particular regard to excretory urography. *J Urol* 120:685, 1978.

Doubilet P, McNeil BJ, Van Houten FX, et al.: Excretory urography in current practice: evidence against overutilization. *Radiology* 154:607, 1985.

Dure-Smith P, McArdle GH: Tomography during excretory urography: technical aspects. *Br J Radiol* 45:896, 1972.

Eklof O, Ringertz H: Kidney size in children. *Acta Radiol Diagn* 17(5):617, 1976.

George DC, Vinnicombe SJ, Balkissoon AR, Heron CW: Bowel preparation before intravenous urography: is it necessary? *Br J Radiol* 66(781):17, 1993.

Gillespie HW, Maile WBD: Routine tomographs with excretion urography. *Br J Radiol* 27:344, 1954.

Goldwasser B, Cohan RH, Dunnick NR, Andriani RT, Carson CC, Weinerth JL: The role of linear tomography in evaluation of patients with nephrolithiasis. *Urology* 23:253, 1989.

Hattery RR, Williamson B Jr, Hartman GW, et al.: Intravenous urographic technique. *Radiology* 167:593, 1988.

Lloyd LK, Witten DM, Bueschen AJ, Daniel WW: Enhanced detection of asymptomatic renal masses with routine tomography during excretory urography. *Urology* 11:523, 1978.

Mellins HZ, McNeil BJ, Abrams HL, et al.: The selection of patients for excretory urography. *Radiology* 130:293, 1979.

Newberg AH, Mindell HJ: Predicting tomographic levels for urography. *Radiology* 118:460, 1976.

Pollack H: Some limitations and pitfalls of excretory urography. *J Urol* 116:537, 1976.

Pollack HM, Banner MP: Current status of excretory urography a premature epitaph? *Urol Clin North Am* 12(4):585, 1985.

Sandler CM, Conley SB, Fogel SR: Splenic compression of the left kidney simulating pathologic unilateral renal enlargement. *J Comput Assist Tomogr* 4(2):248, 1980.

Schuster GA, Nazos D, Lewis GA: Preparation of outpatients for excretory urography: is bowel preparation with laxatives and dietary restrictions necessary? AJR 164(6):1425, 1995.

Simon AL: Normal renal size and absolute criterion. *AJR* 92(2):270, 1964.

Vydareny KH, Stuck KJ, Ellis JH, Ohl DA: Diagnostic usefulness of post-void film in intravenous urogram. *Urology* 38(2):170, 1991.

Wasserman NF, Lapointe S, Eckmann DR, Rosel PR: Assessment of prostatism: role of intravenous urography. *Radiology* 165(3):831, 1987.

Antegrade Pyelography

Hare WS, McOmish: Skinny needle pyelography. *Med J Aust* 2:123, 1981.

Pfister RC, Newhouse JH: Interventional percutaneous pyeloureteral techniques: I. antegrade pyelography and ureteral perfusion. *Radiol Clin North Am* 17:341, 1979.

Pfister RC, Papanicolaou N, Yoder IC: Diagnostic morphologic and urodynamic antegrade pyelography. *Radiol Clin North Am* 24(4):561, 1986.

Urethrography

Kirshy DM, Pollack AH, Becker JA, et al.: Autourethrography. *Radiology* 180:443, 1991.

McCallum RW: The radiologic assessment of the lower urinary tract in paraplegics: a new method. *J Can Assoc Radiol* 25:34, 1974.

McCallum RW: The adult male urethra: normal anatomy, pathology and method of urethrography. *Radiol Clin North Am* 17:227, 1979.

McCallum RW, Colapinto V: *Urological Radiology of the Adult Male Lower Urinary Tract.* Springfield, IL, Charles C Thomas, 1976.

McCallum RW, Colapinto V: The role of urethrography in urethral disease: I. accurate radiological localization of the membranous urethra and distal sphincters in normal male subjects. *J Urol* 122:607, 1979.

Cavernosography

Bookstein JJ: Cavernosal veno-occlusive insufficiency in male impotence: evaluation of degree and location. *Radiology* 164:175, 1987.

Bookstein JJ, Fellmeth B, Moreland S, Lurie AL: Pharmacoangiographic assessment of the corpora cavernosa. *Cardiovasc Intervent Radiol* 11:218, 1988.

Bookstein JJ, Lurie AL: Selective penile venography: anatomical and hemodynamic observations. *J Urol* 140:55, 1988.

Bookstein JJ, Valji K, Parsons L, et al.: Penile pharmacocavernosography and cavernosometry in the evaluation of impotence. *J Urol* 137:772, 1987.

Lue TF, Hricak H, Schmidt RA, et al.: Functional evaluation of penile veins by cavernosography in papaverine-induced erection. *J Urol* 135:479, 1986.

Ultrasonography

Amis ES, Jr, Hartman DS: Renal ultrasound 1984: a practical overview. *Radiol Clin North Am* 22(2):315, 1984.

Bude RO, Rubin JH, Adler RS: Power versus conventional color Doppler sonography: comparison in the depiction of normal intrarenal vasculature. *Radiology* 192(3):777, 1994.

Chang VH, Cunningham JJ: Efficacy of sonography as a screening method in renal insufficiency. *J Clin Ultrasound* 13:414–417, 1985.

Coleman B: Ultrasonography of the upper genitourinary tract. *Urol Clin North Am* 12(4):633, 1985.

Fowler RC, Chennells PM, Ewing R: Scrotal ultrasound: a clinical evaluation. *Br J Radiol* 60(715):649, 1986.

Haller JO, Cohen HL: Pediatric urosonography: an update. *Urol Radiol* 9:99, 1987.

Ralls PW, Larsen D, Johnson MB, Lee KP: Color Doppler sonography of the scrotum. *Semin Ultrasound CT MR* 12(2):109, 1991.

Rifkin MD: Scrotal ultrasound. *Urol Radiol* 9:119, 1987.

Rubin JM, Bude RO, Carson PL, et al.: Power Doppler US: a potentially useful alternative to mean frequency-based color Doppler US. *Radiology* 190(3):853, 1994.

Scoutt LM, Zawin ML, Taylor KJW: Doppler US: Part II. clinical applications. *Radiology* 174:309, 1990.

Taylor KJ, Burns PN: Duplex Doppler scanning in the pelvis and abdomen. *Ultrasound Med Biol* 11(4):643, 1985.

Taylor KJW, Holland S: Doppler US: Part I. basic principles, instrumentation and pitfalls. *Radiology* 174:297, 1990.

Computed Tomography

Dunnick NR, Korobkin M: Computed tomography of the kidney. *Radiol Clin North Am* 22(2):297, 1984.

Einstein DM, Herts BR, Weaver R, et al: Evaluation of renal masses detected by excretory urography: cost-effectiveness of sonography versus CT. *AJR* 164(2):371, 1995.

Love L, Churchill RJ, Reynes CJ, et al.: CT of the kidney and perinephric space. *Semin Roentgenol* 16(4):277, 1981.

McClennan B, Lee JKT, Peterson RR: Anatomy of the perirenal area. *Radiology* 158:555, 1986.

Rubin GD, Dake MD, Napel SA, et al.: Three-dimensional spiral CT angiography of the abdomen: initial clinical experience. *Radiology* 186:147, 1993.

Sandler CM, Raval B, David CL: Computed tomography of the kidney. *Urol Clin North Am* 12(4):657, 1985.

Smith RC, Rosenfield AT, Choe KA, et al: Acute flank pain: comparison of non-contrast-enhanced CT and intravenous urography. *Radiology* 194(3):789, 1995.

Wadsworth DE, McClennan BL, Standley RJ: CT of the renal mass. *Urol Radiol* 4:85, 1982.

Zeman RK, Fox SH, Silverman PM, et al.: Helical (spiral) CT of the abdomen. *AJR* 160:719, 1993.

Magnetic Resonance Imaging

Baker LL, Hajek PC, Burkhart TK, et al.: MR imaging of the scrotum: normal anatomy. *Radiology* 163:89, 1987.

Barentsz JO, Ruijs HJ, van Erning LJ: Magnetic resonance imaging of urinary bladder cancer: an overview and new developments. *Magn Reson Q* 9(4):235, 1993.

Cramer BM, Schlegel EA, Thueroff JW: MR imaging in the differential diagnosis of scrotal and testicular disease. *RadioGraphics* 11:9, 1994.

Egglin TK, Hahn PF, Stark DD: MRI of the adrenal glands. *Semin Roentgen* XXIII(4):280, 1988.

Krestin GP, Steinbrich W, Freidmann G: Adrenal masses: evaluation with fast gradient-echo MR imaging and Gd-DTPA-enhanced dynamic studies. *Radiology* 171:675, 1989.

Laissy JP, Faraggi M, Lebtahi R, et al.: Functional evaluation of normal and ischemic kidney by means of gadolinium-DTPA enhanced turboFlash MR imaging: a preliminary comparison with 99m-Tc-MAG3 dynamic scintigraphy. *Magn Reson Imaging* 12(3):413, 1994.

Mitchell DG, Crovello M, Matteucci T, et al.: Benign adrenocortical masses: diagnosis with chemical shift MR imaging. *Radiology* 185:345, 1992.

Rominger MB, Kenney PJ, Morgan DE, et al.: Gadolinium-enhanced MR imaging of renal masses. *RadioGraphics* 12:1097, 1992.

Schiebler ML, Schnall MD, Pollack HM, et al.: Current role of imaging in the staging of adenocarcinoma of the prostate. *Radiology* 189:339, 1993.

Tachibana M, Baba S, Deguchi N, et al.: Efficacy of gadolinium-diethylenetriaminepentaacetic acid-enhanced magnetic resonance imaging for differentiation between superficial and muscle-invasive tumor of the bladder: a comparative study with computerized tomography and transurethral ultrasonography. *J Urol* 145:1169, 1991.

Takeda M, Katayama Y, Tsutsui T, et al.: Does gadolinium-diethylene triamine pentaacetic acid enhanced MRI of the kidney represent tissue concentration of contrast media in the kidney? In vivo and in vitro study. *Magn Reson Imaging* 12:421, 1994.

Tsushima Y, Ishizaka H: Adrenal masses: differentiation with chemical shift, fast low angle shot MR imaging. *Radiology* 186:705, 1993.

Angiography

Ekelund L: Pharmacoangiography of the kidney: an overview. *Urol Radiol* 12:9, 1980.

Harrington DP, Levin DC, Garnick JD, et al.: Compound angulation in the angiographic evaluation of renal artery stenosis. *Radiology* 146:829, 1983.

Johnsrude IS, Jackson D, Dunnick NR: *A Practical Approach to Angiography*. Boston, Little Brown, 1987.

Levin DC, Schapiro RM, Boxt LM, et al.: Digital subtraction angiography: principles and pitfalls of image improvement techniques. *AJR* 143:447, 1984.

Robertson PW, Dyson ML, Sutton PD: Renal angiography: a review of 1,750 cases. *Clin Radiol* 20:401, 1969.

Saddekni S, Sos TA, Sniderman KW, Srur M, Bodner LJ, Kneeland JB, Cahill PT: Optimal injection technique for intravenous digital subtraction angiography. *Radiology* 150:655, 1984.

Lymphography

Dunnick NR: The radionuclide evaluation. In Javadpour N (ed): *Principles and Management of Urologic Cancers*. Baltimore, Williams & Wilkins, 1979.

Dunnick NR, Castelino RA: Pediatric lymphography. *AJR* 129:639, 1977.

Dunnick NR, Javadpour N: Value of CT and lymphography: distinguishing retroperitoneal metastases from nonseminomatous testicular tumors. *AJR* 136:1093, 1981.

Percutaneous Biopsy

Andriole JG, Haaga JR, Adams RB, et al.: Biopsy needle characteristics assessed in the laboratory. *Radiology* 148:659, 1984.

Bret PM, Fond A, Casola G, et al.: Abdominal lesions: a prospective study of clinical efficacy of percutaneous fine-needle biopsy. *Radiology* 159:345, 1986.

Casola G, vanSonnenberg E, Keightley A, et al.: Pneumothorax: radiologic treatment with small catheters. *Radiology* 166:89, 1988.

Charboneau JW, Reading CC, Welch TJ: CT and sonographically guided needle biopsy: current techniques and new innovations. *AJR* 154:1, 1990.

Ferrucci J, Wittenberg J, Mueller P, et al.: Diagnosis of abdominal malignancy by radiologic fine-needle aspiration biopsy. *AJR* 134:323, 1980.

Haaga JR, LiPuma JP, Bryan PJ, et al.: Clinical comparison of small- and large-caliber cutting needles for biopsy. *Radiology* 146:665, 1983.

Jeffrey RB: Coaxial technique for CT-guided biopsy of deep retroperitoneal lymph node. *Gastrointest Radiol* 13:271, 1988.

Kaufman RA: Technical aspects of abdominal CT in infants and children. *AJR* 153:549, 1989.

Matalon TS, Silver B: US guidance of interventional procedures. *Radiology* 174:43, 1990.

Mostbeck GH, Wittich GR, Derfler K, et al.: Optimal needle size for renal biopsy: in vitro and in vivo evaluation. *Radiology* 173:819, 1989.

Nadel L, Baumgartner BR, Bernardino ME: Percutaneous renal biopsies: accuracy, safety and indications. *Urol Radiol* 8:67, 1986.

Parker SH, Hooper KD, Yakes WF, et al.: Image-directed percutaneous biopsies with a biopsy gun. *Radiology* 171:663, 1989.

Sateriale M, Cronan JJ, Savadler LD: A 5-year experience with 307 CT guided renal biopsies: results and complications. *J Vasc Interv Radiol* 2(3):401,k 1991.

Welch TJ, Sheedy PF, Johnson CD, et al.: CT-guided biopsy: prospective analysis of 1,000 procedures. *Radiology* 171:493, 1989.

Whitney W, Dunnick NR: Biopsy techniques in uroradiology. *Radiol Report* 2:302, 1990.

Wittenberg J, Mueller PR, Ferrucci JT Jr, et al.: Percutaneous core biopsy of abdominal tumor using 22 gauge needle: further observations. *AJR* 139:75, 1982.

Yankaskas BC, Staab EV, Craven MB, et al.: Delayed complications from fine-needle biopsies of solid masses of the abdomen. *Invest Radiol* 21(4):325, 1986.

Zornoza J, Wallace S, Goldstein HM, et al.: Transperitoneal percutaneous retroperitoneal lymph node aspiration biopsy. *Radiology* 122:111, 1977.

Radionuclide Evaluation of the Urinary Tract

Blaufox MD, Kalika V, Scharf S, et al.: Applications of nuclear medicine in genitourinary imaging. *Urol Radiol* 4:155, 1982.

Dubovsky EV, Russel CD: Quantitation of renal function with glomerular and tubular agents. *Semin Nucl Med* 12:308, 1982.

Eshima D, Taylor A Jr: Technetium 99m (99mTC) mercaptoacetyl-triglycine: update on the new 99mTC renal tubular function agent. *Semin Nucl Med* 22(2):61, 1992.

Itoh K, Tsukamoto E, Kakizaki H, et al.: Phase II study of Tc99m MAG3 in patients with nephrourologic diseases. *Clin Nucl Med* 18(5):387, 1993.

Kirchner PT, Rosenthal L: Renal transplant evaluation. *Semin Nucl Med* 12:370, 1982.

Lutzker LG: The fine points of scrotal scintigraphy. *Semin Nucl Med* 12(4):387, 1982.

Mettler FA Jr, Guiberteau MJ: *Essentials of Nuclear Medicine Imaging,* ed 2. Orlando, FL, Grune and Stratton, 1986.

O'Malley JP, Ziessman HA, Chantarapitak N: Tc-99m MAG3 as an alternative to Tc-99m DTPA and I-131 Hippuran for renal transplant evaluation. *Clin Nucl Med* 18(1):22, 1993.

Taux WN, Dubovsky EV, Kidd T, et al.: New formulas for the calculation of effective renal plasma flow. *Eur J Nucl Med* 7:51, 1982.

Taylor A Jr, Nally JV: Clinical aspects of renal scintigraphy. *AJR* 164:31, 1995.

Percutaneous Nephrostomy

Dunnick NR, Illescas FF, Mitchell S, et al.: Interventional uroradiology. *Invest Radiol* 24:831, 1989.

Hopper KD, Yakes WF: The posterior intercostal approach for percutaneous renal procedures: risk of puncturing the lung, spleen, and liver as determined by CT. *AJR* 154:115, 1990.

Kay KW, Reinke DB: Detailed caliceal anatomy for endourology. *J Urol* 132:1085, 1984.

Matalon TAS, Silver B: US guidance of interventional procedures. *Radiology* 174:43, 1990.

Pfister RC: Percutaneous nephrostomy. In Lang EK (ed): *Percutaneous and Interventional Urology and Radiology.* Berlin, Springer Verlag, 1986, pp. 1–28.

Sherman JL, Hopper KD, Greene AJ, et al.: The retrorenal colon on computed tomography: a normal variant. *J Comput Assist Tomogr* 9(2):339, 1985.

Seldinger, SI: Catheter replacement of needle in percutaneous arteriography: new technique. *Acta Radiol Stockh* 39:368, 1953.

Silverman SG, Mueller P, Pfister RC: Hemostatic evaluation before abdominal interventions: an overview and proposal. *AJR* 154:233, 1990.

Spies JB, Rosen RJ, Liebowitz AS: Antibiotic prophylaxis in vascular and interventional radiology: a rational approach. *Radiology* 166:381, 1988.

Stables DP, Ginsberg NJ, Johnson ML: Percutaneous nephrostomy: a series and review of the literature. *AJR* 130:75, 1978.

Stanley P, Bear JW, Reid BS: Percutaneous nephrostomy in infants and children. *AJR* 141:473, 1983.

Winfield WC, Kirchner SG, Brun ME, et al.: Percutaneous nephrostomy in neonates, infants and children. *Radiology* 151:617, 1984.

4

Functional Renal Anatomy, Renal Physiology, and Contrast Media

FUNCTIONAL RENAL ANATOMY AND RENAL PHYSIOLOGY

The main function of the kidney is to maintain the homeostasis of body fluids. A number of specialized tasks are involved in this homeostasis. These include the excretion of metabolic end products and toxins, the regulation of body fluid volume, blood pressure regulation, and the regulation of mineral and acid-base balance. Body fluids are divided into two discrete compartments.

Approximately two thirds of the fluid is located within cell membranes, and this is termed the *intracellular fluid*. The remaining one third is contained in the *extracellular compartment* (extracellular fluid [ECF]). Approximately one third of the volume of the ECF is contained within the vascular space and two thirds is in the interstitium. The regulatory function of the kidney directly effects the fluid that is located in the vascular compartment, however, because there is free movement of water between the intracellular and extracellular fluid compartments, the effect of this function is to regulate the composition of all body fluids.

Functional Renal Anatomy

On gross inspection, a bisected kidney can be divided into two major regions (Fig. 4.1): (*a*) the inner renal medulla, and (*b*) the outer renal cortex.

The functional unit of the kidney is the nephron (Fig. 4.2). Each kidney contains approximately 1 million nephrons. Each nephron consists of a specialized capillary vascular network called the *glomerulus,* which is surrounded by Bowman's capsule, a balloon-like structure into which the capillary tufts of the glomerulus protrude. Each glomerulus is connected to a series of specialized epithelial segments that collectively are known as the *renal tubule*.

The tubule, in turn, is divided into several segments. The first segment is called the proximal tubule, which in turn is subdivided into a convoluted and a straight portion; the second segment, the loop of Henle, is subdivided into the thin descending, the thin ascending, and the thick ascending limbs; and the third segment, the distal tubule, is subdivided into the distal convoluted tubule and the cortical, medullary, and papillary collecting ducts. The cortex contains the glomeruli, the proximal tubule, the distal tubule, and the cortical collecting duct. The medulla is made up of the loops of Henle, the medullary and papillary collecting ducts, and renal pyramids, the apices of which project into the minor calyces. The nephrons that are located close to the corticomedullary junction have larger glomeruli and their loops of Henle descend deeper into the renal papilla than those located more superficially in the renal cortex.

The main renal artery branches into interlobar arteries that branch into the arcuate arteries located at the

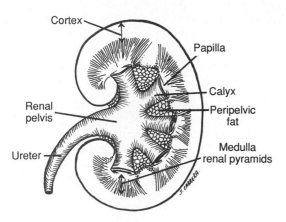

Figure 4.1. Bisected section of the kidney showing the relationship of the cortex, the medulla, and the renal collecting system. Fat in the renal sinus surrounds the calyces and the renal pelvis.

corticomedullary junction. These, in turn, branch into the interlobular arteries, and finally, the afferent arterioles, each of which leads to a glomerulus. The glomerulus is drained by an efferent arteriole that subdivides to form a peritubular capillary network known as the vasa

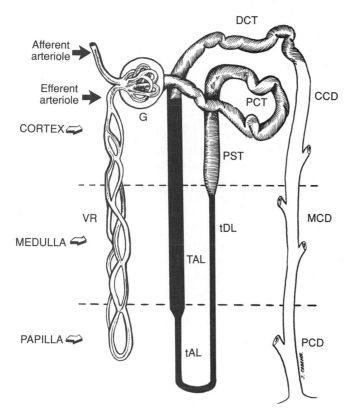

Figure 4.2. The nephron. A = afferent arteriole; CCD = cortical collecting duct; DCT = distal convoluted tubule; E = efferent arteriole; G = glomerulus; MDC = medullary collecting duct; PCD = papillary collecting duct; PCT = proximal convoluted tubule; PST = proximal straight tubule; TAL = thick ascending limb of the loop of Henle; tAL = thin ascending limb of the loop of Henle; VR = vasa recta.

recta. The vasa recta then anastomose to form venous channels. This unique arrangement in the kidney, in which the glomerulus is located between two resistive capillary networks as opposed to the arteriole-capillary-venule arrangement of the other tissues of the body, helps to maintain constant hydrostatic pressure at the level of the glomerulus despite changes in blood pressure (Fig. 4.3) and is the driving force for glomerular filtration.

The *macula densa* is a distinctive portion of the tubule between the ascending loop of Henle and the distal convoluted tubule that courses between the afferent and efferent arterioles. The macula densa represents the tubular component of a specialized area of the nephron called the juxtaglomerular apparatus. The juxtaglomerular apparatus is the site of renin synthesis and plays a major role in the blood pressure regulation function of the kidney.

Basic Renal Physiology

The homeostatic functions of the kidney are achieved through two simultaneous processes: (*a*) glomerular filtration, and (*b*) tubular resorption/secretion. Glomerular ultrafiltration occurs as a result of the net Starling forces across the glomerular capillary wall. The net filtration pressure (NFP) is equal to the sum of the glomerular hydrostatic pressure and the colloid osmotic pressure in Bowman's capsule (which favors fluid movement from the capillary space into Bowman's space) minus the sum of the mean glomerular capillary oncotic pressure and the hydrostatic pressure in Bowman's space (the principal forces opposing ultrafiltration). Because protein is not filtered by the glomerulus, the fluid of Bowman's space is protein-free, and thus, the colloid os-

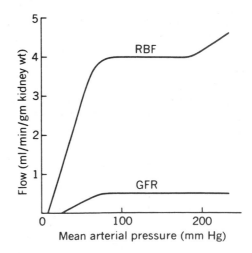

Figure 4.3. Renal blood flow and glomerular filtration remain constant over a wide range of blood pressure. This helps to maintain a constant level of glomerular filtration. (From Gottschalk CW, Lassiter WE: Mechanisms of urine formation. In Mountcastle VD (ed): *Medical Physiology,* vol 2, ed 14. St. Louis, CV Mosby, 1980).

motic pressure in Bowman's space is negligible. The glomerular filtration rate (GFR) is determined by the net filtration pressure and the surface area available for filtration, as well as the permeability of the glomerular capillary bed. Thus, GFR can be expressed as

$$GFR = Kf \times NFP$$

where Kf is a constant expressing the product of the capillary permeability and the surface area of the capillary bed, and NFP is the net filtration pressure. The average glomerular filtration rate in a human is approximately 125 ml/min, which is equal to 180 L/day or approximately 12 times the volume of the ECF.

Although 180 L of fluid is filtered in a day, only 1 to 2 L of urine is produced per day in which wastes and toxins may be concentrated 100- to 200-fold above their plasma concentration. This concentration of the final urine product is the result of tubular reabsorption and secretion. Under normal conditions, approximately two thirds of the ultrafiltrate volume is reabsorbed by the proximal tubule by a process linked to the active secretion of hydrogen ions and the active reabsorption of sodium, glucose, amino acids, and other solutes. Isotonicity of the fluid in the proximal tubule with the plasma is maintained, because the cells of the proximal tubule are freely permeable to water.

In the loop of Henle, which begins at the corticomedullary junction, differential absorption of sodium chloride occurs so that the fluid in the tubular lumen, initially isotonic with the interstitium, becomes progressively more concentrated in the descending limb, reaching its maximum concentration at the bend of the loop and then becomes progressively more hypotonic with respect to plasma as it reaches the thick ascending limb of the loop. This differential absorption of sodium chloride occurs because the cells in the descending limb have a high permeability for water, but a low permeability for salt; whereas, in the thick ascending limb, the cells are impermeable to water, but have a high permeability for salt, which is actively reabsorbed. This process, known as the *renal counter-current mechanism,* results in progressive interstitial hypertonicity in the medulla and is required for final concentration of the urine by the distal tubules.

The distal tubule continues the water dilution of urine through the active transport of sodium and chloride coupled with relative water impermeability. The collecting ducts are the primary site of action of antidiuretic hormone (ADH). The final 15% of water absorption is achieved within the collecting ducts. The collecting ducts are virtually impermeable to water in the absence of ADH, but when ADH is present, water passes freely across the tubular wall, allowing the tubular fluid to achieve the same tonicity as the fluid in the surrounding interstitium. Thus, a hypertonic urine is produced without the active transport of water. The distal nephron also reabsorbs sodium and secretes hydrogen ions and potassium under the influence of aldosterone. Parathyroid hormone also acts on the distal tubule to conserve calcium.

Clearance

The rate at which a substance is removed from the plasma in a given period is termed the clearance of that substance. For a substance that is freely filtered and not reabsorbed or secreted by the tubule, the rate of clearance of that substance is equal to the GFR. The rate of clearance is expressed as the urinary volume per unit time, multiplied by the urine concentration of that substance, divided by the plasma concentration of the substance. Thus

$$GFR = \frac{U \times V}{P}$$

where U is the urine concentration of the substance, V is the urine volume produced per unit time, and P is the plasma concentration of the substance.

The polysaccharide, inulin, meets the criteria expressed above, and therefore, can be used to determine GFR. Creatinine, an endogenous product of muscle metabolism, is produced by the body in relatively constant amounts per day, is present in the plasma, and is excreted by glomerular filtration. Measurement of creatinine clearance is therefore convenient, although it is not as exact as the inulin clearance, because a small amount of creatinine is secreted by the tubules.

Renal Plasma Flow

If a substance were freely filtered and removed from the blood completely in one pass through the kidney, then clearance of that substance should represent the renal plasma flow. The substance paraminohippurate (PAH) is freely filtered and that portion that is not filtered is virtually completely secreted by the proximal tubule, so that at low plasma concentrations of PAH, all plasma supplying nephrons is completely cleared of the substance. The clearance of PAH, therefore, should represent the renal plasma flow (RPF); however, because 10–15% of renal blood flow supplies non-nephron-bearing portions of the kidney (i.e., the renal capsule and the peripelvic fat), the clearance of PAH is referred to as the effective renal plasma flow (ERPF). The normal value for ERPF is 650 ml/min/1.73 m^2 in males and 600 ml/min/1.73 m^2 in females. Once the ERPF has been calculated, the effective renal blood flow (ERBF) can be calculated by the formula:

$$ERBF = \frac{ERPF}{1 - hematocrit}$$

The filtration fraction is the ratio of the clearance of inulin to that of PAH or C_{inulin}/C_{PAH}. In humans, this ratio is normally 0.2.

CONTRAST MEDIA: HISTORICAL BACKGROUND

Attempts at radiography in the urinary tract began shortly after Roentgen's discovery of x-rays in 1895 with the retrograde insertion of rigid metal stylets into the ureters to demonstrate their course. In 1905, the techniques of retrograde cystography and pyelography using Kollargol, a colloidol preparation of silver, were introduced by Voelcker and Von Lichtenberg. The first report of opacification of the urinary tract using excreted contrast media came in 1923 when Osborne, Sutherland, Scholl, and Rowntree, from the Mayo Clinic reported that there was discernible opacification of the bladder on abdominal radiographs in patients who had received a 10% solution of sodium iodine, either orally or intravenously, for the treatment of syphilis. This report represented the initial discovery that iodine could be used as a radiopaque contrast medium. It is remarkable that in the more than 70 years since this discovery, no other element has proven suitable for this purpose. Successful opacification of the urinary tract using sodium iodide, however, was not routinely possible, because it proved to be far too toxic in sufficient quantities to achieve diagnostic opacification.

The next significant breakthrough came in 1925 and 1926, when the German chemists Kurth Rath and Arthur Binz synthesized several organic pyridine compounds containing a single atom of iodine per molecule. They had been seeking to devise therapeutic agents that would be useful in the treatment of bacterial infections of the kidney and gallbladder. One of these pyridine compounds was found to be excreted by both the kidney and the liver, and was called Selectan neutral (Fig. 4.4).

Clinical therapeutic trials of Selectan neutral were performed in Hamburg, Germany under the direction of Professor Leopold Lichtwitz. Dr. Moses Swick, a young American urologist, was working with him and became interested in the potential of Selectan neutral for imaging the urinary tract. Professor Lichtwitz was so impressed with Swick's preliminary investigation that he suggested that the investigation be continued in Berlin with Professor Von Lichtenberg, the eminent German urologist, who several years earlier had described retro-

Figure 4.5.   Uroselectan.

grade pyelography and cystography. Von Lichtenberg also had been working on developing a satisfactory contrast medium for intravenous injection that would allow visualization of the urinary tract. After several discussions among Von Lichtenberg, Binz, and Swick, modifications of Selectan neutral designed to increase its water solubility and decrease its neurotoxicity were proposed. This collaboration resulted in the synthesis of Uroselectan (Iopax) (Fig. 4.5), which contained 42% iodine. Swick found that Uroselectan was the first agent to produce reliable opacification of the urinary tract after intravenous administration and that it was much better tolerated than the previously available compounds. Shortly thereafter, a further modification of the compound was made by Binz that was known as Uroselectan B in Europe and as Neo-Iopax (Fig. 4.6) in the United States. Neo-Iopax represented a significant improvement over Iopax in that it contained two iodine atoms per molecule, and therefore, the radioopacity of the compound was significantly greater. In addition to Neo-Iopax, Binz and Rath also synthesized an additional diiodo compound known as iodopyracet, which was marketed as Diodrast (Fig. 4.7). These two products became the radiologic contrast media of choice and were used successfully for the next 20 years.

In 1933, Swick, who by then was working at Mt. Sinai Hospital in New York, proposed that the six-carbon benzene ring serve as the carrier of iodine instead of the heterocyclic five-carbon atom and one-nitrogen-atom pyridine ring that had been used by Binz and Rath. The product that was introduced, sodium monoiodo hippu-

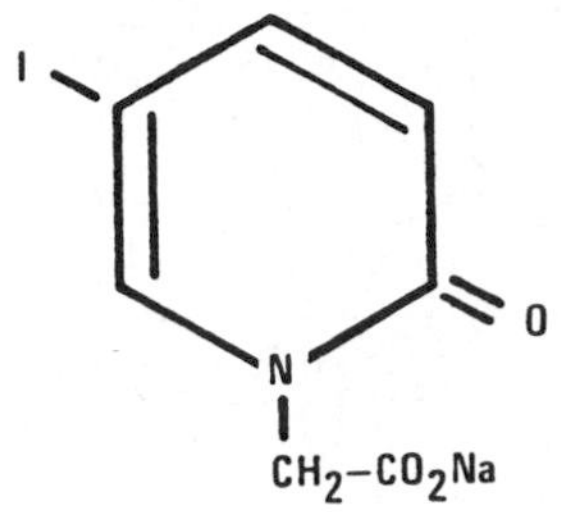

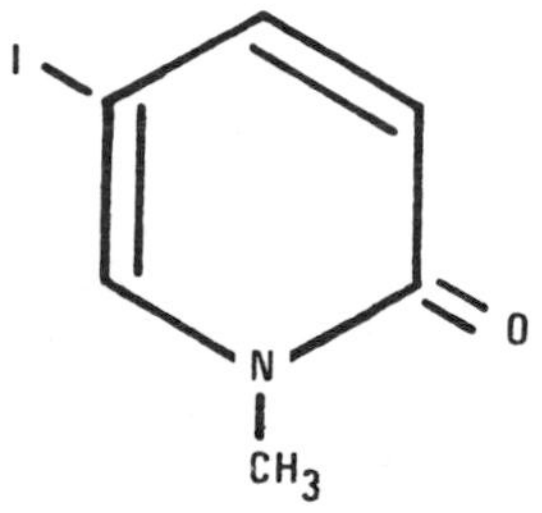

Figure 4.4.   Selectan—neutral.

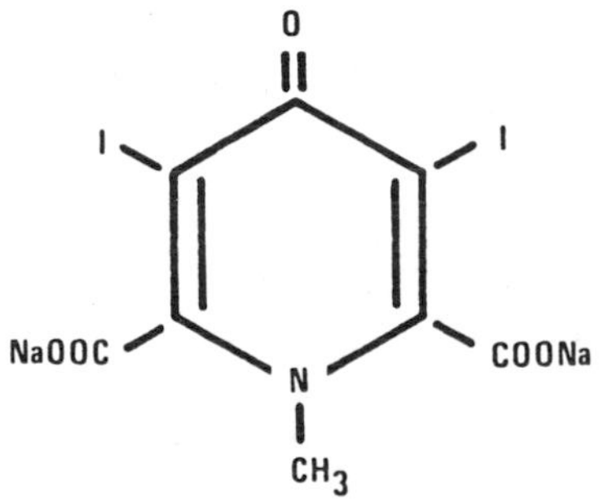

Figure 4.6.   Sodium iodomethamate (Neo-Iopax).

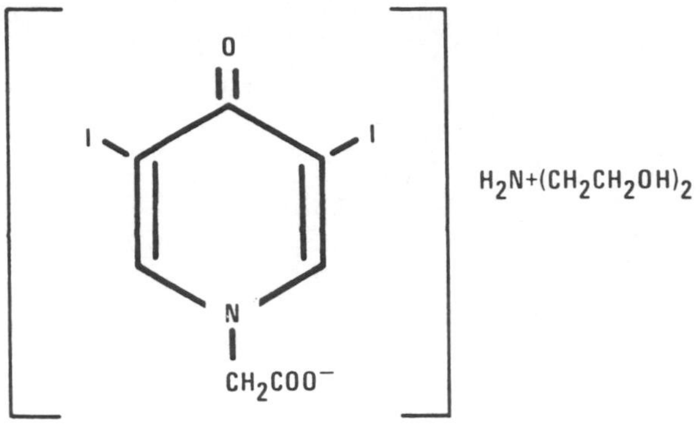

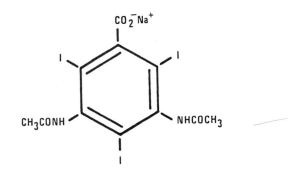

Figure 4.7. Iodopyracet (Diodrast).

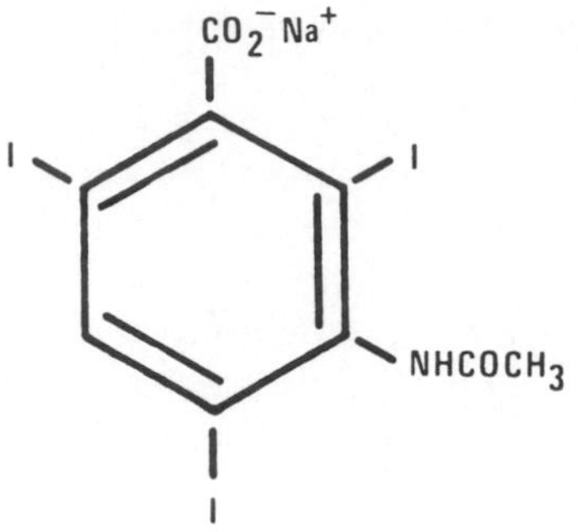

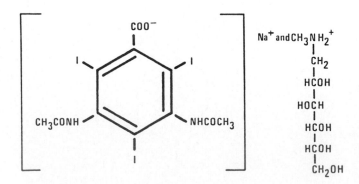

Figure 4.9. Sodium acetrizoate (Urokon).

rate (Fig. 4.8) did not prove, however, to be a significant improvement over Diodrast or Neo-Iopax. However, the principle of using the six-carbon benzene ring as the carrier of iodine was established by this investigation.

The six-carbon molecule was not perfected as a contrast medium for approximately another 20 years. In the late 1940s, Wallingford and colleagues at the Mallinckrodt Chemical Works of St. Louis synthesized acetrizoate, which became the first triiodo derivative of benzoic acid to have proven clinical efficacy. This product, marketed as Urokon (Fig. 4.9), contained 65.8% iodine, and showed distinct advantages over the diiodo products because of its improved radioopacity, decreased toxicity, and high water solubility. Initial physiologic studies indicated that it was excreted principally by glomerular filtration, and thus, better urinary tract opacification was achieved.

In 1955, Hoppe and coworkers at Sterling Winthrop Research Institute produced further modification of the triiodo benzoic acid ring by the addition of a side chain in the five position. This compound was known as sodium diatrizoate and was given the brand name Hypaque (Fig. 4.10). This product and its derivatives, including sodium/meglumine diatrizoate (Fig. 4.11) and meglumine iothalmate (Fig. 4.12) became the standard urographic contrast media for the next 30 years.

During this period, many came to realize that while these ionic contrast media were much safer than the previously used materials, a great portion of the remaining toxicity of the compounds was related to their high osmolality (greater than 1500 mosm/kg of water or

approximately 5 times greater than plasma). In 1968, Torsten Almen of Malmö, Sweden, a radiologist, theorized that the high osmolality of ionic contrast could be reduced by synthesizing a product that would be nondissociating. He suggested that the ionizing carboxyl group of conventional contrast be replaced with a nondissociating group such as an amide. This would theoretically reduce the osmolality by 50% by reducing the number of particles in solution without loss of iodine content. Almen's hypothesis was pursued by a Norwegian company, Nyegaard AS and Company, which produced the first nonionic contrast medium, metrizamide (Fig. 4.13). Metrizamide, while readily excreted by the kidneys, was never used in the United States as a urographic agent, because of its considerable cost and

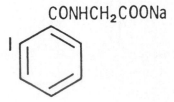

Figure 4.10. Sodium diatrizoate (Hypaque).

$$CONHCH_2COONa$$

Figure 4.8. Sodium monoiodo hippurate.

Figure 4.11. Sodium/meglumine diatrizoate (Renografin 60).

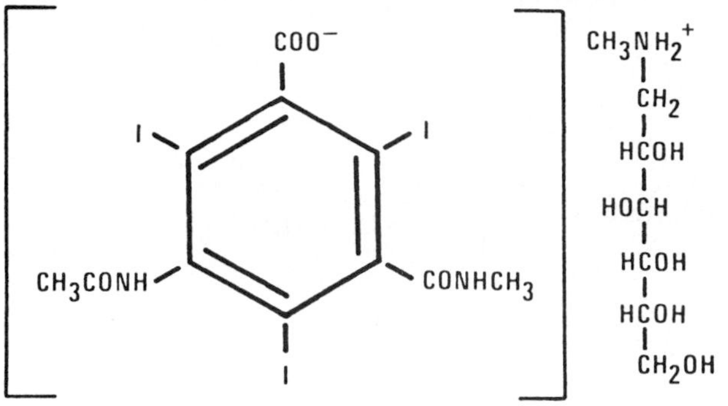

Figure 4.12.   Meglumine iothalamate (Conray).

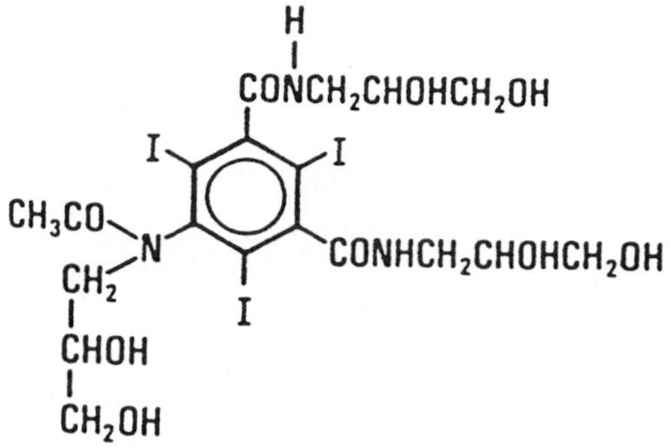

Figure 4.14.   Iohexol (Omnipaque).

the inability to sterilize the product by autoclave. It was necessary to package the media as a freeze-dried lypholized powder that needed to be reconstituted with water immediately before use.

Several years after the introduction of metrizamide, second-generation low-osmolality contrast media were introduced into clinical practice. These products developed along two general lines. In the first group, hydrophilic nonionizing radicals are introduced in positions one, three, and five of the benzene ring, while positions two, four, and six remain the position of the iodine atoms. Because the number one position does not dissociate, the number of iodine atoms relative to the number of particles in solution is increased from 1.5 to 3 as compared to ionic contrast media. Compounds in this category that have been approved for clinical use in the United States include iohexol (Omnipaque—Nycomed Inc., NY, NY) (Fig. 4.14), iopamidol (Isovue—Bracco Inc., Princeton, NJ) (Fig. 4.15), and ioversol (Optiray—Mallinckrodt Chemical Works, St. Louis, MO) (Fig. 4.16). These products are generically known as *nonionic monomers*. The second line of development

of low osmolality contrast has been directed toward the linkage of two triiodinated benzene rings sharing one ionizing carboxyl group. These compounds have a ratio of six iodine atoms to two molecules in solution, and therefore, also produce a ratio of 3. They are generally known as *monoacidic dimers*. Sodium-meglumine ioxaglate (Hexabrix—Mallinckrodt Chemical Works, St. Louis, MO) (Fig. 4.17) is a monoacidic dimer that has been introduced into clinical practice and represents the only approved contrast medium in this class.

The next line for development for contrast media was the introduction of *nonionic monoacidic dimers,* which have a ratio of six iodine atoms to one particle in solution, and therefore, represent ratio 6 compounds. This modification reduces the osmolality of the contrast medium approximately to that of plasma. Iodixanol (Visipaque—Nycomed Inc., NY, NY), a ratio 6 dimer, the first of the agents to be brought to the United States,

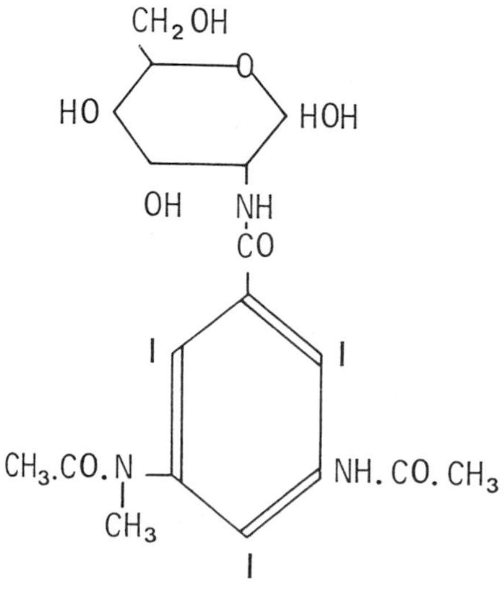

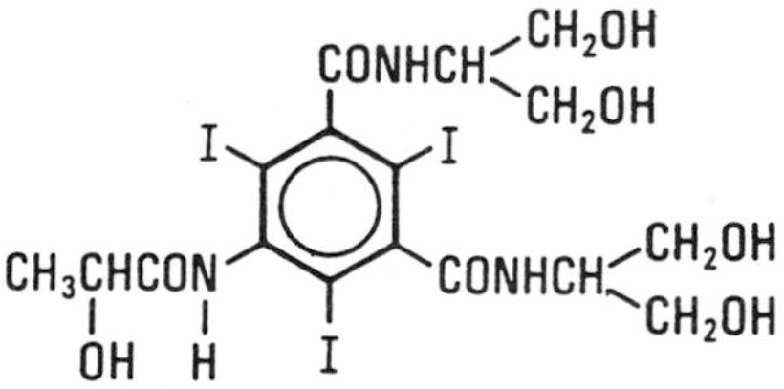

Figure 4.15.   Iopamidol (Isovue).

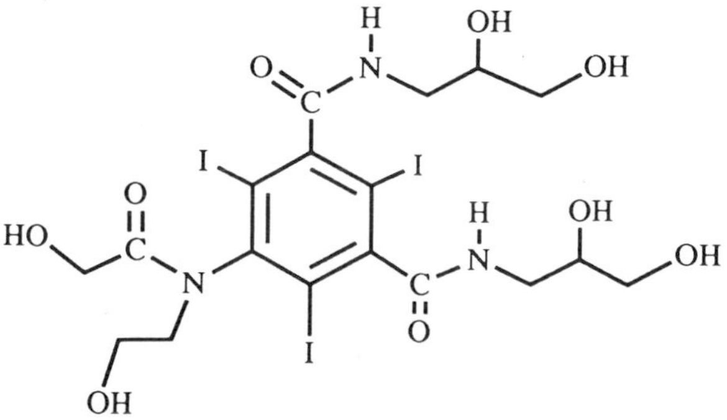

Figure 4.13.   Metrizamide.

Figure 4.16.   Ioversol (Optiray).

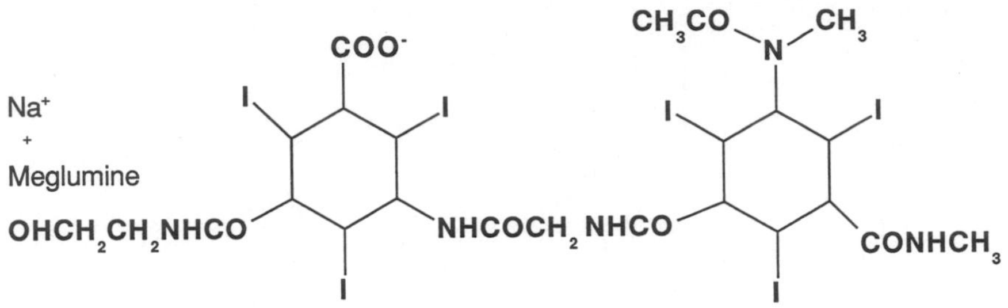

Figure 4.17.   Sodium/meglumine ioxaglate (Hexabrix).

has recently been approved in the United States by the Food and Drug Administration (FDA) (Fig. 4.18).

The late 1980s and early 1990s brought several changes to manufacturers of contrast media in the United States. Sterling Drug Inc., the parent of Winthrop Pharmaceuticals, was bought by the Eastman Kodak Company and subsequently sold to Nycomed, the successor to Nyegaard AS, the original developer of metrizamide and iohexol. E.R. Squibb and Company was bought by Bristol-Meyers and then was sold to Bracco, the Italian pharmaceutical company that developed iopamidol. Schering AG, the German pharmaceutical company that produced diatrizoate for both Winthrop and Squibb in their own contrast formulations, became an important U.S. contrast company in its own right with the introduction of gadolinium DTPA for use in magnetic resonance imaging by its American subsidiary, Berlex. Berlex re-entered the radiographic contrast market in the United States with the introduction of iopromide, a second-generation nonionic contrast medium after many years of successful European use.

PHYSIOLOGY OF CONTRAST EXCRETION

Principles

A knowledge of the basic physiology of contrast media excretion is crucial to the optimal performance of the urogram and its interpretation.

In 1960, Woodruff and Malvin demonstrated that the modern triiodobenzoic acid derivative contrast media were excreted by glomerular filtration without a significant component of tubular secretion. This is in contrast to the diiodo pyridone–based contrast media (Diodrast and Neo-Iopax) in which a significant component of tubular secretion is present.

In 1964, Schwartz and colleagues described using a "double dose" of contrast medium to perform urography in patients with impaired renal function. The authors theorized that if contrast medium is excreted by glomerular filtration, excretion of the contrast should be governed by its plasma concentration. They reasoned that with depressed renal function (i.e., a depressed GFR), raising the plasma concentration of contrast by increasing the administered dose would compensate for the depressed renal function, and therefore, would improve the quality of the urogram that could be obtained in patients with azotemia. Their study demonstrated the efficacy of such an approach and was the first attempt to improve the quality of urography using basic physiologic principles. This report thus became the first description of "high-dose" urography.

In the same year, Schenker popularized the technique of drip infusion pyelography in which a large volume (150 ml) of contrast medium diluted with an equal volume of dextrose and water was infused by gravity through an 18-gauge needle. This technique was touted as a method of achieving better visualization of the collecting system. Schenker theorized that the majority of improvement in opacification of the collecting system was due to a diuretic effect achieved by mixing the contrast medium with the dextrose and water. He believed that this would obviate the need for abdominal compression and dehydration, and that better visualization would be achieved by "flooding the collecting system from above."

In the late 1960s, Purkiss and associates developed an ultraviolet spectrographic absorption technique by which

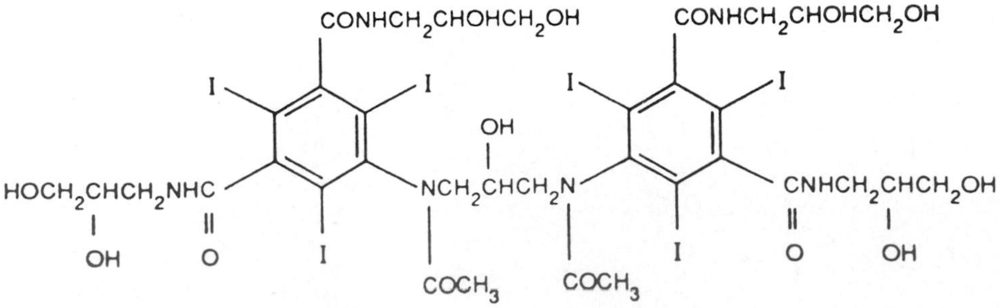

Figure 4.18.   Iodixanol (Visipaque)

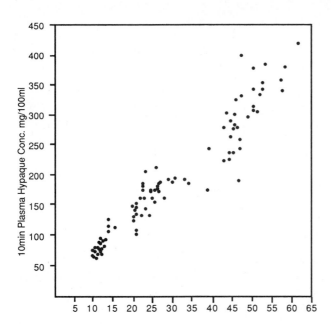

Figure 4.19. Graph showing that a linear relationship between plasma contrast concentration normalized to body surface area and administered dose is present 10 minutes after intravenous injection. (From Cattell WR, Fry IK, Spencer AG, et al.: Excretory urography I: factors determining the excretion of Hypaque. *Br J Radiol* 40(476):561–571, 1967).

plasma and urine contrast concentrations could be directly measured. In 1967, Cattel and colleagues at St. Bartholomew's Hospital in London used the technique to perform the first direct physiologic studies of contrast excretion in humans. They demonstrated a direct relationship between the plasma concentration of contrast and the dose of contrast administered (Fig. 4.19). In addition, they reported that the urinary contrast concentration is directly related to its rate of glomerular filtration. They further demonstrated that after intravenous injection of contrast medium, there is a rapid increase followed by a rapid decrease in plasma concentration of contrast. However, only 12% of the decrease in plasma concentration in the first 10 minutes after injection of contrast is caused by renal excretion; the remainder (88%) of the rapid decline is due to equilibration of the contrast throughout the ECF.

These studies were later amplified by Dure-Smith, who emphasized that while only 12% of the decrease in contrast concentration was due to excretion of the contrast by the kidneys, this 12% represents the critical amount of contrast that produces the diagnostic opacification of the urinary tract during urography, because during this period the glomerular filtration of the contrast medium is at its maximum (Fig. 4.20). It is therefore within the first few moments after injection that the nephrogram, representing

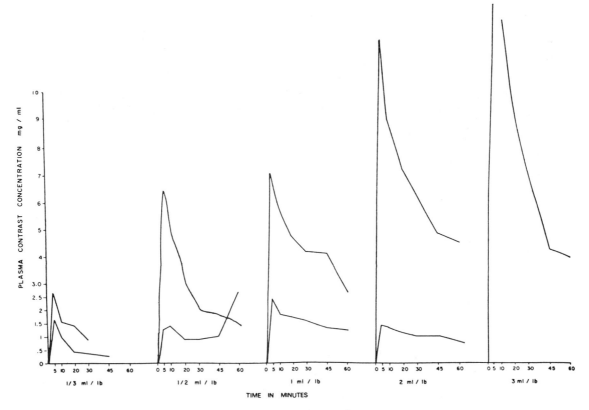

Figure 4.20. Minimum and maximum plasma concentration of contrast medium at various dose levels plotted against the time after injection. Approximately 12% of the rapid decrease is caused by excretion of the contrast in the urine. (From Dure-Smith P, Simenhoff M, Zimskind PD, et al.: The bolus effect in excretory urography. *Radiology* 101:29–34, 1971.)

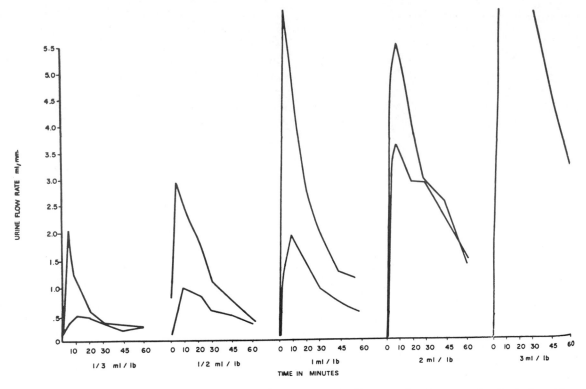

Figure 4.21. Minimum and maximum urine flow rates after varying doses of contrast medium. (From Dure-Smith P, Simenhoff M, Zimskind PD, et al.: The bolus effect in excretory urography. *Radiology* 101:29–34, 1971.)

contrast within the renal tubules, is at its peak intensity. Dure-Smith also pointed out that the degree of opacification of the urinary tract is not a function of the concentration of the contrast medium in the urine alone, but rather that it is the total amount of contrast (urinary contrast concentration times the volume of urine produced) on which opacification depends. Thus, opacification depends on the total number of iodine atoms in the path of the x-ray beam, rather than their concentration in the urine. Both Dure-Smith and Cattel demonstrated that there is a dose-related increase in urine flow rate that occurs after contrast administration related to the fact that the contrast medium acts as an osmotic diuretic (Fig. 4.21).

As we previously noted, the formula for glomerular filtration is

$$GFR = \frac{U_c V_c}{P_c}$$

Opacification of the urinary tract can be described by rearranging the equation so that

$$U_c V_c = GFR \times P_c$$

where U_c is the urinary contrast concentration, V_c is the volume of urine produced, P_c is the plasma concentration of contrast, and GFR is the patient's glomerular filtration rate. The product, $U_c V_c$, therefore, represents the total amount of contrast medium in the urine. Because

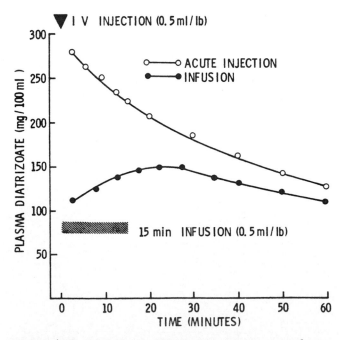

Figure 4.22. Comparison of plasma concentration of contrast medium from equivalent doses of diatrizoate administered by infusion and by bolus injection. The bolus injection produces a higher contrast concentration throughout the entire study. (From Cattell WR: Excretory pathways for contrast media. *Invest Radiol* 5(6):473–497, 1970.)

the GFR is fixed in any given patient, the only factor over which the radiologist has control is the plasma concentration, and this is directly related to the dose of contrast medium and the speed with which it is administered. Thus, the intensity of the nephrogram is directly related to these two factors. As a corollary, in a patient with a reduced GFR, P_c must be raised proportionately to achieve the same U_cV_c that would give satisfactory opacification in a patient with normal renal function. Therefore, the improvement in opacification described by Schenker with the drip infusion technique was not related to the method of administration of contrast, but rather to the total dose of contrast administered (Fig. 4.22). While the rate of excretion of contrast medium is greatest in the first 10 minutes after injection, it falls logarithmically thereafter. With increasing time, the contrast that had equilibrated with the ECF, returns to the vascular space and is excreted. Approximately 24 hours is required to excrete 100% of the administered dose (Fig. 4.23).

The sequential change in computed tomography (CT) attenuation value for the renal cortex that occurs after bolus administration of contrast medium intravenously directly correlates with the amount of iodine administered. Indeed, a plot of CT number against time (Fig. 4.24) produces a curve similar in appearance to the plot of plasma contrast concentration against time. Therefore, the change in CT number in the renal cortex following contrast administration accurately reflects the physiology of contrast excretion.

Physiologic Considerations

Body Size and Dose

The dose of contrast administered is the greatest single factor affecting the quality of opacification achieved

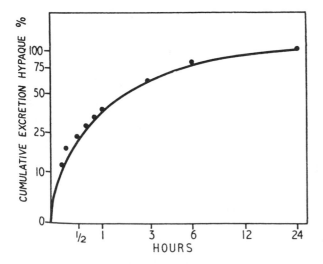

Figure 4.23. Graph demonstrating cumulative excretion of Hypaque. (From Cattell WR, Fry IK, Spencer AG, et al.: Excretory urography 1—factors determining the excretion of Hypaque. *Br J Radiol* 40(476):561–571, 1967.)

during excretory urography. It is generally useful to relate the dose administered to the body weight of the patient and to quantitate the dose in terms of the amount of iodine administered. In this fashion, contrast media of varying concentrations can be equated. In an average patient with normal renal function, a dose of 15 to 20 g of iodine will generally produce a satisfactory study. In obese patients, a proportionately larger dose is customarily employed; although the size of the vascular compartment is unrelated to body weight, there is such rapid equilibration of the contrast medium between the vascular compartment and ECF, that a higher dose contrast medium is desirable.

Age and Dose

There is a progressive decrease in GFR with age; this is generally attributed to nephron loss as a result of nephrosclerosis (Table 4.1). This nephron loss may not be reflected in the serum creatinine level, because there is a corresponding loss of muscle mass, as well. In addition, atheromatous disease results in nephron loss from multiple small cortical infarcts. As a result, it is prudent to administer a higher dose of contrast medium to patients in an older age group.

Correspondingly, in the pediatric age group, there is an inverse relationship between age and the GFR; at birth, the absolute GFR is under 5 ml/min which, when corrected for body surface area, represents a GFR of 20–30 ml/min/1.73 m^2. By the age of 1 year, however, the GFR corrected for body surface area has reached a level comparable to that of the adult patient; however, the absolute GFR in children remains diminished until adolescence. It is customary, therefore, to use a larger dose related to body weight in the pediatric age group than is commonly used for adult examinations.

It is customary in adult patients to round off the administered dose to the nearest 25 ml; for children, except infants, the dose is usually rounded off to the nearest 5 ml.

Other Considerations

TYPE OF CONTRAST MEDIUM.   With conventional ionic contrast media, the various anions in use are all derivatives of benzoic acid, and the differences in these anions usually does not significantly affect the renal handling of the medium.

The cations, sodium or methylglucamine, however, do affect the physiologic property of the contrast. The sodium-based media result in a higher urinary contrast concentration, because the sodium is resorbed actively by the tubules. Some authors have suggested that this factor results in a detectably greater density in the pyelogram when compared with studies performed with methylglucamine. Methylglucamine, however, is not resorbed by the tubules, and therefore contributes to the osmotic di-

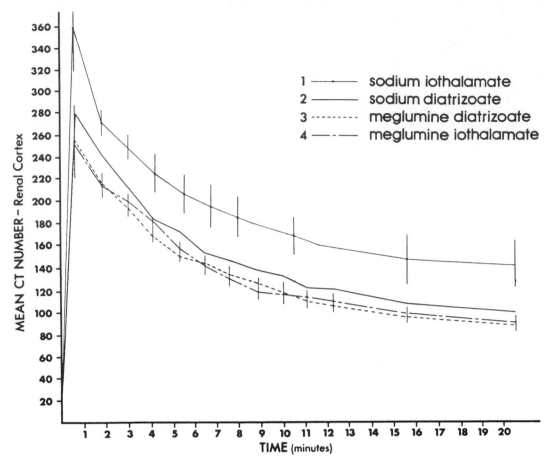

Figure 4.24. The sequential change in CT numbers measured in the renal cortex after an acute injection of contrast material shows a rapid decline similar to that shown in Figure 4.18. (From Brennan RE, Curtis JA, Pollack HM, et al.: Sequential changes in the CT numbers of the normal canine kidney following intravenous contrast administration: I. the renal cortex. *Invest Radiol* 14(2):141–148, 1979.)

uresis that is obtained after contrast administration. Theoretically, this should result in slightly improved distention of both the renal tubules and the collecting system. This increased distention, therefore, may result in slightly denser opacification of the nephrogram. In practice, how-

ever, the differences between sodium and methylglucamine are very slight, and in the vast majority of patients, do not significantly affect urographic quality.

With low-osmolar contrast media, a significantly higher urinary contrast concentration is produced and is accompanied by a significantly reduced osmotic diuresis compared with ionic contrast media. Total iodine excretion rates, however, are similar (Fig. 4.25). It has been demonstrated that urography using low-osmolar contrast media produces perceptibly greater opacification of the collecting system, but that abdominal compression is required to achieve satisfactory distention. There is little perceptible difference in the quality of the tubular phase (nephrogram) of the urogram.

STATE OF HYDRATION.   In the past, overnight fluid restriction often was recommended to improve the diagnostic quality of urography. The rationale of this approach was based on solid physiologic principles—namely, that in a dehydrated state, ADH production is stimulated and this results in a more concentrated urine. At the same time, however, a lower urine volume is produced. Ex-

Table 4.1.
Contrast Dose Schedule for Excretory Urography[a]

Patient Group	Dose
Adults	
Less than 40 years of age	100–150 mg I_2/lb (⅓–½ ml/lb)
40–55 years	150–200 mg I_2/lb (½–¾ ml/lb)
55 years and older	200–300 mg I_2/lb (¾–1 ml/lb) up to a maximum initial dose of 125 ml)
Pediatric patients	
Infant	400 mg I_2/lb (1½ ml/lb)
Childhood	300 mg I_2/lb (1 ml/lb)
Adolescence	150–200 mg I_2/lb (½–¾ ml/lb)

[a]Dosage in parentheses is calculated using standard urographic media containing 300 mg I_2/ml.

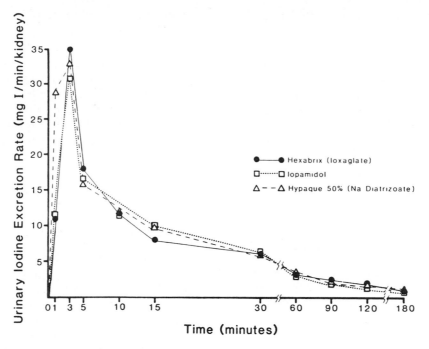

Figure 4.25. The total excretion rates for nonionic, ionic low-osmolar, and conventional contrast media are similar. (From Spataro RF, Fischer HW, Boylan L: Urography with low-osmolality contrast media: comparative urinary excretion of iopamidol, Hexabrix, and diatrizoate. *Invest Radiol* 5(17): 494–500, 1982.)

perimental studies in animals show that, with dehydration, the urinary contrast concentration is indeed increased compared with the nondehydrated state. However, when higher doses of contrast medium are used, the relative contribution of increased urinary concentration to total opacification is diminished. Furthermore, it has been shown that the usual period of overnight fluid restriction is ineffective in producing a statistically significant change in preinjection urinary osmolality. In addition, the increment of increased contrast concentration that is needed to be visible radiographically at the usual contrast concentrations in the collecting system approaches 80 to 100%. This level of increase is unlikely to be approached by fluid restriction alone.

While these data demonstrate little evidence in support of the practice of fluid restriction before urography, there is little doubt that inadvertent dehydration may occur as a result of bowel preparation, the diuresis that occurs from the contrast medium itself, and overnight fluid restriction. This inadvertent dehydration may pose an increased risk to the patient, particularly, the so-called high-risk debilitated patient or the patient with multiple myeloma. Whether dehydration plays a role in contrast-induced nephrotoxicity remains an open question, and this will be discussed later in this chapter (*see* Contrast-Induced Renal Dysfunction). For all these reasons, however, deliberate fluid restriction before contrast administration cannot, therefore, be recommended.

It is clear, however, that deliberate overhydration may have an adverse effect on pyelographic density when the hydration is sufficient in and of itself to produce a sustained diuresis. It is unlikely that such a diuresis could be achieved in the average patient with routine oral hydration, but in patients being hydrated with intravenous fluids, a "washout" of the pyelogram can occur. This is often the case, for example, when an emergency urogram is performed in surgery. The quality of the nephrogram, however, is usually unaffected.

The ideal patient for urography, therefore, is one in a state of euhydration, and this is probably best achieved by giving the patient or the referring physician no specific instructions on fluid intake before a urographic study.

TYPE OF EXAMINATION. Much of the foregoing discussion has centered on the physiologic factors affecting the quality of opacification in excretory urography. As has been discussed, the greatest single factor affecting the quality of the urogram is the dose of contrast administration, and it is usually necessary to increase the dose of contrast in patients with reduced renal function. The same considerations, however, do not apply when the contrast is to be administered for other types of examinations. When the purpose of contrast administration is to achieve generalized organ opacification in head or body CT in patients with depressed renal function, a proportionately lower dose of contrast may be used, because there will be less renal excretion. With angiographic examinations, the type of contrast used and the dose administered is usually governed by the type of examination and by the maximum dose of contrast that may be safely administered.

The optimal method of contrast administration for body CT has been studied extensively. After contrast administration, three distinct phases of contrast enhancement can be identified: (*a*) a bolus phase (an attenuation difference of 30 Hounsfield units [HU] or greater between the aorta and the inferior vena cava); (*b*) a nonequilibrium phase (aorto-caval difference of between 10–30 HU); and (*c*) an equilibrium phase (aorto-caval difference of less than 10 HU). Studies have suggested that enhancement and thus tissue differentiation is greatest in all three phases for body CT when the contrast medium is administered as a bolus rather than by infusion technique. During spiral CT examination, three distinct phases of contrast enhancement of the kidneys can be seen after a bolus of contrast medium has been administered by a mechanical injector: these are termed (*a*) the corticomedullary phase, (*b*) the nephrographic phase, and (*c*) the excretory phase.

Extrarenal (Vicarious) Excretion

In patients with normal renal function, less than 1% of a dose of injected contrast medium is excreted via a nonrenal route. The primary routes of nonrenal excretion are through the biliary tract and the small bowel. Under normal circumstances, this excretion is not detectable on plain radiographs, even when a high dose of contrast medium is employed. Contrast may be visible, however, in the gallbladder on CT scans made 15 to 48 hours after a large dose of contrast medium is administered. This visibility is presumed to be related to the high contrast sensitivity of CT and is not a manifestation of renal or hepatic disease.

In patients with depressed renal function, however, excretion of the contrast via the biliary and small bowel routes is markedly increased and may be visible on plain films. Such excretion has been termed *vicarious excretion*. The exact mechanism for this phenomenon is not certain, but it is speculated that in such patients protein binding of the contrast medium occurs and that this results in increased hepatic excretion. As a corollary, contrast administration is believed to be contraindicated in patients with hepatic and renal disease, because both the hepatic and renal routes for excretion may be impaired. In addition to biliary excretion, there is evidence that there is direct transmural excretion of contrast through the small bowel. Such excretion is usually not visible until the contrast reaches the colon, where water absorption increases the concentration of the contrast medium. Direct colon excretion of the contrast medium is not thought to occur.

The phenomenon of vicarious excretion may occasionally be seen in patients with unilateral ureteral obstruction but a functioning opposite kidney, and in whom overall renal function is normal. The explanation for such cases is poorly understood; there is speculation that this is related to decreased total renal blood flow and prolonged recirculation of the contrast medium.

There has been a concern that the administration of contrast media to patients with little or no renal function might have adverse hemodynamic effects, and therefore, immediate hemodialysis after contrast administration should be instituted. It has been shown, however, that dialysis is not necessary and that even functionally anephric patients can be given nonionic contrast media without discernible effects. The contrast so administered will be excreted through biliary and small bowel routes.

CONTRAST MEDIA: PHYSICAL PROPERTIES

A variety of physical and chemical properties may be used to describe the contrast media in general use in the United States. With the older, ionic contrast media, the strength of the contrast is frequently expressed in terms of percent concentration. This number represents the number of grams of the contrast per 100 ml of water. For example, Hypaque 50 (Nycomed Inc., NY, NY) is 50 g of sodium diatrizoate in 100 ml of water. This designation does not, per se, describe the amount of iodine in solution; but in general, the higher the percent concentration, the more radioopaque the contrast medium. Some contrast media use the numerical designation to denote the amount of iodine in milligrams per milliliter of the contrast medium. Thus, Conray 325 (Mallinckrodt Chemical Works, St. Louis, MO) contains 325 mg of iodine per milliliter of solution.

The *osmolality* of a contrast solution is equal to the number of particles in solution per kilogram of water. It is determined by the concentration of contrast medium and the molecular size of the compound. Thus

$$Osmolality\ (mOsm/kg) = \frac{mgI/ml}{N \times 127} \times K \times G$$

where N is equal to the number of iodine atoms per molecule; 127 is the molecular weight of iodine; K is the number of particles in solution; and G is the osmotic coefficient of the specific media that varies with concentration and molecular size. Because K is equal to 2 for ionic contrast media and is equal to 1 for nonionic contrast media, one can readily determine that the nonionic agents have approximately one half the osmolality of ionic agents at equal iodine concentrations. The osmolality of differing contrast media must be compared with one another at equal iodine concentrations, because the lower the iodine concentration, the lower the osmolality. In general, the larger the molecular weight of the agent, the lower the osmolality.

Another physical property of contrast media is *viscosity*. This property describes the relative adhesiveness of the molecules of the contrast medium for one another and is important because the viscosity of the contrast

Table 4.2.
Commonly Used Contrast Media in Uroradiology

Trade Name	Generic Name	Manufacturer	Type/Ratio[a]	Percent Solution	Amount of Iodine (mg/ml)	Osmolality (mOsm/kg)	Viscosity at 37°C (CPS)
Conventional Ionic							
Cysto Conray II	Meglumine iothalmate	Mallinckrodt	Ionic monomer/1.5	17.2	81	430	1.5[b]
Cystografin	Meglumine diatrizoate	Bracco	Ionic monomer/1.5	18.0	85	349	1.44
Conray 30	Meglumine iothalmate	Mallinckrodt	Ionic monomer/1.5	30.0	141	681	1.43
Hypaque 30%	Meglumine diatrizoate	Nycomed	Ionic monomer/1.5	30.0	141	633	1.43
Reno-M-DIP	Meglumine diatrizoate	Bracco	Ionic monomer/1.5	30.0	141	644	1.44
Conray 43	Meglumine iothalmate	Mallinckrodt	Ionic monomer/1.5	43.0	202	1025	2.24
Conray	Meglumine iothalmate	Mallinckrodt	Ionic monomer/1.5	60.0	282	1539	4.13
Reno-M-60	Meglumine diatrizoate	Bracco	Ionic monomer/1.5	60.0	282	1404	4.44
Renografin-60	Sodium 8% meglumine 52% diatrizoate	Bracco	Ionic monomer/1.5	60.0	292	1450	4.27
Hypaque 50%	Sodium diatrizoate	Nycomed	Ionic monomer/1.5	50.0	300	1515	2.43
Conray 325	Sodium iothalmate	Mallinckrodt	Ionic monomer/1.5	54.3	325	1797	2.83
Hypaque 60%	Meglumine diatrizoate	Nycomed	Ionic monomer/1.5	60.0	282	1415	4.10
Hypaque 76%	Sodium 10% meglumine 66% diatrizoate	Nycomed	Ionic monomer/1.5	76.0	370	2016	8.32
Renografin 76	Sodium 10% meglumine 66% diatrizoate	Bracco	Ionic monomer/1.5	76.0	370	1940	8.40
Conray 400	Sodium iothalmate	Mallinckrodt	Ionic monomer/1.5	66.8	400	2348	4.49
Low-Osmolar							
Omnipaque 240	Iohexol	Nycomed	Nonionic monomer/3.0	51.8	240	520	3.40
Optiray 240	Ioversol	Mallinckrodt	Nonionic monomer/3.0	50.9	240	502	3.00
Ultravist 240	Iopromide	Berlex	Nonionic monomer/3.0	51.8	240	483	2.80
Isovue 250	Iopamidol	Bracco	Nonionic monomer/3.0	51.0	250	524	3.00
Visipaque 270	Iodixanol	Nycomed	Nonionic dimer/6	55.0	270	290	5.90
Isovue 300	Iopamidol	Bracco	Nonionic monomer/3.0	61.2	300	616	4.70
Oxilan 300	Ioxilan	Cook Imaging	Nonionic monomer/3.0	62.0	300	585	5.10
Ultravist 300	Iopromide	Berlex	Nonionic monomer/3.0	64.7	300	607	4.90
Omnipaque 300	Iohexol	Nycomed	Nonionic monomer/3.0	64.7	300	672	6.30
Optiray 320	Ioversol	Mallinckrodt	Nonionic monomer/3.0	67.8	320	702	5.80
Visipaque 320	Iodixanol	Nycomed	Nonionic dimer/6	65.2	320	290	10.30
Hexabrix	Sodium 19.6% meglumine 39.3% ioxaglate	Mallinckrodt	Monoacidic ionic dimer/3.0	58.9	320	600	7.50

Table 4.2.—*continued*

Trade Name	Generic Name	Manufacturer	Type/Ratio[a]	Percent Solution	Amount of Iodine (mg/ml)	Osmolality (mOsm/kg)	Viscosity at 37°C (CPS)
Omnipaque 350	Iohexol	Nycomed	Nonionic monomer/3.0	75.5	350	844	10.4
Optiray 350	Ioversol	Mallinckrodt	Nonionic monomer/3.0	75.5	350	792	9.00
Oxilan 350	Ioxilan	Cook Imaging	Nonionic monomer/3.0	73.0	350	695	8.10
Isovue 370	Iopamidol	Bracco	Nonionic monomer/3.0	75.5	370	796	9.40
Ultravist 370	Iopromide	Berlex	Nonionic monomer/3.0	76.0	370	774	10.0

[a]Ratio is number of iodine atoms per molecule/number of particles in solution.
[b]at 25°C

determines how rapidly the contrast may be injected. The viscosity of contrast media decreases with increasing temperature. The unit of viscosity is the poise; the commonly used unit is the centipoise (CPS), which is equal to 0.01 poise.

A list of several of the contrast media commonly used in uroradiology in the United States is presented in Table 4.2.

Drug Incompatibilities

Conventional ionic contrast medium forms a precipitate when mixed with some drugs, including some antihistamines and amobarbital sodium. Ioxaglate has been reported to be incompatible with vasodilators such as papaverine. To prevent such incompatibilities, it is important that intravenous lines or catheters be thoroughly flushed before injecting pharmacologic agents after contrast medium has been injected.

ADVERSE REACTIONS TO CONTRAST MEDIA

Reactions to contrast media, while uncommon, continue to constitute a significant hazard to patients despite considerable research into their nature, incidence, and mechanism. Minor side effects including flushing, a metallic taste in the mouth, and tachycardia are common; they usually resolve within a few minutes and should not be considered reactions in the usual sense.

Adverse effects of contrast media can generally be divided into two groups: (*a*) idiosyncratic or anaphylactoid reactions, those which mimic an allergic response to contrast media; and (*b*) chemotoxic effects, those thought to be secondary to a direct toxic effect of the contrast medium. Since many of the known reactions to contrast media mimic those produced by known allergens (i.e., urticaria or bronchospasm) but are not mediated by immunoglobulins, these reactions are sometimes referred to as *anaphylactoid*.

Idiosyncratic Reactions

Idiosyncratic reactions are generally classified as: (*a*) mild, (*b*) moderate, (*c*) severe, and (*d*) death. Mild reactions are defined as those having physiologic side effects requiring no therapy. Moderate reactions are those that are transient and not life-threatening, but usually require therapy. Severe reactions are defined as those that are life-threatening and that require intensive therapy. The symptoms of these reactions are listed in Table 4.3.

In separate studies, Shehadi (1975) and Ansell (1970) cite an overall incidence of 4.7% of contrast reactions with conventional ionic high-osmolar contrast media

Table 4.3.
Symptoms of Contrast Medium Reactions

Minor
  Nausea
  Mild vomiting, retching
  Heat sensation
  Mild urticaria
  Flushing
  Arm pain
  Tachycardia
  Sneezing
Intermediate
  Faintness, mild hypotension
  Severe vomiting
  Generalized urticaria
  Bronchospasm, laryngospasm (mild)
  Dyspnea
  Facial edema
  Vasovagal reaction
Severe
  Hypotension (systolic blood pressure <70 mm Hg)
  Loss of consciousness
  Pulmonary edema
  Epiglottic edema, severe bronchospasm
  Cardiac arrest
  Sustained cardiac arrhythmia

(HOCM) in unselected series after intravenous injection. Of these, mild reactions represent the great majority (3.3%). Moderate reactions comprise 1 to 2%. Severe reactions occur in only 0.009% of patients after intravenous contrast injection.

Objective data on the incidence of contrast reactions with low-osmolar contrast media (LOCM) have mostly been based on trials outside the United States. Katayama evaluated more than 300,000 patients who received intravenous contrast media for a variety of examinations in Japan. The overall incidence of an adverse drug reaction was 12.7% in those who received ionic contrast media; in patients who received nonionic contrast media, the overall incidence was 3.1%. More importantly, the incidence of severe and very severe contrast reactions was 0.26% for ionic media and 0.04% for nonionic media. Katayama estimated that nonionic media could be considered safer by a factor of 6 compared with conventional contrast. In another study, Palmer reviewed 106,000 patients for the Royal Australian College of Radiology. Their patients were stratified into high- and low-risk categories and were given ionic or nonionic contrast media at the discretion of the attending radiologist. Adverse reactions occurred 5 times more commonly in low-risk patients who received ionic media compared with those who received nonionic contrast. Reactions were 3 times more common in low-risk patients who received ionic contrast media when compared with high-risk patients who received nonionic contrast media. Severe reactions were 4.5 times as common in the ionic group for all patients. While the methodology of this study has been criticized, the results are generally consistent with the findings of other large-scale trials.

The incidence of death after intravenous injection of conventional ionic contrast media has generally been reported to range from 1:14,000 to 1:75,000; 1:40,000 is the most consistently reported figure. The death rate in patients who receive nonionic contrast media has been difficult to estimate. There were only two deaths in Palmer's study (both in the ionic group), and only one death in each group in the Katayama study.

Because so few deaths have been reported in these large-scale comparative studies, Caro and associates undertook to examine the relative frequency of death after contrast injection using metaanalysis, a technique whereby data from independent studies can be combined for statistical analysis. This study indicated that the risk of death is very low with either type of contrast media and that there is no statistically significant difference between LOCM and HOCM. For severe reactions, it was estimated that a risk reduction of 126 per 100,000 contrast examinations could be achieved by using LOCM. Thus, the authors concluded that 80% of severe reactions associated with HOCM could be prevented

with LOCM. Other large-scale studies also have confirmed that the difference in death rate for the two classes of contrast media is small.

Lalli, in a survey based on data reported by manufacturers involving deaths due to contrast media, found that the majority of deaths involved a cardiovascular event including acute myocardial infarction, ventricular fibrillation, or pulmonary edema. The initial symptoms in patients who subsequently had a fatal contrast reaction was frequently nausea and vomiting or respiratory distress. Other common initial symptoms include hypotension, cardiac arrhythmia, seizures, restlessness, and chills. Only one patient in this series presented with urticaria as the initial manifestation of a subsequently fatal reaction.

Risk Factors

Factors that may predispose a patient to developing an idiosyncratic reaction to contrast medium have been extensively studied. In general, patients at greatest risk are in the older age groups and have significant preexisting disease.

Patients with a history of allergy to food, drugs, and ragweed (i.e., hayfever) or asthma have an increased chance of having a contrast reaction, but the magnitude of this increased risk varies somewhat in the reported series (Table 4.4). Witten and colleagues indicate a minimal increased risk for most types of allergies when compared with the overall 4.7% incidence of reactions in the general public, while Shehadi indicates that the risk may be increased as much as threefold. The data are of special interest with respect to seafood allergy which is popularly believed to correlate highly with a sensitivity to contrast. Using Shehadi's (1975) data, 85% of such patients will undergo a contrast examination without an adverse reaction.

A history of a previous reaction to the administration of contrast media is the greatest single predictor of an

Table 4.4.
Incidence of Reactions Related to Type of Allergic History

	Incidence of Reaction (%)	
Type of Allergy	Witten	Shehadi
Asthma	6	11.2
Hayfever	4	10.3
Seafood	6	15.0
Other food	6	14.0
Other allergies	7	13.0
Penicillin, sulfa	—	7.5

Data from Witten DM, Hirsch FD, Hartman GW: Acute reactions to urographic contrast medium. *AJR* 119:832–840, 1973; Shehadi, WH: Adverse reactions to intravascularly administered contrast media. *AJR* 124:145–152, 1975.

untoward reaction. In the series by Witten and colleagues, 20% of patients giving a history of mild or moderate reaction to contrast on reexamination suffered a contrast reaction; in Shehadi's (1975) series, the number varied between 16 and 22%. No patient in Witten's series experienced a reaction that was more serious than was the case on the prior exposure to the contrast medium, although this occurrence has been reported by others. A history of prior exposure to contrast media without difficulty in the past does not confer immunity to a subsequent contrast reaction. Multiple cases have been reported in which patients suffered a contrast reaction after several prior studies without difficulty. In Shehadi's most recent report (1982) from the cooperative study of the International Society of Radiology, approximately 1% of the reactions reported occurred in patients with a history of no reaction to a prior examination. Thus, a history of prior mild or moderate reaction to contrast media should not be taken as an absolute contraindication to reexamination when a repeated study is grounded on sound medical indications. At worst, only 20% of such patients will experience a contrast reaction on re-challenge. A history of a severe reaction to contrast media, however, is considered a contraindication to reexamination in all but the most urgent cases.

In a randomized prospective study designed to identify which risk factors were important predictors of an increased risk of a contrast reaction, Barrett (1992a) concluded that a history of prior contrast medium reaction and a history of allergy to food or drugs were the only independent risk factors associated with a statistically important increased risk of reaction. This study was unable to validate the previous observation that a history of asthma also places the patient at increased risk.

Other Factors

Sex

The incidence of reactions is virtually identical overall in men and women.

Age

The incidence of moderate and severe reactions is approximately equal in all age groups. The data do not validate the commonly held notion that reactions are virtually unknown in the pediatric population. Ansell's (1980) data indicate that the majority of deaths, however, occur in the older (greater than 50 years) age group. Most of the deaths occur in patients with significant preexisting cardiac or vascular disease. This observation also has been substantiated by Shehadi (1985).

Dose

The incidence of reactions is unrelated to the dose for mild and moderate reactions; for severe reactions,

the incidence appears to be slightly higher when larger doses (greater than 20 g of iodine) are used. In fact, Ansell (1980) reported the incidence of reactions to be 3 times greater when infusion pyelography was compared with conventional urography.

Rate of Administration of the Contrast

Several studies have shown no difference in the rate of reactions when rapid administration of the contrast was compared to slow injection. These data contrast with the popular opinion that rapid administration of the contrast increases its side effects.

Type of Examination

Intraarterial contrast injection appears to reduce the overall incidence of reactions by approximately one half to an incidence of 2.3%; however, it may be associated with a higher percentage of severe reactions than the intravenous route. With nonvascular examinations, (e.g., retrograde pyelography) the exact incidence of reactions is very difficult to determine, but anaphylactoid reactions and deaths have been reported. In these cases, it is assumed that a small amount of contrast has been absorbed into the vascular system.

Type of Contrast

There appears to be little difference among the HOCM in the overall rate of reactions. Ansell (1970) reports, however, that bronchospasm appears to be 4 times as common when the methylglucamine salts are used compared with the pure sodium salts. The data for LOCM have been described in the previous section. Ioxaglate (Hexabrix), however, appears to produce nausea and vomiting with frequency comparable to that of HOCM. This is in contrast to the nonionic media in which the incidence of nausea and vomiting is less than 1.5%.

Timing of Reactions

Most contrast reactions occur within the first 10 minutes after injection of the contrast medium; some patients have symptoms almost immediately, while in others, the reaction is not noted until the end of the examination. A few patients report the development of arm pain or urticaria several hours after the examination has been completed.

Late reactions to contrast media (defined as those occurring between 30 minutes and 2 days after contrast administration) also have been reported with LOCM and HOCM. For the most part, such reactions are not severe and most often are manifested by headache or a skin eruption; they are usually described as self-limiting.

An atypical form of late reaction to contrast medium has also been reported in patients receiving interleukin-2 for chemotherapy. The majority of such reactions occur 1 to 8 hours after contrast exposure and consist of erythema, diarrhea, flu-like symptoms, flushing, joint pain, pruritus, and other nonspecific symptoms. Such reactions recall or mimic those produced by the chemotherapy itself. In an occasional patient, such symptoms may be sufficiently severe to require hospitalization.

Miscellaneous Factors

Patients receiving β-adrenergic blockers or those with severe underlying cardiovascular disease have been shown to be at increased risk for developing an anaphylactoid reaction manifested as bronchospasm.

Mechanism of Contrast Reactions

At present, there is no universally accepted mechanism that acceptably explains the diverse manifestations of idiosyncratic contrast reactions. Possible mechanisms are listed in Table 4.5

Brasch has been the principal proponent of an antigen-antibody mediated mechanism. There are a few case reports in which IgE or IgM antibodies to contrast have been reported in patients suffering severe contrast reactions. Brasch also has demonstrated significantly greater binding of serum immune globulins in patients who have had contrast reactions when compared with nonreactors. Analogues of contrast media, when chemically linked to a carrier protein, can act as a haptene and induce antibodies in rabbits. Indeed, the most suggestive evidence, albeit indirect, in support of the antigen-antibody hypothesis is the immune-like nature of some contrast reactions, and thus the designation anaphylactoid.

Despite these data, there is overwhelming evidence that in the majority of cases, contrast reactions are not mediated by the immune system. The fact that some patients react on their first exposure to contrast (and thus, before any sensitization) and that most repeat reactions are not progressive militate against the immune theory. In addition, no circulating antibody can be demonstrated in the sera of the vast majority of patients studied after contrast reactions. Finally, rats immunized with diatrizoate conjugated to albumin do not manufacture anticontrast immunoglobin (IgE).

Lalli (1980) has proposed that anxiety, mediated through the hypothalamus, plays a significant role in the pathogenesis of contrast reactions. He believes that small amounts of contrast medium cross the blood-brain barrier, and in the presence of anxiety on the part of the patient or the patient's perception of anxiety on the part of radiology personnel, provoke a contrast reaction by activation of the limbic system. In support of this hypothesis are data that show that diazepam, which depresses the limbic system, significantly increases the lethal median dose (LD_{50}) of iothalmate (see definition of LD_{50} under Chemotoxic Effects, below).

Histamine release has been implicated in the pathogenesis of contrast reactions. It is known that contrast can induce histamine release from mast cells and basophils, but whether this can occur in sufficient quantities to produce the type of reaction seen with contrast sensitivity has been questioned. Activation of the complement system has been shown to occur after contrast administration, and this mechanism is implicated by other authorities. Whether a cause-and-effect relationship between complement activation and the clinical syndrome of contrast sensitivity exists remains in doubt, however.

Attention also has been directed toward the contact system as a cause of reactions to contrast media. This system begins with activation of clotting factor XII (possibly by local disruption of the vascular endothelium as a result of the needle puncture and the introduction of the contrast medium) and continues as a cascade involving the activation of kallikrein from prekallikrein and kinins from high-molecular-weight kinogens. Lasser (1980) has demonstrated a higher rate of prekallikrein-kallikrein transformation in patients who have suffered contrast reactions than in nonreactors.

Still other factors have been implicated. Clustering of reactions has at times suggested that these adverse effects are the result of contamination of the contrast medium itself, rather than as the result of an untoward reaction to the contrast on the part of the patient. Chemical tests of contrast medium from the same lot of contrast implicated in a contrast reaction, however, have almost always proven fruitless. It has been suggested that such clustering may be the result of contamination of the contrast medium by lubricants or other contaminants in the rubber seals of the plastic syringes used to inject the contrast. This observation prompted the recommendation that contrast media be drawn into the syringe immediately before use rather than in advance, as is done in many departments. It is further recommended that contrast media be stored upright, so as to avoid contamination from the rubber stoppers used to seal the

Table 4.5.
Possible Mechanisms for Idiosyncratic Contrast Reactions

Antigen-antibody reaction
Anxiety
Cholinesterase inhibition
Calcium binding
Complement activation
Disruption of the blood-brain barrier
Hemodynamic alterations
Histamine release
Injection of impurities
Protein binding

Modified from Katzberg RW (Ed). *The Contrast Media Manual 1992.* Baltimore, Williams and Wilkins, 1992.

contrast vials. Finally, additives, preservatives, or chelators added to the contrast media by the manufacturers have been implicated as a possible source of untoward contrast reactions.

The observation that LOCM are associated with a lower rate of contrast reactions has directed attention toward osmolality as an important factor in the genesis of contrast reactions. Although many hemodynamic effects of contrast are reduced with LOCM (see Chemotoxic Effects below) it is difficult to attribute a reduction in idiosyncratic reactions to this factor alone. LOCM also reduce the binding of ionized calcium, which has been implicated as a possible mechanism for the induction of ventricular fibrillation during coronary angiography. In addition, since LOCM are associated with a lower degree of lipid binding, there is a lower degree of neurotoxicity because of reduced penetration of the blood-brain barrier. Some have speculated that this mechanism might explain the reduced incidence of reactions seen with LOCM if such reactions are mediated by a central nervous system mechanism.

Iodism, an acute reaction to the iodine itself, is a syndrome characterized by sialadenitis, diarrhea, and occasionally pulmonary edema that has been reported after contrast administration. Such cases are referred to as "iodine mumps." Such cases are reported with both LOCM and HOCM. Contact allergy to iodine-containing products is thought to be unrelated to contrast sensitivity. As such, sensitivity to such iodine containing products such as povidone-iodine solution (Betadine—The Purdue Frederick Co., Norwalk, CT) should not be considered a contraindication to the administration of contrast media.

Prevention of Anaphylactoid Contrast Reactions

Attempts to predict or modify anaphylactoid reactions to contrast media have been attempted with varying degrees of success for a number of years. Predictions of those who will have an adverse reaction to contrast media have largely centered around the use of a test dose of contrast. At various times, intradermal, subcutaneous, intraoccular, and intravenous test doses of contrast have been used. The most widely used procedure has been the intravenous test dose; however, it has not been shown reliably to predict a subsequent adverse reaction to the full dose of contrast medium, and its use has largely been abandoned. In Lalli's (1980) series of fatal contrast reactions, 29 of 32 patients given a test dose showed no adverse affect, but subsequently died after administration of the full dose; the remaining 3 patients died after the test dose itself. In Witten's series, the test alone induced nausea and vomiting in 28 patients; in all 28 patients, the administration of the full dose of contrast continued after the initial symptoms subsided. Only 6 of the 28 patients experienced nausea

and vomiting after receiving a full dose of contrast medium.

The inability of a test dose to accurately predict a subsequent adverse reaction to contrast medium was recently reaffirmed in a large-scale study conducted by the Japanese Committee on the Safety of Contrast Media in a study which involved 337,647 patients.

The routine use of antihistamines, either mixed with the contrast media or administered immediately before the contrast study, was described more than 40 years ago. No data, however, show that this technique in any way modifies the overall incidence of severe adverse reactions to contrast medium. At least one double-blind study has demonstrated a protective effect against minor reactions for hydroxyzine, an ataraxic agent with antihistaminic activity given at least 12 hours before exposure to ioxaglate. Others have demonstrated a similar effect for both H_1 and H_2 antihistamines.

Because of the anaphylactoid-like nature of idiosyncratic reactions, the empirical use of corticosteroids to prepare "high-risk" patients for contrast studies has been used for many years. Lasser (1977) has presented theoretical and limited experimental evidence in an animal model that pretreatment with steroids may help in preventing some minor contrast reactions, when the steroids were administered more than 12 hours before the contrast study.

A multi-institutional randomized prospective study reported by Lasser (1987) showed that two doses of orally administered corticosteroids (methylprednisolone, 32 mg) at 12 and 2 hours prior to a contrast examination significantly reduced the incidence of contrast reactions of all types in a group of patients who received conventional ionic contrast media. There was no such protective effect in a group of patients who received a single dose of steroids 2 hours before examination. In this study, Lasser found that the incidence of contrast reactions using conventional ionic media with steroid pretreatment approached the overall incidence of reactions using nonionic media without pretreatment. In another study, Wolf, Arenson, and Cross (1989), using an identical protocol to the one used by Lasser, found an overall incidence of reactions of 4.4% in those who received ionic contrast, 4.0% in those who received ionic contrast and steroid premedication, and 0.6% in those who received iohexol. In an update of the above study which involved almost 9000 patients, Wolf (1991) reported that iohexol reduced mild reactions by sixfold, moderate reactions by sixfold to ninefold, and severe reactions by tenfold when compared with ionic contrast alone or in combination with steroid premedication.

Greenberger has presented data on clinical trials of pretreatment with corticosteroids in patients who have a history of a prior contrast reaction. In this study, 10 of 150 patients experienced mild reactions on re-challenge with contrast medium, an incidence well below that which would have been predicted if no pretreatment regimen had been used. There were no serious contrast reactions in this series. The regimen they used consisted of prednisone, 50 mg orally, every 6 hours, for three doses ending 1 hour before the contemplated examination and diphenhydramine, 50 mg intramuscularly, 1 hour before the study. In an expanded series, Greenberger reports that a pretreatment regimen consisting of prednisone, diphenhydramine, and ephedrine reduced the overall rate of reaction on re-challenge to 5%. Ephedrine should be withheld in patients with hypertension or unstable angina.

Severe reactions have been reported despite pretreatment regiments. In Lalli's (1980) series of contrast media–associated deaths, 3 of the 140 patients who died during urography had received pretreatment with corticosteroids.

In patients with a documented prior reaction to ionic contrast medium, Siegle and colleagues (1991) have shown that only 5.5% of patients given nonionic contrast medium (iohexol) suffered a repeat reaction. The majority of such reactions were mild, and only one patient in the series suffered a repeat reaction more serious than the prior reaction. This incidence is in contrast to the expected 20% incidence of repeat reactions without premedication. In a small subset of the series, patients who were given steroid preparation and nonionic contrast media were not shown to have a significantly lower repeat reaction rate than those given iohexol alone. The authors of this study warned that this data should be interpreted with caution, because this portion of the study was not randomized.

In a randomized controlled study, Lasser (1994) demonstrated that pretreatment with 32 mg of prednisolone significantly decreased the incidence of mild reactions in patients receiving intravenous nonionic contrast examinations. Although there also was a decrease in the number of moderate and severe reactions, this difference did not reach statistical significance.

Chemotoxic Effects

Chemotoxic effects are those effects of the contrast medium thought to be due to direct organ toxicity of the contrast medium. The LD_{50} is a number commonly used in toxicology to describe the dose of a compound that will kill 50% of the affected test animals. The LD_{50} values for various contrast media in mice are provided in Table 4.6.

In humans, the primary manifestation of contrast overdosage is neurotoxicity, including the induction of seizures. The exact dose in humans at which this occurs is not known, but systemic doses of contrast medium exceeding 5 to 6 ml/kg should be exceeded only in special circumstances. The neurotoxicity of nonionic con-

Table 4.6.
Lethal Median Dose (LD_{50}) of Various Contrast Agents

Contrast Medium	LD_{50} (g I/kg)
Sodium/meglumine diatrizoate	7.6
Sodium iothalmate	8.0
Ioxaglate	10.2–13.5
Metrizamide	18.1
Iopamidol	21.8–22.1
Iohexol	24.3

Modified from McClennan BL: Low osmolality contrast media: premises and promises. *Radiology* 162:1–8, 1987.

trast media has been shown to be less than that of ionic media in in vitro experiments. In addition, the second-generation nonionic contrast media (iohexol and iopamidol) show less neurotoxicity than metrizamide, perhaps because there is less interference with glucose metabolism in the brain with these agents.

Hyperosmolar Effects

Conventional ionic media (HOCM) cause vasodilatation, vascular spasm, hemodilution, changes in red cell morphology, and changes in vascular permeability, all of which are related to their high osmolality. Changes in the permeability of the blood-brain barrier also are likely related to osmolality and may be responsible for some of the neurotoxicity of HOCM. As would be expected, LOCM markedly reduce these effects in human and animal studies.

Cardiovascular Effects

Several studies have demonstrated that significant electrocardiographic abnormalities may occur during the intravenous administration of contrast media. These changes, which consist of tachycardia, minor or major cardiac arrhythmias, and ischemic changes, are transient and may occur in a small number (5%) of patients with normal baseline electrocardiograms and in up to 25% of patients with preexisting cardiac abnormalities. These changes are usually asymptomatic and are only discovered if electrocardiographic monitoring is employed. These abnormalities have been attributed to a direct toxic effect of the contrast medium on the heart, but whether these changes play a role in the development of hypotensive contrast reactions is not known. Recent studies using LOCM have demonstrated a marked reduction in the frequency of such changes, and for this reason, the use of LOCM in patients with significant underlying cardiac disease has been advocated.

Ionic contrast media reduce free ionic calcium levels and subsequently increase serum parathormone levels. The decrease in serum calcium levels is presumed to be caused by divalent cation chelators that the manufacturers add to the contrast media. The magnitude of the decrease in serum calcium is so small as to be clinically insignificant, except in a small number of patients with pre-existing cardiac disease in whom the contrast medium is administered for coronary angiography. In these patients, this mechanism has been implicated in the development of cardiac arrhythmias.

HOCM are known to exert negative inotropic and chronotropic actions on the heart; both of these effects are diminished with LOCM.

Hematologic Effects

HOCM inhibit platelet aggregation and cause a prolongation of the thrombin time by inhibition of fibrin monomer polymerization. These anticoagulant properties have a beneficial effect in angiography by helping to prevent thrombus formation in catheters and syringes. In addition, red cell deformation has been reported after incubation with HOCM. This phenomenon may explain the pulmonary hypertension that occasionally complicates pulmonary angiography. In patients with sickle cell anemia, contrast medium is known to provoke sickling and occasional development of sickle cell crisis. LOCM cause less inhibition of platelet aggregation than HOCM. Caution must be exercised when using LOCM in angiographic procedures, because clots may form in contrast-containing syringes and then may be inadvertently injected into patients.

Thrombophlebitis

A chemical phlebitis may develop after injection of contrast medium, particularly when it is used for venography of the lower extremities. This complication has been reported in up to 30% of patients when 60% contrast is used and is most likely the result of prolonged contact of the contrast medium with the venous endothelium as the result of slow flow. The clinical syndrome can be markedly reduced by using diluted contrast medium and other measures including use of a heparinized saline flush following the procedure. It may rarely be seen in patients in whom the contrast medium has been injected in the upper extremity for other imaging studies. The incidence of thrombophlebitis is markedly reduced with LOCM.

Extravasation of Contrast Medium

Subcutaneous or intradermal extravasation of some contrast medium is not uncommon, particularly since the advent of mechanical injectors used in CT to produce consistent organ enhancement. Such extravasation may result in local pain, erythema, and swelling, but these symptoms usually resolve with local therapy and without sequelae, even when amounts as large as 150 ml are extravasated.

Rarely, significant tissue necrosis and dermal sloughing can occur unpredictably with even very small amounts of extravasation. In some cases, the extravasation may be so small as to be inapparent until the complication develops. When severe sloughing and local necrosis develops, the extremity may turn cold with severe ecchymosis and edema. The pulses in the extremity may vanish. These features are typical of a compartment syndrome and may require extensive releasing incisions and subsequent skin grafting. Most of the reported cases in which this extensive reaction develops are in children or in the elderly. Such reactions also occur more commonly when the injection was made in either the hand or the foot. This phenomenon may occur with LOCM or HOCM.

INDICATIONS FOR THE USE OF LOW-OSMOLAR CONTRAST MEDIA

Accumulated data indicate that LOCM have a significantly lower incidence of adverse drug reactions (ADRs) than do HOCM. Overall, the rate of reactions after intravenous use is reduced by a factor ranging from four- to eightfold, and the chemotoxic effect of contrast is significantly lowered. For urography, physiologic studies indicate a higher excretion rate for LOCM and urographic quality that is at least as good as that obtained with HOCM. In addition, there is a marked improvement in patient tolerance for LOCM, particularly for previously painful angiographic procedures. These data would seem to indicate that LOCM should completely replace HOCM for most imaging studies. In parts of Canada and Europe, this has largely been the case. In the United States, two schools of thought have been developed. The first group has argued that the available data justify a complete switch to LOCM, at least for intravenous use. The second group have advocated a policy of "selective use" of LOCM, largely because LOCM costs significantly more than HOCM, and have suggested that a cost-benefit analysis justifies using LOCM only for "high-risk" patients.

Those who argue for universal use of nonionic contrast media point to evidence suggesting that the largest identifiable risk factor is the contrast medium itself, and that were cost not a factor, LOCM would completely replace HOCM. Assignment of "high risk" cannot be made without a certain degree of subjectivity; indeed in one study that was designed to enforce a policy of selective use, it was found that during the study period, the use of LOCM increased from 26.5% to 55.3% despite unchanging criteria. In addition, studies designed to identify which factors would place a patient into a high-risk category have identified previous reaction to contrast material as the only factor that can be consistently identified from study to study. Although when LOCM were first introduced the price differential was 10 to 25 times that of HOCM, over the years the price differential has narrowed so that presently, LOCM only costs five to eight times more than HOCM.

The arguments for selective use also are persuasive. Wolf (1986) has estimated that approximately 5.2 million contrast-assisted procedures are performed in the United States per year and that a total switch to LOCM will increase the yearly expenditures for contrast studies in this country by over $300 million. Jacobson and Rosenquist estimate that the annual expenditure for contrast would be $80 million if only HOCM were used in the United States; a complete switch to low-osmolar contrast media would cost $1.5 billion.

Barrett and coworkers (1992a) performed a study in which nearly 2,000 patients perceived to be at high risk for the administration of HOCM were randomized into two groups; one received LOCM and the other received HOCM. While there was indeed a reduction in the number of ADRs from 3.9% to 0.9% in the LOCM group, if one looked at the outcome of the reaction rather than the incidence, the number of therapeutic interventions requiring the attention of a physician only increased from 0.5% with LOCM to 1.4% with HOCM. Furthermore, almost all of the difference was due to a reduction in the number of urticarial reactions. There were no life-threatening reactions or deaths in either group. Gertsman reviewed the findings in the Katayama study and concluded that epidemiologic flaws in the study may have biased the results to show a greater difference in ADRs between LOCM and HOCM than should be present. The most serious of these flaws was the failure to precisely define an ADR and a possible selection bias, because patients in the study were not randomly assigned. Gertsman further argued that serious reactions and deaths were rare in either group, despite the large number (more than 300,000) of patients studied. Other studies have confirmed that the death rate is low in both groups.

Other investigators have found that it is possible to enforce a policy of selective use. Using criteria developed locally or modified from recommendations of the American College of Radiology's Manual on Iodinated

Table 4.7.
Indications for the Use of Low-Osmolar Contrast Media

Previous reaction to contrast medium
History of asthma or allergy
History of cardiac disease or dysfunction
Generalized debilitation
Blood dyscrasia
Risk of aspiration
Age less than 1 year
Other[a]

[a]Situations in which the supervising radiologist believes that the patient would benefit from low-osmolar contrast media. Such cases might include patients with poor communication skills, severe anxiety, or a patient preference for low-osmolar contrast media.
Modified from the *Manual on Iodinated Contrast Media,* ©1991 American College of Radiology.

Contrast Media or from the Society of Cardiovascular and Interventional Radiology, it has been found in separate studies that use of LOCM could be limited to between 21 to 38% of the total number of intravenous contrast examinations, with considerable cost savings. Suggested criteria are listed in Table 4.7.

Despite these statistics, manufacturers' data indicate that the percent share of LOCM of the total iodinated contrast media market has grown from less than 5% in 1986 to more than 75% in 1994.

CONTRAST-INDUCED ACUTE RENAL DYSFUNCTION

Reports linking contrast media with the development of acute renal failure began to appear with increasing frequency in the early 1970s. In one of the initial studies, Krumlovsky and colleagues reported eight patients in whom acute renal dysfunction (ARD) developed following exposure to radiographic contrast media identified during a period in which 7125 contrast procedures were performed at their institution, an incidence of 0.112%. In other reported series, the incidence of contrast-induced renal failure has ranged from 0 to 100%, when only selected patients who were retrospectively identified as being at high risk for the development of this complication are considered.

At least part of this discrepancy in incidence is related to varying definitions of what constitutes ARD and to reports based on poorly controlled retrospective data. There is no doubt that contrast medium has been held responsible for ARD in some cases that are multifactorial in etiology. This impression is substantiated in a report by Cramer in which patients undergoing cranial CT were evaluated for the presence of ARD. Their study included three patients who experienced ARD after head CT, but who had not received contrast medium.

The definition of ARD has varied widely in the reported series. Most authors define ARD as an increase in blood urea nitrogen (BUN) of 50% or 20 mg/dl and/or an increase in serum creatinine of 50% or 1 mg/dl within 48 hours of the procedure. Others have required an absolute rise in creatinine of 1 mg/dl or have required the rise to occur within 24 hours of the administration of the contrast. In some series, when GFR has been measured, ARD has been defined as a 25% change in GFR.

ARD associated with contrast material is usually non-oliguric and in the typical case, the serum creatinine peaks in 3–5 days and returns to baseline values within 7–10 days. In the rare case, the renal failure is oliguric and in these cases the damage is more likely to be permanent.

Most studies have identified specific risk factors for the development of contrast-induced ARD. However, conflicting data are often present in other studies.

Risk Factors

Preexisting Renal Insufficiency

Preexisting renal insufficiency has been identified as a major risk factor. In most studies, the higher the baseline level of serum creatinine, both the risk for developing ARD and the magnitude of the renal compromise that was present were increased. D'Elia and coworkers in a study of 378 patients undergoing angiography defined the risk of ARD as 33% for patients with baseline serum creatinine levels more than 1.5 mg/dl or serum BUN levels more than 30 mg/dl; for the remainder of the patients in their series, the incidence was 2%. An even higher incidence of ARD (41.7%) in patients with preexisting azotemia was cited by Martin-Paredero and colleagues. Of their patients, 8.3% required dialysis.

Preexisting renal insufficiency has not been found to predispose patients to ARD in other studies. In a prospective study, Parfrey and coworkers concluded that there was little risk of clinically important nephrotoxicity after use of contrast material in patients with preexisting renal insufficiency. Mason studied 120 patients who underwent angiography and found an overall incidence of ARD of 31%; however, there was no difference between those with preexisting renal insufficiency and those without. Cruz and coworkers studied 125 patients, including 11 with baseline creatinine values greater than 4 mg/dl, and did not find a single case of ARD. Preexisting renal insufficiency, when secondary to obstructive uropathy, has not been associated with an increased risk of contrast-induced ARD.

These data are of particular interest because, prior to 1960, renal dysfunction was considered a contraindication to the use of contrast media. In 1963, Schwartz and colleagues introduced "high-dose" urography specifically for the purpose of identifying those patients in whom there was a correctable cause of renal insufficiency. They concluded that contrast administration was safe and efficacious in patients with renal insufficiency. Other early studies by Gup, MacEwan, and others showed no deleterious effect of contrast media on renal function. The precise factors that have contributed to the apparent dramatic change in the appreciation of the nephrotoxic potential of contrast media are not known.

Diabetes Mellitus

Harkonen and coworkers found that 76% of 29 diabetic patients with baseline creatinine levels greater than 2 mg/dl had deterioration of renal function after exposure to contrast medium; in 9 of these patients, the deterioration was irreversible. He found the risk of nephrotoxicity to be greatest in patients with long-standing diabetes (particularly of juvenile onset) and in those requiring insulin. VanZee and colleagues found the presence of diabetes to be a major risk factor regarding contrast-induced ARD. There was deterioration of renal function in 50% of diabetics with baseline creatinine values of 1.5 to 4.5 mg/dl and in 100% of the small number studied with baseline creatinine values greater than 4.5 mg/dl. In neither series were diabetic patients without renal insufficiency at greater risk than the general population for development for ARD.

Conflicting data concerning the risk of diabetes for the development of contrast-induced ARD also can be found. In a study by Mason and coworkers, diabetics were at no increased risk compared to the remainder of the study group. Parfrey and associates concluded in a prospective study that the risk for diabetic patients with preexisting renal insufficiency for ARD was 9%, much lower than previously reported.

Dehydration

Some authors speculate that dehydration from the contrast study itself or from the preparation for the study may play a role in the development of contrast-induced ARD. Harkonen and coworkers found that the state of hydration did not appear to play a role, however. Eisenberg and colleagues believed that vigorous hydration with normal saline could prevent the development of ARD. In his series of 537 patients in whom hydration was maintained before and during angiography, no patients with ARD were identified. Other authors, however, have reported conflicting data. Martin-Paredero and Gomes both report that hydration during and after a contrast study did not prevent the development of ARD in their patients. Others have reported that volume expansion with mannitol or the use of furosemide may be beneficial in protecting high-risk patients from the development of ARD.

Dose of Contrast

Lang and colleagues thought that the dose of contrast administered was a major factor in the development of ARD. In his series, the incidence of ARD increased with increasing dose of contrast material. In other series, however, ARD has been described in patients receiving contrast containing as little as 30 g of iodine. Cruz and coworkers did not find an increased incidence of ARD in the subgroup of their study who received a dose of contrast medium containing greater than 48 g of iodine. Hayman and colleagues found no difference in the incidence of ARD after contrast-enhanced cranial CT when a dose of 43 g of iodine was compared to a dose of 80 g. Miller and associates reported no consistent effect on renal function with increasing doses of ionic or nonionic contrast media.

Type of Contrast

Multiple studies have addressed the relative nephrotoxicity of LOCM compared to HOCM. Some authorities had speculated that because of lower osmolality, decreased chemotoxicity would be observed. Indeed, LOCM have been shown to cause less of an effect on renal blood flow, reduced proteinuria, less damage to proximal tubular epithelial cells in vitro, and a smaller increase compared to HOCM in urinary excretion of proximal tubular enzymes like alkaline phosphatase and N-acetyl-b-glucosaminidase (NAG), considered to be sensitive indicators of proximal tubular damage. In addition, LOCM can experimentally be shown to produce less nephrotoxicity than HOCM in several animal models. Nonetheless, several clinical studies initiated and reported shortly after the approval of LOCM in the United States, showed no difference in ARD between LOCM and HOCM. Several studies reported more recently, however, have shown that the LOCM may be associated with lower nephrotoxicity under certain conditions. Harris and coworkers prospectively studied 101 adult patients with preexisting renal insufficiency undergoing CT and found that serum creatinine increased by at least 25% in 2% of patients receiving LOCM compared to a similar increase in 14% of patients receiving HOCM. No patient, however, in either group experienced clinically significant ARD. Katholi and colleagues studied 70 patients with normal or mildly depressed renal function undergoing coronary angiography in a prospective, randomized, double-blind fashion and found a decrease in creatinine clearance of 19% in patients receiving LOCM compared with a decrease of 40% in those receiving HOCM. Barrett prospectively studied 117 patients undergoing cardiac catheterization in a nonrandomized fashion and found that the increase in serum creatinine after the study was associated with the severity of the preexisting renal disease and the presence of diabetes, but not the type (LOCM vs HOCM) of contrast medium. Subsequently, the same author reported on the relative nephrotoxicity of high- and low-osmolar contrast media by pooling data from 31 different trials reported in the literature using metaanalysis, a technique that determines whether data from different studies can be meaningfully added together to increase its statistical power. He concluded that a statistically meaningful benefit of LOCM on renal function could only be shown in patients with preexisting renal impairment (serum creatinine > 120μmol/L) who received intraarterial contrast material. A beneficial effect for LOCM could not be demonstrated for patients with normal renal function (with or without diabetes) or for those receiving intravenous contrast administration.

Other Factors

A multitude of other factors have been implicated in the development of other contrast-induced ARD. These include advanced age, hypertension, the presence of peripheral vascular disease, digitalis requiring congestive heart failure, proteinuria, and liver dysfunction. Multiple contrast studies within a short interval (72 hours or less) also have been implicated.

Patients with multiple myeloma have long been thought to be at increased risk for ARD because of precipitation of myeloma proteins in the renal tubules. This mechanism for renal dysfunction associated with myeloma after contrast administration has recently been questioned. Some investigators now believe that dehydration, hypercalcemia, infection, and Bence-Jones proteinuria are the most important risks for the development of ARD in patients with myeloma. Most authorities now feel contrast studies in patients with myeloma can be performed with safety, provided dehydration is avoided.

The mechanism for contrast-induced ARD remains obscure, and our understanding of the pathogenesis of this disorder is hampered by the lack of a reproducible animal model. Speculation has centered around structural changes in the proximal tubule epithelium, contrast-induced vasoconstriction of renal blood vessels, and increased tubular pressure caused by the osmotic diuresis associated with contrast media. In support of this theory is the observation that calcium antagonists may mitigate some of the deleterious effect of contrast medium on the kidney. Such agents are known potent renal vasodilators. Other investigators have demonstrated that contrast medium can cause lysis of proximal tubule cells in vitro in the presence of ischemia and that this damage is reduced when nonionic contrast medium is used.

Still other investigators have focused on intratubular obstruction, perhaps caused by contrast-induced precipitation of Tamm-Horsfall proteins, or by other causes. In support of this theory, Older and coworkers report that a persistent nephrogram will be seen 24 hours after the contrast medium has been administered in approximately 50% of the patients subsequently shown to develop contrast-induced ARD. A similar phenomenon has recently been reported on CT. Several studies have shown that contrast medium acts as a powerful uricosuric agent, and this mechanism has been implicated in the development of acute urate nephropathy in patients with hyperuricemia. This syndrome also may be encountered in patients with myeloproliferative disorders or leukemia after chemotherapy. The role of the uricosuric effect of contrast in other cases of ARD is probably small.

TREATMENT OF ADVERSE REACTIONS TO CONTRAST MEDIA

Every physician using contrast media must be prepared to deal with a contrast-induced emergency. These preparations should be thorough, but not so extensive as to cause undue alarm on the part of the patient. An organized plan to deal with the emergency, so that the physicians and technical staff work together in a coordinated fashion, is desirable. All personnel in the department must be familiar with the location of emergency drugs and equipment.

A common sense approach to dealing with the emergency should be used, because overtreatment may be as disastrous as undertreatment. Familiarity with the basic principles of cardiopulmonary resuscitation (including A—airway, B—breathing, C—circulation) is mandatory. The physician responsible for the contrast study must be immediately available for at least 10 minutes after the injection and should be generally available for the next 30 minutes. Equipment for resuscitation, including blood pressure monitoring equipment, drugs, and oxygen, must be immediately available. Access to other equipment such as ventilators, cardiac monitors or electrocardiograph machines, and defibrillators is desirable. It is prudent to inject the contrast medium through a secure intravenous line that is then left in place for the first several minutes after the injection so that immediate venous access is available should the need arise.

The radiologist should be prepared to deal with mild and moderate reactions, as well as the initial therapy of severe reactions. However, life-threatening reactions occur so infrequently in the career of an average radiologist that it is prudent to have available the assistance of physicians who deal with resuscitative emergencies on a more frequent basis. Therefore, only general principles for the initiation of therapy will be offered here.

At the first sign of a significant reaction, the patient's pulse and blood pressure should be assessed. It is also prudent to perform chest auscultation to assess the adequacy of ventilation.

Appropriate therapy for acute reactions to contrast media is summarized in Table 4.8.

Minor Reactions

Minor reactions, by definition, are not serious and for the most part do not require therapy.

Nausea and vomiting is the most common adverse reaction encountered with HOCM. The cause for such reactions is poorly understood; because it is commonly

Table 4.8.
Treatment of Acute Contrast Media Reactions

Type of Reaction	Drug	Dose/Route	Comments
Nausea and vomiting	None	—	Supportive measures; usually transient
Urticaria, mild	None	—	Self-limiting; supportive therapy only
Urticaria, generalized	Diphenhydramine *or* Cimetidine *or* Ranitidine	25–50 mg slow IV or IM 300 mg diluted in 10 ml 50 mg diluted in 10 ml	Observe for drowsiness Administer slowly Administer slowly
Bronchospasm/wheezing Mild Moderate or severe	Epinephrine 1:1000 metaproterenol *or* terbutaline *or* albuterol *or* aminophylline	0.1–0.3 cc subcutaneous Deep inhalations 2 times 6 mg/kg in D5W loading dose IV infused over 10–20 minutes 0.4–1.0 mg/kg/hr maintenance	β-agonist inhaler Onset slow and somewhat unpredictable; may potentiate hypotension
Facial edema	Epinephrine 1:1000	0.1–0.3 cc subcutaneous	May be repeated 3 times
Laryngospasm/edema	Epinephrine 1:1000	0.1–0.3 cc subcutaneous	If severe, may require intubation
Bradycardia w/wo hypotension	Atropine IV fluids (NS)	0.6–1.0 mg IV slowly Rapid infusion	Caution in patients on β-blockers (i.e., propranolol)
Hypotensive tachycardia	IV fluids (LR>NS) Epinephrine 1:1000 1:10,000 Dopamine Hydrocortisone	Rapid infusion 0.1–0.3 cc subcutaneous 1.0–3.0 ml IV 2.0–20.0 μg/kg/min IV 0.5–1.0 gm IV	Place patient in Trendelenburg; O₂ use in young patients; use IV if in circulatory collapse; caution in elderly or those on nonselective β-blockers use in patients unresponsive to above questionable value acutely; may prevent delayed symptoms
Seizures	Diazepam	2.0–10.0 mg IV	
Ventricular arrhythmias	Lidocaine 1%	1.0–1.5 mg/kg (5.0–10 ml loading dose IV) 1.0–4.0 mg/min maintenance	Must have cardiac monitor, defibrillator; if not quickly reversed prepare to call a code

seen after intravenous administration of ioxaglate, a low-osmolar ionic contrast medium, some have speculated that it is related to the ionicity of the contrast medium itself. Others have speculated it is a vasomotor effect, but it may occur after only a few milliliters of the contrast medium has been injected. Nausea and vomiting is generally self-limited; it is normally treated by slowing or temporarily stopping the contrast infusion. In most cases, the nausea will pass and the contrast administration may be safely resumed; the patient should be continually monitored, because nausea and vomiting can be the precursors of a major anaphylactoid reaction.

Occasionally, limited urticarial reactions may benefit from the administration of antihistamines, primarily for their antipruritic effect. Caution should be exercised when using antihistamines, particularly in outpatients, because of their tendency to cause drowsiness. Some authors have found that the H_2 antagonist, cimetidine, is of value in the treatment of contrast-induced urticarial reactions and have recommended their use in addition to or in place of the H_1 antagonist, diphenhydramine.

More extensive dermal reactions usually respond to antihistamines (i.e. diphenhydramine 50 mg IV given over 1 or 2 minutes or cimetidine 300 mg IV, diluted in 10 ml of 5% dextrose solution administered slowly. Epinephrine (1:1000), 0.1 to 0.3 ml administered subcutaneously, may be necessary if the urticaria is so extensive that generalized edema is present.

Respiratory Reactions

Bronchospasm and mild laryngospasm should be treated with epinephrine (1:1000) 0.3–0.5 ml administered subcutaneously. For mild reactions, a lower dose of 0.1–0.3 ml may be employed. The dose of epinephrine may be repeated in 15 minutes if no response is obtained. Alternatively, a β-agonist inhaler (i.e., metaproteranol, albuterol, or terbutaline) may be used. In severe cases, it may be necessary to add aminophylline, 5 to 6 mg/kg intravenously infused over 20 to 30 minutes as a loading dose, followed by a maintenance dose of 0.4 to 1.0 mg/kg/hr. Aminophylline, however, may accentuate hypotension and should only be used if the bronchospasm fails to respond to epinephrine, or in patients in whom epinephrine is contraindicated. Corticosteroids probably have no immediate impact on respiratory distress, but can be administered as a supplemental agent to prevent a secondary recurrence of the clinical symptoms.

Vasovagal Reactions

It is crucial to distinguish hypotensive bradycardia from hypotensive tachycardia. Vasovagal reactions are characterized by sinus bradycardia and may be present with or without hypotension. If the reaction is vagal in origin, atropine 0.6 to 1.0 mg intravenously should be administered. An additional dose of 0.5 mg may be administered every 5 minutes until a heart rate of 60 beats/min is achieved or a maximum dose of 3 mg has been given. If accompanied by hypotension, the patient should be placed in the Trendelenburg position, and large volumes of intravenous fluids such as lactated Ringer's solution or normal saline solution also should be administered.

Hypotensive Tachycardia

The vast majority of patients experiencing hypotensive anaphylactoid contrast reactions will have hypotensive tachycardia. Supportive measures such as placing the patient in the Trendelenburg position or elevating the legs as well as the administration of oxygen should begin immediately. In addition, electrocardiographic monitoring should be started.

Patients experiencing hypotensive tachycardia are manifesting circulatory hypovolemia resulting from a variety of factors including decreased venous return, decreased cardiac filling, peripheral vasodilatation, and most importantly, sequestration of fluid in nonvital compartments. In this circumstance, an effective circulatory hypovolemia ensues. Administration of large volumes of intravenous fluid has been shown to be a highly effective therapy. Isotonic saline or lactated Ringer's solution (500–1000 ml or more) should be administered intravenously as quickly as possible. The use of a second intravenous line may facilitate this therapy.

In younger patients, epinephrine (1:1000) 0.3 ml subcutaneously or 1 to 3 ml of 1:1000 diluted in 10 ml of saline (1:10,000) intravenously can be used if the hypotension is severe and if it fails to respond to fluid therapy alone. In older patients, especially those with significant underlying cardiovascular disease, epinephrine is fraught with hazard because of the tendency of this drug to produce cardiac arrhythmias. If an older patient fails to respond to fluid therapy alone, dopamine 10 to 20 mg/kg/min may be added. The rate of infusion should be titrated to the blood pressure response. Dopamine also should be used in younger patients who fail to respond to epinephrine.

The use of older pressor agents, such as levarterenol (Levophed—Sanofi-Winthrop Pharmaceuticals, Des Plaines, IL) and metaraminal (Aramine—Merck & Co., Inc., West Point, PA) as first-line agents should probably be avoided.

Patients taking β-adrenergic blocking agents (i.e., propranolol) may present a special problem in diagnosis, should hypotension develop during the course of a contrast reaction. β-blockers produce a sinus bradycardia that may not vary in the face of shock, making the distinction of a vasovagal reaction from an anaphylactoid reaction difficult. In addition, because epinephrine is both an α- and a β-adrenergic agonist, the β-blocker may successfully neutralize the β-effect of epinephrine, leaving its α effect unopposed. This combination of circumstances can result in a precipitous increase in blood pressure. In such cases, fluid therapy alone should probably be used until more specialized help becomes available. This is much less of a problem in patients receiving cardioselective blockers such as atenolol. Calcium channel blocking agents such as nifedipine and diltiazem are potent peripheral vasodilators and also may complicate the therapy of a contrast reaction.

Ventricular Arrhythmias

In the event that significant ventricular arrhythmias such as multifocal premature ventricular contractions, couplets, or ventricular tachycardia develop, immediate consultation with a qualified specialist should be obtained. A loading dose of lidocaine of 1 mg/kg may be administered, followed by an infusion at the rate of 1 to 4 mg/min. If sustained ventricular tachycardia with hypotension or ventricular fibrillation develops, electrical defibrillation will be necessary. If a full-scale cardiac arrest develops, cardiopulmonary resuscitation should immediately be instituted.

SUGGESTED READINGS

Functional Renal Anatomy and Renal Physiology

Andreoli TE, Culpepper RM, Thompson CS, Weinman EJ: Essentials of normal renal function. In Andreoli TE, Carpenter CCJ, Plum F, Smith LH (eds): *Cecil's Essentials of Medicine.* Philadelphia, WB Saunders, 1986.

Gottschalk CW, Lassiter WE: Mechanisms of urine formation. In Mountcastle VB (ed): *Medical Physiology,* vol 2, ed 14. St. Louis, CV Mosby, 1980.

Meschan I: Background physiology of the urinary tract for the radiologist. *Radiol Clin North Am* 3(1):13, 1965.

Vander AJ: *Renal Physiology,* ed 3. New York, McGraw-Hill, 1985.

Contrast Media: Historical Background

Almén T: Development of nonionic contrast media. *Invest Radiol* 20(suppl):S2, 1985.

Elkin M: Stages in the growth of uroradiology. *Radiology* 175: 297, 1990.

Gavant ML, Seigle RL: Iodixanol in excretory urography: initial clinical experience with a nonionic, dimeric (ratio 6:1) contrast medium. *Radiology* 183:515, 1992.

Grainger RG: Intravascular contrast media: the past, the present and the future. *Br J Radiol* 55(649):1, 1982.

Katzberg RW, Donahue LA, Morris TW, et al.: Ioxilan, a third generation low osmolality nonionic contrast medium. systemic and renal hemodynamic effects. *Invest Radiol* 25(1):46, 1990.

Luker GD, McAlister WH: High costs of low-osmolality contrast media. *AJR* 165(3):732, 1995.

Morris TW: X-ray contrast media: where are we now, and where are we going? *Radiology* 88:11, 1993.

Renwick IG, Fowler RC: A double blind comparison of iopromide and iopamidol in intravenous urography. *Clin Radiol* 41(6):405, 1990.

Svaland MG, Haider T, Langseth-Manrique K, et al.: Human pharmacokinetics of iodixanol. *Invest Radiol* 27(2):130,1992.

Physiology of Contrast Excretion

Becker JA, Gregoire A, Berdon W, Schwartz D: Vicarious excretion of urographic media. *Radiology* 90:243, 1968.

Benamor M, Aten EM, McElvany KD, et al.: Ioversol clinical safety summary. *Invest Radiol* 24(1):S67, 1989.

Benness GT: Urographic excretion study. *Invest Radiol* 11:261, 1967.

Benness GT: Urographic contrast agents: a comparison of sodium and methylglucamine salts. *Clin Radiol* 21:150, 1970.

Cattell WR: Excretory pathways for contrast media. *Invest Radiol* 5:473, 1970.

Cattell WR, Fry IK, Spencer AG, Purkiss P: Excretory urography I: factors determining the excretion of Hypaque. *Br J Radiol* 40(476):561, 1967.

Dure-Smith P: The dose of contrast medium in intravenous urography: a physiologic assessment. *AJR* 108(4):691, 1970.

Dure-Smith P, Simenhoff M, Brodsky S, Zimskind PD: Opacification of the urinary tract during excretory urography: concentration vs. amount of contrast medium. *Invest Radiol* 7:407, 1972.

Dure-Smith P, Simenhoff MB, Zimskind PD, Kodroff M: The bolus effect in excretory urography. *Radiology* 101:29, 1971.

Dyer RB, Gilpin JW, Zagoria RJ, et al.: Vicarious contrast material excretion in patients with acute unilateral ureteral obstruction. *Radiology* 177(3):739, 1990.

Lautin EM, Friedman AC: Vicarious excretion of contrast media. *JAMA* 247(11):1608, 1982.

Purkiss P, Lane RD, Cattel WR, et al.: Estimation of sodium diatrizoate by absorption spectrophotometry. *Invest Radiol* 3:271, 1968.

Schencker B: Drip infusion pyelography. *Radiology* 83:12, 1964.

Schwartz WB, Hurwit A, Ettiger A: Intravenous urography in the patient with renal insufficiency. *N Engl J Med* 269(6):277, 1963.

Sherwood T, Doyle FH: Value of fluid deprivation in large dose urography. *Lancet* 2:754, 1968.

Woodruff MW, Malvin RL: Localization of renal contrast media excretion by stop flow analysis. *J Urol* 84(5):677, 1960.

Younathan CM, Kaude JV, Cook MD, et al.: Dialysis is not indicated immediately after administration of contrast agents in patients with end-stage renal disease treated by maintenance dialysis. *AJR* 163(4):969, 1994.

Adverse Reactions to Contrast Media

Ansell G: Adverse reactions to contrast agents: scope of problem. *Invest Radiol* 5:374, 1970.

Ansell G, Tweedie MCK, West CR, et al.: The current status of reactions to intravenous contrast media. *Invest Radiol* 15(6 suppl): S32, 1980.

Barrett BJ, Parfrey PS, McDonald JR, et al.: Nonionic low osmolality versus ionic high osmolality contrast material for intravenous use in patients perceived to be at high risk: randomized trial. *Radiology* 183:105, 1992(a).

Barrett BJ, Parfrey PS, Vavasour HM, et al.: A comparison of nonionic, low osmolality radiocontrast agents with ionic, high osmolality agents during cardiac catheterization. *N Engl J Med* 326(7):431, 1992.

Berman HL, Delaney V: Iodide mumps due to low osmolality contrast material. *AJR* 159:1099, 1992.

Bernadino ME, Fishman EK, Jeffrey RB Jr, et al.: Comparison of iohexol 300 and diatrizoate meglumine 60 for body CT: image quality, adverse reactions and aborted/repeated examinations. *AJR* 158:665, 1992.

Bertrand PR, Soyer RM, Rouleau RJ, et al.: Comparative randomized double-blind study of hydroxyine versus placebo as premedication before injection of iodinated contrast media. *Radiology* 184:383, 1992.

Bettmann MA: Guidelines for use of low-osmolality contrast agents. *Radiology* 172:901, 1989.

Bettmann MA: Ionic versus nonionic contrast agents for intravenous use: are all the answers in? *Radiology* 175:616, 1990.

Bettmann MA, Holzer JF, Trombly ST: Risk management issues related to the use of contrast agents. *Radiology* 175:629, 1990.

Beyer-Enke SA, Zeitler E: Late adverse reactions to non-ionic contrast media: a cohort analytic study. *Eur Radiol* 3:327, 1993.

Brasch RC: Allergic reactions to contrast media: accumulated evidence. *AJR* 134:797, 1980.

Brasch RC: Evidence supporting an antibody mediation of contrast media reactions. *Invest Radiol* 15(6 suppl):S29, 1980.

Brismar J, Jacobsson BF, Jorulf H: Miscellaneous adverse effects of low-versus high-osmolality contrast media: a study revised. *Radiology* 179:19, 1991.

Caro JJ, Trindade E, McGregor M: The cost-effectiveness of replacing high-osmolality with low-osmolality contrast media. *AJR* 159:869,1992.

Caro JJ, Trindade E, McGregor M: The risks of death and of severe nonfatal reactions with high vs low osmolality contrast media: a meta-analysis. *AJR* 156:825, 1991.

Cashman JD, McCredie J, Henry DA: Intravenous contrast media: use and associated mortality. *Med J Aust* 155(4):618, 1991.

Carr DH: Contrast media reactions: experimental evidence against the allergy theory. *Br J Radiol* 57:469, 1984.

Choyke PL, Miller DL, Lotze MT, et al.: Delayed reactions to contrast media after interleukin-2 immunotherapy. *Radiology* 183:111, 1992.

Christensen J: Iodide mumps after intravenous administration of a nonionic contrast medium: case report and reveiw of the literature. *Acta Radiol* 36(1):82, 1995.

Cohan RH, Dunnick NR: Intravascular contrast media: adverse reactions. *AJR* 149:665, 1987.

Cohan RH, Ellis JH, Dunnick NR: Use of low osmolar agents and premedication to reduce the frequency of adverse reactions to radiographic contrast media: a survey of the Society of Uroradiology. *Radiology* 194(2):357, 1995.

Cohan RH, Dunnick NR, Leder RA, et al.: Extravasation of nonionic radiologic contrast media: efficacy of conservative treatment. *Radiology* 176(1):65, 1990.

Curry NS, Schabel SI, Reiheld CT, et al.: Fatal reactions to intravenous nonionic contrast material. *Radiology* 178:361, 1991.

Debatin JF, Cohan RH, Leder RA, et al.: Selective use of low-osmolar contrast media. *Invest Radiol* 26(1):17, 1991.

Dunnick NR, Cohan RH: Cost, corticosteroids, and contrast media. *AJR* 162(3):527, 1994.

Dyer R, Cohan RH: What is the risk of reaction on repeat exposure to contrast material, and how should the patients be premedicated? *AJR* 165(6):1543, 1995.

Fareed J, Walenga JM, Saravia GE, Moncada RM: Thrombogenic potential of nonionic contrast media? *Radiology* 174:321, 1990.

Fischer HW: Occurrence of seizure during cranial computed tomography. *Radiology* 137:563, 1980.

Fischer HW, Siegel R: Value of non-ionic contrast medium in previous reactors: experience thus far. *AJR* 154:195, 1990.

Fink U, Fink BK, Lissner J: Adverse reactions to non-ionic contrast media with special regard to high risk patients. *Eur Radiol* 2:317, 1992.

Gertsman BB: Epidemiologic critique of the report on adverse reactions to ionic and nonionic media by the Japanese Committee on the Safety of Contrast Media. *Radiology* 178:787, 1991.

Greenberger PA, Patterson R, Tapio CM: Prophylaxis against repeated radiocontrast media reactions in 857 cases. *Arch Intern Med* 145: 2197, 1985.

Hartman GW, Hattery RR, Witten DM, Williamson B Jr: Mortality during excretory urography: Mayo Clinic experience. *AJR* 139:919, 1982.

Higashi TS, Takizawa K, Nagashima J, et al.: Prospective two phase study of delayed symptoms after intravenous injection of low osmolality contrast media. *Invest Radiol* 26:S37, 1991.

Hirshfeld JW Jr: Low osmolality contrast agents-who needs them? *N Engl J Med* 326(7):482, 1992.

Hunter TM, Dye J, Duval JF: Selective use of low osmolality contrast agents for IV urography and CT: safety and effect on cost. *AJR* 163:965, 1994.

Johenning PW: Reactions to contrast material during retrograde pyelography. *Urology* 16(4):442, 1980.

Jensen N, Dorph S: Adverse reactions to urographic contrast medium: rapid versus slow injection rate. *Br J Radiol* 53:659, 1980.

Jacobson PD, Rosenquist CJ: The introduction of low-osmolar contrast agents in radiology: medical, economic, legal and public policy issues. *JAMA* 260:1586, 1988.

Katayama H, Yamaguchi K, Kozuka T, et al.: Adverse reactions to ionic and nonionic contrast media: a report from the Japanese Committee on the Safety of Contrast Media. *Radiology* 175:621, 1990.

Lalli AF: Contrast media reactions: data analysis and hypothesis. *Radiology* 134:1, 1980.

Lalli AF, Greenstreet R: Reactions to contrast media: testing the CNS hypothesis. *Radiology* 138:47, 1981.

Lang DM, Alpern MB, Visintainer PF, et al.: Elevated risk of anaphylactoid reaction from radiographic contrast media is associated with both beta-blocker exposure and cardiovascular disorders. *Arch Intern Med* 153(17):2033, 1993.

Lasser EC, Lang J, Sovak M, et al.: Steroids: theoretical and experimental basis for utilization in prevention of contrast media reactions. *Radiology* 125:1, 1977.

Lasser EC, Lang JH, Lyon SG, Hamblin AE: Changes in complement and coagulation factors in a patient suffering a severe anaphylactoid reaction to injection of contrast material: some considerations of pathogenesis. *Invest Radiol* 15(6 suppl):S6, 1980.

Lasser EC: A coherent biochemical basis for increased reactivity to contrast material in allergic patients: a novel concept. *AJR* 149:1281, 1987.

Lasser EC, Berry CC, Talner LB, et al.: Pretreatment with corticosteroids to alleviate reactions to intravenous contrast material. *N Engl J Med* 317(14):845, 1987.

Lasser EC, Berry CC: Adverse reactions to contrast media. ionic and nonionic media steroids. *Invest Radiol* 26:402, 1991.

Lasser EC, Berry CM Mishkin MM, et al.: Pretreatment with corticosteroids to prevent adverse reaction to nonionic contrast media. *AJR* 162:523, 1994.

Lawrence V, Matthai W, Hartmaier S: Comparative safety of high-osmolality and low-osmolality radiographic contrast agents. *Invest Radiol* 1:2, 1992.

Leung PC, Cheng CY: Extensive local necrosis following the intravenous use of x-ray contrast medium in the upper extremity. *Br J Radiol* 53:361, 1980.

Levin DC, Gardiner GA Jr, Karasick S, et al.: Cost containment in the use of low-osmolar contrast agents: effect of guidelines, monitoring, and feedback mechanisms. *Radiology* 189:753, 1993.

Madowitz JS, Schweiger MJ: Severe anaphylactoid reaction to radiographic contrast media: recurrence despite premedication with diphenhydramine and prednisone. *JAMA* 241(26):2813, 1979.

McCarthy CS, Becker JA: Multiple myeloma and contrast media. *Radiology* 183:519, 1992.

McClennan BL: Low osmolality contrast media: premises and promises. *Radiology* 162:1, 1987.

Michaelson A, Franken EA, Smith W: Cost-effectiveness and safety of selective use of low-osmolality contrast media. *Acad Radiol* 1:59, 1994.

Mikkonen R, Kontkanen T, Kivisaari L: Acute and late adverse reactions to low-osmolar contrast media. *Acta Radiol* 36(1):72, 1995.

Palmer FJ: The RACR survey of intravenous contrast media reactions: final report. *Australas Radiol* 32:426, 1988.

Panto PN, Davies P: Delayed reactions to urographic contrast media. *Br J Radiol* 59:41, 1986.

Pfister RC, Hutter AM Jr: Cardiac alterations during intravenous urography. *Invest Radiol* 15(6 Suppl):S239, 1980.

Powe NR: Low versus high-osmolality contrast media for intravenous use: a health care luxury or necessity? *Radiology* 183:21, 1992.

Powe NR, Steinberg EP, Erickson JE, et al.: Contrast medium-induced adverse reactions: economic outcome. *Radiology* 169:163, 1988.

Rivera M, Teruel JL, Castano JC, et al.: Iodine-induced sialadenitis: report of 4 cases and review of the literature. *Nephron* 63:466, 1993.

Robertson HJF: Blood clot formation in angiographic syringes containing nonionic contrast media. *Radiology* 163:621, 1987.

Sadler DJ, Parrish F, Coulthard A: Intravenous contrast media reactions: how do radiologists react? *Clin Radiol* 49(12):879, 1994.

Shehadi WH: Adverse reactions to intravascularly administered contrast media. *AJR* 124:145, 1975.

Shehadi WH: Contrast media adverse reactions: occurrence, recurrence, and distribution patterns. *Radiology* 143:11, 1982.

Shehadi WH: Death following intravascular administration of contrast media. *Acta Radiol (Diagn)* 26(Fasc 4):457, 1985.

Shehadi WH, Toniolo G: Adverse reactions to contrast media. *Radiology* 137:299, 1980.

Siegle RL: Current problems of contrast materials. *Invest Radiol* 21(10):779, 1986.

Siegle RL, Halvorsen RA, Dillon J, et al.: The use of iohexol in patients with previous reactions to ionic contrast material. a multicenter clinical trial. *Invest Radiol* 26(5):411, 1991.

Siegle RL, Lieberman P, Jennings BR, Rice MC: Iodinated contrast material: studies relating to complement activation, atopy, cellular association and antigenicity. *Invest Radiol* 15(6 suppl):513, 1980.

Thomsen HS. Dorph S: High-osmolar and low-osmolar contrast media. an update on frequency of adverse drug reactions. *Acta Radiologica* 34(fasc 3):205, 1993.

Stadalnik RC, Vera Z, DaSilva O, et al.: Electrocardiographic response to intravenous urography: prospective evaluation of 275 patients. *AJR* 129:825, 1977.

Stovsky MD, Seftel AD, Resnick MI: Delayed hypersensitivity reaction after infusion of nonionic intravenous contrast material for an excretory urogram: a case report and review of the literature. *J Urol* 153(5):1641, 1995.

Weese DL, Greenberg HM, Zimmern PE: Contrast media reactions during voiding cystourethrography or retrograde pyelography. *Urology* 41(1):81, 1993.

White RI, Halden WJ Jr: Liquid gold: low osmolality contrast media. *Radiology* 159:559, 1986.

Witten DM, Hirsch FD, Hartman GW: Acute reactions to urographic contrast medium. *AJR* 119:832, 1973.

Wolf GL: Safer, more expensive iodinated contrast agents: how do we decide? *Radiology* 159:557, 1986.

Wolf GL, Arenson RL, Cross AP: A prospective trial of ionic vs. nonionic contrast agents in routine clinical practice: comparison of adverse effects. *AJR* 152:939, 1989.

Wolf GL, Mishkin MM, Roux SG, et al.: Comparison of the rates of adverse drug reactions. ionic contrast agents, ionic agents combined with steroids and nonionic agents. *Invest Radiol* 26(5):404, 1991.

Yamaguchi K, Katayama H, Takashima T, et al.: Prediction of severe adverse reactions to ionic contrast media in Japan: evaluation of pretesting. A report from the Japanese Committee on the Safety of Contrast Media. *Radiology* 178:363, 1991.

Contrast-Induced Acute Renal Dysfunction

Barrett BJ, Carlisle EJ: Metaanalysis of the relative nephrotoxicity of high and low osmolality iodinated contrast media. *Radiology* 188:171,1993.

Barrett BJ, Parfrey PS, Vavasour HM, et al.: Contrast nephropathy in patients with impaired renal function: high versus low osmolar media. *Kidney Int* 41:1274, 1992.

Bursztyn M: Contrast nephrotoxicity [letter]. *N Engl J Med* 321(6):395, 1989.

Cramer BC, Parfrey PS, Hutchinson TA, et al.: Renal function following infusion of radiologic contrast material. *Arch Intern Med* 145:87, 1985.

Cruz C, Hricak H, Samhouri F, et al.: Contrast media for angiography: effect on renal function. *Radiology* 158:109, 1986.

D'Elia JA, Gleason R, Alday M, et al.: Nephrotoxicity from angiographic contrast material. A prospective study. *Am J Med* 72:719, 1982.

Eisenberg RL, Bank WO, Hedgock MW: Renal failure after major angiography can be avoided with hydration. *AJR* 136:859, 1981.

Gomes AS, Baker JD, Martin-Paredero V, et al.: Acute renal dysfunction after major arteriography. *AJR* 145:1249, 1985.

Gomes AS, Lois JF, Baker JD, et al.: Acute renal dysfunction in high-risk patients after angiography: comparison of ionic and nonionic contrast media. *Radiology* 170:65, 1989.

Gup AK, Fischman JI, Aldridge G, Schlegel JU: The effect of drip infusion pyelography on renal function. *AJR* 98:102, 1966.

Harkonen S, Kjellstrand CM: Exacerbation of diabetic renal failure following intravenous pyelography. *Am J Med* 63:939, 1977.

Harris KG, Smith TP, Cragg AH, et al.: Nephrotoxicity from contrast material in renal insufficiency: ionic versus nonionic agents. *Radiology* 179:849, 1991.

Hayman LA, Evans RA, Fahr LM, Hinck VC: Renal consequences of rapid high dose contrast CT. *AJR* 134:553, 1980.

Hunter JV, Kind PRN: Nonionic iodinated contrast media: potential renal damage assessed with enzymuria. *Radiology* 183:101, 1992.

Jakobsen JA, Lundby B, Kristoffersen DT, et al.: Evaluation of renal function with delayed CT after injection of nonionic monometic and dimeric contrast media in healthy volunteers. *Radiology* 183:419, 1992.

Katholi RE, Taylor GH, Woods WT, et al.: Nephrotoxicity of nonionic low osmolality versus ionic high osmolality contrast media: a prospective double blind randomized comparison in human beings. *Radiology* 186:183, 1993.

Krumlovsky FA, Simon N, Santhanam S, et al.: Acute renal failure: association with administration of radiographic contrast material. *JAMA* 239(2):125, 1978.

Lang EK, Foreman J, Schlegel JU, et al.: The incidence of contrast medium induced acute tubular necrosis following arteriography. *Radiology* 138:203, 1981.

Love L, Lind JA, Olson MC: Persistent CT nephrogram: significance in the diagnosis of contrast nephropathy. *Radiology* 172:125, 1989.

MacEwan DW, Dunbar JS, Nogrady MB: Intravenous pyelography in children with renal insufficiency. *Radiology* 78:893, 1962.

Martin-Paredero V, Dixon SM, Baker JD, et al.: Risk of renal failure after major angiography. *Arch Surg* 118:1417, 1983.

Myers GH Jr, Witten DM: Acute renal failure after excretory urography in multiple myeloma. *AJR* 113:583, 1971.

Older RA, Korobkin M, Cleeve DM, et al.: Contrast-induced acute renal failure: persistent nephrogram as clue to early detection. *AJR* 13:339, 1980.

Parfrey PS, Griffiths SM, Barrett BJ, et al.: Contrast material-induced renal failure in patients with diabetes mellitus, renal insufficiency, or both. *N Engl J Med* 320(3):143, 1989.

Postlethwaite AE, Kelley WN: Uricosuric effect of radiocontrast agents: a study in man of four commonly used preparations. *Ann Intern Med* 74:845, 1971.

Schwab SJ, Hlatky MA, Pieper KS, et al.: Contrast nephrotoxicity: a randomized controlled trial of a nonionic and ionic radiographic contrast agent. *N Engl J Med* 320(3):149, 1989.

Schwartz WB, Hurwit A, Ettinger A: Intravenous urography in the patient with renal insufficiency. *N Engl J Med* 269(6):277, 1963.

Stacul F, Carraro M, Magnaldi S, et al.: Contrast agent nephrotoxicity: comparison of ionic and nonionic contrast agents. *AJR* 149:1287, 1987.

Talner LB: Does hydration prevent contrast material renal injury? *AJR* 136:1021, 1981.

VanZee BE, Hoy WE, Talley TE, Jaenike JR: Renal injury associated with intravenous pyelography in nondiabetic and diabetic patients. *Ann Intern Med* 89:51, 1978.

Treatment of Adverse Reactions to Contrast Media

Bush WH, Swanson DP: Acute reactions to intravascular contrast media: types, risk factors, recognition, and specific treatment. *AJR* 157:1153, 1991.

Cohan RH, Dunnick NR, Bashore TM: Treatment of reactions to radiographic contrast material. *AJR* 151:263, 1988.

Freitag JJ, Miller LW (eds): *Washington Manual of Medical Therapeutics,* ed 23. Boston: Little, Brown, 1980.

Hamilton G: Severe adverse reactions to urography in patients taking beta-adrenergic blocking agents. *Can Med Assoc J* 133:122, 1985.

Katzberg RW: *The Contrast Media Manual.* Baltimore, Williams & Wilkins, 1992.

Manual on Iodinated Contrast Media. American College of Radiology, 1991.

Siegle RL: Iodinated contrast material reactions: treatment and prevention. *Contemp Diagn Radiol* 9(16):1, 1986.

vanSonnenberg E, Neff CC, Pfister RC: Life-threatening hypotensive reactions to contrast media administration: comparison of pharmacologic and fluid therapy. *Radiology* 162:15, 1987.

5

··

Renal Cystic Disease

·········

Renal cysts, cystic disease, and cystic masses are the most common abnormalities encountered in uroradiology. In some cases, the renal cysts are part of a systemic process that also involves the kidneys. In most patients, however, one or several cystic masses are detected, and the question is whether the lesion is benign or malignant. In the vast majority of cases, the radiographic findings are sufficiently characteristic that surgery is not required. However, use of various radiographic modalities may be necessary before a confident diagnosis can be reached.

The classification of renal cystic diseases reflects both morphologic features and pathophysiology. In 1964, Osathanondh and Potter used microdissection studies to divide renal cysts into four groups. Although this classification helped to understand the pathophysiologic basis of cystic disease, it is no longer commonly used. Other investigators, including Gleason and coworkers and Grossman and colleagues, have developed classification systems based on radiologic–pathologic correla-

tion or the appearance at urography. In 1969, Elkin and Bernstein suggested a classification of renal cysts based on genetic, clinical, and morphologic criteria. A modification of this classification is used here.

CORTICAL CYSTS

Simple Cysts

The most common renal mass lesion is a simple cortical cyst. Cortical cysts are uncommon in children or young adults, but are detected by excretory urography (IVP) in as many as 20% of men with prostatic enlargement. Many more cysts can be detected with computed tomography (CT) and ultrasound than with urography. In fact, with more routine use of CT and ultrasound, renal cysts are estimated to occur in 50% of the population older than 50 years of age. Thus, they are considered acquired lesions and probably arise from obstructed ducts or tubules.

Simple cysts are composed of fibrous tissue and are lined by flattened cuboidal epithelium. They contain clear serous fluid and do not communicate with the collecting system.

Most patients with a simple cyst are asymptomatic, and the cyst is detected as an incidental finding. Hematuria is occasionally attributed to a benign cyst, but this occurs so infrequently that other lesions must be sought in patients who bleed (Table 5.1). Rarely a large cyst may obstruct the collecting system or cause hypertension. Local pain may be caused by distention of the cyst wall or spontaneous bleeding into the cyst. Occasionally, a simple cyst may become infected.

Although simple cysts have been described in all age groups, they are unusual in children. A cyst in a child must be carefully examined to differentiate a benign cyst from a cystic Wilms' tumor.

Cortical cysts can occasionally be detected on plain abdominal radiographs. The water-density cyst is seen as a cortical bulge projecting into the perinephric fat. Calcification is seen in the wall of a simple cyst in only 1% of cases.

During urography, a simple cyst is seen as a lucent mass in the renal parenchyma. Radiographs obtained soon after intravenous contrast injection (1 or 2 minutes) optimize visualization of cortical masses, because

Table 5.1. Benign Cyst Features

Well defined (sharp interface with normal parenchyma)
Round, often peripheral
Homogeneous
Lucent on IVP; water density on CT
Thin wall (imperceptible)
No contrast enhancement

this is the peak parenchymal opacification (*see* Chapter 4). A cyst is well defined and has a sharp interface with the normal renal cortex (Fig. 5.1). The cyst does not enhance, but does distort the adjacent parenchyma. If the cyst extends beyond the surface of the kidney, the parenchyma is extended to produce a "beak" or "claw sign." The margin of the cyst with the kidney is smooth and the cyst wall is too thin to be seen during urography. If the cyst is entirely intrarenal, its wall cannot be distinguished from the adjacent renal parenchyma and its thickness cannot be assessed. Exophytic cysts that displace perinephric fat instead of renal parenchyma may appear relatively dense at urography.

These same findings are present on CT examination. Computed tomography has superior contrast resolution, allowing measurement of the density of the cyst fluid, which should approximate that of water (Fig. 5.2). A density greater than 15 Hounsfield units (HU) is suspi-

cious for a complicated cyst or even for a solid mass lesion. There should be no contrast enhancement of a simple cyst. Renal cysts often are detected as an incidental finding during a contrast-enhanced CT examination of the abdomen, and there is no opportunity to test for contrast enhancement. However, if the density of the cyst fluid is less than 15 HU and other criteria of a simple cyst are present, the lesion will almost certainly be benign.

The wall of a benign cortical cyst is too thin to be seen on CT. However, when evaluating wall thickness with CT, it is important to look at a portion of the cyst that extends well away from the parenchyma so that a portion of adjacent renal tissue ("beak") is not included in the section. If the cyst is completely intrarenal, wall thickness cannot be assessed.

Although these same features also are seen using ultrasound, the terminology is different because sound waves are used rather than x-rays. A simple cyst is still a rounded homogeneous mass with a sharp interface with the normal renal parenchyma (Fig. 5.3). However, rather than being lucent, a simple cyst is echo-free with enhanced through-transmission. Thin septations that are too fine to be detected with CT may be seen with ultrasound.

Cysts may be seen with renal scintigraphy as a photopenic region because of the displacement of functioning parenchyma by the cyst. If the cyst is small or exo-

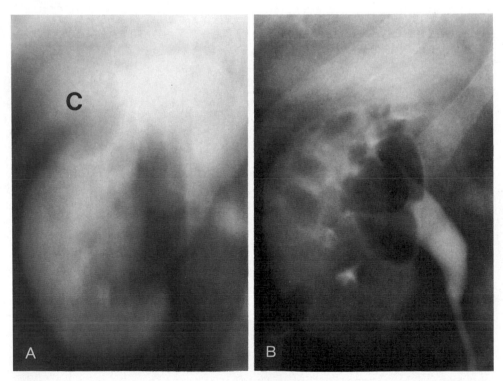

Figure 5.1.   Simple cyst. **A,** The early nephrotomogram demonstrates a rounded, peripheral mass (**C**) which has an imperceptibly thin wall and sharp interface with the normal renal parenchyma. **B,** The cyst is obscured by bowel gas and cannot be seen on the plain radiograph obtained 5 minutes after contrast injection.

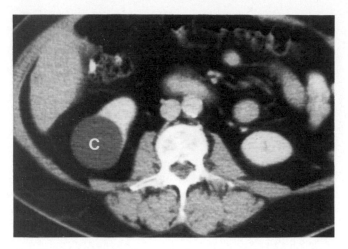

Figure 5.2.   Simple cyst. An enhanced computed tomography scan reveals a left renal mass (*C*) with the same cystic characteristics seen with urography. The cyst fluid measured 4 Hounsfield units.

phytic, scintigraphy may be normal. Parapelvic cysts may cause photopenic regions in the renal sinus that mimic hydronephrosis. The correct diagnosis is reached if the isotope can be identified in the ureter, even though the photopenic region persists.

Angiography is not routinely used to evaluate a suspected renal cyst. However, if performed, the cyst is seen as an avascular mass displacing adjacent blood vessels. A few tiny vessels may be seen supplying the cyst wall.

Simple cortical cysts also are readily detected with magnetic resonance imaging (MRI) (Fig. 5.4). The appearance of a homogeneous rounded mass with a thin wall and sharp interface with normal renal parenchyma is similar to that on CT. The long T1 values result in a low signal intensity on T1-weighted images. However, they have a very high signal intensity on T2-weighted images, which reflects the long T2 value of water.

The accuracy of the radiographic diagnosis of a renal cyst depends on how well it is seen with each modality. When all of the criteria of a benign simple cyst are present, it is highly unlikely to be anything else and further evaluation is not warranted. However, cysts often are not visualized well enough by IVP to make this determination. Because of cost considerations, ultrasound is the most efficient method of confirming the presence of a simple cyst that is poorly seen during urography. Ultrasound has the added advantages of not requiring ionizing radiation and avoiding the potential adverse reactions associated with intravenous contrast injection.

Computed tomography is the gold standard for the evaluation of renal mass lesions, but it is a more expensive examination than ultrasound and requires intravenous contrast medium. It is indicated when the ultrasound examination is indeterminate or is technically inadequate due to the patient's obesity or overlying gas. It is also appropriate to proceed directly to CT if the uro-

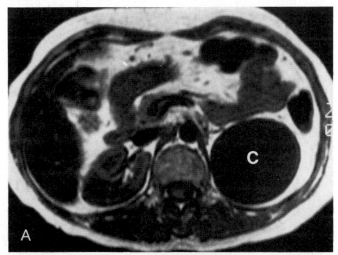

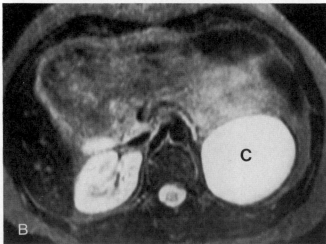

Figure 5.4.   Simple cyst. **A,** T1-weighted (TR = 500 ms; TE = 15 ms) images demonstrate a low signal intensity (*C*) which is much higher on **B,** T2-weighted (TR = 2000 ms, TE = 40 ms) images.

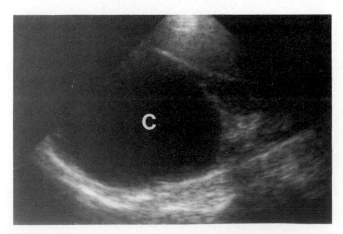

Figure 5.3.   Simple cyst. A well-defined, echo-free mass (*C*) is seen in the upper pole of the kidney.

gram indicates that the mass is complex or likely to be solid. Although seldom needed for the evaluation of renal cystic masses, MRI is used in patients with a contraindication to the use of intravenous contrast medium.

Renal cysts occasionally regress in size or disappear completely. Although this phenomenon may be caused by resorption of a hematoma misdiagnosed as a cyst, most cases are probably due to spontaneous cyst rupture. An increase in pressure within the cyst relative to the collecting system or the perinephric space may result in rupture. Such a pressure increase could be caused by hemorrhage into the cyst or by a change in the composition of the cystic fluid.

The most common clinical manifestations of cyst rupture are hematuria and flank pain. The diagnosis can be made by IVP or retrograde pyelography if the cyst communicates with the collecting system. The cyst cavity was opacified by urography in 88% of cases reported by Papanicolaou and colleagues. In most cases, the communication of the cyst with the collecting system closes spontaneously. Once the diagnosis is made, management is conservative.

Unilateral Cystic Disease

Unilateral or localized renal cystic disease is characterized by replacement of all or a portion of one kidney by multiple cysts. Although sometimes described as unilateral polycystic kidney disease, it is not familial. The disease is not progressive, and there is no association with renal failure or cysts in other organs.

Complicated Cysts

Cystic masses that do not satisfy the criteria of a benign simple cyst must be further evaluated to exclude malignancy. Various abnormalities are now recognized that exclude the diagnosis of a simple cyst.

Septations

Thin internal septations can be detected by ultrasound, but their presence alone does not suggest malignancy. Many of these thin septations are not seen during urography or CT, and they will likely be classified as typical simple cysts.

Other septations are thick enough to be seen during CT examination. If the septa are thin, smooth, and do not have localized areas of thickening or irregularity, a diagnosis of benign cyst can be made (Fig. 5.5). However, if there is an associated solid mass, the lesions must be considered malignant.

Calcification

The presence of calcification also is a nonspecific finding (Fig. 5.6). When evaluation of the kidney depended primarily on urography, the presence of calcification, especially central calcification, was an ominous

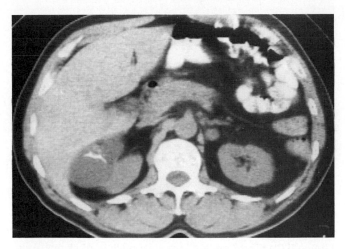

Figure 5.5. Septated cyst. Calcified septations are seen in this cystic mass which otherwise has the characteristics of a benign cyst.

sign. However, CT has made the presence or absence of calcification almost irrelevant, because wall thickening and soft tissue masses can easily be detected without the help of calcification. Thin calcification in the wall of a cyst or in a septation does not, in itself, warrant surgical exploration.

Thick Wall

A thick wall is incompatible with a simple cyst. It indicates that the lesion is another cystic mass or that the cyst has become complicated by some process such as infection or hemorrhage. Inflammatory or infectious cavities may result in this appearance, or the lesion may be a cystic renal adenocarcinoma (*see* Chapter 6). These lesions must be considered indeterminate, and surgical exploration is indicated (Fig. 5.7). The presence of an associated soft tissue tumor mass is an even more ominous finding and is highly suspicious for a malignancy.

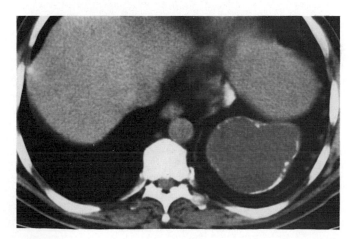

Figure 5.6. Calcified cyst. Calcification is seen in the wall of this benign cyst.

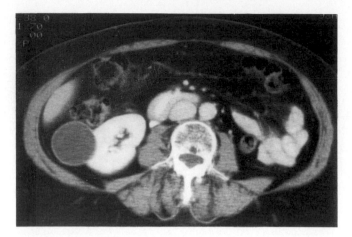

Figure 5.7. Thick-walled cyst. The thick wall in this cystic mass indicates a complicated cyst or other cystic mass. Further evaluation is warranted.

Increased Density

A cystic mass with a density above water must contain more than simple cystic fluid. A density greater than 15 HU is worrisome, but this reading should be checked against the water bath phantom, as there may be considerable drift in the CT numbers. If an increased density is present, further evaluation with US, precontrast- and postcontrast–enhanced CT, or aspiration is warranted.

One category of atypical renal cyst that has an increased attenuation coefficient is the hyperdense cyst. These lesions look like typical simple cysts on CT examination in that they are rounded, well-defined, homogeneous masses that do not enhance with intravenous contrast injection. They are usually small, peripheral lesions, measuring less than 3 cm in diameter (Fig. 5.8). However, instead of having a density near water, they measure 60 to 90 HU. They are easily recognized on an unenhanced CT examination, but often are masked by the enhanced renal parenchyma, because their densities are similar. Thus, these lesions are probably more common than is appreciated, inasmuch as most abdominal CT scans are performed after intravenous contrast injection.

There are several possible etiologies for a hyperdense renal cyst. The most common etiologies are hemorrhage and a high protein content of the cyst fluid. However, a diffuse paste-like calcified material also has been found. The vast majority of these hyperdense cysts are benign, but they must be carefully examined for other atypical features. Computed tomography examination before and after intravenous contrast injection often is helpful. A cyst will not enhance, whereas a solid tumor will increase in density.

Ultrasonography is another useful modality in the evaluation of the hyperdense renal mass. It enables the examiner to distinguish between a cystic and solid lesion. With ultrasound, blood elements can sometimes be seen floating within the cyst. However, if the lesion cannot be clearly evaluated, surgical exploration may still be needed.

Hemorrhagic cysts also can be identified with MRI. Simple cysts have a low signal intensity on T1-weighted images, whereas hemorrhagic cysts may have a high signal intensity on all pulse sequences. Because the blood elements tend to settle out, the more intense signal of the paramagnetic methemoglobin can be seen in the dependent portion of the cyst on T1-weighted images. The relative intensity of the two cyst layers may reverse on

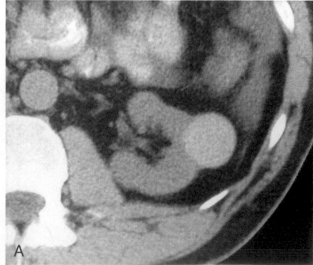
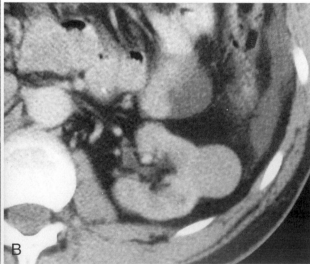

Figure 5.8. Hemorrhagic cyst. **A,** A rounded, well-defined, homogeneous mass is seen in the lateral aspect of the left kidney. It has a density of 58 HU and shows no contrast enhancement (**B**).

T2-weighted sequences. A renal adenocarcinoma can usually be distinguished by its inhomogeneity, indistinct or irregular margins, and lack of a fluid-hemoglobin level.

Classification

To clarify the need for further evaluation or treatment of complicated cystic lesions, Bosniak has classified cystic renal masses into four categories.

Class I lesions are cysts that have no atypical features. No further evaluation is needed.

Class II lesions are those with some atypical features, but are most likely benign. This group includes a subset of patients with findings such as an increased density or calcification that require follow-up evaluation in 3 months, 6 months, and 12 months to make sure the lesion is not growing.

Class III lesions cannot be distinguished from malignancies; they often require surgical exploration. Features of lesions in class III include increased density, complex septations, multiloculated cysts, and dense calcification. Many of these lesions will be benign, and it may be appropriate to perform a biopsy or simple enucleation rather than the more formal radical nephrectomy.

Class IV lesions have features that strongly suggest malignancy. Although there may be a large cystic component, there is an enhancing solid component or thick irregular walls. These are treated as presumed renal carcinomas.

Milk of Calcium Cyst

Milk of calcium is a collection of small calcific granules in the cystic fluid. The granules, usually calcium carbonate, are in suspension and layer out in the dependent portion of the cyst (Fig. 5.9). They are seen most frequently in calyceal diverticulae (*see* Chapter 13), but also may be present in simple cysts or polycystic kidneys. Milk of calcium cysts have no sex predilection, but are more common in the upper poles of the kidneys.

The milk of calcium nature of these calculi may not be appreciated on a supine radiograph, but the fluid-calcium layer is easily detected on upright films or CT examination. A horizontal line of calcium density also can be detected using ultrasound, regardless of the patient's position. Most of these cysts are detected as an incidental finding, and intervention is unnecessary.

MEDULLARY CYSTIC DISEASE

This disease complex includes medullary cystic disease and related diseases, such as juvenile nephronophthisis and retinal-renal dysplasia. The kidneys are small to normal in size, and maintain a normal configuration and smooth contour. A variable number of small cysts, up to 2 cm in diameter, are located primarily in the medulla. The cortex is thin but does not contain cysts.

Biopsy shows interstitial and periglomerular fibrosis as well as tubular atrophy. However, the diagnosis cannot be made if cysts are not included in the biopsy specimen, because the fibrotic changes are nonspecific.

The uremic medullary cystic diseases can be classified by the age of onset. The adult form is transmitted by autosomal-dominant inheritance. Patients usually present as young adults with anemia, which may be severe, and have progressive renal failure. These patients have a salt-wasting nephropathy that is not corrected with mineralocorticoids. Other than a fixed low specific gravity, the urine sediment is normal. Hypertension may develop near the end of the disease course.

Patients with juvenile nephronophthisis typically present at 3 to 5 years of age with polydipsia and polyuria. The clinical course with anemia and progressive renal failure is similar to the adult-onset variety, but progression is slower, with 8–10 years before terminal uremia. Juvenile nephronophthisis is transmitted by autosomal-recessive inheritance.

Abdominal radiographs may demonstrate small kidneys without calcification. High-dose nephrotomography reveals a thin renal cortex. Linear contrast collections radiating from the renal pyramids may be seen. However, excretory urography is not likely to be helpful and is seldom performed because of the renal failure. Computed tomography demonstrates small smooth kidneys and may reveal the small medullary cysts.

High-resolution ultrasound may be the examination of choice in these patients. The corticomedullary differentiation is lost, and the parenchyma appears isoechoic or hypoechoic with the liver or spleen. In patients with severe uremia, medullary cysts can usually be demonstrated, but they may not be detectable in milder cases.

POLYCYSTIC RENAL DISEASE

Autosomal Recessive Polycystic Disease

Autosomal-recessive or infantile polycystic disease (IPCD) is transmitted by autosomal-recessive inheritance and is frequently referred to as autosomal-recessive polycystic kidney disease. IPCD includes a spectrum of abnormalities ranging from newborns with grossly enlarged spongy kidneys to older children with medullary ductal ectasia. The older children also develop hepatic fibrosis that progresses to portal hypertension and esophageal varices.

Congenital hepatic fibrosis (CHF) may represent yet another disease transmitted by autosomal-recessive inheritance in which the renal disease is different and milder than IPCD. Other entities associated with CHF include adult polycystic disease (APCD), multicystic dysplastic kidneys, choledochal cyst, and Caroli's disease. However, medullary ductal ectasia is found in all forms of IPCD, with or without CHF.

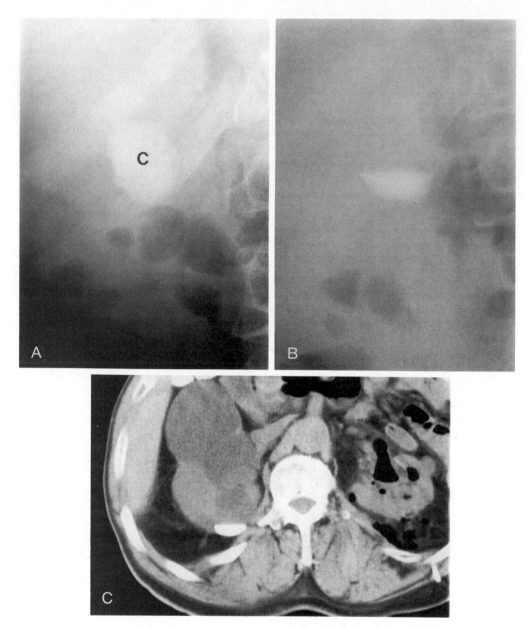

Figure 5.9. Milk of calcium cyst. **A,** A homogeneous calcific density (*C*) is identified on this supine abdominal radiograph. **B,** A "fluid/calcium" level is seen on an upright film. **C,** This level is also appreciated on an unenhanced computed tomography scan.

Patients with IPCD have renal failure at birth and most die within the first few days of life. Patients with the juvenile form have a milder renal disease characterized by tubular ectasia and renal cysts. They often present with symptoms arising from hepatic fibrosis with portal hypertension and varices rather than renal failure.

The radiographic manifestations reflect the age of onset and the severity of renal involvement. In the neonatal form, there is massive enlargement of the kidneys, which maintain their reniform shape. The kidneys are enlarged, but function poorly. The nephrogram is faint with blotchy opacification. Linear striations due to stasis of contrast medium in the dilated renal tubules have been described. The numerous small (1- to 2-mm) cysts in both the cortex and medulla result in increased echogenicity on sonography. However, with high-resolution scanners a peripheral sonolucent rim can be seen representing compressed renal cortex (Fig. 5.10). A prominent renal pelvis and calyces may result in a sonolucent central zone.

Polycystic Disease of Childhood

Among older children, fewer than 10% of the renal tubules are affected and hepatic fibrosis dominates the clinical course. This is sometimes referred to as congen-

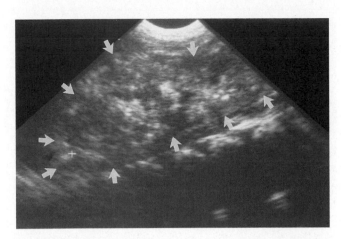

Figure 5.10. Autosomal recessive polycystic disease. The kidney is enlarged (*arrows*). Numerous small cysts create disorganized echogenicity and loss of corticomedullary differentiation. (From Amis ES Jr, Newhouse JH: *Essentials of Uroradiology,* Boston, Little, Brown & Company, 1991).

ital hepatic fibrosis. The clinical presentation is usually a result of portal hypertension with splenomegaly, gastric, and esophageal varices. The kidneys are only mildly enlarged, but contain variably sized cysts that are predominantly medullary in location. The appearance of tubular ectasia in these children is similar to that seen in medullary sponge kidney in adults (*see* Chapter 13). An increased echogenicity with loss of the normal corticomedullary junction is demonstrated on ultrasound. The sonolucent rim of compressed renal parenchyma also may be seen in the juvenile form.

Autosomal-Dominant Polycystic Kidney Disease

Autosomal-dominant or adult polycystic kidney disease (APCD) is the most common form of cystic kidney disease and is responsible for 10 to 12% of patients on chronic dialysis. It is transmitted by autosomal-dominant inheritance. However, because of variable expressivity and spontaneous mutations, as many as 50% of patients with APCD may have no family history of renal disease. Although the etiology is unknown, the cysts seem to arise from nephrons that initially were able to function normally.

Patients with APCD present most commonly in the third or fourth decade. However, APCD may be seen in children or in older adults. The initial complaint is usually lumbar, inguinal, or upper abdominal pain. The enlarged kidneys may be palpable as abdominal masses.

Hypertension, which occurs in almost two thirds of patients with APCD, is caused by increased renin production by the kidneys. Hematuria may be caused by rupture of one of the renal cysts into the renal pelvis or by the presence of a stone.

Patients with APCD often suffer from flank pain due to a variety of etiologies. Acute pain may result from swelling of one of the cysts due to hemorrhage or infection. Colicky pain may arise from ureteral obstruction by stone, blood clot, or rarely a cyst. Chronic pain is more likely caused by progressive enlargement of the cysts with stretching of the renal capsule.

All patients with APCD have progressive renal failure. The rate of progression of the azotemia is related to the age of onset; those patients whose symptoms begin after 50 years of age have a better prognosis. Although the incidence is variable, approximately one half of patients with APCD have cerebral (berry) aneurysms in the circle of Willis, and stroke from rupture of a berry aneurysm is a significant cause of morbidity and mortality. Renal stones occur more frequently in patients with APCD than in the general population. Because more than one half of these stones are predominantly uric acid, they may be radiolucent and may be overlooked on an abdominal radiograph or conventional tomography. Using CT, Levine and Grantham found renal calculi in 36% of patients with APCD.

Excretory urography is seldom used to evaluate patients with known APCD. However, new cases may be diagnosed with IVP because the findings are characteristic. The plain abdominal radiograph is remarkable for the poor visualization of the renal outlines. Three quarters of the renal outline is seen in less than 10% of patients with APCD compared with 80% of patients with unilateral renal enlargement due to other causes. Calcification in the cyst walls is common, and nephrolithiasis may be detected. If renal function is adequate, the urogram will demonstrate enlarged kidneys with a mottled renal parenchyma due to the many cysts. The collecting system is splayed by the parenchymal cysts (Fig. 5.11), which may cause infundibular obstruction. Although its appearance is typical for APCD, it may not be distinguishable from the renal involvement by multiple cysts and hamartomas in patients with tuberous sclerosis or from other conditions with multiple space-occupying lesions in the kidney such as von Hippel–Lindau disease, multiple simple cysts, renal metastases, or renal lymphoma.

Sonography and CT have replaced nephrotomography as the standard method of examination of patients with APCD. Innumerable renal cysts are seen with either modality. The kidneys are markedly enlarged, but maintain their basic reniform shape.

Computed tomography has the advantage of clearly demonstrating the cysts and collecting systems of both kidneys. Precontrast scans are needed to demonstrate renal stones and facilitate the diagnosis of hemorrhagic cysts (Fig. 5.12). Because the kidneys are typically riddled with innumerable cysts that abut each other, the cysts are not round in shape, but assume a variety of irregular contours.

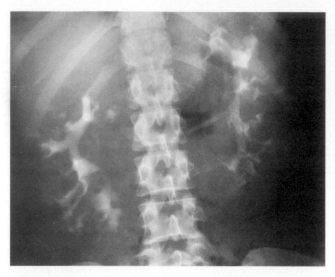

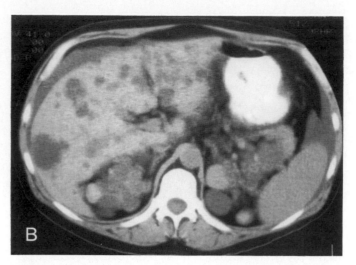

Figure 5.11. Autosomal dominant polycystic kidney disease. Urography demonstrates bilateral enlarged kidneys and splaying of the collecting systems by multiple masses. (From Amis ES Jr, Newhouse JH: *Essentials of Uroradiology,* Boston, Little, Brown & Company, 1991).

Figure 5.13. Autosomal dominant polycystic kidney disease. Several hyperdense renal cysts as well as multiple hepatic cysts are seen on this abdominal computed tomography image.

Computed tomography also is useful in demonstrating hepatic cysts, which are present in 54 to 74% of patients with APCD. These liver cysts develop from dilatation of aberrant bile ducts that embryologically failed to establish communication with the biliary tree (Fig. 5.13). The cysts gradually accumulate fluid secreted by the lining cuboidal epithelial cells. Fewer than 10% of patients have associated cysts in other organs, such as the spleen or pancreas.

Multiple renal cysts are easily identified on MRI. Uncomplicated cysts resemble simple cortical cysts with a homogeneous low signal intensity on T1-weighted images and a high signal intensity on T2-weighted images.

Complicated cysts reflect the presence of infection or age of the hemorrhage. Acute bleeding results in a hyperintense image regardless of the pulse sequence. However, the appearance varies with the age of the bleed. The high protein content of an infected cyst results in a signal intensity between a simple cyst and one with an acute hemorrhage.

Bleeding into renal cysts is common and may be the source of acute flank pain. If the cyst ruptures into the renal pelvis, hematuria will occur. Cyst hemorrhage may be more common in patients with APCD because of the associated hypertension or the increased bleeding tendency of uremia or heparinization during dialysis. Hemorrhagic renal cysts may be seen in 70% of patients with APCD. Perinephric hemorrhage has been reported, but is rare.

Both kidneys are affected in patients with APCD, but involvement may be asymmetric. Rare cases of unilateral APCD are reported, but these may represent manifestations too small for macroscopic imaging.

There is no treatment for APCD, and patients often must be sustained by dialysis or transplantation. By informing patients of the heritability of APCD, genetic counseling can help them with family planning. Thus, it is important for the diagnosis to be made before the patients reach child-bearing age. Excretory urography with nephrotomography and sonography are both able to detect changes of APCD among children of affected families. Because ultrasound is less invasive, it is the preferred screening examination.

MULTICYSTIC DYSPLASTIC KIDNEY

A multicystic dysplastic kidney (MCDK) consists of a collection of irregularly sized cysts and fibrous tissue, but no functioning renal parenchyma. The cysts do not

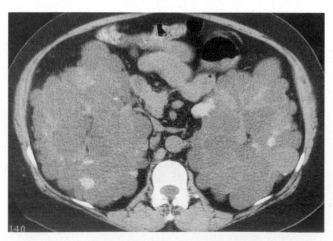

Figure 5.12. Autosomal dominant polycystic kidney disease. Bilateral renal enlargement due to numerous cysts is demonstrated on this enhanced computed tomography examination. Several high-density cysts indicate hemorrhage.

communicate, the renal collecting system is small or absent, and there are atretic ipsilateral renal vessels. The anomaly results from occlusion of the fetal ureters usually before 8 to 10 weeks of gestation.

A variant, the hydronephrotic type of multicystic dysplasia, may result from incomplete ureteral obstruction later in gestation. In such cases, the cysts communicate with the renal pelvis.

In rare cases, MCDK may be confined to one segment of the kidney. Most of these cases occur in the upper-pole moiety of a duplicated collecting system.

Most renal dysplasias are detected as an abdominal mass in infancy. MCKD is the second most common cause of an abdominal mass in the neonate, trailing only hydronephrosis in frequency. Males are more commonly affected than females, and there is a predilection for the left kidney.

Malformations including bilateral MCDK, uretero-pelvic junction (UPJ) obstruction, hypoplasia of the opposite kidney, and horseshoe kidney are commonly associated with MCKD. These occurred in 41% of fetuses examined ultrasonographically by Kleiner and colleagues. Because some of these contralateral anomalies are fatal, less severe changes are more common, and UPJ obstruction is the most common malformation seen in children or adults. If the MCDK is not detected in infancy, it may remain asymptomatic and may be detected as an incidental finding in an adult.

Abdominal radiographs may demonstrate a soft tissue flank mass. In adults, calcification is common, usually in the cyst walls (Fig. 5.14). There is no functioning renal parenchyma on the affected side, but excretory urography demonstrates compensatory hypertrophy of the contralateral kidney.

If retrograde pyelography is performed, an atretic ureter may be demonstrated (Fig. 5.15). Atresia may be found at various levels, or there may be no ureter at all. Extravasation is common because cannulation of the small ureteric opening may be difficult.

The multiple cysts with thick septa are nicely demonstrated by CT (Fig. 5.16). Mural calcifications can be demonstrated in the cyst walls, but there is no evidence of contrast excretion.

Sonography is particularly valuable in assessing infants and demonstrates multiple cysts of varying sizes (Fig. 5.17). There is no connection between adjacent cysts or renal parenchyma surrounding the cysts. If angiography is performed, no ipsilateral renal artery will be seen (Fig. 5.16).

Segmental multicystic renal dysplasia in an upper-pole moiety may be seen in patients with obstruction from an ectopic ureterocele. The dysplastic segment has the same features as the multicystic dysplastic kidney and causes compression of the normally functioning lower-pole moiety.

Focal multicystic renal dysplasia also has been reported. This presumably results from in utero infundibular obstruction. This entity is fortunately rare,

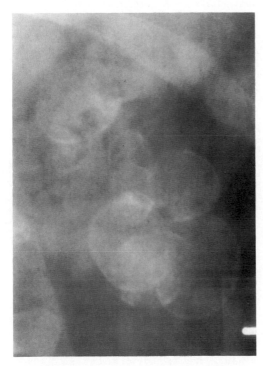

Figure 5.14.   Multicystic dysplastic kidney. Calcification can be seen in cyst walls.

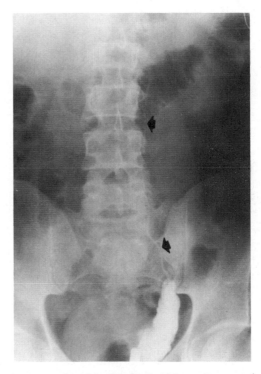

Figure 5.15.   Multicystic dysplastic kidney. Retrograde pyelography demonstrates a small atretic ureter (*arrows*) which does not reach the kidney. Extravasation is present around the distal ureter.

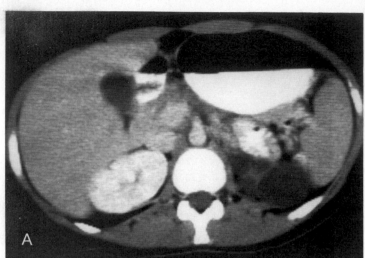

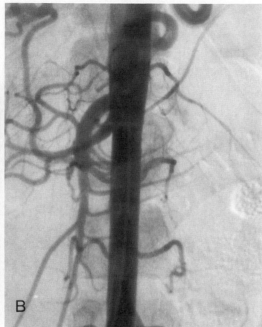

Figure 5.16. Multicystic dysplastic kidney. **A,** On computed tomography, multiple cysts, but no functioning renal tissue, are present on the left. The right kidney is normal. **B,** An abdominal aortogram demonstrates absence of the left renal artery.

since it cannot be distinguished radiographically from other renal cystic masses.

The classic multicystic dysplastic kidney must be distinguished from the "hydronephrotic" type of multicystic dysplasia. This hydronephrotic form probably results from incomplete obstruction of the ureter after the tenth week of gestation. In this form, a renal pelvis communicates with the multiple cysts. Function may be demonstrated by excretion of contrast medium during urography or CT, or excretion of radionuclide during nuclear medicine studies. If the diagnosis is uncertain, percutaneous aspiration with antegrade pyelography may be required. Surgery is indicated in patients with the hydronephrotic type of disease, because significant renal function often can be preserved.

Treatment

Our knowledge of the natural history of MCDK is increasing with the use of in utero ultrasound. As many as 41% of fetuses with MCDK have a contralateral renal anomaly, which is much higher than the 11 to 15% incidence seen in neonates. Many of these associated anomalies are fatal, and in some cases, there is involution of MCDK to what appears in the neonate as renal agenesis.

This involution also may occur after birth. In a review of 30 patients with MCDK by Vinocur and coworkers, 13.5% of the cystic masses decreased in size or disappeared. This decrease is presumably due to leakage or reabsorption of cyst fluid. The majority of MCDKs (73%) did not change in size and 13.5% increased. Surgery is needed if there is significant growth during the first year of life, if the diagnosis is inconclusive, or if complications arise that require nephrectomy.

MULTILOCULAR CYSTIC NEPHROMA

This uncommon lesion has been described by various names including multilocular renal cyst, cystic adenoma, lymphangioma, segmental multicystic kidney,

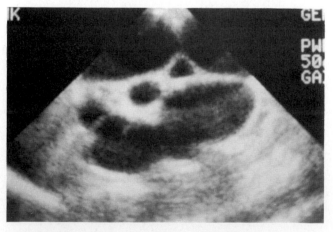

Figure 5.17. Multicystic dysplastic kidney. Multiple cysts of varying sizes are seen in an infant. (Courtesy of Kate Feinstein, M.D.)

segmental polycystic kidney, cystic hamartoma, benign cystic nephroma, and Perlman's tumor. It is a congenital renal lesion that is not genetically transmitted.

Multilocular cystic nephroma (MLCN) is a well-circumscribed lesion containing many cysts of variable sizes. The cystic mass is surrounded by a thick fibrous capsule that compresses adjacent renal parenchyma and often projects into the renal pelvis. The cysts are lined by flattened or cuboidal epithelium and contain clear fluid. Hemorrhage and necrosis are uncommon.

Two forms of MLCN, which are distinct histologically but not grossly, have been described. A cystic nephroma is a multiseptated cystic mass composed entirely of differentiated tissues. A cystic partially differentiated nephroblastoma is similar, but embryonal cells are found in the septations. These two subtypes of MLCN cannot be distinguished radiographically and are treated the same.

The presenting signs and symptoms depend on the patient's age. Male patients with MLCN are usually younger than 4 years of age and present with a palpable abdominal mass. Female patients with MLCN typically present with symptoms between 4 and 20 years of age or after 40 years of age. Among children presenting younger than 4 years of age, 73% are male; of patients older than 4 years of age at presentation, 89% are female. In the adult, MLCN may be found during examination of an unrelated complaint or during the investigation of pain, hematuria, or urinary tract infection.

Calcification is uncommon, especially in pediatric patients. However, radiographically detected calcifications were found in 7 of 12 adult patients reported by Banner and colleagues. Such calcifications are usually found in the cyst walls or intervening stroma. The pattern of calcification is nonspecific and may be central or peripheral. A large renal mass is seen with excretory urogra-

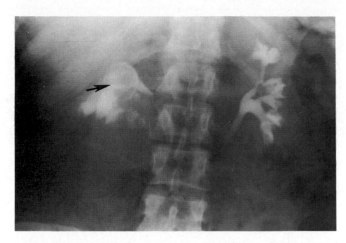

Figure 5.18.   Multilocular cystic nephroma. A large mass in the lower pole of the right kidney is projecting into the renal pelvis (*arrow*).

phy. The cystic mass occurs with equal frequency on either side, but is more common in the lower pole. Projection of the mass into the renal pelvis often can be demonstrated (Fig. 5.18). The mass is hypovascular and mottled in appearance.

The multiple cystic spaces are best demonstrated using ultrasound. Large, multiple locules separated by echogenic stroma suggest the diagnosis of MLCN (Fig. 5.19). If the cysts are small, they may not be defined by ultrasound, and the echogenic stroma may suggest a complex or solid renal mass.

The CT appearance is usually characteristic. The masses are large, averaging approximately 10 cm in diameter. They are sharply delineated from the normal renal parenchyma. MLCN is hypovascular, but the septations enhance after intravenous contrast injection (Fig. 5.19). When large cysts are present, the internal septa-

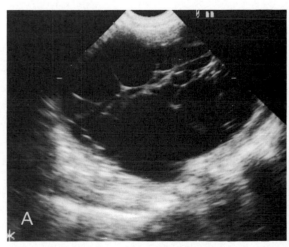
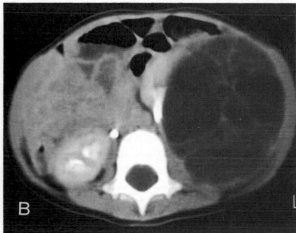

Figure 5.19.   Multilocular cystic nephroma. **A,** Multiple cysts are separated by echogenic stroma on ultrasound. **B,** A large cystic mass with multiple septations is seen on computed tomography.

tions are well defined. If the cysts are small, the mass may have a pitted appearance.

Angiography demonstrates most lesions to be hypovascular, but the degree of vascularity depends on the size of the cysts and the amount of intervening stroma. Tortuous vessels and modest neovascularity can be seen, but signs of frank tumor vascularity, such as encasement, arteriovenous shunting, or vascular pooling are not present.

MLCN must be differentiated from a cystic renal adenocarcinoma. Although adenocarcinoma arising in MLCN has been reported, Madewell and coworkers at the Armed Forces Institute of Pathology believe these cases are multiloculated renal adenocarcinoma, because the pathologic features of MLCN are not present.

Radiologic imaging studies are not adequate to exclude malignancy, and further evaluation is needed. Cyst aspiration is usually inadequate because the locules do not communicate and because an excessive number of punctures would be required to evaluate all portions of the lesion. Thus, surgical excision is indicated.

Because MLCN is a benign lesion and often can be suggested preoperatively, local excision may be appropriate. Frozen sections should be obtained, however, to exclude malignancy. If malignant tissue is seen, a radical nephrectomy could be performed.

CYSTS ASSOCIATED WITH SYSTEMIC DISEASE

The phakomatoses are a group of neurologic disorders that include congenital abnormalities of the skin and other organs. Two of these disorders, tuberous sclerosis and von Hippel–Lindau (VHL) disease, are associated with renal cysts.

Tuberous Sclerosis Complex

The complex of tuberous sclerosis (Bourneville's disease) includes small cutaneous angiofibromas on the face (adenoma sebaceum) and hamartomas in a variety of organs, such as the brain, eyes, heart, and kidneys. The disease is transmitted by autosomal-dominant inheritance, but with incomplete penetrance. Sporadic cases, presumably due to spontaneous mutation, also may occur.

Patients may present with mental retardation, seizures, or characteristic skin lesions. Approximately 80% of patients have renal angiomyolipomas, which may cause hematuria.

In addition to the angiomyolipomas found in patients with tuberous sclerosis (*see* Chapter 6), there is an increased incidence of renal cysts. These cysts are small and seldom exceed 3 cm in diameter. They have a distinctive microscopic appearance with hyperplastic epithelium. Severe renal involvement can lead to renal failure, which is second only to involvement of the central nervous system (CNS) as a cause of death in these patients. Multiple enlarging renal cysts and retroperitoneal hemorrhage from an angiomyolipoma are the most common causes of renal failure. Computed tomography may demonstrate only hamartomas, hamartomas and cysts (Fig. 5.20), or only cysts.

Sonography clearly distinguishes the anechoic cysts from angiomyolipomas, which are typically very echogenic. The appearance of the cysts is the same as simple cortical cysts. The appearance of an angiomyolipoma reflects the proportion of each tissue element within the tumor.

Computed tomography often is used to confirm the presence of an angiomyolipoma by demonstrating the

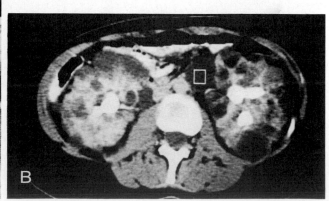

Figure 5.20.   Tuberous sclerosis. Ultrasound and computed tomography both demonstrate multiple mass lesions. **A,** On ultrasound, echogenic masses represent hamartomas while the echo-free areas are cysts. **B,** Computed tomography reveals fatty density hamartomas and water density cysts.

Table 5.2. Bilateral Renal Cysts

Acquired cystic disease
Autosomal dominant polycystic disease
Multiple simple cysts
Tuberous sclerosis
von Hippel-Lindau disease

fatty nature of the tumor. Tumors without fat will be indistinguishable from renal adenocarcinomas.

von Hippel–Lindau Disease

This syndrome consists of cerebellar and retinal hemangioblastomas, renal carcinomas, pheochromocytomas, and a variety of visceral cysts, including renal cysts. It is transmitted by autosomal-dominant inheritance, but with only moderate penetrance.

Patients with VHL disease present most commonly with symptoms of a cerebellar hemangioblastoma. Capillary angiomas involve the retina and may cause progressive visual loss. Renal cysts occur in approximately three fourths of patients, and renal adenocarcinomas develop in 25 to 45% of patients (*see* Chapter 6). The renal tumors often are bilateral and are usually multifocal. Other urologic manifestations include adrenal pheochromocytomas and papillary cystadenomas of the epididymis.

Three distinct phenotypes of VHL disease are now recognized. The most common pattern (type I) includes retinal and CNS hemangioblastomas, renal cysts and cancers, and pancreatic cystic disease (Fig. 5.21). The second most common pattern (type IIA) includes retinal and CNS hemangioblastomas, as well as pheochromocytomas and islet cell tumors of the pancreas. Renal cysts and cancers are not present in type IIA. The least common phenotype of VHL (type IIB) includes retinal and CNS hemangioblastoma, pheochromocytoma, and renal and pancreatic disease.

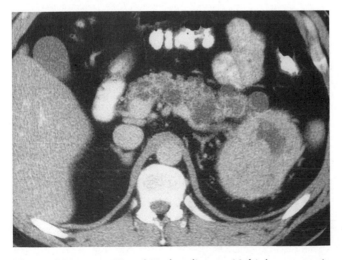

Figure 5.21. von Hippel Lindau disease. Multiple pancreatic cysts and a left renal carcinoma are visualized.

The renal cysts, which usually range in size from 0.5 to 3.0 cm, are reported in approximately 60% of patients with VHL. However, if families with pheochromocytomas (type IIA) are excluded, the prevalence increases to 85%. They demonstrate a continuum from simple cysts to carcinoma manifesting as complex papillary projections into the cystic lumen. However, the hyperplastic epithelial lining may be a precursor of malignancy.

Radiographic evaluation of patients with VHL disease is difficult. The numerous cysts distort the normal renal architecture. Tumors develop in the cyst wall, so careful evaluation is essential. Narrowly collimated CT is the most useful modality for this purpose. However, the tumors often are small and difficult to distinguish from cysts. Levine and coworkers recommend annual follow-up CT examination of any lesions that do not satisfy the criteria for a benign cyst or a frank neoplasm.

Renal arteriography is less sensitive than CT in detecting the small renal tumors (*see* Chapter 6). However, angiography is valuable if surgical resection is contemplated, and precise knowledge of the vascular anatomy is needed to remove the tumor and spare as much renal parenchyma as possible.

MISCELLANEOUS RENAL CYSTS

Acquired Renal Cystic Disease

Since the initial description in 1977, many investigators have documented the progressive development of renal cysts and solid tumors in patients with renal failure. Although the mechanism of cyst formation in these uremic patients is unknown, it is postulated that dialysis incompletely removes toxins and that their build up may induce these changes. The cysts are thought to develop as a result of fusiform dilations of the proximal renal tubules. The involution of these cysts after successful renal transplantation supports this hypothesis.

Renal cysts occur in approximately 8% of patients at the initiation of dialysis and increases proportional to the duration of dialysis. After 3 years, 10 to 20% of patients have acquired renal cystic disease (ARCD). This increases to 40% of patients after 3 years of dialysis and to 90% after 5 to 10 years. ARCD is seen equally among patients receiving hemodialysis or peritoneal dialysis.

Solid tumors also are seen with increased frequency, up to 7%. These solid neoplasms include adenomas, oncocytomas, and adenocarcinomas. From pathologic examination it is not easy to determine the biologic behavior of these tumors, but the incidence of malignant adenocarcinomas is probably small. Many of these tu-

Table 5.3. Multiple Solid and Cystic Renal Masses

Acquired cystic kidney disease
Tuberous sclerosis complex
von Hippel-Lindau disease

mors which are classified as malignant histologically do not demonstrate malignant behavior. In a review of 14 long-term dialysis series, Grantham and colleagues found that only 2 of 601 (0.33%) patients developed metastatic cancer. Prospective longitudinal studies indicate that the annual incidence of metastatic or locally invasive renal carcinoma among dialysis patients is three to six times that of the general population.

Although the renal cysts tend to regress after successful renal transplantation, the effect on the risk of developing renal cancer is less clear. Any nondialyzable carcinogenic factors are likely removed by the functioning renal allograft, and the risk of renal cancer would then be reduced. However, transplant recipients have an increased risk of developing renal carcinoma, presumably due to immunosuppression. The net result is that these patients remain at increased risk for developing renal carcinoma, even after successful transplantation.

The ultrasonographic examination of native kidneys is difficult because they often are small, distorted, and surrounded by highly echogenic fat. There is an increased incidence of hemorrhage into renal cysts or perinephric space. Calcification frequently occurs in the cyst walls or in the renal interstitium, making ultrasonographic evaluation even more difficult.

A renal mass with internal echoes, neural nodules, or no distal acoustic enhancement is likely to be a renal carcinoma. Tumor enhancement has been described with ultrasonographic angiography.

It is easier to examine the native kidneys with CT (Fig. 5.22) than with ultrasound, and the sensitivity of CT using thin-section techniques to detect small lesions is greater than with ultrasound. Multiple small cysts are seen by CT in virtually all patients with acquired cystic disease. Dystrophic calcifications are common in the renal parenchyma or cyst walls. Bleeding is a common complication, so hemorrhagic cysts and subcapsular or

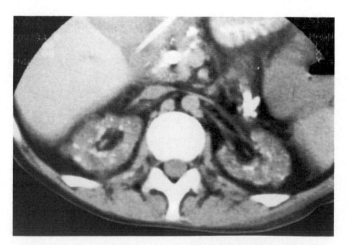

Figure 5.22. Acquired renal cystic disease. Dystrophic calcification and multiple renal cysts are present on this unenhanced computed tomography scan.

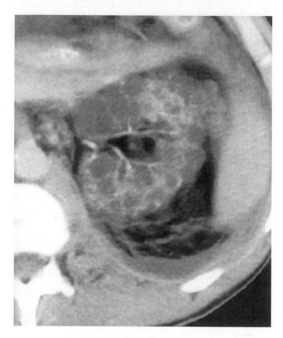

Figure 5.23. Acquired renal cystic disease. Multiple renal cysts and a perinephric hematoma are identified on this contrast-enhanced computed tomography scan.

perinephric hematomas are common (Fig. 5.23). Carcinomas are seen as masses with a density similar to the unenhanced parenchyma. If large (greater than 3 cm), the masses may be inhomogeneous, which is better seen with contrast enhancement.

Orofaciodigital Syndrome

This rare x-linked inherited disorder includes malformations of the mouth, face, and digits. It is lethal in utero in males, and therefore, all patients are female. Multiple renal cysts may mimic autosomal-dominant or autosomal-recessive polycystic kidney disease. Many patients develop progressive renal insufficiency and eventually require dialysis.

Hydatid Disease

Hydatid disease in humans is usually caused by infection with *Echinococcus granulosus*, but also may be caused by *E. multilocularis*.

The adult worm lives in the intestine of a dog (definitive host) and discharges the egg-containing proglottid into the feces. The intermediate host is usually a sheep that ingests the eggs while grazing on contaminated ground. The protective chitinous layer is dissolved in the duodenum, and the hydatid embryo passes through the intestinal wall into the portal vein. Thus, the liver is the most commonly involved organ. The embryo develops into a slowly growing cyst. The cycle is completed when the intermediate host (sheep) dies and the larva are eaten by the definitive host (dog). The human being is infected as an accidental host by eating contaminated food.

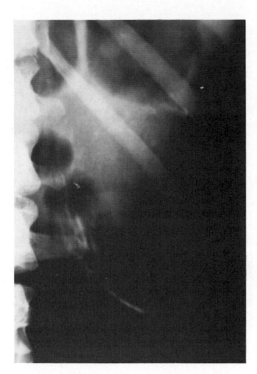

Figure 5.24. Hydatid disease. A calcified cyst wall is appreciated on the plain radiograph.

Hydatid cysts are composed of three layers. (*a*) an outer protective pericyst, (*b*) an easily broken middle membrane, and (*c*) a thin inner germinal layer that produces the scolices. The organs most commonly involved in humans are the liver (75%) and lung (15%). Other organs, such as brain, bone, and kidney are infected in less than 10% of cases.

Although most cases are acquired in childhood, they are not usually detected until adulthood. The symptoms of renal hydatid disease are nonspecific, and many patients are asymptomatic. Flank pain, hematuria, or signs of urinary tract infection may be present. A serologic test is available for patients suspected of having hydatid disease, on the basis of contact or radiologic findings.

Curvilinear calcifications in the wall of the hydatid cyst may be detected on plain radiographs (Fig. 5.24). A hypovascular mass can be detected with urography. However, the thick rim distinguishes the hydatid cyst from a simple cortical cyst.

Thick wall cysts also are well demonstrated by CT or ultrasound. If daughter cysts are present, they can be detected by internal echoes or a high-density component next to the clear, water-density cystic fluid.

Communicating Cysts

Occasionally a renal cyst communicates with the collecting system and opacifies with intravenous contrast medium on IVP, CT, or retrograde pyelography. Any cystic renal mass, such as a benign cortical cyst, inflammatory cyst, or even cystic carcinoma may rupture into the collecting system and produce this appearance. However, the most common etiology is a pyelogenic cyst or calyceal diverticulum (*see* Chapter 13).

A pyelogenic cyst is lined with transitional epithelium and communicates with the collecting system through a narrow isthmus. The connection is usually at the fornix, but can be at any portion of the calyx. Most cysts are small, usually less than 2 cm in diameter. Pyelogenic cysts are usually asymptomatic, but occasionally may contain calculi or milk of calcium.

Since excreted contrast medium enters the calyces from the tubules of Bellini, the calyces opacify before the calyceal diverticulum. This useful differentiating feature distinguishes the calyces from papillary necrosis or focal hydronephrosis. Communicating cysts also are well demonstrated by CT, in which contrast accumulation can be clearly seen (Fig. 5.25).

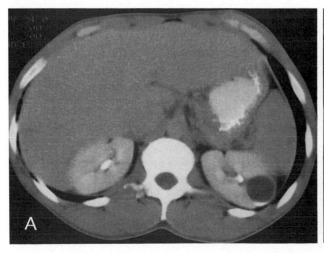
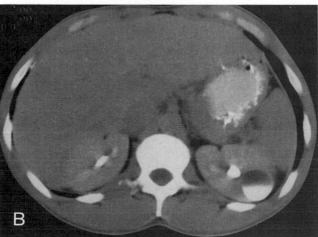

Figure 5.25. Communicating cyst. **A,** A small amount of contrast material is seen in the left renal cyst. The thick wall suggests it is most likely a calyceal diverticulum. **B,** Later images demonstrate further contrast accumulation.

EXTRAPARENCHYMAL CYSTS

Various investigators have used different terms to describe extraparenchymal cysts. To minimize this ambiguity, we consider cysts in two anatomic locations. The term *parapelvic cyst* is applied to cysts lying in the region of the renal sinus and the term *perinephric cyst* is used to describe those just beneath the renal capsule.

Amis and Cronan have suggested that cysts in the renal sinus are further subdivided into etiologies. They use the term parapelvic cyst for a renal parenchymal cyst that projects into the renal sinus. Cysts that develop in the renal sinus, probably from lymphatics, are termed peripelvic cysts. Using this terminology, parapelvic cysts are usually large but solitary, whereas peripelvic cysts more often are small and multiple.

Renal Sinus Cysts

These benign cysts lie in the region of the renal hilum and cause extrinsic compression on the collecting system. Smooth bowing or displacement of the infundibuli is seen on the IVP (Fig. 5.26). The CT appearance is that of a benign cyst located in the hilar area (Fig. 5.27) rather than the cortex of the kidney.

Renal sinus or parapelvic cysts may not be renal in origin, but could be lymphocysts or may arise from embryologic remnants in the renal hilum. With increased use of CT and ultrasound, they are frequently recognized and often are multiple and bilateral (Fig. 5.27). Problems arise when renal sinus or parapelvic cysts are confused with other entities.

On urography, the mass effect of the renal sinus cyst

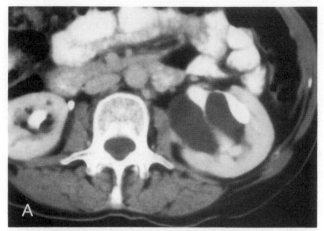

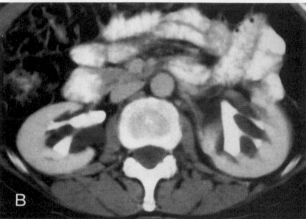

Figure 5.27.   Renal sinus cyst. **A,** A large cyst in the left renal hilus is bowing the collecting system. **B,** Computed tomography demonstrates that these cysts are often multiple and bilateral.

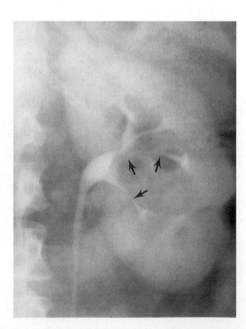

Figure 5.26.   Renal sinus cyst. A mass is seen displacing the renal pelvis and major infundibuli (*arrows*) on excretory urography.

on the collecting system also could be caused by a renal tumor or metastases to lymph nodes in the hilar region. Ultrasound demonstrates their benign cystic nature (Fig. 5.28). However, on ultrasound, the multiple echo-free areas in the central portion of the kidney may suggest hydronephrosis. Care must be taken to demonstrate that a dilated calyx is continuous with an enlarged infundibulum and pelvis before hydronephrosis is diagnosed.

Renal sinus cysts should not be confused with renal sinus fat (sinus lipomatosis). Both of these entities produce extrinsic compression on the renal collecting system and may be indistinguishable by urography. However, CT and ultrasound can easily distinguish between these processes. The low-density fat is clearly different from the water density cysts on CT examination. Fat is highly echogenic on ultrasound, through which it can be easily differentiated from the echo-free parapelvic cysts.

Perinephric Cysts

A perinephric cyst is renal in origin, but is not a true cyst. It represents a collection of fluid, presumably ex-

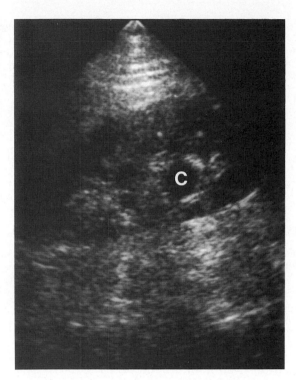

Figure 5.28. Renal sinus cyst. A cyst (*C*) in the region of the renal hilus is seen with ultrasound.

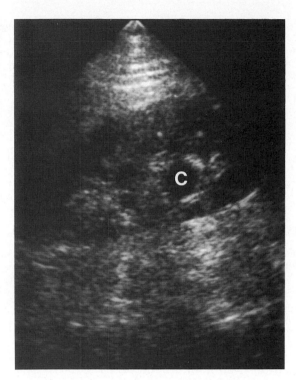

travasated urine, that is formed, often after renal trauma, but trapped beneath the renal capsule. Perinephric cysts also may be seen in infants with congenital lower urinary tract obstruction. The cyst walls are composed of fibrous tissue and do not have an epithelial lining. They are seldom of any clinical significance but, if large, could result in hypertension due to the compressive force on the renal parenchyma (Page kidney).

RENAL CYST PUNCTURE

During the early 1970s, renal cyst puncture gained great popularity as the definitive procedure, short of surgery, for the diagnosis of a renal cyst. By the late 1970s and early 1980s, however, there was widespread acceptance of CT and ultrasound as noninvasive studies that demonstrated accuracy similiar to cyst puncture. In addition to its use as a diagnostic procedure, renal cyst puncture may be used as a therapeutic maneuver in selected patients.

Approximately 5 to 8% of all renal lesions will not be adequately characterized by ultrasound or CT. When there is a discrepancy between imaging studies or between the radiographic appearance of the lesion and the clinical symptoms for which the initial studies were obtained, renal cyst puncture may be helpful. In the majority of cases, the true nature of the lesion can be ascertained using thin-collimation CT performed with and without contrast enhancement. If, after such a study, a

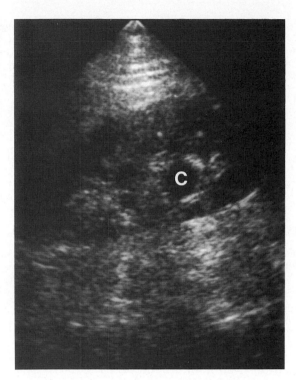

mass remains indeterminate, many authorities now feel that cyst puncture is unlikely to give a definitive answer. In these patients, short-term follow-up or exploratory surgery should be considered.

Ultrasound, CT, or fluoroscopic guidance may be used to guide the cyst puncture. With the fluoroscopic technique, intravenous contrast medium is needed to identify the lesion. The cyst is generally punctured with a 22-gauge Chiba needle, and cystic fluid is aspirated and sent to the laboratory for analysis. If a double-contrast study of the cyst is desired, the remainder of the cystic fluid is aspirated and exchanged for air and contrast medium on an equal volume basis until approximately 50% of the cyst volume has been replaced by air, approximately 25% has been replaced by contrast medium, and approximately 25% remains as cystic fluid. Once the air and contrast medium have been injected into the lesion, the needle is withdrawn and radiographs are obtained in multiple horizontal beam projections so that all of the walls of the cyst can be demonstrated with double-contrast images.

If after needle placement no fluid or only grossly bloody fluid can be aspirated, and if proper needle position has been verified, the mass can be presumed to be solid. A small amount of contrast medium may be injected to verify the needle position. This will result in a "tumorogram" that will demonstrate extravasation of the contrast medium within the interstices of the lesion.

Complete aspiration of the cystic fluid is necessary before therapeutic sclerosis of the cyst. To accomplish this, a pigtail catheter is placed into the cyst over a guidewire and the cyst is evacuated as completely as possible.

The radiographic assessment of the renal cystogram begins with a comparison of the size of the lesion as demonstrated by the cystogram to the mass that has been discovered on the preceding imaging examination. If the exact dimensions of the mass are not entirely explained by the cyst, the presence of an additional cyst or a cyst adjacent to another mass must be considered.

The walls of a simple renal cyst should be entirely smooth, without evidence of nodules or masses. On the horizontal beam radiographs, a sharp demarcation between the injected air and the contrast medium should be demonstrated. Any irregularity of this surface should suggest the possibility that the lesion does not represent a simple cyst. Occasionally, internal septations may be demonstrated within the lesion that may explain the presence of internal echoes that may have been present on a preceding ultrasound examination.

Fluid aspirated from a renal cyst may be analyzed for the following: (*a*) appearance, (*b*) biochemical profile, and (*c*) the histology of the cellular content. A clear, straw-colored cystic aspirate is strongly correlated with an entirely benign cyst. Thus, some authorities believe that cytologic and biochemical examination of clear cystic fluid is unnecessary.

If murky, dark, or frankly bloody cystic fluid is aspirated, biochemical studies (protein, lactic dehydrogenase, and fat content) have been reported to be of value in differentiating benign and inflammatory lesions from necrotic malignancies, but in practice, such studies are rarely obtained. Negative cytology does **not** exclude malignancy; such studies are therefore helpful only if the results are positive.

In the occasional patient, diagnostic puncture and therapeutic sclerosis may be indicated. Patients in this category include those with unexplained pain, hydronephrosis as a result of compression of the collecting system by the cyst, and rarely, the presence of renin-mediated hypertension caused by the renal cyst.

The majority of symptomatic cysts can be treated by percutaneous drainage or a combination of percutaneous drainage and sclerosis. Drainage without scleral therapy will result in a recurrence of 30 to 78% of cases. A number of sclerosing agents have been used to prevent cyst fluid reaccumulation. The most commonly used is 95% ethanol. With alcohol sclerosis, a minimum of 25% of the original cyst volume should be replaced with 95% ethanol. The patient is then placed in the prone, supine, and decubitus positions for a minimum of 5 minutes each to allow adequate contact of the alcohol with all areas of the cyst. The alcohol is then aspirated through the pigtail catheter. Using this technique, Bean has shown a 0.5% incidence of recurrence in 34 cysts followed for 3 months.

SUGGESTED READINGS

Cortical Cysts

Bosniak MA: The current radiological approach to renal cysts. *Radiology* 158:1, 1986.

Coleman BG, Arger PH, Mintz MC, et al.: Hyperdense renal masses: a computed tomographic dilemma. *AJR* 143:291, 1984.

Dunnick NR, Korobkin M, Clark WM: CT Demonstration of hyperdense renal carcinoma. *J Comput Assist Tomogr* 8(5):1023, 1984.

Dunnick NR, Korobkin M, Silverman PM, et al.: Computed tomography of high density renal cysts. *J Comput Assist Tomogr* 8(3):458, 1984.

Elkin M, Bernstein J: Cystic diseases of the kidney: radiological and pathological considerations. *Clin Radiol* 29:65, 1969.

Friedland GW: Shrinking and disappearing renal cysts. *Urol Radiol* 9:21, 1987.

Hartman DS: Cysts and cystic neoplasms. *Urol Radiol* 12:7, 1990.

Levine E, Grantham JJ: High-Density renal cysts in autosomal dominant polycystic kidney disease demonstrated by CT. *Radiology* 154:477, 1985.

Osathanondh V, Potter EL: Pathogenesis of polycystic kidneys. *Arch Pathol* 77:459, 1964.

Papanicolaou N, Pfister RC, Yoder IC: Spontaneous and traumatic rupture of renal cysts: diagnosis and outcome. *Radiology* 160:99, 1986.

Reynolds WF, Goldstein AMB, Williams EJ, et al.: Uncommon radiologic observations in renal milk-of-calcium stone. *Urology* 11(4):419, 1978.

Rosenberg ER, Korobkin M, Foster W, et al.: The significance of septations in a renal cyst. *AJR* 144:593, 1985.

Sussman S, Cochran ST, Pagani JJ, et al.: Hyperdense renal masses: a CT manifestation of hemorrhagic renal cysts. *Radiology* 150:207, 1984.

Unilateral Cystic Disease

Curry NS, Chung CJ, Gordon B: Unilateral renal cystic disease in an adult. *Abdom Imaging* 19:366, 1994.

Extraparenchymal Cysts

Amis ES Jr, Cronan JJ: The renal sinus: an imaging review and proposed nomenclature for sinus cysts. *J Urol* 139:1151, 1988.

Cronan JJ, Yoder IC, Amis ES Jr, et al.: The myth of anechoic renal sinus fat. *Radiology* 144:149, 1982.

Elkin M, Bernstein J: Cystic diseases of the kidney: radiological and pathological considerations. *Clin Radiol* 29:65, 1969.

Hidalgo H, Dunnick NR Rosenberg ER, et al.: Parapelvic cysts: appearance on CT and sonography. *AJR* 138:667, 1982.

Polycystic Renal Disease

Hayden CK Jr, Swischuk LE, Smith TH, et al.: Renal cystic disease in childhood. *Radiographics* 6:97, 1986.

Higashihara E, Aso Y, Shimazaki J, et al.: Clinical aspects of polycystic kidney disease. *J Urol* 147:329, 1992.

Kirks DR: *Practical Pediatric Imaging: Diagnostic Radiology of Infants and Children*. Boston, Little, Brown, 1991.

Levine E, Cook LT, Grantham JJ: Liver cysts in autosomal-dominant polycystic kidney disease: clinical and computed tomographic study. *AJR* 145:229, 1985.

Levine E, Grantham JJ: Perinephric hemorrhage in autosomal dominant polycystic kidney disease: CT and MR findings. *J Comput Assist Tomogr* 11(1):108, 1987.

Levine E, Grantham JJ: Calcified renal stones and cyst calcifications in autosomal dominant polycystic kidney disease: clinical and CT study in 84 patients. *AJR* 159:77, 1992.

McCallum RW, Gildiner M: Diminished visualization of renal outlines in adult renal polycystic disease. *J Can Assoc Radiol* 32:13, 1981.

Segal AJ, Spataro RF: Computed tomography of adult polycystic disease. *J Comput Assist Tomogr* 6(4):777, 1982.

Walker FC Jr, Loney LC, Root ER, et al.: Diagnostic evaluation of adult polycystic kidney disease in childhood. *AJR* 142:1273, 1984.

Younathan CM, Kaude JV: Renal peripelvic lymphatic cysts (lymphangiomas) associated with generalized lymphangiomatosis. *Urol Radiol* 14:161, 1992.

Cysts Associated with Systemic Disease

Choyke PL, Glenn GM, Walther MM, et al.: The natural history of renal lesions in von Hippel-Lindau disease: a serial CT study in 28 patients. *AJR* 159:1229, 1992.

Choyke PL, Glenn GM, Walther MM, et al.: von Hippel-Lindau disease: genetic, clinical, and imaging features. *Radiology* 194:629, 1995.

Chonko AM, Weiss SM, Stein JH, et al.: Renal involvement in tuberous sclerosis. *Am J Med* 56:124, 1974.

Hough DM, Stephens DH, Johnson CD, Binkovitz LA: Pancreatic lesions in von Hippel-Lindau disease: prevalence, clinical significance, and CT findings. *AJR* 162:1091, 1994.

Levine E, Collins DL, Horton WA, et al.: CT screening of the abdomen in von Hippel-Lindau disease. *AJR* 139:505, 1982.

Loughlin ER, Gittes RF: Urologic management of patients with von Hippel-Lindau's disease. *J Urol* 136:789, 1986.

Miller DL, Choyke PL, Walther MM, et al.: von Hippel-Lindau disease: inadequacy of angiography for identification of renal cancers. *Radiology* 179:833, 1991.

Mitnick JS, Bosniak MA, Hilton S, et al.: Cystic renal disease in tuberous sclerosis. *Radiology* 147:85, 1983.

Shinohara N, Nonomura K, Harabayashi T, et al.: Nephron sparing surgery for renal cell carcinoma in von Hippel-Lindau disease. *J Urol* 154:2016, 1995.

Torres VE, King BF, Holley KE, et al.: The kidney in the tuberous sclerosis complex. *Adv Nephrol* 23:43, 1994.

Acquired Renal Cystic Disease

Chandhoke PS, Torrence RJ, Clayman RV, Rothstein M: Acquired cystic disease of the kidney: a management dilemma. *J Urol* 147:969, 1992.

Grantham JJ, Levine E: Acquired cystic disease: replacing one kidney disease with another. *Kidney Int* 28:99, 1985.

Levine E: The query corner: acquired cystic kidney disease. *Abdom Imaging* 20:569, 1995.

Levine E, Grantham JJ, Slusher SL, et al.: CT of acquired cystic kidney disease and renal tumors in long-term dialysis patients. *AJR* 142:125, 1984.

Levine LA, Gburek BM: Acquired cystic disease and renal adenocarcinoma following renal transplantation. *J Urol* 151:129, 1994.

Levine E, Slusher SL, Grantham JJ, Wetzel LH: Natural history of acquired renal cystic disease in dialysis patients: a prospective longitudinal CT study. *AJR* 156:501, 1991.

Mindell HJ: Imaging studies for screening native kidneys in long-term dialysis patients. *AJR* 153:768, 1989.

Takase K, Takahashi S, Tazawa S, Terasawa Y, Sakamoto K: Renal cell carcinoma associated with chronic renal failure: evaluation with sonographic angiography. *Radiology* 192:787, 1994.

Taylor AJ, Cohen EP, Erickson SJ, et al.: Renal imaging in long-term dialysis patients: a comparison of CT and sonography. *AJR* 153:765, 1989.

Medullary Cystic Disease

Garel LA, Habib R, Pariente D, et al.: Juvenile nephronophthisis: sonographic appearance in children with severe uremia. *Radiology* 151.93, 1984.

Rego JD Jr, Laing FC, Jeffrey RB: Ultrasonographic diagnosis of medullary cystic disease. *J Ultrasound Med* 2:433, 1983.

Steele B, Lirenman DS, Beattle CW: Nephronophthisis. *Am J Med* 68:521, 1980.

Multicystic Dysplastic Kidney

Kleiner B, Filly RA, Mack L, et al.: Multicystic dysplastic kidney: observations of contralateral disease in the fetal population. *Radiology* 161:27, 1986.

Pedicelli G, Jequier S, Bowen A, Boisvert J: Multicystic dysplastic kidneys: spontaneous regression demonstrated with US. *Radiology* 160:23, 1986.

Sanders R, Hartman D: The sonographic distinction between neonatal multicystic kidney and hydronephrosis. *Radiology* 151:621, 1984.

Vinocur L, Slovis TL, Perlmutter AD, et al.: Follow-up studies of multicystic dysplastic kidneys. *Radiology* 167:311, 1988.

Multilocular Cystic Nephroma

Agrons GA, Wagner BJ, Davidson AJ, Suarez ES: From the archives of the AFIP. *RadioGraphics* 15:653, 1995.

Banner MP, Pollack HM, Chatten J, et al.: Multilocular renal cysts: radiologic-pathologic correlation. *AJR* 136:239, 1981.

de Wall JG, Schroder FH, Scholtmeijer RJ: Diagnostic workup and treatment of multilocular cystic kidney. *Urology* 28(1):73, 1986.

Madewell JE, Goldman SM, Davis CJ, et al.: Multilocular cystic nephroma: a radiographic-pathologic correlation of 58 patients. *Radiology* 146:309, 1983.

Parienty RA, Pradel J, Imbert MC, et al.: Computed tomography of multilocular cystic nephroma. *Radiology* 140:135, 1981.

Orofaciodigital Syndrome

Curry NS, Milutinovic J, Grossnickle M, Munden M: Renal cystic disease associated with orofaciodigital syndrome. *Urol Radiol* 13:153, 1992.

Hydatid Disease

Beggs I: Therapy of multilocular cystic nephroma. *AJR* 145:639, 1985.

Lewall DB, McCorkell SJ: Rupture of echinococcal cysts: diagnosis, classification and clinical implications. *AJR* 146:391, 1986.

Cyst Aspiration

Amis ES Jr, Cronan JJ, Pfister RC: Needle puncture of cystic renal masses: a survey of the Society of Uroradiology. *AJR* 148:297, 1987.

Bean WJ: Renal cysts: treatment with alcohol. *Radiology* 138:329, 1985.

Lang EK: Renal cyst puncture and aspiration: a survey of complications. *AJR* 128:723, 1977.

Sandler CM, Houston GK, Hall JT, et al.: Guided cyst puncture and aspiration. *Radiol Clin North Am* 24(4):527, 1986.

6

Renal Tumors

• • • • • • • • • •

Because any cell type found in the kidney or renal capsule has the potential to become neoplastic, there are many types of renal tumors. Unfortunately, few of these tumors have a radiographic appearance sufficiently characteristic to make a confident diagnosis. Thus, the majority of solid renal masses must be considered malignant until proven otherwise.

RENAL PARENCHYMAL TUMORS

Adenocarcinoma

Renal adenocarcinoma is a malignant neoplasm that arises from proximal convoluted tubular epithelial cells. The many synonyms that have been applied to this tumor, such as hypernephroma, Grawitz's tumor, clear cell carcinoma, and malignant nephroma, are misleading or inadequate and are best ignored.

Renal carcinoma is twice as common among men than women. The tumor may occur at any age, but the incidence peaks in the sixth decade. No etiologic agents are recognized, but there is an increased incidence in patients who use tobacco. Patients with von Hippel-Lindau disease often develop renal carcinomas that are smaller but frequently multiple and bilateral. There also is a familial renal cell carcinoma unrelated to von Hippel-Lindau disease.

Patients on chronic hemodialysis or peritoneal dialysis develop acquired renal cystic disease (*see* Chapter 5). These patients have an overall incidence of renal carcinoma of approximately 7%, although not all of these tumors behave in a biologically aggressive manner. These tumors begin to appear in patients as early as 3 years after initiation of dialysis, but are difficult to detect because these patients' kidneys are not functioning and usually contain multiple cysts and dystrophic calcifications. The incidence of renal tumors seems to parallel the development of acquired cystic disease, such that more tumors are seen the longer the patients are maintained on dialysis. The effect of renal transplantation on the development of renal cancer is unclear. Although it is likely that successful transplantation reduces the risk of renal carcinoma by removing undialyzable carcinogens, this is counter-balanced by the increased risk of malignancy with immunosuppression.

The classic clinical presentation with a flank mass, pain, and hematuria occurs in only a minority of patients. Often patients first complain of nonspecific symptoms such as weight loss, fatigue, or even gastrointestinal or neurologic symptoms. Less common presenting complaints include fever or a new varicocele. Fatigue may be caused by a normochromic normocytic anemia. A variety of other hormones may be secreted by renal adenocarcinomas in sufficient quantity to cause distinct clinical manifestations (Table 6.1). These hormones include renin, erythropoietin, parathormone, adrenocorticotropic hormone, prolactin, and gonadotropin. Thus, renal adenocarcinoma has sometimes been called the "internist's tumor."

Hematuria is the most common sign, occurring in more than 50% of patients. It is usually gross, but is occasionally only microscopic. Flank pain, present in more

Table 6.1. Endocrine Manifestations of Renal Adenocarcinoma

Hormone	Manifestation
Renin	Hypertension
Erythropoietin	Erythrocytosis
Parathormone	Hypercalcemia
Prolactin	Galactorrhea
Gonadotropin	Gynecomastia
ACTH	Cushing's syndrome

ACTH = corticotrophin

than one third of patients, is probably caused by distension of the renal capsule. A flank mass is palpable at presentation in approximately one third of patients. As abdominal computed tomography (CT) and ultrasound examinations are being performed more commonly, there has been an increase in the discovery of small, asymptomatic renal carcinomas.

It is difficult to predict the natural history of renal adenocarcinoma. Some tumors demonstrate aggressive behavior by growing rapidly and metastasizing early. However, occasionally patients may live for years with an untreated primary tumor. Metastases have been reported as late as 31 years after nephrectomy and spontaneous regression of metastases or a primary tumor may occur.

Radiology

The radiologic investigation of patients suspected of having renal carcinoma usually begins with excretory urography. However, urography is not as sensitive as CT in the detection of renal masses. Urography detects only one half of the renal masses between 2 and 3 cm in diameter that are seen by CT. In a retrospective review of 65 consecutive patients with renal tumors, Demos and colleagues found that excretory urography missed four (6%) tumors. Curry found only 3 (33%) of 9 small renal neoplasms (less than 3 cm) using screening urography. Thus, CT is needed in patients with a strong clinical suspicion of a renal tumor, even if excretous inography (IVP) is unrevealing.

Calcification, which can be detected on the preliminary radiograph in as many as 20% of renal adenocarcinomas (Fig. 6.1), is even easier to detect on an unenhanced CT examination (Fig. 6.2). However, calcification also may be seen in other renal masses, including common lesions such as benign cysts.

The character of the calcification is helpful in determining the etiology of a renal mass. Peripheral curvilinear calcification is more commonly seen in a cyst, whereas central calcification means the lesion is more likely a renal carcinoma. However, the importance of calcification has decreased since CT, ultrasound, and magnetic resonance (MR) can be used to more clearly define the nature of a renal mass (*see* Fig. 6.1). Any of these cross-sectional imaging modalities can directly detect a soft tissue mass or tumor nodule within a cystic mass without relying on the presence of a central calcification. Furthermore, calcification of a central septation within a cyst may give the misleading impression of a solid mass on urography.

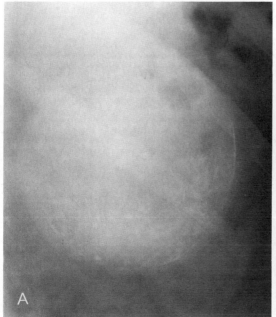
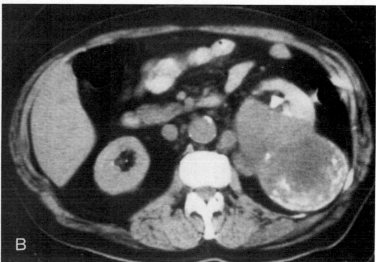

Figure 6.1.   Renal carcinoma. **A,** Calcification is appreciated in a left renal mass on the preliminary radiograph. **B,** Computed tomography confirms a large calcified renal tumor.

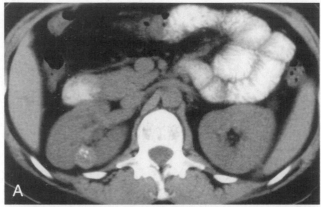

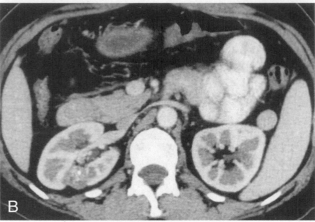

Figure 6.2. Renal carcinoma. **A,** Calcification is seen in a small mass in the right kidney on this unenhanced CT examination. **B,** During the cortical phase of contrast administration, the mass enhances, but less than the normal renal cortex.

In all but very large tumors, renal function is preserved. In fact, diminished renal function suggests tumor thrombosis in the renal vein. The carcinoma is identified as a vascular mass with mottled density that causes a focal bulge in the renal contour. Involvement of the collecting system is seen as irregularity of the urothelial surface or complete occlusion of a calyx or infundibulum. A filling defect within the collecting system may represent blood clot or tumor invasion.

Hypovascular or cystic renal carcinomas may be difficult to distinguish from benign cysts on IVP. Benign cortical cysts are sharply defined and have an imperceptibly thin wall (*see* Chapter 5). If the wall of a cystic mass can be detected by IVP or CT, the lesion is not a simple cyst and further evaluation is warranted.

Even with routine nephrotomography, it often is impossible to define a renal mass well enough by IVP to make a diagnosis of a benign lesion. Further study with ultrasound or CT is needed. Those lesions that are most likely benign cysts are most efficiently confirmed by ultrasound. However, if the lesion is complex or solid,

CT will probably be needed, and it may be more expeditious to omit ultrasound and proceed directly to CT.

Ultrasound is particularly helpful in distinguishing solid from cystic renal masses. A renal adenocarcinoma is usually seen as a solid mass, although cystic regions representing areas of hemorrhage or necrosis are common.

The echogenicity of renal carcinomas is variable. They may be more echogenic, less echogenic (Fig. 6.3), or isoechoic with the normal renal parenchyma. Highly echogenic tumors, which are more frequently small tumors, may mimic the increased echogenicity of fat-containing tumors such as angiomyolipomas. With the increased recognition of small renal carcinomas, more hyperechoic tumors mimicking angiomyolipomas are found. However, an anechoic rim often is present in hyperechoic renal carcinomas and is not seen in angiomyolipomas. Isoechoic tumors may be difficult to detect with ultrasound, especially if they are small and do not displace the collecting system or produce a contour deformity. Less echogenic tumors simulate more homogeneous tumors such as lymphomas or may be confused with renal cysts. However, these solid tumors have poorly defined margins and do not have the increased sound transmission seen with cysts. A few renal adenocarcinomas are frankly cystic. However, even these tumors can usually be distinguished from simple cysts by their irregularly thick walls and the presence of some internal echoes.

Doppler ultrasound provides a noninvasive measure of the vascularity of a renal mass. High velocity-signals, which are presumably due to arteriovenous shunting, are frequently seen in renal carcinomas. Kuijpers and colleagues report that a Doppler shift of 2.5 kHz or more indicates a renal carcinoma or inflammatory mass, whereas a shift of less than 2.5 kHz supports the diagnosis of a benign cyst.

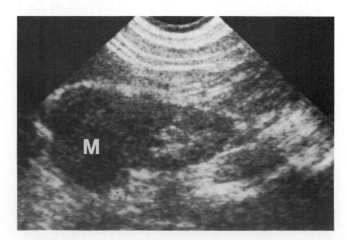

Figure 6.3. Renal carcinoma. Ultrasound reveals a mass (*M*) in the upper pole that is slightly less echogenic than the normal renal parenchyma.

Computed tomography is the single most valuable modality in assessing a renal mass. It is the most sensitive radiographic examination for the detection of renal masses, although reports of equal sensitivity with MR are beginning to appear. Computed tomography also can isolate simple cysts with a high degree of accuracy. Other mass lesions that are indeterminate or clearly solid must be considered renal adenocarcinoma until proven otherwise.

Renal adenocarcinomas are readily detected by CT. Their density is variable and depends on the presence of tissue necrosis, hemorrhage, or calcification. Although a contour bulge often may be appreciated, smaller masses may easily be missed on precontrast images (Fig. 6.4).

After intravenous contrast injection, renal carcinomas usually demonstrate an inhomogeneous enhancement. Portions of the tumor become nearly as dense as the normal renal cortex, whereas other areas show little enhancement (Fig. 6.5). Cystic carcinomas are recognized by their thick irregular wall or the presence of a tumor nodule (Fig. 6.6).

The speed of spiral (helical) CT allows imaging of the kidneys during corticomedullary (CMP) and nephro-

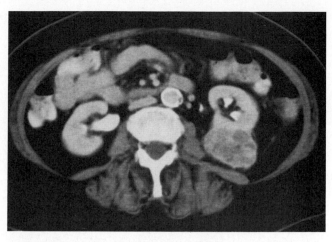

Figure 6.5.   Renal carcinoma. Computed tomography reveals inhomogeneous enhancement of the tumor.

graphic (NP) phases of contrast enhancement. Cohan and colleagues found more renal masses during the NP than the CMP, especially for masses in the medulla.

The use of angiography as a method of diagnosing renal carcinoma has decreased, because CT has assumed this role. However, arteriography may be employed to identify small vascular tumors when CT is equivocal. Arteriography has been used when the renal parenchyma is abnormal or distorted, which may occur in patients with von Hippel-Lindau disease. The definition of the tumor vascularity, and identification of the number and location of the renal arteries may contribute to a safer surgical resection, particularly when a segmental or wedge resection is being considered in a pa-

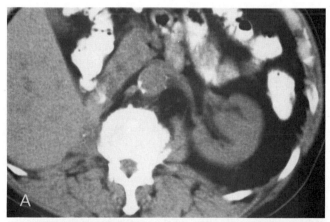

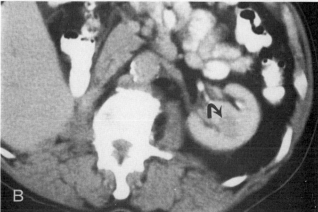

Figure 6.4.   Renal carcinoma. **A,** The precontrast image is unremarkable. **B,** After contrast injection, a small low-density mass (*arrow*) is seen.

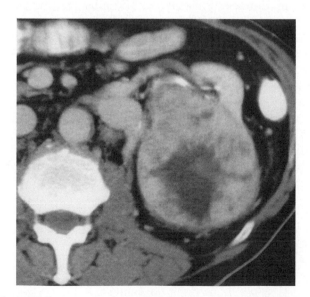

Figure 6.6.   Cystic renal carcinoma. The low-density center of this left renal mass represents tumor necrosis. The thick irregular wall indicated renal carcinoma rather than a complicated cyst.

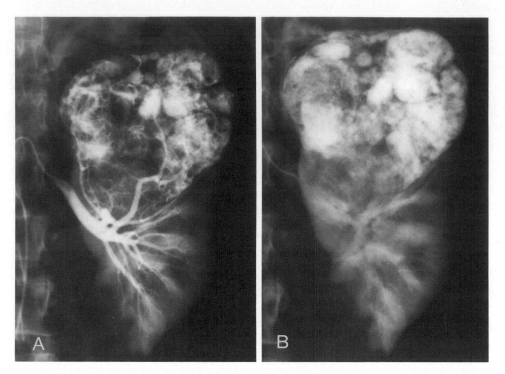

Figure 6.7.   Renal carcinoma. **A** and **B,** The arteriographic findings of neovascularity, encasement, and venous laking indicate renal carcinoma.

tient with one kidney. However, careful examination of excised kidneys has shown poor sensitivity for angiography in detecting small tumors, because the tumors were less vascular than expected and occasionally had the angiographic appearances of a complicated cyst.

Most renal adenocarcinomas are vascular tumors and display tumor neovascularity. The most specific vascular appearance is encasement, whereby a vessel decreases in caliber as it is entrapped by tumor but then increases in caliber farther along its course (Fig. 6.7). This phenomenon is rarely seen in inflammatory masses. Arteriovenous shunting is common and there may be a dense tumor stain, vascular puddling, or the formation of venous lakes.

These changes may be less obvious in the minority of renal carcinomas which are hypovascular. Such tumors often have large areas of hemorrhage or tumor necrosis but still demonstrate some abnormal vessels.

Small tumors whose vascularity is similar to that of the normal renal parenchyma also may be difficult to detect with arteriography. In this setting, epinephrine injected before the arteriogram may demonstrate a tumor not seen on the routine films. Five to 10 μgm of epinephrine is injected through the catheter into the renal artery. This constricts the normal renal arteries and diminishes blood flow to the normal renal parenchyma. However, tumor vessels do not have a muscular wall and are unable to constrict. Thus, more blood (and con-

trast medium) go to the tumor, making it easier to identify (Fig. 6.8).

Arteriography is seldom needed to stage renal carcinoma, but may be employed as a diagnostic tool or as part of a therapeutic technique with vascular occlusion. Arteriography may be used occasionally to evaluate the liver, especially to distinguish a hemangioma from a metastasis. A hepatic dysfunction syndrome associated with renal adenocarcinoma has been reported. It consists of nonspecific constitutional symptoms, hepatomegaly, and abnormal liver function tests. The liver is hypervascular with accentuation of the normal fine granular pattern. The hepatomegaly and abnormal liver function tests return to normal after nephrectomy.

Magnetic resonance imaging has become a valuable modality for evaluating renal masses. The improved signal-to-noise ratios of higher (1.5-Tesla) field strength units combined with fat suppression techniques to make lesions more conspicuous and the use of intravascular contrast agents have improved MR sensitivity for detecting renal masses to approximately equal that of contrast-enhanced CT. Furthermore, the higher field-strength magnets have made breath-hold techniques that remove respiratory-induced artifacts more practical.

Yamashita and coworkers recently reported finding a pseudocapsule in 66% of renal carcinomas 4 cm in diameter or smaller. This may be useful in surgical plan-

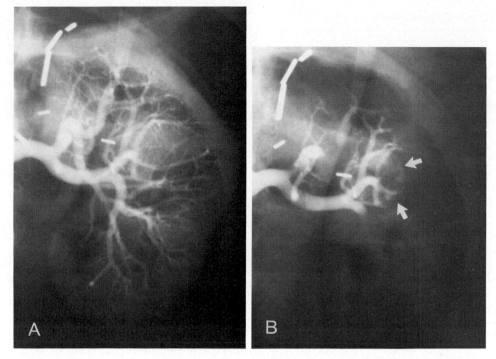

Figure 6.8.   Renal carcinoma. Previous surgery makes evaluation of the kidney difficult in this patient with von Hippel-Lindau disease. **A,** A renal arteriogram is suggestive of a solid renal mass. **B,** After epinephrine, the normal renal arteries constrict, making the tumor vessels more conspicuous (*arrows*).

ning, because the presence of a pseudocapsule may make enucleation easier.

The signal characteristics of renal carcinomas vary with the vascularity of the tumor and the presence or absence of central necrosis, calcification, hemorrhage, and iron deposits. Homogeneous tumors are relatively isointense, with the renal parenchyma on T1- and T2-weighted sequences. Intravenous contrast (Gd-DTPA) administration enhances the vascular tumors. This is usually done with spin-echo or T1-weighted sequences. Hypovascular tumors are better detected with fat-saturation techniques. Although recent studies have shown the sensitivity of MR to be similar to CT for detecting renal masses, CT remains the primary imaging modality for the detection of renal tumors. Magnetic resonance has advantages for staging, especially tumor extension into the vein, and can be used as a problem-solving technique for specific situations. Magnetic resonance also may be substituted for CT in patients in whom iodinated intravascular contrast medium is contraindicated.

Staging

The two most commonly used staging systems are the classic system described by Robson and colleagues in 1969 and the TNM system described by the American Joint Committee for Cancer Staging (Table 6.2).

The Robson classification is simpler, has been in use longer, and provides anatomic and prognostic information.

In the Robson system, stage I disease is confined to the kidney. Tumor does not extend beyond the renal capsule. The 5- and 10-year survival rates for these patients are 67% and 56%, respectively.

Tumor that has grown through the renal capsule into the perinephric space is considered stage II disease. The ipsilateral adrenal gland may be involved. Because the entire contents of Gerota's fascia are removed during radical nephrectomy, the distinction between stage I and stage II disease does not usually affect surgical treatment. The 5- and 10-year prognoses are 51% and 28%, respectively.

Stage III disease is subdivided into A, B, and C categories. Tumor that involves the main renal vein is classified as stage IIIA. The tumor may grow into the inferior vena cava (IVC) and up to the right atrium. The precise delineation of the tumor thrombus is critical to planning the surgical approach.

Involvement of regional lymph nodes indicates stage IIIB, whereas in stage IIIC disease, the tumor involves the main renal vein and regional lymph nodes. The 5- and 10-year prognoses for stage III disease are 34 and 20%, respectively. Because the tumor thrombus often can be surgically removed, patients with stage IIIA dis-

Table 6.2. Renal Carcinoma Staging

Robson Stage	Disease Extent	TNM
I	Confined within renal capsule	T1 (<2.5 cm)
		T2 (>2.5 cm)
II	Penetrates beyond renal capsule but remains within Gerota's fascia	T3A
IIIA	Extends into renal vein and may progress into inferior vena cava	T3B
IIIB	Involves regional lymph nodes	N1–3
IIIC	Includes both venous extension and lymph node involvement	T3B, N1–3
IVA	Tumor growth through Gerota's fascia into adjacent tissues	T4
IVB	Distant metastases	M1

ease have a much better prognosis than those with stage IIIB disease.

Stage IV disease indicates disseminated tumor. Direct extension through Gerota's fascia into the adjacent organs is classified as stage IVA. Hematogenous or lymphatic metastases to distant sites results in a stage IVB classification. The 5- and 10-year prognoses for stage IV disease are 14 and 3%, respectively. Interestingly, patients with solitary metastases do better than those with multiple metastatic deposits.

Once a renal mass suspicious for renal carcinoma is found, staging is needed. A standard posteroanterior and lateral chest radiograph will detect most pulmonary metastases. If the patient has bone pain or an elevated serum alkaline phosphatase level, a radionuclide bone scan is indicated to detect bone metastases. Metastases to the skeleton or thorax is classified as stage IV disease and is treated with palliation.

If the patient is a surgical candidate, the abdomen is best evaluated using CT (Fig. 6.9). The overall accuracy

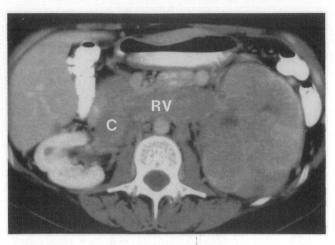

Figure 6.10. Renal carcinoma. A large left renal carcinoma is seen extending into the renal vein (*RV*) and inferior vena cava (*C*) on this enhanced computed tomography scan.

of CT in staging renal carcinoma is greater than 90%. However, some distinctions are more crucial than others. In most patients, for instance, a radical nephrectomy is performed, and it is inconsequential whether or not there is penetration of the renal capsule by tumor. Because it is difficult to make this distinction by CT, the elimination of this category raises the accuracy of CT staging to more than 95%.

Because CT is highly sensitive for the detection of adrenal metastases, a negative CT examination virtually excludes all but microscopic involvement. Thus, urologists may elect to spare the adrenal gland during nephrectomy in patients whose CT examinations show a normal-appearing ipsilateral adrenal gland.

Precise delineation of any venous extension is essential to plan the surgical approach and to gain vascular control of the kidney (Fig. 6.10). Inferior vena cavography has been used to delineate precisely the venous extension of a renal adenocarcinoma. However, it is an invasive technique that may require a second catheter to visualize the cephalad extent of a tumor thrombus (Fig. 6.11). If the CT examination is equivocal, MR imaging may be required.

Magnetic resonance imaging can precisely define venous extension of tumor thrombus. Because flowing blood does not impart a signal, a patent vein can easily be distinguished from the higher signal intensity of tumor extending into the vein. Furthermore, gradient-recalled echo techniques rapidly assess the status of the major veins (Fig. 6.12).

Magnetic resonance imaging also may prove accurate in assessing the small opacities seen in the perinephric space in many of these patients on CT examination. Some of these opacities represent inflammatory changes, whereas others may be caused by involved lymph nodes or collateral vessels. Magnetic resonance

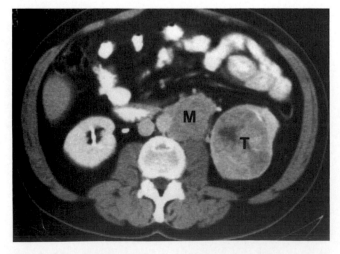

Figure 6.9. Renal carcinoma. A large tumor (*T*) is seen in the lower pole of the left kidney. Regional lymph node metastases (*M*) indicate stage IIIB disease.

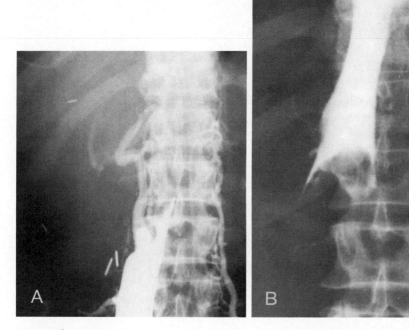

Figure 6.11.   Renal carcinoma. **A,** An inferior vena cavogram demonstrates complete occlusion. **B,** A cavogram "from above" delineates the cephalad extent of the tumor.

imaging can clearly identify patent vessels and can distinguish them from lymphadenopathy (Fig. 6.13).

Papillary Adenocarcinoma

Renal adenocarcinomas may be subdivided into papillary and nonpapillary types based on the pattern of cellular architecture. Papillary carcinomas comprise only 5 to 15% of all renal adenocarcinomas, but are character-

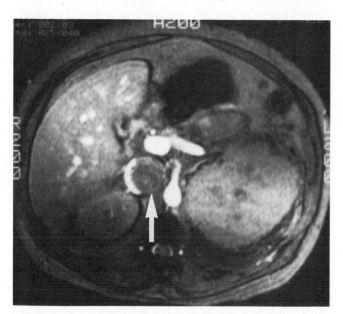

Figure 6.12.   Renal carcinoma. Gradient-recalled echo techniques are useful in identifying tumor extension into the inferior vena cava (*arrow*).

ized by a lower stage at presentation, slower growth, and a better prognosis than nonpapillary carcinomas.

Papillary tumors are less vascular than nonpapillary types, as seen by CT (Fig. 6.14) or angiography. They show less vascular enhancement and often do not have the frankly malignant hypervascular pattern seen with nonpapillary tumors. Calcification also is seen more commonly in papillary tumors, presumably reflecting slower growth.

Bellini Duct Carcinoma

Bellini duct carcinoma, a rare tumor that arises from the collecting duct (of Bellini) is considered a varient of renal cell carcinoma. Because it is usually found in the medullary portion of the kidney or renal sinus, the cortical margin is preserved. The tumor is hypovascular and shows only modest contrast enhancement on CT.

Sarcomatoid Carcinomas

Sarcomatoid renal cell carcinomas contain elements of renal adenocarcinoma, transitional cell carcinoma, and sarcoma. They occur more frequently in elderly patients, but are radiographically indistinguishable from renal adenocarcinoma.

Treatment

Surgical resection is the primary mode of therapy for patients with renal adenocarcinoma. Most patients undergo radical nephrectomy, which is why the distinction between stage I and stage II is seldom of value other

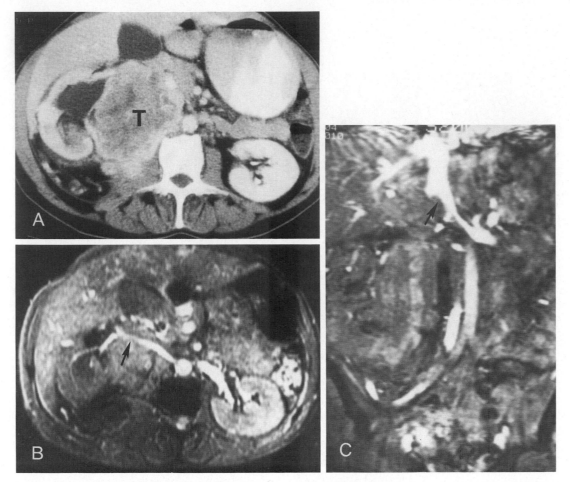

Figure 6.13.   Renal carcinoma. **A,** A large right renal tumor (*T*) is obstructing the upper-pole collecting system and is obscuring the inferior vena cava on computed tomography. **B,** On magnetic resonance imaging a gradient-recalled echo image demonstrates encasement of the right renal artery (*arrow*) by the tumor. **C,** On a coronal image, tumor (*arrow*) extends into the inferior vena cava.

than for assessing prognosis. In this operation, the entire contents of the perirenal space are removed without opening Gerota's fascia. The regional lymph nodes, paraaortic for left-sided tumors and paracaval for tumors of the right kidney, also are resected. Tumor extending into the renal vein and IVC often can be removed, because this tumor is usually well-encapsulated and is not attached to the vessel wall.

Patients with stage IV disease also may be treated with surgical resection. This may be done as palliation or to prevent complications such as hematuria, pain, or even congestive heart failure due to large arteriovenous fistulae. Occasional cases of regression of metastatic disease after removal of the primary tumor have been reported.

Angiography also may play a valuable role in the therapy of renal adenocarcinoma. Presurgical embolization of the tumor may dramatically reduce the vascularity of the tumor, making resection easier by di-

minishing blood loss. Research conducted at the M.D. Anderson Cancer Center suggested that a delay in surgical resection after embolization would improve survival because of an enhanced immunologic response to the tumor antigen. However, these results have not been supported by long-term studies, and surgical resection is usually performed within 24 hours of embolization.

Arterial embolization also can be used to treat complications in patients who are not surgical candidates. Hematuria often can be stopped with embolization of particulate materials such as Gelfoam (Upjohn, Kalamazoo, MI) and steel coils. Absolute ethanol also may be used to occlude the renal artery. However, this should be done with an occlusion balloon to prevent reflux and unwanted damage to other vessels.

Disease monitoring is usually performed with CT, which can precisely define existing disease as well as detect new lesions. Tumor recurrence in the renal fossa

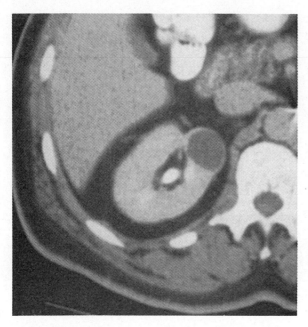

Figure 6.14. Renal carcinoma. The homogeneous low density is typical of papillary adenocarcinoma.

is difficult to recognize clinically, but is readily detected on CT (Fig. 6.15).

Renal Medullary Carcinoma

Recently, Davis and colleagues reported a previously unrecognized renal neoplasm in young black patients with sickle cell trait. The dominant tumor mass was in the medulla, with satellite lesions in the cortex. Venous and lymphatic invasion was usually present.

The patients ranged from 11 to 39 years of age, and there was a male preponderance, especially among the younger patients. Although almost all patients had sickle cell trait, none had sickle cell disease.

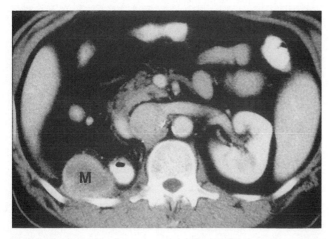

Figure 6.15. Recurrent tumor. This follow-up enhanced computed tomography scan after nephrectomy demonstrates a mass (*M*) in the right renal fossa.

The tumor is centrally located, grows in an infiltrative pattern, and is usually very large at presentation. The renal sinus is typically invaded, and caliectasis without pelviectasis often is present. The contrast enhancement and echotexture are heterogeneous.

The differential diagnosis for lesions with this appearance includes an infiltrative transitional cell carcinoma, acute pyelonephritis, or possibly, lymphoma. However, the clinical setting should allow the presumptive diagnosis of renal medullary carcinoma.

Adenoma

These benign tumors often are confused with and may be difficult to distinguish from renal adenocarcinoma. Both renal adenomas and adenocarcinomas develop in the proximal convoluted tubule and cannot be distinguished by histologic or histochemical means. They both occur in the same age groups, and both show a marked male predominance. Many authors believe that an adenoma is a small renal carcinoma that has not yet metastasized.

Because most of these small renal adenomas are detected at autopsy, they have little clinical significance. However, when they are detected at surgery, the nomenclature used to describe these cortical glandular tumors implies prognostic significance. It may be best to describe these tumors as renal adenocarcinomas, but with a low likelihood of metastasis. Search for evidence of metastases and arranging appropriate follow-up may be beneficial.

Oncocytoma

An *oncocyte* is a large transformed epithelial cell that has a finely granular eosinophilic cytoplasm. Oncocytes increase in number with age and are found in a variety of organs, including salivary glands, thyroid, pancreas, and kidney. In the kidney, oncocytomas develop in the distal tubule or collecting ducts.

Oncocytomas have a male predilection and a mean age of presentation in the seventh decade. They comprise approximately 5% of renal tumors. Oncocytomas most often are detected as an incidental finding and average more than 7 cm in diameter. Occasionally patients may complain of a flank mass, pain, or hematuria.

The gross appearance of an oncocytoma is a well-defined tan to brown tumor. Oncocytomas are homogeneous and do not show necrosis or hemorrhage, but often contain a prominent central stellate scar. In contrast, renal carcinomas are orange-yellow and often have areas of hemorrhage and tumor necrosis.

Although there are occasional reported cases of involvement of regional lymph nodes and tumor extension into the vein, the vast majority of oncocytomas are well-differentiated and benign. In the series reported by Lieber and coworkers, the actuarial survival curve for

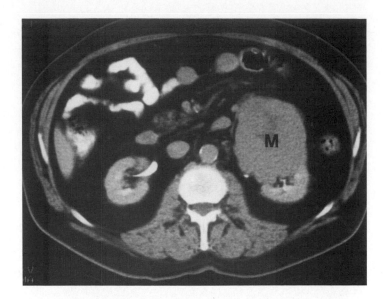

Figure 6.16. Oncocytoma. A large left renal mass (*M*) has a well-defined interface with the normal renal parenchyma.

the 90 patients with an oncocytoma was not significantly different from an age- and sex-matched cohort.

Oncocytomas can be detected as solid renal masses by excretory urography. They are moderately vascular tumors and cannot be distinguished from renal adenocarcinomas.

On CT, an oncocytoma often is well-defined with a relatively sharp interface with the normal renal parenchyma (Fig. 6.16). The central stellate scar is best seen with CT, but is not pathognomonic for an oncocytoma because it can be seen in renal adenocarcinoma. The initial enthusiasm for these criteria to distinguish an oncocytoma from a renal carcinoma has waned.

MRI reveals a low-signal-intensity mass on T1-weighted images, which differs from the intermediate to high signal intensity often seen in renal cell carcinomas. On T2-weighted images, oncocytomas show a high signal intensity.

Angiography demonstrates a vascular renal tumor with a dense tumor blush. A "spoke wheel" pattern of vessels penetrating into the center of the tumor is common. Although this vascular configuration often is described in an oncocytoma, it is not pathognomonic because it also can be seen in renal adenocarcinoma.

Because an oncocytoma cannot be reliably diagnosed radiographically, treatment is surgical. If typical radiographic features of an oncocytoma, such as a central stellate scar and a spoke wheel vascular pattern are present, an oncocytoma may be suggested. However, neither appearance is pathognomonic, and surgery is required (Fig. 6.17). Alerting the surgeon to the possible diagnosis of oncocytoma may encourage inspection and biopsy or local excision. Thus, more normal renal parenchyma may be preserved than if the more radical formal nephrectomy is performed.

Wilms' Tumor

Wilms' tumor (nephroblastoma) arises from metanephric blastema and most commonly is found in young children; 50% of cases are diagnosed in patients younger than 2 years of age, and 75% of cases are diagnosed in patients younger than 5 years of age. There is no sex predilection, but there is a high association with several malformation syndromes.

Wilms' tumor develops in approximately one third of children with sporadic aniridia. Patients with aniridia and Wilms' tumor present at an earlier age and more frequently have bilateral tumors than patients with Wilms' tumor in general. An anomaly localized to the short arm of chromosome 11 has been found in 33% of patients with aniridia and Wilms' tumor.

Patients with hemihypertrophy have an increased in-

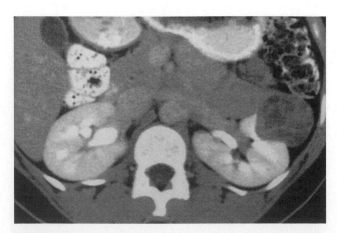

Figure 6.17. Renal carcinoma with oncocytic changes. The well-defined margins of this left renal mass suggest a benign etiology. Pathology revealed a renal carcinoma with oncocytic changes.

cidence of nephroblastomas, adrenal cortical neoplasms, and hepatoblastomas. The side of hypertrophy and the tumor are unrelated.

In 1970, Drash reported the association of male pseudohermaphroditism, glomerulonephritis, and Wilms' tumor. The components of this syndrome may not occur at the same time. Thus, the development of any two should alert physicians to the possibility of the third component arising.

The Beckwith-Wiedemann syndrome also is related to Wilms' tumor. This syndrome, comprising macroglossia, omphalocele, adrenal cytomegaly, and visceromegaly, often includes a proliferation of nephrogenic blastema (from which Wilms' tumors develop). Other anomalies including microcephaly, malformed ears, a variety of genitourinary anomalies (e.g., horseshoe kidneys), and developmental retardation also are associated with Wilms' tumor.

Wilms' tumor is usually a mixed tumor containing epithelial, blastemal, and stromal elements. The nonepithelial elements may differentiate into striated muscle, adipose, cartilage, or bone. This may explain the rare case in which the detection of fat may cause confusion with an angiomyolipoma. There is usually a pseudocapsule that separates the tumor from the rest of the kidney.

Most children with Wilms' tumor present with a palpable abdominal mass. Abdominal pain, anorexia, fever, and hypertension also are commonly present. Gross hematuria occurs in less than 10% of cases. Improved accuracy in staging has allowed more specific therapy and has resulted in improved survival.

Wilms' tumors are usually large (averaging 12 cm) by the time they are detected. Because they develop in the renal cortex, much of the tumor growth may be exophytic. Thus, the splaying of the collecting system seen with intrarenal masses may not be present. However, the large size of these tumors makes them more readily detected. The expansile tumor mass compresses the normal kidney, but maintains a relatively sharp margin.

Ultrasound has become the preferred examination for young children presenting with an abdominal mass (Fig. 6.18). The solid nature and renal origin of the tumor mass can be determined. Most tumors will be hypo- to hyperechoic solid masses, are usually well-defined, and may be demarcated from the normal parenchyma by a tumor pseudocapsule or compressed renal cortex.

Hypoechoic areas within the tumor may represent regions of hemorrhage or tissue necrosis. Dystrophic calcification is uncommon, but may cause hyperechoic foci with shadowing when it occurs. Ultrasound also is useful in detecting tumor extension into the renal vein or IVC and for identifying hepatic metastases. The renal vein may be difficult to image, but identification of tu-

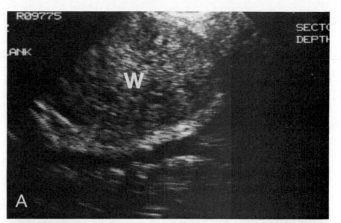

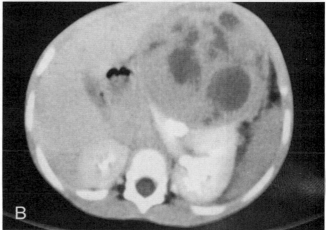

Figure 6.18.   Wilms' tumor. **A,** On ultrasound, a large solid tumor (*W*) is detected in the upper pole of the left kidney. **B,** Splaying of the renal parenchyma and distortion of the collecting system on computed tomography confirm its renal origin.

mor thrombus in the IVC is of greater importance. The surgeon can examine the renal vein during surgery, but the extent of tumor thrombus determines the operative approach. Color flow Doppler ultrasound is especially useful in detecting tumor thrombus in the IVC.

The paucity of retroperitoneal fat in young children makes CT evaluation of Wilms' tumor more difficult than adult renal neoplasms. Furthermore, the ionizing radiation and need for intravenous contrast medium makes this examination less desirable than ultrasound in children.

Wilms' tumor is seen as a large mass that enhances less than the normal renal parenchyma. The degree of heterogeneity depends on the presence of tissue necrosis or hemorrhage. The tumor mass is usually large, causing compression of the remainder of the kidney (Fig. 6.19).

Computed tomography is valuable, however, in contributing to the staging evaluation and in providing precise delineation of the size of the tumor mass. Computed tomography with contiguous narrow collimation

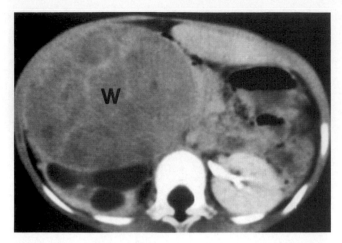

Figure 6.19. Wilms' tumor. A huge Wilms' tumor (*W*) is obstructing the collecting system.

(5 mm) is superior to ultrasound in detecting local invasion of the Wilms' tumor into adjacent lymph nodes or muscle. It also is useful in evaluating the contralateral kidney when ipsilateral nephrectomy is contemplated.

Arteriography is seldom necessary to evaluate patients with Wilms' tumor. The tumors are moderately vascular, with splaying of intrarenal branches. Neovascularity is common and areas of vascular puddling may be seen. The angiographic appearance is not specific and is not helpful in making the diagnosis, other than confirming the presence of a vascular mass.

Magnetic resonance imaging appears to be no more valuable in Wilms' tumor than in adult renal neoplasms. Although ionizing radiation is spared, the children require sedation and monitoring to undergo an MRI examination. The most promising application of MRI is in defining the venous extent of tumor, but it also may prove to be useful in detecting hepatic metastases.

The most common sites for metastases are the lung and liver. Involvement of the adjacent retroperitoneum, the peritoneum, or mediastinum is not uncommon. Tumor staging is similar to renal adenocarcinoma (Table 6.3).

Approximately 5% of patients have bilateral renal involvement (stage V). These patients usually present at a younger age and the tumors may be synchronous or metachronous. Patients at increased risk for bilateral in-

Table 6.3. Staging Wilms' Tumor

Stage	Disease extent
I	Limited to kidney
II	Extends beyond kidney but is completely resected
III	Residual nonhematogenous tumor confined to the abdomen
IV	Hematogenous metastases to lung, liver, bone, or brain
V	Bilateral renal involvement

volvement include those with a family history of Wilms' tumor, multifocal lesions in the index kidney, nephroblastomatosis, and those with other associated congenital anomalies.

Nephroblastomatosis

Nephroblastomatosis is a group of pathologic entities characterized by persistent nephrogenic blastema. It results from an arrest in normal nephrogenesis, with persistence of residual blastema. Although nephroblastomatosis is not malignant, it is associated with Wilms' tumor and those conditions with a high incidence of Wilms' tumor.

Nephroblastomatosis may be diffuse, or more commonly, multinodular. The radiographic features are dependent on the size and distribution of the embryologic remnants. The lesions in the multifocal form are usually microscopic nodules and are difficult to image. In the diffuse form, the kidneys are enlarged and the collecting system may be deformed by parenchymal nodules.

The lesions often are hypoechoic, but also may be iso- or hyperechoic. Their subcapsular location suggests nephroblastomatosis and helps to distinguish this condition from polycystic renal disease or lymphoma. This distribution also is seen on CT. Nephroblastomatosis is clearly distinguished from normal renal tissue by the difference in contrast enhancement (Fig. 6.20).

Typical angiographic features include a normal-caliber main renal artery. Peripheral nodules are hypovascular and do not blush with contrast, and the kidney has a scalloped appearance.

Patients with nephroblastomatosis are at increased risk of developing Wilms' tumor. Many are treated with antineoplastic drugs, which often decrease the renal size. However, such patients remain at risk and should be followed to detect the subsequent development of a Wilms' tumor.

Mesoblastic Nephroma

This benign tumor is usually present at birth and has been described as a congenital Wilms' tumor or fetal mesenchymal hamartoma. Mesoblastic nephromas are comprised of interlacing sheets of fibromatous cells. Small bundles of these fibromatous cells are characteristically found diffusely interspersed in the adjacent renal parenchyma.

The tumor is large, averaging over 6 cm in diameter, and often replaces almost the entire renal parenchyma. The cut surface has a whorled appearance resembling leiomyoma of the uterus. It is not encapsulated, and finger-like extensions of the tumor may penetrate the adjacent kidney. Although the tumor may penetrate the capsule and may involve the perinephric space, it rarely extends into the renal vein or renal pelvis. Cases with a low grade of malignancy have been reported and may be confused with Wilms' tumor.

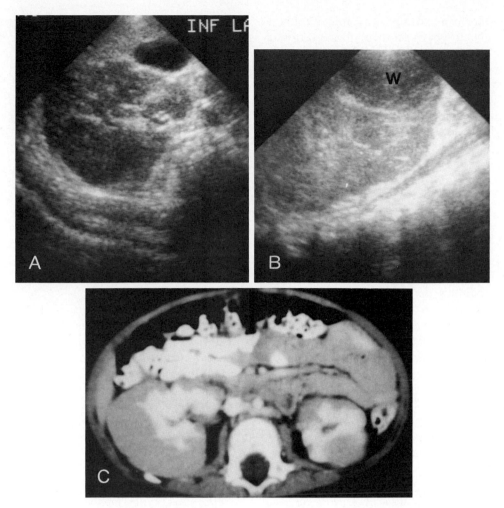

Figure 6.20. Nephroblastomatosis. **A,** A lobulated kidney with indistinct corticomedullary junction is seen on ultrasound. **B,** A Wilms' tumor (*W*) is seen as a hypoechoic mass in the lower pole. **C,** On computed tomography, the diffuse confluent nephroblastomatosis is clearly demarcated from the functioning renal parenchyma. (From Fernback SK, Feinstein KA, Donaldson JS, Baum ES: Nephroblastomatosis: comparison of CT with US and urography. *Radiology* 166:153, 1988.)

Patients with mesoblastic nephroma typically present with a nontender abdominal mass. It is detected at birth or the first few months of life, and there is no sexual predilection.

If urography is performed, a large mass replacing most of the ipsilateral kidney will be seen. Calcification is uncommon.

Ultrasound is the most commonly used modality in the evaluation of these patients. The most common pattern, homogeneously echoic, reflects the smooth mass of fibromatous cells. Occasionally hyperechoic foci are seen. Although uncommon, areas of necrosis or hemorrhage are readily detected as hypoechoic regions. A fairly uniform, solid, intrarenal mass has been reported on CT. Angiography may occasionally be needed for preoperative evaluation. Most mesoblastic nephromas are moderately vascular and demonstrate tumor vascularity.

Treatment is by surgical excision, and cure is usually achieved with nephrectomy. In some patients, extensive tumor necrosis, extrarenal infiltration, and mesenchymal immaturity suggest more aggressive behavior of the tumor. In these patients, who usually present beyond 3 months of age, adjunctive chemotherapy or radiation therapy may be given.

MESENCHYMAL TUMORS

Angiomyolipoma

These hamartomatous tumors are composed of mature adipose tissue, thick-walled blood vessels, and sheets of smooth muscle. The amount of each component varies in each tumor. Some pathologists prefer to use the name reflecting the predominant tissue to describe the tumor. Thus, a *myoangiolipoma* comprises primarily smooth muscle. Other tumors may have only two of the three tissue elements and may be referred to as myolipoma, angiomyoma, etc.

Angiomyolipomas more often are found in women

than in men, and the mean age at presentation is 41 years. Most patients are asymptomatic, however, intra- or perirenal hemorrhage may cause flank pain. Hematuria and hypertension are occasionally reported.

A strong association exists between angiomyolipomas and tuberous sclerosis. However, sporadic angiomyolipomas are being recognized with increasing frequency on CT and ultrasound examinations. Although 80% of patients with tuberous sclerosis have an angiomyolipoma, less than 40% of patients with an angiomyolipoma have an element of the tuberous sclerosis complex.

Tuberous sclerosis, or Bourneville's disease, is caused by an autosomal-dominant gene with variable expressivity. Only approximately 50% of patients with tuberous sclerosis have family members with one or more manifestations of the disease. The tuberous sclerosis syndrome includes epilepsy, mental retardation, and various hamartomas. In addition to renal angiomyolipomas and multiple renal cysts, patients often develop retinal phakomas and cerebral hamartomas. Adenoma sebaceum may be seen in the malar areas of the face. In some patients, the clinical syndrome is incompletely manifest.

Among patients with tuberous sclerosis, the angiomyolipomas are usually multiple and bilateral. In patients without tuberous sclerosis, the tumors are usually solitary. As the spatial resolution of CT and ultrasound continues to improve, tiny angiomyolipomas are being detected in asymptomatic patients as incidental findings.

Lymphangiomyomatosis is an idiopathic disease that occurs in young women consisting of smooth muscle hamartomas along the lymphatic system. It most commonly involves intrathoracic lymphatics, but abdominal involvement can be extensive. Lymphangiomyomatosis is considered by many to be a "forme fruste" of tuberous sclerosis. Renal hamartomas are found in approximately 15% of patients with lymphangiomyomatosis.

Plain abdominal radiographs may demonstrate a relatively lucent mass if there is a large fatty component to the tumor. Calcification is seldom seen, but may be caused by previous hemorrhage. Urography may demonstrate a renal mass. However, the urogram often is unrevealing, because the tumors frequently have an exophytic growth pattern.

The typical ultrasonographic finding of a highly echogenic renal mass (Fig. 6.21) depends on the fat content of the tumor. If there is relatively little fat, the ultrasonographic pattern will be indistinguishable from other renal masses. Even the very echogenic appearance can occasionally be mimicked by renal adenocarcinoma. If there has been hemorrhage, sonolucent areas may be seen.

The most reliable imaging modality for angiomyolipoma is CT. The detection of a renal mass of fat den-

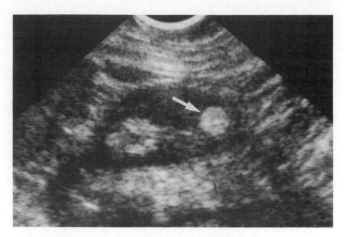

Figure 6.21.   Angiomyolipoma. The highly echogenic pattern (*arrow*) is typical of an angiomyolipoma.

sity virtually assures the diagnosis of angiomyolipoma (Fig. 6.22). Although a Wilms' tumor, oncocytoma, metastasis, and renal adenocarcinoma have all been reported with macroscopic fat demonstrable in the tumor mass, these are rare occurrences and should only add a note of caution to the presumptive diagnosis of an angiomyolipoma. Both lipomas and liposarcomas also may be fatty density, and thus are indistinguishable from an angiomyolipoma by imaging techniques; however, they are rare renal tumors. Because some angiomyolipomas may contain little or no fat, the absence of fat does not exclude the diagnosis of angiomyolipoma.

Examination of a fatty renal mass by CT must be performed carefully to avoid volume-averaging adjacent perinephric fat and a false low-density reading. In small tumors, narrow collimation is essential. Lesions smaller than 1 cm are commonly seen in the kidneys during enhanced CT examinations of the abdomen. These lesions are often cysts, but are too small for adequate analysis

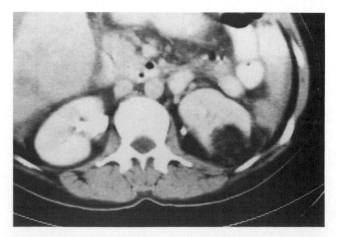

Figure 6.22.   Angiomyolipoma. An angiomyolipoma can be diagnosed by the macroscopic fat detected by computed tomography.

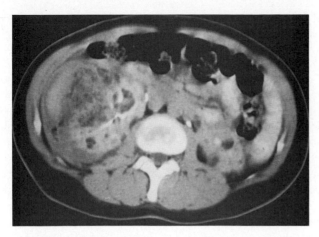

Figure 6.23. Angiomyolipoma. Multiple fatty-density renal lesions are seen in this patient with tuberous sclerosis.

and are considered indeterminate. However, re-scanning through these lesions with narrow collimation, such as 1.5-mm sections, may demonstrate the fatty component and may allow the diagnosis of angiomyolipoma. The presence of multiple angiomyolipomas or associated renal cysts suggests tuberous sclerosis (Fig. 6.23). Patients with tuberous sclerosis may have intrahepatic angiomyolipomas as well.

Magnetic resonance imaging also can detect fat within an angiomyolipoma. A high signal intensity is seen on both T1- and T2-weighted images. When clearly imaged, MRI should have the same accuracy as CT in diagnosing an angiomyolipoma. However, MRI is probably not as sensitive as CT in detecting fat in small tumors.

Arteriography may demonstrate tortuous, almost aneurysmally dilated vessels. Vascular encasement found in malignant tumors is not present in angiomyolipomas. Arteriography may be helpful in defining the vascular supply to tumors in which local resection is planned. Growth of angiomyolipomas is usually expansile, but venous extension into the IVC has been reported.

Treatment of angiomyolipomas has traditionally been surgical. This reflects the predominance of symptomatic and large lesions detected. Because a benign diagnosis can be made with confidence, tumorectomy or partial nephrectomy is appropriate. When angiomyolipomas, especially small lesions, are detected in asymptomatic patients, no therapy is needed. Should hemorrhage occur, surgery or catheter embolization may be performed. Selective arterial embolization also may be performed in patients with large tumors not amenable to partial nephrectomy. Some investigators, however, recommend elective exploration with renal-sparing surgery, as there is a slightly increased incidence of renal adenocarcinoma in patients with an angiomyolipoma.

Fibrous Tumors

Fibromas are usually small tumors that occur more frequently in the renal medulla than in the renal cortex. Although occasionally large enough to cause symptoms, most fibromas are detected as incidental findings at autopsy and are not imaged ante mortem. Fibrosarcomas are rare tumors that usually develop in the renal capsule.

Osteosarcoma

This tumor is rarely a primary renal neoplasm, but may arise from a fibrosarcoma undergoing metaplasia to tumor osteocytes. Diagnosis is based on the presence of formed bone. The main differential diagnosis is a metastasis to the kidney from a primary skeletal osteosarcoma. The age of the patient helps with this distinction, because patients with primary renal osteosarcoma are usually elderly, whereas primary skeletal osteosarcomas occur in adolescents and young adults.

Lipoma

Intrarenal lipomas are rare tumors that are usually small and seldom symptomatic. All but 1 of the 18 cases reviewed by Dineen and colleagues involved middle-aged women. They should be easily detected by CT, but may not be distinguishable from an angiomyolipoma.

Leiomyoma and Leiomyosarcoma

Smooth muscle tumors may arise from vessel walls or scattered muscle fibers of the renal capsule, and most are found in the lower poles. Most leiomyomas are small and asymptomatic. There is a female preponderance and an increased incidence in patients with tuberous sclerosis.

Leiomyosarcomas are usually large and locally invasive by the time they become clinically apparent. These tumors tend to metastasize widely, and the prognosis for patients is poor. Treatment is surgical resection and focal recurrence is common.

Malignant Fibrous Histiocytoma

Although malignant fibrous histiocytoma (MFH) is common elsewhere in the body, it is rarely seen as a primary renal tumor. It has been reported in patients ranging from 13 to 68 years of age. Symptoms are nonspecific, and most tumors are large by the time they are detected. Common metastatic sites include liver, lung, and bone. Local recurrence is common, and the prognosis is poor.

Hemangioma

Hemangiomas are uncommon renal tumors of endothelial cells and capillary size vessels. If the vessels are dilated, the tumor may be called a *cavernous hemangioma*. The tumors are usually small, ranging from several millimeters to 5 cm in diameter and are most frequently located at the apex of the renal pyramids.

The most common presenting complaint is hematuria, and some patients may experience colicky pain due to passage of blood clots. Men and women are affected equally and present most often during the third or fourth decade.

The plain radiograph and urogram are usually normal, although sometimes a small defect can be appreciated in the urothelium. The lesions are usually too small to be detected by ultrasound or CT.

Selective renal angiography is the most useful modality in the diagnosis of these small vascular tumors. The ipsilateral renal artery is not usually enlarged. A dense tangle of vessels that may allow arteriovenous shunting is seen. Because these endothelial-lined spaces lack contractile elements, they do not react to vasoactive stimuli. Thus, vasoconstrictive drugs may improve the diagnostic capability by constricting normal renal arteries and by shunting contrast into the hemangioma.

Treatment has traditionally been surgical for symptomatic lesions. However, transcatheter ablation should be effective therapy and may minimize loss of renal tissue.

Juxtaglomerular Tumors

Robertson first described this tumor of the juxtaglomerular apparatus in 1967. Although a rare tumor, it is a curable cause of significant hypertension. Patients with juxtaglomerular tumors (reninomas) are usually younger than those with essential hypertension, and there is a marked female preponderance.

The juxtaglomerular tumor is composed of small uniform cells with little nuclear pleomorphism or mitotic activity. The presence of renin can be confirmed with an immunofluorescence antibody test. Juxtaglomerular cells are similar to smooth muscle and may be difficult to distinguish from hemangiopericytomas.

Juxtaglomerular tumors range from 3 to 7 cm in diameter when they are detected. The tumors are benign; local invasion or distant metastases have not been reported.

Patients usually present with symptoms of moderate to severe hypertension. Elements of secondary aldosteronism such as hypokalemia also may be present. Rarely, acute flank pain, hypotension, or anemia may reflect hemorrhage from the tumor.

The plain abdominal radiograph is unrevealing, because juxtaglomerular tumors are not calcified. Excretory urography can demonstrate a mass in the majority of cases. The tumor often is peripheral in location and may not distort the collecting system unless it is quite large.

Sonography reveals an echogenic mass owing to the abundant small vascular channels within the tumor. This is most helpful in distinguishing the tumor from a cortical cyst.

The CT findings are nonspecific, because a juxtaglomerular tumor can not be distinguished from most other solid neoplasms. Contrast enhancement is necessary, because the tumor is isodense with normal renal parenchyma.

Arteriography often is performed in patients with juxtaglomerular tumors. Many patients undergo aortography to look for stenosis of the main renal artery. It is essential, however, to study both kidneys as well as the main renal arteries to detect these tumors. Despite the abundant vascular spaces, juxtaglomerular tumors are hypovascular (Fig. 6.24). Thus, selective renal arteriography should be performed even if aortography is normal.

A small amount of tumor vascularity often can be appreciated, but splaying of adjacent vessels by a hypovascular mass is the most obvious finding. The nature of the tumor can be confirmed by measuring selective renal-vein renin levels.

Treatment of juxtaglomerular tumors is surgical. Since the tumors are benign, local tumorectomy or partial nephrectomy often is performed to preserve as much normal renal parenchyma as possible.

RENAL PELVIC TUMORS

Most of the tumors arising from the renal pelvis are malignant, and transitional cell carcinomas are the most common type. Less often, squamous cell, undifferentiated, or adenocarcinomas may occur. Papillomas comprise approximately 50% of the benign tumors, and the remaining 50% consist of angiomas, fibromas, myomas, or polyps.

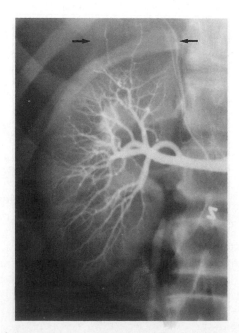

Figure 6.24. Juxtaglomerular tumor. A hypovascular mass (*arrows*) is seen in the upper pole of the right kidney. (From Amis ES Jr, Newhouse JH: *Essentials of Uroradiology*. Boston, Little Brown & Co, 1991.)

Transitional Cell Carcinoma

Primary tumors of the renal pelvis are relatively uncommon, because they comprise less than 10% of renal tumors. The most common tumor, transitional cell carcinoma, occurs twice as often in men than women and peaks in occurrence in the seventh decade.

Transitional cell carcinoma may occur anywhere along the urothelium. The incidence of carcinoma is roughly proportional to the surface area. For every 50 bladder tumors, there are 3 transitional cell carcinomas in the renal pelves or intrarenal collecting systems and 1 tumor in the ureters.

Metabolites of aminophenols may cause carcinoma of the renal pelvis, ureter, or bladder. The incidence of renal pelvic carcinoma is markedly increased in patients who consume large amounts of phenacetin, which is metabolized to aminophenol. Similarly, acrolein, a metabolite of cyclophosphamide, is excreted in the urine and is toxic to the urothelium. Infection with *Schistosoma hematobium* is associated with squamous cell carcinoma of the bladder or ureter, but the parasite does not usually reach the renal pelvis. An increased incidence of carcinoma of the renal pelvis is seen in patients with Balkan nephropathy.

Transitional cell carcinomas may be flat or papillary, and approximately 20% also contain metaplastic squamous changes. Papillary carcinomas are more common, tend to be of low-grade malignancy, and have a relatively benign course. Nonpapillary tumors (including squamous cell carcinoma) tend to be flat and may be more difficult to detect radiographically. These tumors are generally of high-grade malignancy and spread by direct extension as well as lymphatic and hematogenous metastases. Multicentric lesions are seen in approximately 30% of renal pelvic carcinomas and are even more common among transitional cell carcinomas of the bladder.

Hematuria is the most common presentation, present in approximately 80% of patients. Flank pain, dysuria, and abdominal mass or pyuria are infrequent. Obstruction of the collecting system may be caused by the tumor mass, sloughed pieces of tumor, or blood clot.

The plain abdominal radiograph is usually unrevealing because transitional cell carcinomas are rarely calcified. It is important, however, to exclude a radiopaque renal stone that may be the etiology of a filling defect seen with urography. During excretory urography or retrograde pyelography, the tumor is seen as a filling defect arising from the wall of the renal pelvis (Fig. 6.25). Transitional cell carcinomas, especially nonpapillary types, may be flat. Papillary tumors often grow in a frond-like pattern that allows contrast medium into the interstices of the tumor.

If the tumor has obstructed the ureteropelvic junction or an infundibulum, the entire collecting system or a calyx may be dilated and may display diminished opacification. Retrograde pyelography may reveal an "amputated" (nonopacified) calyx (Fig. 6.26) or a completely obstructed proximal ureter.

An intraluminal filling defect must be distinguished from the smooth extrinsic compression defect of crossing vessels. A sloughed papillae or fungus ball (myce-

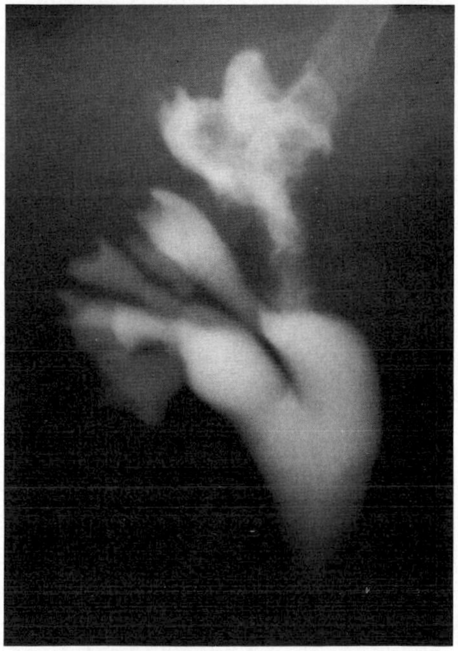

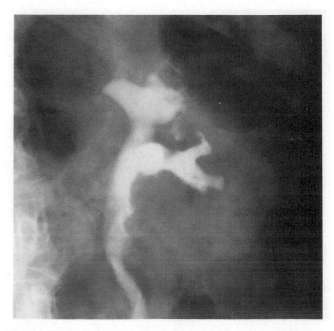

Figure 6.25. Transitional cell carcinoma. An irregular filling defect involves the upper-pole infundibulum and calyces.

Figure 6.26. Transitional cell carcinoma. The lower-pole collecting system does not fill ("amputated") on this retrograde pyelogram. (From Amis ES Jr, Newhouse JH: *Essentials of Uroradiology*. Boston, Little, Brown & Co, 1991.)

toma) should be detected by radiographic evidence of papillary necrosis or by the clinical findings of fungus infection. One common problem is distinguishing a renal pelvic tumor from a radiolucent stone such as a urate calculus. This can easily be accomplished with CT, because even uric acid stones are much denser than soft tissue tumors.

Ultrasound is not routinely used in the evaluation of patients with renal pelvic tumors, but it can distinguish them from the highly echogenic appearance of renal stones. A transitional cell carcinoma may be detected as a soft tissue mass within the lumen of the collecting system.

It may be difficult to image small renal pelvic tumors with CT, but larger lesions are well-defined after intravenous contrast injection (Fig. 6.27). They are seen as soft tissue masses causing filling defects in the collecting system. The greatest contribution of CT in this setting is the identification of renal stones that are not sufficiently opaque to be seen on the plain abdominal radiograph.

Preoperative staging of transitional cell carcinoma is an important aspect of determining whether or not the tumor can be locally resected. Because the tumors tend to be multifocal, renal sparing surgery is desirable. Computed tomography is useful in detecting regional invasion and lymph node metastases if the nodes are enlarged. Metastases to normal-sized lymph nodes cannot be detected by CT.

Although transitional cell carcinomas can be imaged with MRI, this modality has little role in either the detection or staging of these neoplasms. The MR findings of transitional cell carcinoma are similar to those of other renal tumors, with an increased signal intensity on T2-weighted images. However, small lesions may be missed, especially if there is motion artifact.

Angiography is seldom used to diagnose or evaluate renal pelvic tumors. Transitional cell carcinomas are usually hypovascular, but neovascularity and encasement may be seen. Invasion of the main renal vein and/or IVC is uncommon.

Percutaneous biopsy of a suspected transitional cell carcinoma should be performed only after other methods of confirming the diagnosis have been done. Transitional cell carcinoma has a tendency to spread by surface shedding and may seed the track of a percutaneous biopsy or percutaneous nephrostomy.

Treatment of transitional cell carcinoma of the renal pelvis is nephroureterectomy. Because these tumors often are multifocal, the rest of the urothelium must be closely examined for additional tumors. The entire ipsilateral ureter and a cuff of bladder must be removed, because the distal ureter is a common site for recurrent disease.

Squamous Cell Carcinoma

Squamous cell carcinomas constitute only about 7% of tumors of the renal pelvis. They are frequently associated with leukoplakia or chronic irritation from stones or urinary tract infection. Squamous cell carcinomas are also associated with schistosomiasis when there is involvement of the upper urinary tracts. Most are flat and extend along the urothelium and ulcerate.

Although multifocal lesions are less common than with papillary types, squamous cell carcinomas tend to be a high-grade malignancy, and local invasion is common. The presence of renal stones or infection makes these tumors difficult to recognize.

Radiographically, squamous cell carcinomas are difficult to detect. A renal stone often is present and an associated mass may be indistinguishable from xanthogranulomatous pyelonephritis.

SECONDARY TUMORS OF THE KIDNEY

Lymphoma

Since the kidneys do not contain lymphoid tissue, primary renal lymphoma is rare. However, the kidneys may become involved by hematogenous dissemination or direct extension from adjacent retroperitoneal disease. Thus, renal lymphoma is usually part of a generalized process involving multiple sites.

Renal involvement is much more common in non-Hodgkin's lymphomas than in Hodgkin's disease. When present, involvement more often is bilateral than unilateral. At presentation, involvement of the kidneys by non-Hodgkin's lymphoma is seen in 5.8% of cases; at autopsy, the frequency of renal involvement increases to 41.6%.

Renal involvement is more frequent among certain subgroups of non-Hodgkin's lymphoma. Poorly differentiated Burkitt's lymphoma often is described as an ex-

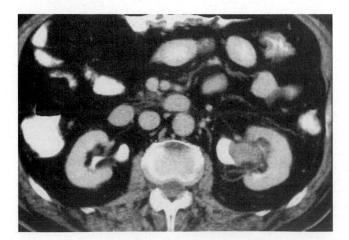

Figure 6.27. Transitional cell carcinoma. A soft tissue mass in the left renal pelvis is defined after intravenous contrast injection.

tranodal tumor, and the kidneys are affected in approximately 10% of cases at presentation. AIDS-related lymphomas were found by CT to involve the kidneys in 11% of patients in one recent series.

Renal lymphoma is more common among patients with immune deficiencies, including those with AIDS. The incidence of renal lymphoma has increased among patients with graft-versus-host disease, iatrogenic immunosuppression, and renal transplantation, in whom it is 350 times more frequent than in the general population.

Most patients with renal lymphoma have disease in other locations that dominates the clinical presentation. Fever, weight loss, and palpable adenopathy are common complaints. Occasionally, diffuse involvement of both kidneys or ureteral obstruction by adenopathy may compromise renal function. Renal lymphoma is usually clinically silent and occurs late in the course of the disease.

Renal lymphoma may have several different appearances. Multiple lymphomatous masses are the most common and are seen in more than 50% of cases of renal lymphoma. A solitary mass or diffuse infiltration of the kidney by lymphoma also may be seen. Although most renal lymphoma has spread by hematogenous dissemination (Fig. 6.28), CT may demonstrate local extension from paraaortic disease in some cases.

The plain abdominal radiograph is seldom revealing. Lymphadenopathy or renal enlargement may occasionally be detected in patients with abundant retroperitoneal fat. Excretory urography may demonstrate diffuse renal enlargement or one or more discrete renal masses. If there is extensive involvement, there may be delayed contrast excretion or even absent renal function. Lymphadenopathy may cause obstruction anywhere from the ureter to the renal pelvis. Bulky lymphadenopathy often will displace the ureters. Because the proximal ureters lie lateral to the paraaortic lymph nodes, they are displaced laterally. The distal ureters are pushed medially, since the external iliac lymph nodes are lateral to the ureters.

On ultrasound, lymphoma is usually hypoechoic, reflecting the homogeneous nature of the tumor (Fig. 6.29). However, a lymphomatous mass shows little sound through transmission, which helps to distinguish it from a cyst. Ultrasound often is helpful in identifying hydronephrosis and is the examination of choice in patients with renal failure or other contraindications to intravenous contrast media.

Computed tomography is routinely used to stage and monitor patients with malignant lymphoma and is an excellent method of detecting renal involvement. Lymphomatous masses are homogeneous and rounded. Renal lymphoma is difficult to detect on unenhanced examinations unless the masses are large. After intravenous contrast injection, lymphoma is usually well-demarcated from the normal parenchyma by its diminished enhancement (Fig. 6.30). The CT pattern reflects the pathologic involvement as a solitary mass, multiple nodules, or diffuse involvement. Adjacent lymphadenopathy and direct tumor extension to the kidney also are well depicted with CT (Fig. 6.31). Renal or perirenal involvement (Fig. 6.32) without evidence on CT of other retroperitoneal disease is common.

Magnetic resonance imaging is seldom needed in the evaluation of renal lymphoma. Lymphomatous masses have a medium signal intensity on T1-weighted sequences and a high intensity on T2-weighted sequences. With diffuse infiltration, there is loss of the corticomedullary junction.

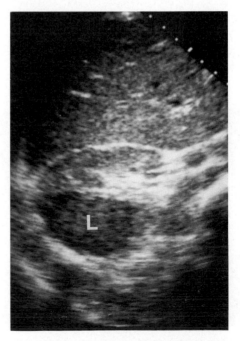

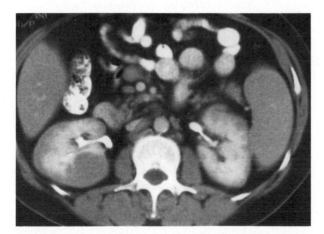

Figure 6.28. Lymphoma. Multiple lymphomatous nodules are seen in the periphery of the renal cortex after contrast enhancement.

Figure 6.29. Lymphoma. On ultrasound, a hypoechoic mass (*L*) is seen in the posterior aspect of the right kidney.

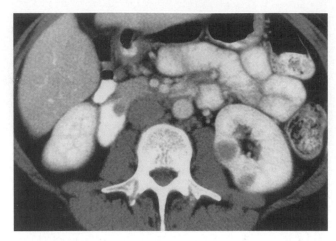

Figure 6.30. Lymphoma. Two homogeneous soft tissue masses are seen in the left kidney on an enhanced CT examination.

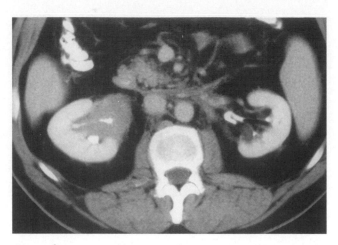

Figure 6.32. Lymphoma. A soft tissue mass is encasing the right renal pelvis.

Angiography is seldom needed in the evaluation of patients with renal lymphoma, but may be used if a primary renal carcinoma with regional lymph node metastases is suspected. Renal lymphoma is typically hypovascular, but may show encasement and modest neovascularity. The major renal arteries are displaced by the tumor masses, which also efface the nephrogram.

Leukemia

Kidney involvement in patients with leukemia is usually due to diffuse infiltration by leukemic cells. It occurs more often with lymphocytic than granulocytic forms. Occasionally a discrete mass, such as a chloroma, may be produced. Intrarenal hemorrhage and hematuria are common.

With leukemic infiltration, both kidneys are symmetrically enlarged. The collecting system is attenuated, and filling defects may be seen due to blood clots. Occasionally acute urate nephropathy occurs.

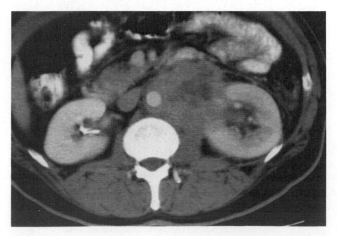

Figure 6.31. Lymphoma. Extension of paraaortic tumor invades the left kidney.

Multiple Myeloma

Multiple myeloma is a disorder of older adults characterized by proliferation of plasma cells and abnormal serum and urine proteins. Renal failure results from precipitation of Bence-Jones proteins in the tubules that may cause mechanical obstruction or damage of tubular cells. Intravascular contrast media causes in vitro precipitation of these proteins and may worsen renal failure in these patients. However, many patients undergo contrast studies without difficulty, and underlying renal disease is probably necessary before contrast-induced nephropathy occurs.

Hypercalcemia results from bone lesions and causes nephrocalcinosis. The kidneys are smoothly enlarged, and the collecting system is attenuated. Precipitation of abnormal proteins in the tubules or uric acid nephropathy may impair contrast excretion.

Solid Tumor Metastases

Metastatic disease involving the kidneys is relatively common in autopsy series, where it may be seen in as many as 20% of patients. The most common primary tumors are carcinomas of the lung, breast, colon, and malignant melanoma. Approximately 50% of these patients have metastases to both kidneys, and the remaining 50% have involvement of only one kidney.

The patient's symptoms are usually dominated by manifestations of the primary tumor, but hematuria and proteinuria are common. Tumors that are especially vascular may cause significant renal hemorrhage resulting in gross hematuria or a perinephric hematoma. Unless extensive metastases involve both kidneys, the renal function is normal. Occasionally urine cytology may be positive.

Although renal metastases are common in autopsy

series, where they outnumber primary renal malignancy 4:1, they are not commonly seen clinically. Most patients with renal metastases have widespread metastatic disease, and imaging studies are not needed to demonstrate renal involvement as well. In the series reported by Choyke and colleagues, more than 50% of the patients died within 3 months of the demonstration of renal metastases.

More recent use of CT to stage and monitor patients with an underlying malignancy has made detection of metastases more common. In a patient with extensive metastases, a renal mass is most likely another metastasis. However, among patients whose disease is in remission, a new renal mass is more likely to be a primary renal tumor. Perirenal metastases are readily detected by CT, because the soft tissue density mass is easy to see within the perirenal fat. The metastases have been reported in patients with underlying lung cancer, melanoma, and lymphoma. Lymphatic connections may be responsible for this pattern of spread.

Plain radiographs are seldom revealing in patients with renal metastases. A solid renal mass may be detected with excretory urography, especially if the tumor is 2 cm or more in size.

Ultrasound often is used to monitor patients with an underlying malignancy for the development of hydronephrosis. Renal metastases are seen as a solid renal mass. Echo-free areas may represent tumor necrosis or local hemorrhage.

Renal metastases are most commonly detected by CT, since this modality is most frequently used to stage and monitor oncology patients (Fig. 6.33). Unenhanced scans are seldom useful in detecting metastases, but may be helpful in excluding renal calculi. Metastases often are small and multiple, but certain primary tumors such as colonic carcinomas may produce a solitary large renal

metastasis. These may be indistinguishable from primary renal adenocarcinomas. Renal biopsy may be required to make this distinction (Fig. 6.34). Tumor invasion of the renal vein and extension into the IVC is commonly seen in renal adenocarcinoma, but is rare in renal metastases. Although vascular lesions may enhance as much as the normal renal parenchyma during the early vascular phase, they later become hypodense. Small lesions may resemble cysts but can be differentiated by their higher density.

Renal metastases demonstrate high signal intensity on T2-weighted images. However, MR imaging is seldom useful, as other entities such as primary renal malignancy or an inflammatory process may have similar signal characteristics.

Arteriography has been used to help distinguish a metastasis from a primary renal adenocarcinoma. The vascularity of the metastasis reflects the vascularity of the primary tumor. Furthermore, selective angiography may reveal small tumors that may be missed by CT, ultrasound, or MR imaging. Multiple tumors make metastatic disease more likely. A definitive diagnosis can usually be made with fine-needle biopsy.

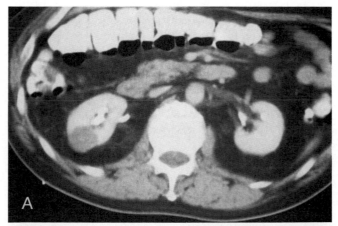

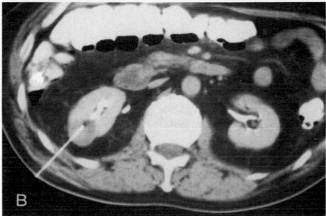

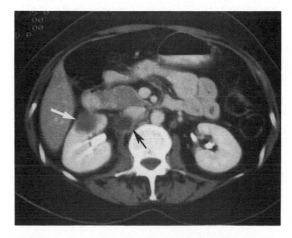

Figure 6.33.   Metastasis. The low-density mass in the right kidney (*light arrow*) is a metastatic tumor. Another metastasis is just posterior to the inferior vena cava (*dark arrow*).

Figure 6.34.   Metastasis. **A,** A solitary renal mass is detected in this man with lung carcinoma. **B,** A renal biopsy confirmed metastatic disease rather than a second primary tumor.

RENAL CAPSULAR TUMORS

The renal capsule is composed of fibrous tissue, nerves, smooth muscle, blood vessels, and perirenal fat. A benign or malignant tumor may develop in any of these tissues. However, tumors of the renal capsule are rare.

Malignant capsular tumors often are quite large at the time of diagnosis. Presenting complaints include a flank mass, abdominal pain, and weight loss. Unless the renal parenchyma is invaded, hematuria is uncommon. The prognosis for these patients is usually poor.

If the tumor is large, a soft tissue mass may be appreciated on the plain abdominal radiograph. Calcification is uncommon, but a lipoma or liposarcoma may be recognized by the fat density. Extrinsic compression or displacement of the kidney is seen on urography. If the kidney is invaded, distortion of the collecting system or poor function may be present.

Computed tomography is helpful in identifying the mass, especially if the growth is exophytic. Preservation of the collecting system suggests an extrarenal mass, but a capsular tumor cannot be distinguished from an exophytic renal neoplasm in this manner.

Angiography is very helpful in the diagnosis of renal capsular tumors, because the mass is fed by enlarged capsular arteries (Fig. 6.35). The intrarenal arteries remain intact, although they may be compressed by a large capsular tumor. The capsular vessels often are stretched and separated from the kidney, while the renal parenchyma is displaced inwardly.

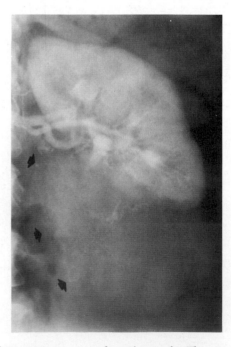

Figure 6.35. Leiomyoma of renal capsule. The capsular nature of this tumor is revealed by the feeding capsular vessels (*arrows*).

INDETERMINATE RENAL MASS

Renal masses with the typical features of a benign simple cyst or renal adenocarcinoma present little difficulty in diagnosis. However, the differential diagnosis for a cystic mass extends from a simple cyst to a cystic renal adenocarcinoma and includes benign cysts with atypical features, and inflammatory or hemorrhagic masses. Lesions that require further evaluation or follow-up fall into one of two general categories. Either the lesion has atypical features that do not allow a confident diagnosis, or the lesion is too small to assess the imaging features reliably.

Cystic Masses

Before the advent of CT and ultrasound, excretory urography was the primary method of identifying a renal mass. Because a confident diagnosis of a benign cyst could seldom be made, many were surgically explored. Angiography, cyst aspiration, and cystography were sometimes used to distinguish a malignant lesion from a benign cyst. However, these invasive tests have now given way to CT and ultrasound, which are highly accurate in making this distinction. A significant minority of lesions are not obvious cancers, but have some features of malignancy and are, therefore, considered indeterminate.

Excretory urography remains a common imaging modality for patients whose clinical presentation or laboratory findings suggest a renal mass, because it is readily available and relatively inexpensive. However, the majority of lesions detected with excretory urography cannot be assessed well enough to exclude malignancy. Since the vast majority of renal masses are benign simple cysts, ultrasound is the most cost-effective way of further evaluating these lesions. Einstein and coworkers reviewed 225 patients with a renal mass detected on excretory urography. When CT was used as the initial follow-up study, a firm diagnosis was made in 88% of patients and 12% went on to sonography for further evaluation. When ultrasound was used as the initial follow-up study, a firm diagnosis was made in 82% of patients. The sonograms were inconclusive in the remaining 18% who then underwent a CT examination. Using Medicare reimbursement payments as a cost assessment, they determined that 70% of the patients initially studied with ultrasound would have had to go on to CT to justify using CT as the initial follow-up study.

In a few patients, the urographic features are sufficiently suggestive to indicate that the lesion will be at least a complicated cystic mass if not a solid tumor. When the lesion is in the upper pole of the left kidney, it may be technically difficult to obtain an adequate examination. Similarly, if the renal lesion is small or the patient is obese, the ultrasound study may be indeterminate. Although these factors are commonly cited as indications to proceed directly to CT, their use was not supported as being cost-effective in the retrospective study reported by Einstein and coworkers.

The ultrasound criteria of a benign simple cyst include a well-defined, sonolucent mass. The lesion should be homogeneous and have a thin wall. There should be good through-transmission of sound waves with strong posterior enhancement. When all of these criteria are satisfied, a confident diagnosis of a benign cyst can be made. Complex masses that do not satisfy these criteria must be considered indeterminate and should be evaluated with CT.

Computed tomography is best performed by obtaining narrow collimated images both before and after intravenous contrast injection. Narrow collimation improves the reliability of density measurements. A comparison of the density on the enhanced image to that of the unenhanced image allows assessment of contrast enhancement.

The CT criteria of a benign simple cyst include homogeneity, an imperceptibly thin wall, a CT density approximating that of water, and lack of enhancement with intravenous contrast administration. Lesions that satisfy these criteria do not need further evaluation. Some atypical features such as thin septations or thin mural calcification are not worrisome, and these lesions also may be considered benign.

Bosniak suggested and subsequently modified a classification system that places cystic lesions into one of four categories (*see* Chapter 5). These are helpful in determining what follow-up or treatment is most appropriate for patients with these complicated lesions.

Lesions that satisfy the criteria of a benign simple cyst on CT or ultrasound are considered Bosniak category I lesions and do not require further diagnostic studies, patient follow-up, or surgery. Category II lesions smaller than 3 cm are most likely benign and can be followed for 1 or 2 years. If there is no change in the imaging features, they can be considered benign as well. Masses in category III deserve surgical exploration unless there are other mitigating circumstances. Many of these masses will be benign lesions, and for that reason, it may be appropriate to explore the renal mass and obtain surgical biopsy specimens or perform a local excision rather than to perform a formal radical nephrectomy. Surgical biopsy that confirms the benign nature of the lesion or local excision of the lesion may be preferred, since significant renal tissue often can be preserved.

Category IV lesions must be assumed to be malignant. Unless preservation of renal tissue is critical to keeping the patient out of renal failure, a radical nephrectomy will most likely be performed. In some patients, there may be evidence of metastatic disease, in which case, a percutaneous biopsy proving the existence of metastases and defining the renal mass as the etiology may be preferred over surgical resection. In any case, the patient must be fully informed of the likelihood that the lesion is malignant as well as the risks of surgery. The final decision should depend on a compilation of these various factors.

Small Masses

With the routine use of CT and ultrasound, many small (< 3 cm) renal masses are detected. Because chemotherapy has not proven to be effective for renal adenocarcinoma, early detection and surgical removal of malignant tumors is essential for optimal patient outcomes.

However, the majority of all renal masses are benign cysts. Cysts large enough to demonstrate benign features may be confidently diagnosed. However, very small lesions (< 1 cm) can seldom be adequately characterized and are considered indeterminate.

If a renal mass contains fat, it is likely an angiomyolipoma or renal hamartoma. Although there are reports of renal carcinoma containing fat, this occurs with osseous metaplasia, and the calcification is readily recognized. Isolated case reports of other lesions such as an oncocytoma, Wilms' tumor, and metastasis containing fat also have appeared. However, the vast majority of these are angiomyolipomas, and occasional reports should not alter our management protocols.

Fat-containing angiomyolipomas are typically highly echogenic on sonography. However, small renal carcinomas also may be echogenic, and it is essential to confirm the presence of fat with CT. This can best be done by obtaining thin sections through the lesion to minimize partial volume artifact.

Metastases to the kidneys are seen with increased frequency as aggressive cancer treatment with its associated frequent imaging is undertaken. The most common primary tumors are carcinomas of the lung or breast, malignant melanoma, or non-Hodgkin's lymphoma. It is unlikely, however, to have renal metastases without other evidence of metastatic disease or a known primary tumor.

A small solid renal mass without demonstrable fat is most likely a renal adenocarcinoma. Because small cancers seldom metastasize, these small tumors often have been called adenomas. However, many pathologists now consider these small tumors as premalignant or potentially malignant. Approximately 5 to 10% of these small tumors prove to be benign oncocytomas, but their imaging features are not pathognomonic, and a firm diagnosis cannot be made on imaging studies or even percutaneous biopsy.

The prevalence of metastases from a renal carcinoma is roughly proportional to the size of the tumor. It is estimated that fewer than 5% of small tumors have metastasized. Furthermore, improved surgical techniques have made renal-sparing surgery an attractive alternative to nephrectomy for localized problems. With small peripheral tumors, survival with partial nephrectomy is as good as radical nephrectomy. The primary argument against partial nephrectomy or tumorectomy for renal carcinoma is the potential for multifocal lesions.

Continued improvement in our cross-sectional imaging modalities enable us to detect very small renal lesions. Masses less than 1 cm in diameter are usually too small to characterize. Since the overwhelming majority are benign cysts, they can be ignored. Lesions ranging from 1 to 3 cm in diameter must be carefully examined using ultrasound or narrow ($\leq$ 5 mm) collimated CT, ideally before and after intravenous contrast administration. Together, ultrasound and CT are superior to each one individually. In patients with renal insufficiency or an allergy to iodinated contrast media, MR may be substituted for contrast-enhanced CT. In many cases, a confident diagnosis of a benign cyst or angiomyolipoma can be made. If not, the lesion must be considered a potential renal carcinoma and treated accordingly.

Any decision regarding additional examinations, patient follow-up, surgery, or percutaneous biopsy must be made in the context of the patient. In patients with a small renal mass, even if the features suggest malignancy, it may be more appropriate to follow the lesion than to undergo surgery if the patient's life expectancy is relatively short. Many of these small renal carcinomas have a slow growth rate, and the patient may often die of an unrelated problem before the renal carcinoma has metastasized or become locally invasive.

SUGGESTED READING

Renal Parenchymal Tumors

Ambos, MA, Bosniak MA, Valensi QJ, et al.: Angiographic patterns in renal oncocytomas. *Radiology* 129:615, 1978.

Bakal CW, Cynamon J, Lakritz PS, et al.: Value of preoperative renal artery embolization in reducing blood transfusion requirements during nephrectomy for renal cell carcinoma. *J Vasc Interv Radiol* 4:727, 1993.

Bosniak MA: The current radiological approach to renal cysts. *Radiology* 158:1, 1986.

Bosniak MA: Difficulties in classifying cystic lesions of the kidney. *Urol Radiol* 13:91, 1991.

Choyke PL, Filling-Katz MR, Shawker TH, et al.: von Hippel-Lindau disease: radiologic screening for visceral manifestations. *Radiology* 174:815, 1990.

Choyke PL, Glenn GM, Walther MM, et al.: The natural history of renal lesions in von Hippel-Lindau disease: a serial CT study in 28 patients. *AJR* 159:1229, 1992.

Choyke PL, Glenn GM, McClellan MW, et al.: von Hippel-Lindau disease: genetic, clinical, and imaging features. *Radiology* 194:629, 1995.

Cohan RH, Sherman LS, Korobkin M, Bass JC, Francis IR: Renal masses: assessment of the corticomedullary-phase and nephrographic-phase CT scans. *Radiology* 196:445, 1995.

Curry NS: Small renal masses (lesions smaller than 3 cm): imaging evaluation and management. *AJR* 164:355, 1995.

Cushing B, Slovis TL: Imaging of Wilms' tumor: what is important! *Urol Radiol* 14:241, 1992.

Davidson AJ, Hayes WS, Hartman DS, McCarthy WF, Davis CJ: Renal oncocytoma and carcinoma: failure of differentiation with CT. *Radiology* 186:693, 1993.

Demos TC, Schiffer M, Love L, et al.: Normal excretory urography in patients with primary kidney neoplasms. *Urol Radiol* 7:75, 1985.

Drash A, Sherman F, Hartman WH, et al.: A syndrome of pseudohermaphroditism, Wilms' tumor, hypertension and degenerative renal disease. *J Pediat* 76:585, 1970.

Eilenberg SS, Lee JKT, Brown JJ, Mirowitz SA, Tartar VM: Renal masses: evaluation with gradient-echo Gd-DTPA-enhanced dynamic MR imaging. *Radiology* 176:333, 1990.

Einstein DM, Herts BR, Weaver R, et al.: Evaluation of renal masses detected by excretory urography: cost-effectiveness of sonography versus CT. *AJR* 164:371, 1995.

Ekelund L: Pharmacoangiography of the kidney: an overview. *Urol Radiol* 2:9, 1980.

Fernback SK, Feinstein KA, Donaldson JS, et al.: Nephroblastomatosis: comparison of CT with US and urography. *Radiology* 166:153, 1988.

Forman HP, Middleton WD, Melson GL, et al.: Hyperechoic renal cell carcinomas: increase in detection at US. *Radiology* 188:431, 1993.

Foster WL Jr, Halvorsen RA, Jr, Dunnick NR: The clandestine renal cell carcinoma: atypical appearances and presentations. *Radiographics* 5:175, 1985.

Fukuya T, Honda H, Goto K, et al: Computed tomographic findings of Bellini duct carcinoma of the kidney. *J Comput Assist Tomogr* 20:399, 1996.

Gill IS, McClennan BL, Kerbl K, et al.: Adrenal involvement from renal cell carcinoma: predictive value of computerized tomography. *J Urol* 152:1082, 1994.

Guinan PD, Vogelzang NJ, Fremgen AM, et al.: Renal cell carcinoma: tumor size, stage and survival. *J Urol* 153:901, 1995.

Harmon WJ, King BF, Lieber MM: Renal oncocytoma: magnetic resonance imaging characteristics. *J Urol* 155:863, 1996.

Hartman DS: Cysts and cystic neoplasms. *Urol Radiol* 12:7, 1990.

Hartman DS, Lesar MSL, Madewell JE, et al.: Mesoblastic nephroma: radiologic-pathologic correlation of 20 cases. *AJR* 136:69, 1981.

Janis-Dow CA, Choyke PL, Jennings SB, et al.: Small ($\leq$3-cm) renal masses: detection with CT versus US and pathologic correlation. *Radiology* 198:785, 1996.

Johnson CD, Dunnick NR, Cohan RH, et al.: Renal adenocarcinoma: CT staging of 100 tumors. *AJR* 148:59, 1987.

Kioumehr F, Cochran ST, Layfield L, et al.: Wilms' tumor (nephroblastoma) in the adult patient: clinical and radiologic manifestations. *AJR* 152:299, 1989.

Kletscher BA, Qian J, Bostwick DG, et al.: Prospective analysis of multifocality in renal cell carcinoma: influence of histological pattern, grade, number, size, volume and deoxyribonucleic acid ploidy. *J Urol* 153:904, 1995.

Kuijpers D, Kruyt RH, Oudkerk M: Renal masses: value of duplex Doppler ultrasound in the differential diagnosis. *J Urol* 151:326, 1994.

Leo ME, Petrou SP, Barrett DM: Transitional cell carcinoma of the kidney with vena caval involvement: report of 3 cases and a review of the literature. *J Urol* 148:398, 1992.

Levine E, Huntrakoon M, Wetzel LH: Small renal neoplasms: clinical, pathologic, and imaging features. *AJR* 153:69, 1989.

Ljungberg B, Holmberg G, Sjodin JG, et al.: Renal cell carcinoma in a renal cyst: a case report and review of the literature. *J Urol* 143:797, 1990.

Lowe RE, Cohen MD: Computed tomographic evaluation of

Wilms' tumor and nephroblastoma. *Radiographics* 4(6):915, 1984.

Mena E, Bull FE, Bookstein JJ, et al.: Angiography of the nephrogenic hepatic dysfunction syndrome. *Radiology* 111:65, 1974.

Mesrobian HGJ: Wilms' tumor: past, present, future. *J Urol* 149:231, 1988.

Miller DL, Choyke PL, Walther MM, et al.: von Hippel-Lindau disease: inadequacy of angiography for identification of renal cancers. *Radiology* 179:833, 1991.

Morra MN, Das S: Renal oncocytoma: A review of histogenesis, histopathology, diagnosis and treatment. *J Urol* 150:295, 1993.

Nelson JB, Oyasu R, Dalton DP: The clinical and pathological manifestations of renal tumors in von Hippel-Lindau disease. *J Urol* 152:2221, 1994.

Nissenkorn I, Bernheim J: Multicentricity in renal cell carcinoma. *J Urol* 153:620, 1995.

Press GA, McClennan BL, Melson GL, et al.: Papillary renal cell carcinoma: CT and sonographic evaluation. *AJR* 143:1005, 1984.

Rahmouni A, Mathieu D, Berger JF, et al.: Fast magnetic resonance imaging in the evaluation of tumoral obstructions of the inferior vena cava. *J Urol* 148:14, 1992.

Robson CJ, Churchill BM, Anderson W: The results of radical nephrectomy for renal cell carcinoma. *J Urol* 101:297, 1969.

Roubidoux MA, Dunnick NR, Sostman HD, Leder RA: Renal carcinoma: detection of venous extension with gradient-echo MR imaging. *Radiology* 182:269, 1992.

Semelka RC, Shoenut JP, Kroeker MA, MacMahon RG, Greenberg HM: Renal lesions: controlled comparison between CT and 1.5-T MR imaging with nonenhanced and Gadolinium-enhanced fat-suppressed spin-echo and breath-hold FLASH techniques. *Radiology* 182:425, 1992.

Semelka RC, Hricak H, Stevens SK, et al.: Combined Gadolinium-enhanced and fat-saturation MR imaging of renal masses. *Radiology* 178:803, 1991.

Shirkhoda A, Lewis E: Renal sarcoma and sarcomatoid renal cell carcinoma: CT and angiographic features. *Radiology* 162:353, 1987.

Siegel SC, Sandler MA, Alpern MB, et al.: CT of renal cell carcinoma in patients on chronic hemodialysis. *AJR* 150:583, 1988.

Silverman SG, Lee BY, Seltzer SE, et al.: Small (≤ 3 cm) renal masses: correlation of spiral CT features and pathologic findings. *AJR* 163:597, 1994.

Slywotzky C, Maya M: Needle tract seeding of transitional cell carcinoma following fine-needle aspiration of a renal mass. *Abdom Imaging* 19:174, 1994.

Stigsson L, Ekelund L, Karp W: Bilateral concurrent renal neoplasms: report of eleven cases. *AJR* 132:37, 1979.

Wallace S, Chuang VP, Swanson D, et al.: Embolization of renal carcinoma. *Radiology* 138:563, 1981.

Yamashita Y, Honda S, Nishiharu Y, Urata J, Takahashi M: Detection of pseudocapsule of renal cell carcinoma with MR imaging and CT. *AJR* 166:1151, 1996.

Yamashita Y, Takahashi M, Watanabe O, et al.: Small renal cell carcinoma: pathologic and radiologic correlation. *Radiology* 184:493, 1992.

Yamashita Y, Ueno S, Makita O, et al.: Hyperechoic renal tumors: Anechoic rim and intratumoral cysts in US differentiation of renal cell carcinoma from angiomyolipoma. *Radiology* 188:179, 1993.

Zagoria RJ, Bechtold RE, Dyer RB: Staging of renal adenocarcinoma: role of various imaging procedures. *AJR* 164:363, 1995.

Renal Medullary Carcinoma

Davis CJ, Mostofi FK, Sesterhenn IA: Renal medullary carcinoma: the seventh sickle cell nephropathy. *Am J Surg Pathol* 19:1, 1995.

Davidson AJ, Choyke PL, Hartman DS, et al.: Renal medullary carcinoma associated with sickle cell trait: radiologic findings. *Radiology* 195:83, 1995.

Mesenchymal Tumors

Blute ML, Malek RS, Segura JW: Angiomyolipoma: clinical metamorphosis and concepts for management. *J Urol* 139:20, 1988.

Bosniak M, Megibow AJ, Hulnick DH, et al.: CT diagnosis of renal angiomyolipoma: the importance of detecting small amounts of fat. *AJR* 151:497, 1988.

Carmody E, Yeung E, McLoughlin M: Angiomyolipomas of the liver in tuberous sclerosis. *Abdom Imaging* 19:537, 1994.

Curry NS, Schabel SI, Garvin AJ, Fish G: Intratumoral fat in a renal oncocytoma mimicking angiomyolipoma. *AJR* 154:307, 1990.

Davidson AJ, Davis CJ: Fat in renal adenocarcinoma: never say never. *Radiology* 188:316, 1993.

Dunnick NR, Hartman DS, Ford KK, et al.: The radiology of juxtaglomerular tumors. *Radiology* 147:321, 1983.

Kennelly MJ, Grossman HB, Cho KJ: Outcome analysis of 42 cases of renal angiomyolipoma. *J Urol* 152:1988, 1994.

Lemaitre L, Robert Y, Dubrulle F, et al.: Renal angiomyolipoma: growth followed up by CT and/or US. *Radiology* 197:598, 1995.

Lieber MM, Tomera KM, Farrow GM: Renal oncocytoma. *J Urol* 125:481, 1981.

Ochiai K, Onitsuka H, Honda H, et al.: Leiomyosarcoma of the kidney: CT and MR appearance. *J Comput Assist Tomogr* 17:656, 1993.

Radvany MG, Shanley DJ, Gagliardi JA: Magnetic resonance imaging with computed tomography of a renal leiomyoma. *Abdom Imaging* 19:67, 1994.

Rumancik WM, Bosniak MA, Rosen RJ, et al.: Atypical renal and pararenal hamartomas associated with lymphangiomyomatosis. *AJR* 142:971, 1984.

Siegel CL, Middleton WD, Teefey SA, McClennan BL: Angiomyolipoma and renal cell carcinoma: US differentiation. *Radiology* 198:789, 1996.

Soulen MC, Faykus MH, Shlansky-Goldberg RD, Wein AJ, Cope C: Elective embolization for prevention of hemorrhage from renal angiomyolipomas. *J Vasc Interv Radiol* 5:587, 1994.

Srinivas V, Sogani PC, Hajdu SI, et al.: Sarcomas of the kidney. *J Urol* 132:13, 1984.

Steiner MS, Goldman SM, Fishman EK, Marshall FF: The natural history of renal angiomyolipoma. *J Urol* 150:1782, 1993.

Stillwell TJ, Gomez MR, Kelalis PP: Renal lesions in tuberous sclerosis. *J Urol* 138:477, 1987.

Torres VE, King BF, Holley KE, et al.: The kidney in the tuberous sclerosis complex. *Advances in Nephrology* 23:43, 1994.

Van Baal JG, Smits NJ, Keeman JN, Lindhout D, Verhoef S: The evolution of renal angiomyolipomas in patients with tuberous sclerosis. *J Urol* 152:35, 1994.

Renal Pelvic Tumors

Leder RA, Dunnick NR: Transitional cell carcinoma of the pelvicalices and ureter. *AJR* 155:713, 1990.

Levine E: Transitional cell carcinoma of the renal pelvis associated with cyclophosphamide therapy. *AJR* 159:1027, 1992.

Narumi Y, Sato T, Hori S, et al.: Squamous cell carcinoma of the uroepithelium: CT evaluation. *Radiology* 173:853, 1989.

Pollack HM, Arger PH, Banner MP, et al.: Computed tomography of renal pelvic filling defects. *Radiology* 138:645, 1981.

Slywotzky C, Maya M: Needle tract seeding of transitional cell carcinoma following fine-needle aspiration of a renal mass. *Abdom Imaging* 19:174, 1994.

Yousem DM, Gatewood OMB, Goldman SM, et al.: Synchronous and metachronous transitional cell carcinoma of the urinary tract: prevalence, incidence, and radiographic detection. *Radiology* 167:613, 1988.

Secondary Tumors of the Kidney

Choyke PL, White EM, Zeman RK, et al.: Renal metastases: clinicopathologic and radiologic correlation. *Radiology* 162:359, 1987.

Cohan RH, Dunnick NR, Leder RA, Baker ME: Computed tomography of renal lymphoma. *J Comput Assist Tomogr* 14:933, 1990.

Dimopoulos MA, Moulopoulos LA, Costantinides C, et al.: Primary renal lymphoma: a clinical and radiological study. *J Urol* 155: 1865, 1996.

Dunnick NR, Reaman GH, Head GL, et al.: Radiographic manifestations of Burkitt's lymphoma in American patients. *AJR* 132:1, 1979.

Hamper UM, Goldblum LE, Hutchins GM, et al.: Renal involvement in AIDS: sonographic-pathologic correlation. *AJR* 150:1321, 1988.

McCarthy CS, Becker JA: Multiple myeloma and contrast media. *Radiology* 183:519, 1992.

Pagani JJ: Solid renal mass in the cancer patient: second primary renal cell carcinoma versus renal metastasis. *J Comput Assist Tomogr* 7(3):444, 1983.

Richmond J, Sherman RS, Diamond HD, et al.: Renal lesions associated with malignant lymphomas. *Am J Med* 32:184, 1962.

Salem YH, Miller HC: Lymphoma of genitourinary tract. *J Urol* 151: 1162, 1994.

Semelka RC, Kelekis NL, Burdeny DA, et al.: Renal lymphoma: demonstration by MR imaging. *AJR* 166:823, 1996.

Wilbur AC, Turk JN, Capek V: Perirenal metastases from lung cancer: CT diagnosis. *J Comput Assist Tomogr* 16:589, 1992.

Renal Capsular Tumors

Mohler JL, Casale AJ: Renal capsular leiomyoma. *J Urol* 138: 853, 1987.

Myerson D, Rosenfield AT, Itzchak Y: Renal capsular tumors: the angiographic features. *J Urol* 121:238, 1979.

Steiner M, Quinlan D, Goldman SM, et al.: Leiomyoma of the kidney: presentation of four new cases and the role of computerized tomography. *J Urol* 143:994, 1990.

7

··

Renal Inflammatory Disease

··········

Inflammatory conditions involving the urinary tract are among the most common infectious disorders affecting humans. In most cases, the infection is confined to the lower urinary tract and the diagnosis is established by clinical or laboratory studies. Imaging studies are not required when there is prompt resolution after appropriate therapy. However, when the kidney is involved by the inflammatory process or when the precise diagnosis is not known, renal imaging studies play an important role in diagnosis and management.

Pathologically, inflammatory disease involving the kidney can be divided into two broad groups: (*a*) glomerulonephritis, which involves an immunologic injury of the glomerulus; and (*b*) interstitial nephritis, which results from the effect of an infectious or toxic agent on the renal parenchyma. Radiologic studies play a limited role in the diagnosis and management of glomerulonephritis (*see* Chapter 10). Interstitial nephritis is divided into two major subgroups: (*a*) noninfectious interstitial nephritis, which is usually caused by the action of toxic agents on the kidney; and (*b*) infectious interstitial nephritis, the result of the action of a pathogen. Noninfectious interstitial nephritis also will be discussed in Chapter 10. In most cases, infectious interstitial nephritis is caused by a bacterial organism; such cases are commonly called *acute pyelonephritis*.

BACTERIAL INFECTIONS

Pathophysiology

Bacteria usually reach the kidney through the ureter as a result of ascending infection from the lower urinary tract. In children, this commonly occurs as a result of vesicoureteral reflux; in adults, however, frank reflux is uncommon and bacteria are thought to ascend to the kidney via the ureter against the antegrade flow of urine. Some bacteria, for example, *Escherichia coli*, have demonstrated the ability to elaborate a protein termed P. fimbriae that facilitates bacterial adhesion to the cells of the urothelium. Women have a much higher incidence of lower urinary tract infection owing to the short length of the female urethra. Bacterial infections of the kidney are much more common in women than in men younger than 50 years of age. Beyond this age, however, the incidence of urinary tract infection in men increases, as a result of urinary stasis caused by benign prostatic hypertrophy and other factors. Much less commonly, bacterial infections are spread to the kidney hematogenously.

Clinically the patient may present with fever, flank pain, chills, and other systemic symptoms such as nausea, vomiting, and malaise. These symptoms usually help to differentiate infections involving the kidney from those that purely involve the lower urinary tract. In some cases, however, clinical differentiation may be difficult because these symptoms may be present in patients with infection confined to the lower urinary tract. Conditions that predispose patients with lower urinary tract infection to renal involvement include (*a*) vesicoureteral reflux, (*b*) urinary tract obstruction, (*c*) calculi, (*d*) altered bladder function, (*e*) altered host resistance, (*f*) pregnancy, and (*g*) congenital urinary tract anomalies. Nonetheless, there is usually a prompt response to appropriate antibiotic therapy. Diagnostic imaging studies are performed after the fact or are not necessary. Patients with underlying diabetes are of particular concern, because they are more vulnerable to the development of a complication from acute pyelonephritis. It also is more difficult to establish the diagnosis on clinical grounds in patients with diabetes, because as many as 50% of these patients will not present with the typical flank tenderness that helps differentiate pyelonephritis from lower urinary tract infection in an otherwise healthy patient.

Gram-negative enteric pathogens, including *Escherichia coli, Proteus mirabilis, Pseudomonas aeruginosa,* and *Klebsiella spp.* are responsible for the vast majority of bacterial renal infections. In the preantibiotic era, gram-positive urine pathogens including *Staphylococcus* and *Streptococcus spp.* were relatively common; however, today they represent only a small minority of infections.

Pathologically acute pyelonephritis is an acute bacterial infection of the kidney manifested by infiltration of the renal interstitium with neutrophils. On gross examination, the kidney exhibits swelling and the tissues appear hyperemic. Small microabscesses 1 to 5 mm in diameter may be present. These changes tend to occur in foci within the kidney interspersed with zones of unaffected renal tissue.

In the early 1970s, radiologists described a spectrum of patients with acute pyelonephritis in whom there was a significant degree of impairment of contrast medium excretion on urography, a focal area of renal enlargement that simulated a renal abscess or both. Such patients generally had more severe infections and responded more slowly to antibiotic therapy. In an attempt to differentiate such patients from those with uncomplicated pyelonephritis (who generally responded quickly to antibiotic therapy and had normal imaging studies), a variety of terms were coined to describe these severe infections. Such terms included *acute focal pyelonephritis, acute focal bacterial nephritis, acute bacterial nephritis,* and *acute lobar nephronia.* The use of these terms accelerated with the demonstration of subtle changes of renal infection on CT, particularly in patients in whom urography was normal.

The use of this terminology in the literature, however has been inconsistent, and although many of these patients generally had more severe disease, there is no fundamental difference in the *nature* of the disease process. The Society of Uroradiology has recommended, therefore that the terminology used to describe renal inflammatory disease be simplified and that the term *acute pyelonephritis* be used to describe changes in the kidney caused by a renal infection. To characterize the distribution and severity of the infection further, they recommended the modifiers *diffuse, focal,* and with or without *renal enlargement.*

If there is coalescence of the small microabscesses present in acute pyelonephritis with underlying tissue liquefaction, an *acute renal abscess* is formed. After formation of the abscess, fibroblasts migrate into the area of inflammation to build a wall between the normal parenchyma and necrotic tissue. This "walling-off" process is characteristic of more mature abscesses. A *chronic renal abscess,* therefore, represents a walled-off abscess and the remainder of the renal parenchyma returns to normal. If the walling-off process is incomplete and the renal abscess breaks through the renal capsule, a *perinephric abscess* is formed.

If the infection is confined to the collecting system, and the patient also has ureteral obstruction, the process is termed pyonephrosis. In patients with *pyonephrosis,* inflammatory changes may be present throughout the renal parenchyma, but the collecting system itself is filled with pus as a result of inadequate drainage. If pyelosinus extravasation should occur, a perinephric abscess may be formed by this mechanism as well.

Imaging Approach to Renal Inflammatory Disease

Traditionally, excretory urography has been the primary diagnostic modality for imaging patients with acute renal inflammatory disease. The rationale for performing urography is **not** to diagnosis acute pyelonephritis, but to look for an underlying anatomic abnormality (i.e., anomaly) that may have predisposed the patient to the infection, to search for a process such as a calculus, papillary necrosis, or an obstruction, which may prevent a rapid therapeutic response, or to diagnose a complication of the infection such as a renal or perinephric abscess. As such, many urologists routinely order an excretory urogram in all patients with clinical pyelonephritis within the first 24 hours after initiation of therapy.

There is good evidence that routine urography does not alter the clinical care in 90% of patients with pyelonephritis. If investigation is confined to those patients who do not become afebrile after 72 hours of appropriate antibiotic therapy, the number of patients with urographic findings that have immediate clinical significance increases significantly. A fivefold increase in yield from routine urography in patients with underlying diabetes or those infected with a pathogen other than ampicillin-sensitive *E. coli* also has been demonstrated. The validity of the 72-hour period was confirmed by Soulen and associates in a study of the utility of computed tomography (CT) in patients with pyelonephritis. In this series, 95% of patients with uncomplicated pyelonephritis became afebrile within 48 hours of appropriate antibiotic therapy and nearly 100% did so within 72 hours.

There is nearly universal agreement that precontrast and postcontrast CT is the imaging study of choice for the diagnosis of atypical pyelonephritis or to look for a potential complication of the infection such as a renal or perinephric abscess, or renal emphysema. In most of the studies comparing CT to sonography, much of the superiority of CT lies in its ability to detect parenchymal abnormalities in patients with pyelonephritis that are generally missed by ultrasound, but that do not alter the patient's therapy. However, Soulen and associates did report that ultrasound missed 6 of 10 intrarenal and 1 of 5 perinephric abscesses subsequently diagnosed by CT. Only 3 of these 15 cases, however, had the results verified by surgery. The proponents of ultrasound are quick to point out its advantages: namely, low risk, relatively low expense, lack of ionizing radiation, and, most importantly, that it does not require the use of a contrast medium. Ultrasonographic findings in patients with pyonephrosis are relatively specific (i.e., low-level echoes within the collecting system) but this diagnosis also can be suggested by CT. The most specific test for the diagnosis of pyonephrosis, however, is needle aspiration of the collecting system, which is generally performed as a prelude to percutaneous nephrostomy.

Recently there has been increased interest in the diagnosis of acute pyelonephritis in children using technetium-99m-dimercaptosuccinic acid (^{99m}Tc-DMSA) renal scintigraphy. This technique has been shown to be much more sensitive for the detection of pyelonephritis than ultrasonography. Kass and coworkers demonstrated scintigraphic abnormalities in 78% of children with acute pyelonephritis; ultrasonography was positive in only 11% of the same patients. This is important because differentiating lower tract infection from pyelonephritis is more difficult in children and because children are more vulnerable to permanent renal damage from renal inflammatory disease. There are little comparable data, however, regarding the adult population.

Various other imaging studies are of value in selected patients. Magnetic resonance imaging (MRI) has not been shown to have any advantages over other less costly cross-sectional imaging studies. Retrograde pyelography is of value in patients with severe infection and obstruction that can not be demonstrated noninvasively. Antegrade pyelography can be used as an alternative to the retrograde study. Voiding cystourethrography is used to demonstrate vesicoureteral reflux, but is routinely performed only in children.

In summary, otherwise healthy patients with uncomplicated pyelonephritis seldom need a radiologic workup if they respond to antibiotic therapy within 72 hours. If there is no response to therapy, urography is probably the most cost-effective initial examination. Diabetic or other immunocompromised patients should probably be evaluated within 24 hours of diagnosis using precontrast and postcontrast CT as an initial study. Ultrasound should be used as a problem-solving technique, for those in whom pyonephrosis is suspected, and in those patients in whom exposure to contrast media or radiation (i.e., pregnant women) is deemed to be hazardous. In all other patients, (i.e., males, patients with a history of stones or prior urologic surgery, repeated episodes of pyelonephritis, etc.), urography is still the most cost-effective initial study.

Acute Pyelonephritis

Acute uncomplicated pyelonephritis is the most common bacterial infection involving the kidney. The infection responds quickly (within 48–72 hours) to antibiotic therapy and, unlike acute pyelonephritis in children, usually does not lead to any permanent morphologic damage. It is not surprising, therefore, that the results of urography and ultrasonography are normal in three quarters of the cases. In the remainder, abnormal urographic findings include the following (Fig. 7.1): (*a*) diffuse renal enlargement, generally attributed to the edema that accompanies the infection; (*b*) a delay in the appearance of the contrast medium in the renal collecting system; (*c*) attenuation of the calyces, also the result of parenchymal edema; and (*d*) a decrease in the density of the nephrogram in the affected portion of the kidney. In general, the degree of radiographic abnormality and the degree of impairment of contrast excretion reflect the severity of the interstitial inflammatory disease.

Uncommonly, urography may demonstrate severe impairment of contrast excretion in patients with severe pyelonephritis (Fig. 7.2). The nephrogram is typically of normal or increased intensity and persists for several hours after the administration of the contrast medium. This appearance is similar to the nephrogram, which has been described in association with acute tubular necrosis and must be differentiated from the nephrogram of acute extrarenal obstruction. In the latter instance, the nephrogram becomes progressively more intense during the course of the study. The pyelogram typically is markedly delayed in appearance or may be entirely absent. The urographic changes, while generally more pronounced, may be difficult to distinguish from other forms of renal inflammatory disease.

Caliectasis that is not attributable to concomitant obstruction, may occur as the result of acute pyelonephritis, but is rare. This finding has been attributed to an endotoxin elaborated by some gram-negative bacteria that is said to diminish ureteral peristalsis. In the vast majority of cases, however, the finding of caliectasis in association with acute pyelonephritis implies past or present urinary tract obstruction.

Mucosal striations, sometimes referred to as "ridging" of the mucosa, are an uncommon manifestation of acute pyelonephritis in the renal collecting system. These striations are thought to be a manifestation of mucosal edema, but are not specific for acute pyelonephritis; they are found in a variety of other conditions, including vesicoureteral reflux.

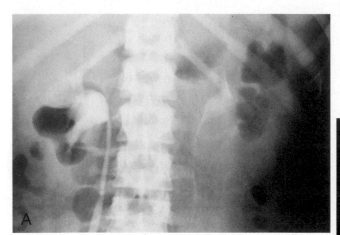

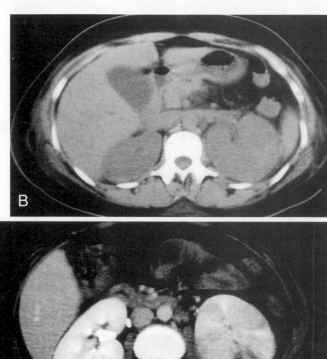

Figure 7.1.   Acute pyelonephritis. **A,** Excretory urography. The left kidney is enlarged; there is a decrease in the density of the nephrogram and pyelogram, and the collecting system is attenuated. **B,** Noncontrast computed tomography demonstrates diffuse parenchymal swelling without a focal parenchymal defect. **C,** Postcontrast computed tomography shows striated nephrographic defects typical of acute pyelonephritis.

Ultrasonographic findings in patients with acute uncomplicated pyelonephritis are normal or show renal enlargement and diffusely hypoechogenic renal parenchyma (Fig. 7.3). Dinkle and colleagues demonstrated an increase in renal size of as much as two standard deviations over normal as determined by ultrasound in children with acute renal inflammatory disease. They reported, however, that renal enlargement appears to be age-dependent, with the youngest children showing the greatest degree of change. When there is renal enlargement with focal pyelonephritis, the "mass" is typically sonolucent, is poorly marginated, and may contain low-level echoes that disrupt the corticomedullary junction. In some patients, areas of involvement have been described as being slightly hyperechoic, but this appearance is uncommon. Differentiating these phlegmatous areas of involvement from true liquefaction may be difficult, even using high-resolution equipment.

There is nearly universal agreement that CT provides the most complete information regarding the nature and extent of the inflammatory process of any imaging study. For the imaging of renal inflammatory disease, CT is best performed using both precontrast and postcontrast scans. Typically in acute pyelonephritis, unenhanced scans are normal or show only renal enlargement. After contrast administration, however, narrow striate areas of decreased contrast enhancement are seen focally or generally in the kidney depending on the degree of involvement (Fig. 7.4). Because of its superior contrast resolution compared with urography, CT may show these changes even in patients in whom urography is normal. These striated areas of decreased contrast enhancement most probably represent areas of decreased excretion of the contrast medium secondary to the inflammatory disease. Gold has postulated that they represent areas of slow urine flow within the tubular lumen secondary to elevated interstitial pressure.

With more focal disease (Figs. 7.5 and 7.6), a wedge-shaped or rounded mass-like lesion secondary to diminished contrast enhancement is demonstrated. This appearance is in contrast to a frank abscess, which is apparent before and after contrast administration.

With increasing severity of involvement, the kidney is diffusely enlarged and nearly homogeneous in density

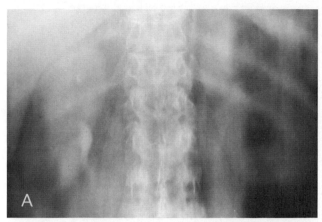

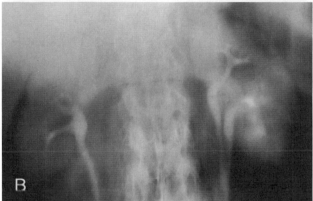

Figure 7.2.   Severe acute pyelonephritis. **A,** Initial study demonstrates swelling of the left kidney with virtually no excretion of contrast medium into the renal collecting system. **B,** Follow-up study after 2 weeks of parenteral antibiotics shows marked improvement. A bifid renal pelvis is now evident.

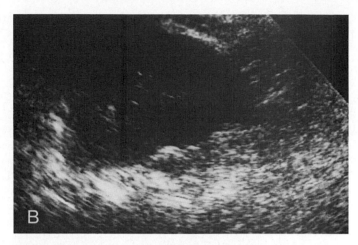

Figure 7.3.   Acute pyelonephritis. Ultrasound shows a diffuse decrease in echogenicity throughout the renal parenchyma. (From Corriere JN Jr, Sandler CM: The diagnosis and immediate therapy of acute renal and perirenal infections. *Urol Clin North Am* 9(2):219, 1982.)

on noncontrast studies. After contrast administration, however, multiple wedge-shaped zones of diminished enhancement can be seen that radiate from the collecting system to the renal capsule (Fig. 7.1). When compared with the attenuation of the kidney before contrast administration, these zones demonstrate a modest increase in density, but less than that present in the unaffected areas of the kidney.

These hypoenhancing areas of diffuse parenchymal involvement are characteristic of the most severe forms of renal infection. Such patients typically respond slowly to antibiotics; may require long periods of therapy for resolution; and may have parenchymal atrophy, scarring, or papillary necrosis as a residua of the infection.

The appearance of pyelonephritis on CT may be modified by antibiotic therapy. Partially treated patients may demonstrate a rounded or ovoid area of decreased enhancement with poorly defined margins (Fig. 7.7).

Long-term follow-up studies in patients with severe renal inflammatory disease may demonstrate generalized wasting of the kidney (Fig. 7.8) and focal calyceal clubbing, suggestive of papillary necrosis. The etiology

of these morphologic changes has been postulated to involve ischemic insult to the kidney as a result of the inflammatory process. Previously scarring from renal infection was thought to be a feature of childhood pyelonephritis only; experience with cross-sectional imaging studies has conclusively demonstrated that scarring may occur in adults after severe infections, as well. Tsugaya suggested that the extent of parenchymal involvement by CT was highly correlated with eventual scar formation.

Radionuclide imaging in patients with acute pyelonephritis has been reported using renal cortical imaging agents such as ^{99m}Tc-DMSA and agents such as gallium

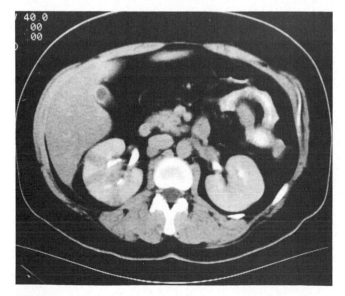

Figure 7.4.   Computed tomography appearance of acute pyelonephritis. Relatively narrow striate zones of decreased contrast enhancement are present in the right renal parenchyma.

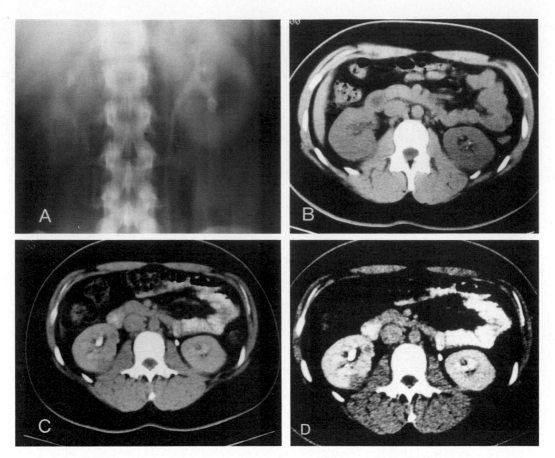

Figure 7.5.   Acute focal pyelonephritis. **A,** Intravenous pyelography demonstrates poor definition of the renal outline with decreased calyceal filling. **B,** Noncontrast computed tomography scan demonstrates slight swelling of the inferomedial portion of the right kidney, but the renal parenchyma appears homogeneous. **C,** After contrast, a poorly defined wedge-shaped area of decreased contrast enhancement is present that is better appreciated at a narrow window setting (**D**).

67 (^{67}Ga) citrate, which image areas of inflammation. Renal cortical imaging studies may show an inhomogeneous distribution of the radionuclide within the affected kidney or polar defects with asymmetric tracer uptake. In some cases, a pattern that was specific for the diagnosis of pyelonephritis, termed the "flare" pattern, representing a striate distribution of decreased radioactivity was present. Ditchfield demonstrated that cortical defects attributed to acute pyelonephritis in children with urinary tract infections were more likely to be present in children less than 2 years of age than in older children. Defects and subsequent scars also were more likely to be present in patients with radiologically demonstrated vesicoureteral reflux; however, defects also were found in 25% of children in whom reflux was not demonstrated.

Gallium 67 will localize in any area of inflammation and is reported to have an accuracy of 86% in distin-

guishing upper-tract from lower-tract infection at 48 hours. Difficulties with gallium imaging for patients with pyelonephritis include the following: (*a*) within the first 24 hours there is normal excretion of the radiotracer by the kidneys, and (*b*) the study cannot differentiate infection within the kidney from that in the surrounding perinephric tissues. In addition, gallium uptake in the kidneys is relatively nonspecific and may be present in a variety of other renal diseases, including acute tubular necrosis and vasculitis. Other investigators have reported using ^{111}indium (^{111}In)-labeled autologous leukocytes in imaging renal inflammatory disease. Indium 111 leukocyte studies have the advantage over ^{67}Ga studies in that the radiopharmaceutical is not normally excreted by the kidneys and that delayed images are not generally required. However, the sensitivity of such studies for the diagnosis of acute pyelonephritis has never been confirmed in large clinical studies.

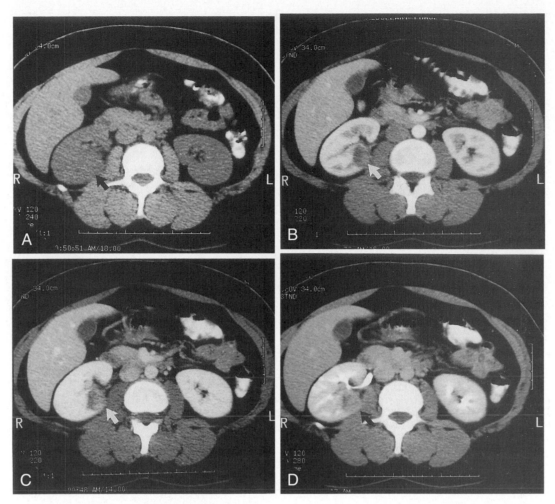

Figure 7.6. Focal acute pyelonephritis (*arrow*). **A,** Noncontrast enhanced; **B,** corti-comedullary phase; **C,** nephrographic phase; **D,** delayed.

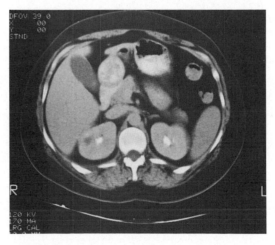

Figure 7.7. Atypical appearance produced by treated pyelonephritis. Computed tomography shows a rounded area of decreased enhancement in the right kidney without significant mass effect; this is in contrast to the striated areas (Fig. 7.4) more typical of untreated acute pyelonephritis.

Acute Renal Abscess

Before the availability of broad-spectrum antibiotics, the majority of renal abscesses formed as a result of hematogenous dissemination of *Staphylococcus aureus,* usually from a site in the skin or bone. Most renal abscesses now form as a result of the coalescence of small microabscesses that are present as a part of acute pyelonephritis. The predominant organisms responsible for abscesses today are gram-negative enteric species and occur in the setting of diabetes mellitus, drug abuse, vesicoureteral reflux, and renal calculus disease. Acute abscesses may be solitary or may form in multiple locations in the kidney simultaneously. Multiple lesions are less common and suggest hematogenous dissemination.

The signs and symptoms of an acute renal abscess are difficult to distinguish from less virulent forms of bacterial infection of the kidney. There is usually a low-grade fever, leukocytosis, and flank pain; urinalysis may demonstrate pyuria, but also may be normal, especially

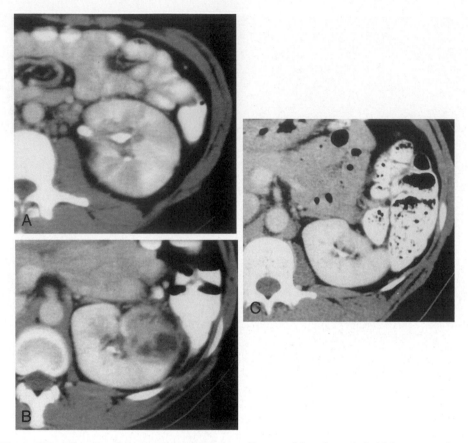

Figure 7.8.   Scarring from pyelonephritis in a 45-year-old patient. **A,** Initial computed tomography scan demonstrates typical findings of acute pyelonephritis. **B,** Follow-up scan demonstrates focal tissue necrosis. **C,** Further follow-up examination shows parenchymal scarring in the area of previous liquefaction.

if some walling-off of the process has occurred. There is frequently a history of prior antibiotic therapy with recrudescence on cessation.

Urography may demonstrate decreased opacification of all or part of the kidney and there is typically decreased calyceal opacification with either compression or amputation of the calyces in the affected segment. Tomography may demonstrate an ill-defined lucency within the renal parenchyma associated with mass effect. The findings on urography are rarely specific, and it may be difficult to distinguish abscess from other forms of inflammatory disease.

Angiography is no longer used to diagnose renal abscesses, but may be performed in an attempt to differentiate an atypical CT appearance of an abscess from that of tumor. The study typically demonstrates pruning of the vascular tree, and there may be draping of vessels around a poorly defined mass, usually best appreciated on the capillary phase.

On sonography, abscesses appear as sonolucent lesions that contain low-amplitude echoes reflecting the necrotic nature of the mass. There is typically poor through-transmission of the ultrasound beam; the findings are usually best characterized as representing a complex mass.

Computed tomography is the imaging study of choice for the diagnosis of an acute renal abscess. The lesion is a low-attenuation (10–20 Hounsfield units [HU]) rounded or ovoid mass which, in contrast to other nonnecrotic inflammatory masses, is present before (Fig. 7.9) and after contrast administration. The attenuation of the mass may increase slightly with contrast administration, but not to the extent that is present with renal tumors. Depending on the degree of the surrounding inflammatory process, the borders of the mass may be relatively sharply defined or indistinct. In some cases, gas may be present within the abscess; when present, this finding is virtually pathognomonic. There is usually thickening of Gerota's fascia, and increased density may be found in the adjacent perinephric and mesenteric fat. This latter finding has been termed "dirty fat" by some investigators, but is not specific for an inflammatory process.

Radionuclide studies performed with ^{67}Ga citrate or ^{111}In-labeled leukocytes will localize in an acute renal

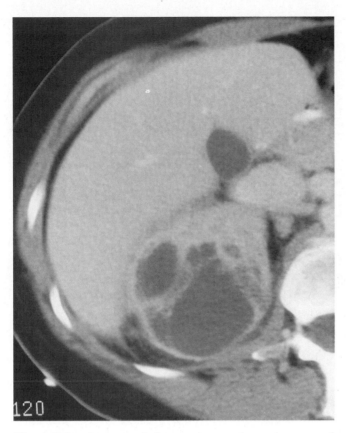

Figure 7.9. Acute renal abscess. An unenhanced computed tomography scan demonstrates an acute multiloculated renal abscess.

abscess. Neither study, however, permits differentiation of a frank abscess from a phlegmon or a focal area of pyelonephritis, nor do they permit separation of those inflammatory masses confined to the kidney from those that have extended into the perinephric space.

Chronic Renal Abscess

When fibroblasts migrate into the area of an acute renal abscess and form a barrier between the abscess and the remainder of the kidney, a chronic renal abscess is formed. Extension of the abscess into the perinephric space may or may not be present.

On imaging studies, a chronic renal abscess is seen as an intrarenal mass. While the interior of the mass is avascular, there is frequently a prominent hypervascular rim on angiography surrounding the avascular center, representing the granulation tissue at the lesion's periphery. This same finding may be seen on CT where the rim of the lesion enhances after contrast administration to a greater extent than does the surrounding normal renal parenchyma. Finding this hypervascular rim helps to identify the lesion as a chronic renal abscess. The presence of a rim, however, is not pathognomonic of a chronic renal abscess; such a pattern of enhance-

ment may be found in some necrotic or cystic renal neoplasms. On ultrasonography, chronic renal abscesses appear as complex intrarenal masses. In some instances, the rim of granulation tissue may be identified by its echogenic nature; however, ultrasonography has not proven to be as reliable as CT in identifying the nature of the lesion. Hoddick and coworkers reported a significant number of false-negative ultrasonograms among 12 patients with renal or perirenal abscesses in whom both modalities were used; there were no false-negative CT studies in this group.

Perinephric Abscess

A *primary* perinephric abscess forms when an intrarenal abscess breaks through the renal capsule into the perinephric space. On discovery, the intrarenal component may be large or may have healed, and the extrarenal component is all that can be identified. Primary perinephric abscesses also may form as a result of pyelosinus extravasation of infected urine. *Secondary* perinephric abscesses may form when infection is spread to the perinephric space hematogenously from an external source. A third mechanism by which perinephric abscesses occur is direct extension into the perinephric space from an infection in an adjacent organ (i.e., a ruptured appendix or diverticulitis).

The signs and symptoms of a perinephric abscess are nonspecific in that clinical differentiation of this process from less advanced forms of renal inflammatory disease is usually not possible. In some patients, however, referred pain to the thorax, the groin, the thigh, or the hip may be a clue that the disease has spread beyond the kidney. In most cases, symptoms of urinary infection are present for periods longer than 2 weeks. Fever is usually present, but tends to be intermittent and low-grade. As many as 25% of patients have normal urinalysis. The development of a perinephric abscess as a complication of renal inflammatory disease is more common in patients with large staghorn calculi (Fig. 7.10), pyonephrosis, diabetes mellitus, and neurogenic bladder disease.

On plain films, a large perinephric abscess may be identified as a soft tissue mass in the perinephric space (Fig. 7.11). A scoliosis of the lumbar spine convex to the opposite side also may be present. The psoas margin may be obscured on the involved side; however, such a finding may be present in up to 10% of healthy patients. Air within the abscess is found in a number of large perinephric abscesses secondary to gas-forming organisms; extensive gas collection, however, may be confused with gas normally present within the colon.

Urography generally demonstrates changes in the renal parenchyma previously described with less severe forms of renal inflammatory disease. With a large abscess, a soft tissue density outside the confines of the kidney may be appreciated. Tomography demonstrates

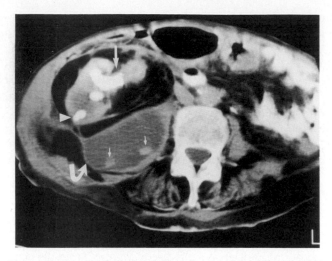

Figure 7.10. A small right kidney containing multiple calculi (*arrow*) is present. A chronic renal abscess containing an extruded calculus is present in the inferior portion of the kidney (*arrowhead*). A perinephric component with an enhancing rim (*curved arrow*) also contains extruded calculi (*small white arrows*).

thickening and displacement of Gerota's fascia (Fig. 7.12). In addition, tomography may demonstrate that the two kidneys are not in focus on the same tomographic section; the affected kidney may be displaced anteriorly because of fluid behind it. In some cases, however, the findings on urography will be subtle, with compression of the kidney by the surrounding soft tissue mass (Fig. 7.11**B**). Loss of the normal mobility of the kidney (Mathe's sign) may be diagnosed by a fixed position of the affected kidney on upright radiographs and by reduced respiratory excursion of the kidney. Maneuvers described in the older literature specifically designed to demonstrate this phenomenon on urography are no longer necessary, because the diagnosis will be established on cross-sectional imaging.

On ultrasonography, perinephric abscesses appear as masses of variable echogenicity adjacent to the kidney. Gas within the abscess will demonstrate acoustic shadowing, but when the abscess is anterior to the kidney, gas may be confused with intestinal gas. Depending on the ultrasonographic characteristics of the abscess, sonography may underestimate the size of or even fail to detect the perinephric fluid collection because its borders may blend into the normally echogenic perinephric fat (Fig. 7.11**D**).

The imaging study of choice for the detection of perinephric abscess is CT. Such abscesses are best detected when contrast-enhanced scans are obtained, but the abnormality is usually readily detected even on unenhanced studies. The strength of CT is its ability to define precisely the boundaries of the process so that extension into the psoas muscle, the posterior pararenal

space, and the true pelvis may all be accurately detected. As in intrarenal abscess, chronic perinephric abscess may demonstrate an enhancing rim (Fig. 7.10).

Percutaneous Drainage of Renal and Perinephric Abscess

Percutaneous drainage of renal and perinephric abscesses using radiologic guidance is the preferred method of therapy, at least initially. Percutaneous drainage provides satisfactory clinical results using only local anesthesia and obviates the need for open surgical drainage.

Fluoroscopic, ultrasonic, or CT guidance (Fig. 7.13) may be used. The method used largely depends on the experience and preference of the radiologist and on the size and location of the cavity to be drained. When possible, we prefer the fluoroscopic method because it allows the drainage to be performed most quickly. Appropriate antibiotic coverage should be started before initiating the procedure. A variety of catheters and techniques may be used, including the placement of a guidewire and catheter using the Seldinger technique and direct placement of the drainage catheter using a trocar catheter combination. Catheters ranging in size from 8 to 16 French may be used depending on the technique that is used for placement and the characteristics of the material to be drained. Self-retaining pigtail, sump, or Malecot catheters may be used with equal degrees of success.

With large perinephric collections, it is preferable to place the drainage catheter in the most dependent portion of the abscess cavity. Loculated collections may require the placement of more than one catheter. When renal and perinephric abscesses coexist, placement of separate drainage catheters in each collection provides the most efficient method of drainage (Fig. 7.14).

In most of the reported series, renal and perinephric abscesses are included in larger series of abdominal and pelvic abscesses. Sacks and associates, however, have reported a series of renal and perirenal abscesses totaling 18 patients. Percutaneous drainage, as the sole therapy, was successful in the management of 61% of the patients; in 39% of patients, successful temporization of the abscess was achieved by percutaneous methods. In these cases, surgery to correct the underlying condition associated with the development of the renal or perirenal abscess was performed. The period of drainage varied and ranged from a few days to 2 months. The drainage catheter may be removed when the patient's clinical condition has improved and drainage ceases.

Complications of renal abscess drainage include the exacerbation of urosepsis and hemorrhage. Migration of the drainage catheter into the gastrointestinal tract also has been described.

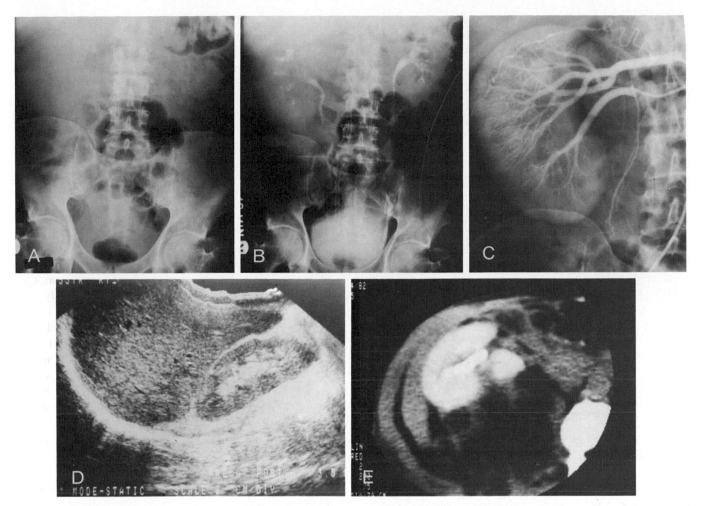

Figure 7.11. Perinephric abscess. **A,** Plain film radiograph shows a large soft tissue mass in the right flank with obliteration of the psoas margin. **B,** Excretory urography shows extrinsic compression of the renal collecting system with generalized renal enlargement. **C,** Selective right renal angiogram shows no evidence of an intrarenal mass, but there is displacement of the capsular vessels from the renal margin, suggesting fluid in the perinephric space. Two renal arteries that have been injected simultaneously are present. **D,** Ultrasound shows anterior displacement of the lower pole of the kidney, but a definite abscess is not seen. **E,** Computed tomography shows a large posterior perinephric abscess with multiple loculations. The abscess displaces the right kidney almost to the anterior abdominal wall.

Pyonephrosis

Pyonephrosis is an obstructed, infected renal collecting system. Most authorities consider it to be one of the few true urologic emergencies in that untreated pyonephrosis leads to sepsis and death. Most patients with pyonephrosis have clinical evidence of urinary tract infection. In one series, however, the aspiration of infected urine under fluoroscopic guidance was the first evidence of urinary tract infection in approximately 10% of the patients. Calculi are the cause of the associated urinary tract obstruction in a majority of cases; metastatic disease, postoperative ureteral strictures, and processes such as retroperitoneal fibrosis account for the remainder.

The role of imaging studies in the diagnosis of pyonephrosis has been reported by Yoder and coworkers in a series of 70 patients. Plain abdominal radiographs demonstrated obvious urinary tract calculi in approxi-

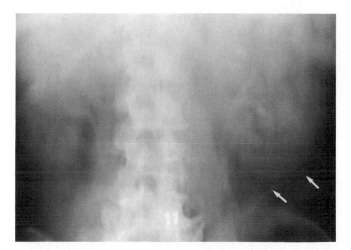

Figure 7.12. Tomogram demonstrates thickening and displacement of Gerota's fascia (*arrows*) secondary to a perinephric abscess.

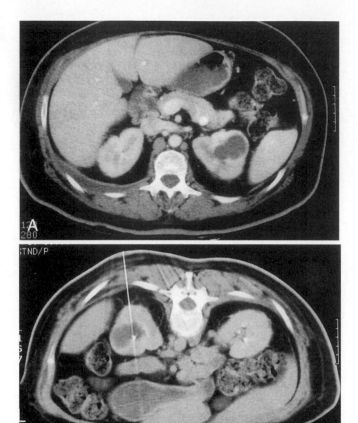

Figure 7.13. Acute renal abscess with computed tomography (CT)–guided aspiration. **A,** CT shows an intrarenal, oval-shaped abscess. **B,** With the patient in the prone position, CT-guided aspiration is performed before drainage.

mately one half of the patients. Urography demonstrated findings typical of acute urinary tract obstruction in those patients in whom sufficient renal function permitted excretion of the contrast material. In approximately one third of the patients in Yoder's study, the involved kidney demonstrated no discernible contrast material excretion. In patients with ileal conduits, loopograms may be helpful by demonstrating partial or complete obstruction of the affected ureter. Radionuclide studies generally demonstrate diminished excretion of technetium-99m diethylenetriaminepentaacetic acid (^{99m}Tc-DTPA), but a dilated renal collecting system may be found on delayed images. Computed tomography usually shows evidence of hydronephrosis and generally demonstrates the cause and level of the associated obstruction. Although rare, layering of contrast medium above purulent material in the collecting system allows a specific diagnosis of pyonephrosis.

Sonography is the most reliable noninvasive method by which pyonephrosis can be distinguished from uninfected hydronephrosis on imaging studies. The findings on sonography include the following: (*a*) persistent dependent echoes within the collecting system, (*b*) shifting urine-debris levels, (*c*) dense peripheral echoes with shadowing secondary to gas in the collecting system, and (*d*) low-level echoes within the dilated collecting system with poor through-transmission (Fig. 7.15). Subramanyam and coworkers reported sonography to have a sensitivity of 90% and an overall accuracy of 96% for this diagnosis among a group of 73 patients. Jeffrey and colleagues, however, reported that while the findings of medium- to coarse-intensity echoes within

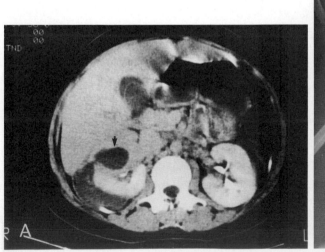

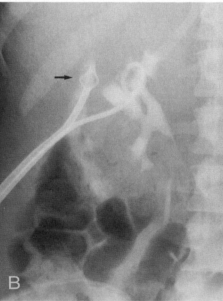

Figure 7.14. **A,** Computed tomography scan demonstrates an acute intrarenal abscess (*arrow*) with a large perinephric component inferior to the kidney. **B,** Two catheters were used for drainage; a pigtail catheter was placed in the intrarenal component, while a Malecot catheter (*arrow*) was placed in the perinephric space.

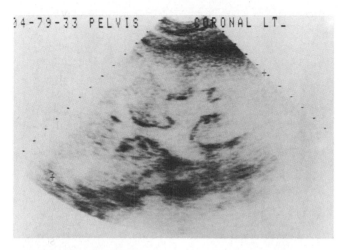

Figure 7.15. Multiple echoes representing pyonephrosis are present within a dilated renal collecting system. (Courtesy of Patricia Athey, M.D.)

the collecting system had a specificity of 100% for pyonephrosis, the sensitivity of the study was only 62%. In this series, 10% of the patients with proven pyonephrosis had ultrasonographic findings indistinguishable from uninfected hydronephrosis. On CT, a grossly dilated collecting system that contains a urine debris level or an air fluid level, suggests the diagnosis (Fig. 7.16).

Percutaneous aspiration of infected urine using radiologic guidance is the definitive diagnostic study in suspected pyonephrosis and is usually performed in association with percutaneous nephrostomy. Yoder has reported that percutaneous nephrostomy and antibiotics were successful as the only therapy for pyonephrosis in 33% of their patients; in 40% of patients, the procedure permitted successful temporization before a surgical pro-

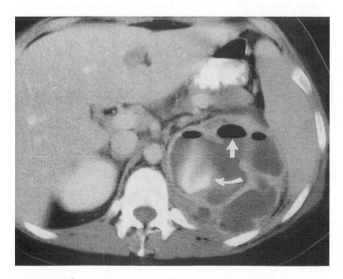

Figure 7.16. Pyonephrosis. A grossly dilated collecting system with some contrast medium excretion (*curved arrow*) and an air fluid level (*arrow*) is present.

cedure to remove the cause of obstruction. Nephrectomy was ultimately required in 20% of patients, whereas 5% of the patients died, commonly from sepsis. Twenty-eight percent of the patients in Yoder's series, however, suffered serious complications from the procedure including the development of temporally related frank sepsis, fever, shaking chills, and hemorrhagic shock.

Gas-Forming Renal Infections

Gas in the kidney or collecting system may be due to a variety of etiologies, including the iatrogenic introduction of air during a surgical or radiologic procedure, or as the result of a renoalimentary fistula, external penetrating trauma, or urinary infection. In the last instance, the presence of gas usually indicates infection with a Gram-negative pathogen (*E. coli* in 70%, followed by *Klebsiella, Aerobacter,* and *Proteus*) and is most common in diabetic patients in whom the presence of glycosuria is said to promote its production through the fermentation of glucose into carbon dioxide and hydrogen. Diabetes, however, is not a necessary precondition for the development of a gas-forming infection. Its rare occurrence, even in diabetic patients, suggests that other factors such as altered host resistance play a role in its pathogenesis. As described earlier, gas may be present in acute or chronic renal abscesses or perinephric abscesses.

A variety of confusing terms have been used to describe gas-forming infections. The term, *emphysematous pyelonephritis* (*EPN*), has generally been reserved for cases in which gas is found diffusely infiltrating the renal parenchyma (Fig. 7.17). More than 90% of these cases are in patients with diabetes mellitus. When the gas is confined to the kidney alone, a mortality rate of 60% has been reported in patients treated with antibiotics with or without surgical drainage. When there is extension of the gas into the perirenal space, the mortality rate on medical therapy alone is said to exceed 80%, however, with nephrectomy, there is a reduction in mortality to the 30–50% range. Gas within the lumen of the renal pelvis with or without an *air pyelogram* (Fig. 7.18) , or gas within the walls of the renal pelvis with or without an air pyelogram, termed *emphysematous pyelitis* (Fig. 7.19), has a less grave implication than does true emphysematous pyelonephritis. Diabetes is present in approximately one-half of this group of patients and the condition has considerably lower mortality, in the range of 15–20%.

In order to standarize the nomenclature regarding gas-forming renal infections and to make comparisons of therapy and outcomes comparable among published seris, Wan and co-workers have suggested that gas-forming renal infections be categorized into two groups. Type I EPN is defined as the classical form of EPN in which gas is found diffusely throughout the renal parenchyma in a streaked or mottled pattern with tissue

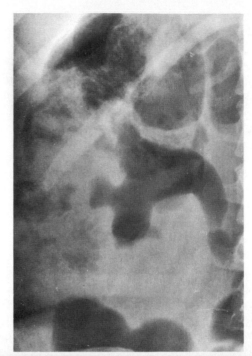

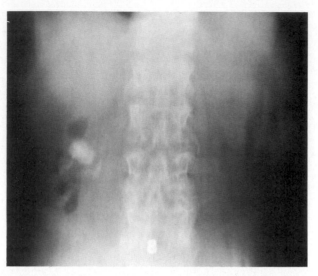

Figure 7.18.   Plain tomogram shows air and several struvite calculi present within the right renal collecting system.

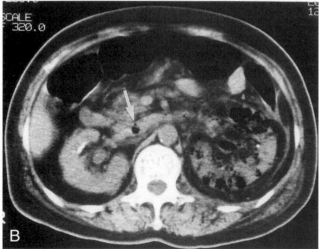

Figure 7.17.   Emphysematous pyelonephritis. **A,** Coned view of the right kidney showing a bubbled appearance within the renal parenchyma secondary to diffuse infiltration of the kidney by gas. An air pyelogram and ureterogram also are present. (Courtesy of Davis S. Hartman, M.D. and the Armed Forces Institute of Pathology.) **B,** Computed tomography in a different patient demonstrating diffuse air infiltrating the left renal parenchyma and extending into the inferior vena cava (*arrow*). A small left renal calculus is also present. (Courtesy of Akira Kawashima, M.D., Hiroshi Honda, M.D., and Kouji Masuda, M.D.)

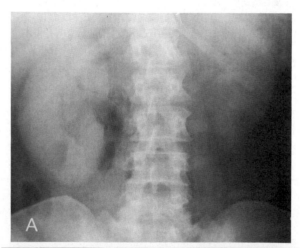

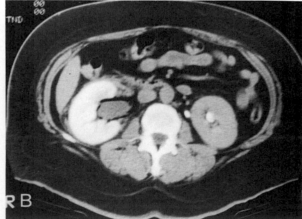

Figure 7.19.   **A,** Twelve-hour delayed film from an excretory urogram demonstrates a persistent nephrogram in the right kidney with air in the walls of the renal pelvis and proximal ureter. **B,** Computed tomography scan clearly demonstrates the mural location of the air.

destruction and little or no fluid (Fig. 7.18). Type II EPN was defined as any renal or perinephric fluid collection with a bubbly or loculated gas collection either in the renal parenchyma or in the collecting system, including air-containing renal and perinephric abscesses. The authors confirmed the grave prognosis for patients with Type I EPN; such patients experienced a more fulminant course

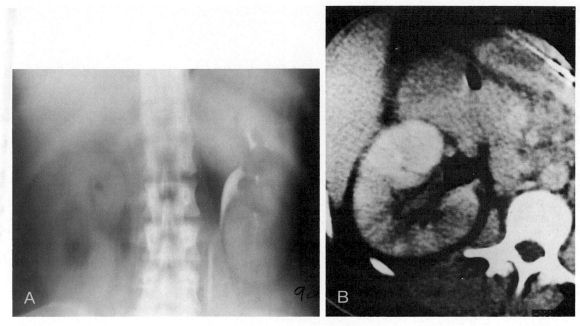

Figure 7.20.   A, Excretory urogram shows a small amount of gas within the poorly functioning right kidney, but it is not possible to distinguish whether this air collection is in the re-nal parenchyma or in the collecting system. **B,** Computed to-mography scan clearly shows the gas is present within the re-nal collecting system.

from the time of onset of symptoms (mean 4.06 days versus 11.16 days for patients with Type II EPN) and had a mortality rate of 69%. In this series all patients with Type I EPN who survived had either nephrectomy or surgical drainage; 46% of the patients who died received medical therapy alone.

Radiologic studies including plain films, excretory urography, and CT aid in the diagnosis of these conditions and especially in distinguishing gas-containing renal abscesses from gas in the collecting system or in the renal parenchyma (Fig. 7.20). Emphysematous pyelonephritis has three sequential stages. Initially, a mottled lucency may be present extending radially along the renal pyramids. In more extensive renal emphysema, air may be found in a bubbled pattern within the parenchyma and associated air is found within the confines of Gerota's fascia. As the process ensues, air diffusely infiltrates the renal parenchyma and extends beyond the confines of Gerota's fascia within the retroperitoneum. These changes are well demonstrated by CT. Intramural gas or gas within the collecting system is usually also well shown on CT, on which it can be distinguished from parenchymal air, even in kidneys that fail to excrete contrast medium.

Renal Fistula

A renoalimentary fistula may result from Crohn's disease, from tumors in the kidney or the gastrointestinal tract, or from severe renal trauma. Most commonly, however, renal fistulas occur as a result of renal inflammatory disease. Usually fistulas develop between the kidney and the colon (Fig. 7.21), but the duodenum (Fig. 7.22), the stomach, and the distal small bowel also may be involved. The site of fistulization is principally determined by the anatomic proximity of the organ to the kidney. Renocutaneous fistulae and fistulae to the pleura or lung also have been described.

Renal fistulae occur in the setting of renal or perinephric abscesses or pyonephrosis, usually complicated by the presence of calculi. In the older literature, renal tuberculosis was described as the causative factor in 25% of the cases.

Although CT will generally be the first study obtained in such patients, CT will rarely demonstrate the fistula directly. Indirect signs, such as the presence of gas within the collecting system, may be found, but the diagnosis of the renal fistula will almost always require retrograde or antegrade pyelography, because the severe inflammatory disease requisite for the development of the fistula will preclude sufficient contrast material excretion for visualization on urography. A single case of a renocolic fistula in association with xanthogranulomatous pyelonephritis diagnosed by CT has been reported.

Xanthogranulomatous Pyelonephritis

Xanthogranulomatous pyelonephritis (XGP) is a relatively uncommon form of renal inflammatory disease

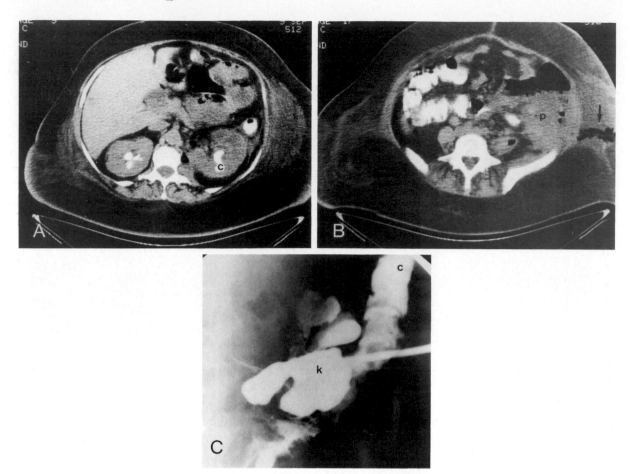

Figure 7.21.   A, Computed tomography scan in an obese diabetic patient shows inflammatory changes involving the left kidney. A renal calculus (*c*) is also present. **B,** A more inferior section reveals a large amount of pus (*p*) in the perinephric space with an air-fluid level. Gas also extends into the soft tissues of the flank (*arrow*). **C,** A percutaneous drainage catheter was placed. Contrast injection reveals a fistula between the renal collecting system (*k*) and the descending colon (*c*).

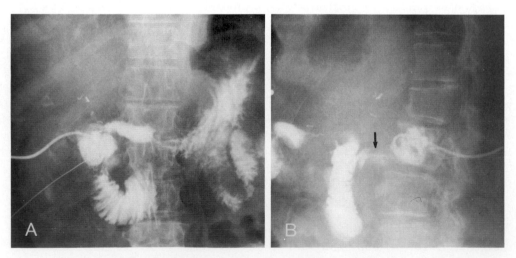

Figure 7.22.   A, Anteroposterior and **B,** lateral radiographs after nephrostomy tube placement demonstrate a pyeloduodenal fistula (*arrow*).

characterized histologically by the presence of lipid-laden macrophages (xanthoma cells), as well as other inflammatory cells including plasma cells, leukocytes, and histiocytes. The classically described triad of findings include: (*a*) a staghorn calculus, (*b*) absent or diminished excretion of contrast medium on urography, and (*c*) a poorly defined renal mass. The signs and symptoms of the disease are nonspecific; fever, malaise, flank pain or tenderness, weight loss, and leukocytosis are the most common presenting complaints. Lower urinary tract symptoms (frequency, dysuria) are present in only one half of the patients. Anemia is present in 70% of the patients, approximately 25% of the patients demonstrate abnormalities in liver function tests, and about 10% of patients have underlying diabetes mellitus. Some series report female preponderance in XGP as high as 4:1. While most patients range from 45 to 65 years of age, patients as young as 5 years of age have been reported. Active urinary tract infection with *E. coli, Proteus mirabilis, Klebsiella,* or *Pseudomonas aeruginosa* alone or in combination is present in virtually every case. Before the advent of cross-sectional imaging, the diagnosis of XGP was rarely established preoperatively.

Xanthogranulomatous pyelonephritis probably represents an uncommon reaction by the kidney to urinary tract obstruction in the presence of urinary tract infection. The obstruction is usually secondary to a calculus (75%), but less commonly may be secondary to a congenital ureteropelvic junction obstruction or a ureteral tumor. Symptoms of XGP are generally of long duration: symptoms are present in 40% of the patients for greater than 6 months, from 1 to 6 months in another 40% of patients, and less than 1 month in only 20% of patients. Rarely, XGP may present as a fulminant illness and may be accompanied by an acute renal abscess. Total or partial nephrectomy is the usual treatment.

Two forms of XGP have been described. The most common form (85%) results in diffuse involvement of the affected kidney. Diffuse XGP may be staged as follows: stage I, involvement is limited to the kidney; stage II, involvement extends to the renal pelvis or the perirenal fat within Gerota's fascia; stage III, involvement extends beyond Gerota's fascia into the retroperitoneum, other organs, or both. A renoalimentary fistula also may rarely be present.

The localized form of XGP (15%) is much less common; in such cases, the inflammatory process is limited to a portion of the kidney. This form is sometimes referred to as the "tumefactive" form of XGP, because the findings are more easily confused with a renal tumor (Fig. 7.23). The majority of cases of both forms of XGP demonstrate extensive perinephric inflammation.

Plain abdominal radiography demonstrates the staghorn calculus, and a poorly defined mass is usually

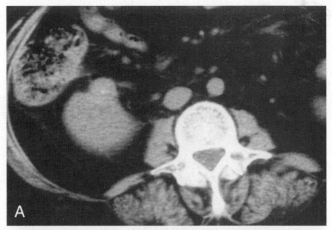

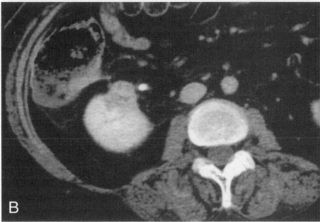

Figure 7.23. Localized xanthogranulomatous pyelonephritis. **A,** Noncontrast computed tomography shows a mass that contains punctate calcification projecting from the anterior margin of the kidney. **B,** After contrast, inhomogeneous enhancement is present. The findings cannot be distinguished from those of a localized renal cell carcinoma.

found in the perinephric space. Loss of the psoas margin may be present but, as in perinephric abscess, is not a reliable sign. Urography demonstrates absent or reduced excretion of the contrast medium in 85% of the cases (Fig. 7.24). Where excretion sufficient for visualization is present, hydronephrosis is generally evident. Retrograde pyelography may be performed to demonstrate the point of obstruction. The calyces may be grossly irregular, with evidence of superimposed papillary necrosis. Angiography, which is no longer routinely employed, shows marked splaying of the intrarenal branch vessels around avascular zones of tissue. In some cases neovascularity, reminiscent of a renal adenocarcinoma, may be found. Enlargement of the capsular branches, reflecting perinephric extension of the inflammatory process, may be present.

Sonography demonstrates diffuse renal enlargement with a central echogenic focus representing the staghorn calculus. Acoustic shadowing from the stone is, however,

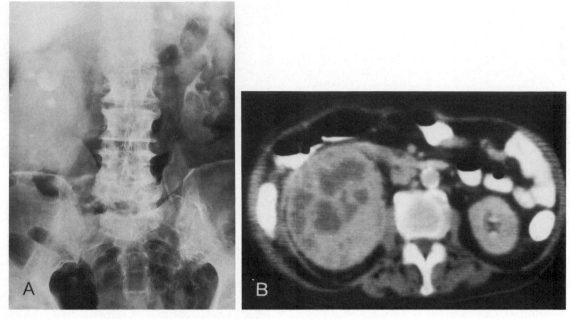

Figure 7.24. Diffuse xanthogranulomatous pyelonephritis. **A,** Excretory urogram shows a swollen, poorly functioning right kidney containing multiple calculi. **B,** Computed tomog- raphy scan demonstrates multiple low-attenuation abscesses; however, the process is confined to the renal capsule.

not always present; this has been attributed to the presence of dense peripelvic fibrosis. The renal parenchyma demonstrates a diffuse anechoic pattern that corresponds to the areas of inflammatory reaction or abscess. In some cases, however, the infected parenchyma may produce an echo pattern similar to that produced by normal renal parenchyma and is a source of potential confusion. The calyces may be seen as multiple fluid-filled masses with echo-producing debris in a picture undistinguishable from pyonephrosis.

While the CT findings in XGP are not specific for the disease, they usually strongly suggest the correct diagnosis. The kidney is diffusely enlarged, but retains its reniform shape. The renal pelvis is characteristically poorly defined or normal in size, unless there is concomitant ureteropelvic junction obstruction. One or more calculi are generally present, and there may be small flecks of parenchymal calcification as well. There are high-density areas at the periphery of the kidney representing atrophic parenchyma with inflamed columns of Bertin rimming low-attenuation central areas representing dilated calyces filled with pus and necrotic material. Subramanyam and coworkers have suggested that the pus in patients with XGP will demonstrate an attenuation that ranges from −15 to +10 HU, where the negative values reflect the lipid-laden macrophages that characterize the disease process. Other investigators have found that the attenuation of the pus in XGP is indistinguishable from that found in conventional renal or perinephric abscesses. Contrast-enhanced scans demon-

strate hyperemia at the periphery of the kidney, around the calyces, and in the renal fascia. The degree of extension to the perinephric space, the posterior pararenal space, the psoas, or the muscles of the back, is well demonstrated (Fig. 7.25). In the tumefactive form of XGP, CT may demonstrate a localized water-density mass that contains a calculus. In other cases, the findings are identical to that produced by diffuse XGP, albeit localized to one portion of the kidney.

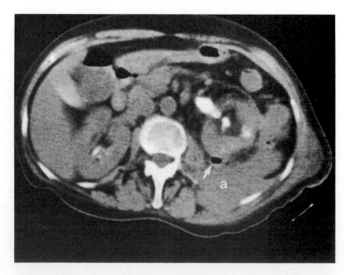

Figure 7.25. Computed tomography scan in a patient with xanthogranulomatous pyelonephritis showing extension of the inflammatory process into the perinephric space (*a*). A gas-containing intrarenal abscess also is present (*arrow*).

Malacoplakia

Malacoplakia is an uncommon form of granulomatous renal inflammatory disease characterized histologically by the presence of distinctive histiocytes (von Hansemann cells) that contain basophilic staining inclusions called Michaelis-Gutmann bodies. These inclusions are thought to represent phagocytized fragments of bacteria. It has been postulated that malacoplakia represents an enzymatic defect within the histiocytes such that intracellular digestion of the phagocytized bacteria is incomplete. Malacoplakia may occur throughout the urinary tract, as well as in a variety of other organs including the gastrointestinal tract, uterus, vagina, adrenal gland, breast, skeleton, and brain. Renal parenchymal malacoplakia (RPM) accounts for 16% of the reported cases in the urinary tract.

Renal parenchymal malacoplakia occurs in women 4 times as frequently as in men. Patients ranging in age from as young as 6 weeks to 85 years have been reported. The peak incidence occurs in patients older than 50 years of age. Fever, flank pain, and a palpable flank mass are the most common presenting complaints. Most patients have active urinary tract infection (*E. coli* in 90%). Patients often have a history of altered host resistance including autoimmune disease, alcoholism, carcinoma, or rheumatoid arthritis.

Two forms of RPM have been described. Multifocal involvement occurs in 75% of the patients and is reported to be bilateral in one half of these. The kidney is enlarged and contains multiple yellow-brown masses that range in size from a few millimeters to a few centimeters. Unifocal RPM (25% of the cases) presents as a solitary mass ranging in size from 2 to 8 cm that is sharply demarcated from the remainder of the kidney.

The radiologic findings depend on the pattern of involvement. With multifocal RPM, diffuse enlargement of the kidney is found frequently. Excretion of contrast medium is diminished in more than one half of the cases, presumably secondary to extensive renal parenchymal replacement. In some cases, the urogram may demonstrate a mass compressing the calyces. Sonography may demonstrate multiple ill-defined masses of varying echogenicity. Computed tomography demonstrates multiple soft tissue masses within the kidney that enhance less than normal renal parenchyma. Extension of the inflammatory process into the retroperitoneum also may be demonstrated (Fig. 7.26**A**). Angiography demonstrates stretching of intrarenal branch vessels with an inhomogeneous angiographic nephrogram (Fig. 7.26**B**). Neovascularity of the parenchymal masses may be present, making differentiation from renal tumors difficult. Renal vein thrombosis complicating multifocal RPM also has been described.

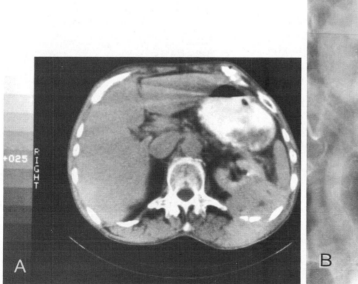
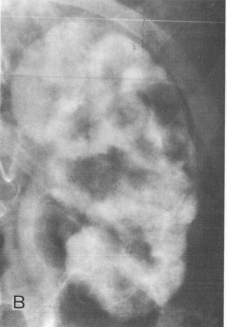

Figure 7.26. Renal parenchymal malacoplakia. **A,** Computed tomography scan shows a large, inhomogeneous, poorly marginated mass arising from the posterior aspect of the left kidney. There is extension into the perinephric space and left flank. **B,** Nephrogram phase from a selective renal angiogram shows a diffusely inhomogeneous nephrogram consistent with the multifocal form of involvement. (Courtesy of Davis S. Hartman, M.D., and the Armed Forces Institute of Pathology.)

With unifocal RPM, the dominant radiographic findings are those of a mass. On urography, the mass is indistinguishable from those produced by renal tumors or other inflammatory conditions. The ultrasonographic features are those of a complex mass.

Because the radiographic findings in malacoplakia are not specific, the diagnosis is only rarely established preoperatively. Major organ involvement is reported to have a 50% mortality. Nephrectomy is the usual treatment for unilateral disease. With bilateral disease, renal failure is common.

Chronic Pyelonephritis

The term chronic pyelonephritis is used to denote a set of morphologic changes in the adult kidney that result from a previous episode of acute renal infection. As such, the term chronic pyelonephritis is a source of confusion in that it implies an indolent or recurrent state of infection. Because this is not the case, many authorities believe that the term chronic atrophic pyelonephritis or the etiologic appellation, reflux nephropathy, is better suited to describe the morphologic changes that occur.

Much of the current understanding of the pathology of chronic pyelonephritis derives from the work of the late C. J. Hodson, who extensively investigated the relationship between renal parenchymal scarring, vesicoureteral reflux, and renal infection. Hodson proposed that the parenchymal scarring that characterizes chronic pyelonephritis is actually the result of vesicoureteral reflux and the subsequent reflux of urine back into the renal tubules, a process known as *intrarenal reflux*. He demonstrated experimentally in pigs that intrarenal reflux of infected urine produced pathologic changes in the kidney identical to those found in chronic pyelonephritis. Thus, chronic atrophic pyelonephritis may be thought of as the residua of a previous episode of acute pyelonephritis.

Ransley and Risdon, expanding on the work of Hodson, discovered that the anatomy of the papilla was the determining factor governing its propensity for intrarenal reflux. In a simple papilla, the openings of the papillary ducts are slit-like; when there is elevated pressure in the collecting system as a result of vesicoureteral reflux, these slit-like orifices close and no intrarenal reflux occurs. However, in the compound calyces found in the polar regions of the kidney, the orifices of the ducts of Bellini tend to be circular; when intrapelvic pressure increases, these circular openings allow intrarenal reflux to occur. Further observations have shown that the shape of the opening of the papillary ducts is not uniform in all compound calyces; some are more prone to reflux than others.

Intrarenal reflux of infected urine causes an acute inflammatory reaction in the renal parenchyma that overlies that papilla. This ultimately results in parenchymal scarring, which extends throughout the thickness of the renal cortex and causes retraction of the overlying calyx. Scarring associated with this intrarenal reflux has a characteristic appearance; it must extend through the entire thickness of the renal parenchyma and must be associated with deformity of the calyx adjacent to the scar. *Scarring associated with reflux nephropathy more commonly occurs in early childhood, usually before the age of 4 years*. Except in severe cases, older children and adults appear to recover from an episode of intrarenal reflux without permanent structural damage to the kidney. Thus, the radiologic picture in the adult often reflects disease in early childhood.

The question regarding whether changes of reflux nephropathy also can develop as a result of reflux of *uninfected* urine is unsettled. Although most authorities believe that urinary tract infection is an essential component of this process, experimental evidence indicates that scarring from high pressure intrarenal reflux can occur with sterile urine. Indeed, reflux of sterile urine in utero has been postulated as the etiology of the Ask-Upmark kidney, a segmental hypoplastic renal anomaly.

A small number of adults with characteristic changes of reflux nephropathy present with a clinical picture of renin-mediated hypertension. If the process is bilateral, renal failure also may occur. Thus, the importance of detecting significant vesicoureteral reflux in children with urinary tract infections is underscored.

The radiologic findings in chronic pyelonephritis on urography include the demonstration of one or more parenchymal scars typically in the upper pole of the kidney overlying a deformed calyx (Fig. 7.27). Focal areas

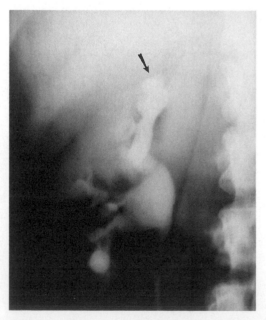

Figure 7.27.   A nephrotomogram from an excretory urogram shows parenchymal scarring (*arrow*) associated with calyceal clubbing as a result of reflux nephropathy.

of compensatory hypertrophy may be seen adjacent to the areas of cortical scarring. The intervening areas of the kidney appear normal. In less severe cases, only an area of parenchymal thickening will be present and no adjoining calyceal abnormality will be found. It is not possible, in such cases, to be certain of the etiology of the parenchymal abnormality, because other causes of parenchymal scarring (i.e., renal infarction) may produce an identical appearance. A definitive diagnosis can be established only when the characteristic radiologic picture is present.

Ultrasound changes in patients with chronic atrophic pyelonephritis include a focal loss of parenchyma, which can be appreciated on longitudinal or cross-sectional images. Increased echogenicity in the area of the scar also may be demonstrated. The central renal sinus echoes may be extended to the periphery of the kidney in the area of abnormality. In contrast to other causes of generalized increased cortical echogenicity, the process appears focal. Similarly, anatomic abnormalities also may be demonstrated on CT, but the degree to which the calyceal deformity is present may not be appreciated on this study.

RENAL TUBERCULOSIS

Renal tuberculosis results from hematogenous dissemination of *Mycobacterium tuberculosis* from a distant site, usually in the lungs or bones. Bacilli lodge in the corticomedullary junction of the kidney, where most heal without sequela. Because the initial lesions occur as a result of hematogenous dissemination, multiple bilateral lesions are initially produced; in approximately three quarters of the cases, however, active tuberculomas form in only one kidney. The lesions then progress along the nephron to rupture into the pelvocalyceal system.

While there has been a decline in the incidence of pulmonary tuberculosis in non-immunosuppressed patients, the incidence of extrapulmonary tuberculosis has remained unchanged. New cases continue to be diagnosed in the United States, particularly among the immigrant population. A history of tuberculosis in another site is present in virtually all cases; however, that site may be inactive at the time of presentation with renal involvement. Kollins and associates report that evidence of pulmonary tuberculosis is found on chest radiography in only about 50% of the patients with active urinary tract infection. Active pulmonary disease is present in coexistence with the renal lesions in approximately 10% of patients.

Within the urinary tract, the renal lesions progress in an indolent fashion, often producing little clinical symptomatology until the entire urinary tract is affected. As such, lower urinary tract symptoms including frequency, dysuria, and nocturia are the most common presenting

Table 7.1
Characteristics of Renal Tuberculosis

Parenchymal calcification
Parenchymal scars
Papillary necrosis
Infundibular strictures
Nonfunction (autonephrectomy)

complaints. About one quarter of the patients have gross hematuria. Approximately 10% of the patients will be completely asymptomatic, but will be found on examination to have the classical laboratory findings of sterile pyuria—the presence of white blood cells in the urine with subsequently sterile cultures on conventional culture media. Generalized constitutional symptoms are unusual; in one series, they were present in less than 10% of the cases.

The radiologic findings in renal tuberculosis depend on the extent of the disease process. In one third of the patients in Kollins' series, plain film examination provided evidence of extraurinary tract tuberculosis that alerted the radiologist to the presence of the disease. Such findings include evidence of skeletal tuberculosis in the hip or sacroiliac joints, or in the spine, with or without a paraspinous abscess, and calcification in abdominal or retroperitoneal lymph nodes.

Radiologic abnormalities (Table 7.1) are demonstrated in the majority of cases of renal tuberculosis. In approximately 10% of the cases in Kollins' series, however, urography was considered normal even when active infection was demonstrated with positive urinary cultures. Urographic abnormalities are described in the following paragraphs.

Papillary Abnormalities

In the earliest stages of renal tuberculosis, the tips of the papilla demonstrate a moth-eaten, irregular appearance. As the disease progresses, extensive papillary necrosis may be present with the formation of frank cavities, which may communicate with each other as a result of caseous necrosis within the renal parenchyma.

Parenchymal Calcification

Calcification occurs throughout the renal parenchyma in approximately one third to one half of the cases. Two types of calcification are described: (*a*) an amorphous granular opacity associated with granulomatous masses, and (*b*) dense, punctate calcifications that represent healed tuberculomas. In addition, approximately 20% of the patients demonstrate renal calculi.

Parenchymal Scarring

Parenchymal scarring may be present in 20% of the cases and may be localized to a single area of the kidney or may involve the entire kidney. The scars are generally associated with underlying calyceal abnormalities and parenchymal calcifications.

Calyceal Abnormalities

The hallmark of renal tuberculosis is the development of multiple irregular infundibular stenoses or strictures with subsequent hydrocalycosis (Figs. 7.28–7.30). When the strictures are complete, the entire calyx may be excluded from the remainder of the collecting system. The renal pelvis is typically small and contracted. These stenoses are the result of fibrosis that accompanies the healing process.

The degree to which these changes will be shown on urography depends on the degree to which renal function is compromised. In more than 50% of the cases, renal function is sufficiently compromised at the time of presentation, so that either antegrade or retrograde pyelography is necessary. Because a majority of cases are associated with inflammatory changes in the urinary bladder as well, retrograde catheterization of the ureteral orifices may be difficult or impossible. Advanced renal tuberculosis presents with a nonfunctioning kidney—the "autonephrectomy" (Fig. 7.31). Extensive parenchymal calcification is typically present in such cases. In other cases where poor excretion of contrast medium is demonstrated, a tuberculous pyonephrosis (Fig. 7.30) will be present as a result of obstruction from extensive ureteral stricture formation.

Because demonstration of the typical calyceal and

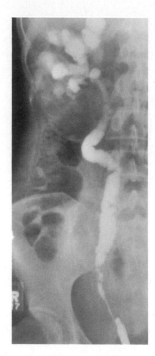

Figure 7.29. Renal tuberculosis. Retrograde pyelogram shows multiple ureteral strictures and infundibular stenoses characteristic of tuberculosis.

ureteral abnormalities is critical to establishing the diagnosis of renal tuberculosis, conventional radiologic contrast studies remain the procedures of choice. While calyceal clubbing may be demonstrated by CT, the delineation of infundibular stenoses may be difficult on cross-sectional imaging. Sonography will also rarely demonstrate specific features of renal tuberculosis. The parenchyma may demonstrate intrarenal masses of varying echogenicity that represent liquefying tuberculous cavities. A sonographic clue to the diagnosis is the demonstration of dilated calyces without commensurate dilatation of the renal pelvis.

UNCOMMON RENAL INFECTIONS

Fungal Infections

Fungal diseases of the kidney develop as opportunistic infections occurring principally in the setting of altered host resistance from such diverse entities as diabetes mellitus, the use of systemic antibiotics, immunosuppressive and chemotherapeutic agents, the use of indwelling intravenous or urinary catheters, acquired immunodeficiency, and renal transplantation. Renal involvement most commonly occurs with infections secondary to *Candida albicans* or other candida species, but has been reported in association with *Coccidiomycosis immitis, Cryptococcus neoformans, Torulopsis glabrata,* and *Aspergillus fumigatus.* Fungal infections also may complicate conventional Gram-negative urinary tract infections.

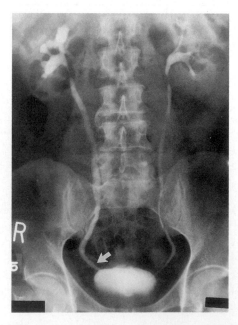

Figure 7.28. Renal tuberculosis. Excretory urography shows mild clubbing of the calyces of the right kidney with subtle strictures of the distal right ureter (*arrow*). Strictures also are present in the proximal ureters bilaterally.

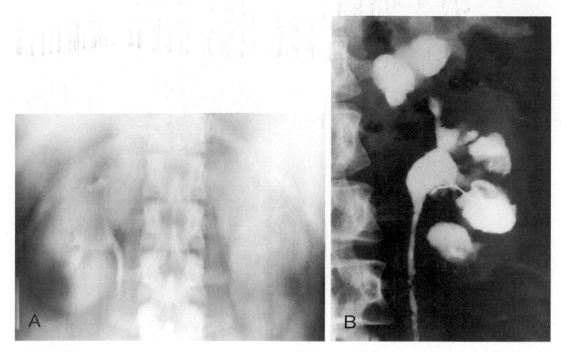

Figure 7.30. Renal tuberculosis. **A,** Excretory urography demonstrates multiple lucencies in the left kidney that represent dilated, but unopacified calyces (negative pyelogram). **B,** Antegrade pyelogram shows characteristic infundibular stenoses, calyceal dilatation, and a contracted renal pelvis. Strictures also are present in the proximal ureter.

Candidiasis

Candida is an ubiquitous organism normally found in the pharynx, the gastrointestinal tract, or vagina. Two patterns of renal involvement with *Candida* have been described. In systemic candidiasis, infection is spread to the kidneys as a result of hematogenous dissemination of the organisms with involvement of the kidneys and multiple other organs, including the brain and lungs. The patient is desperately ill with fever, leukocytosis,

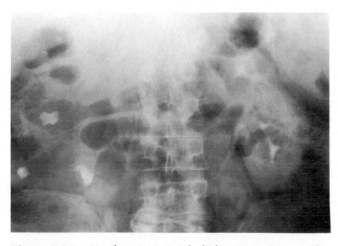

Figure 7.31. Nonfunctioning right kidney containing multiple course calcifications representing a tuberculous autonephrectomy.

splenomegaly, and azotemia. Disseminated candidiasis is invariably fatal if not treated.

Primary renal candidiasis occurs without associated hematogenous or other major organ involvement. It is a less fulminant illness than renal involvement associated with systemic candidiasis. Most of the reported patients with primary renal candidiasis have been women, and there is a strong association with diabetes mellitus. The pathogenesis of primary renal candidiasis also is thought to be a result of hematogenous dissemination of the organism, but in a mild form. Ascending spread from the lower urinary tract also has been implicated. In many of the reported cases, however, asymmetric involvement of the kidneys is present with demonstrable lesions in only one kidney. The fungi are filtered by the glomerulus and lodge in the distal tubules. Proliferation of the fungi results in multiple medullary and cortical abscesses, producing an acute fungal pyelonephritis. There is a diffuse fungal infiltration of the tips of the renal papilla, producing papillary necrosis. The fungi are then extruded into the renal collecting system with subsequent formation of fungus balls (mycetomas), which may then obstruct the renal pelvis or ureter, producing hydronephrosis or renal colic. With severe infection, renal failure may ensue. The diagnosis is established by the demonstration of the fungal hyphae on direct examination of the urine.

Radiologic findings include diminished excretion of

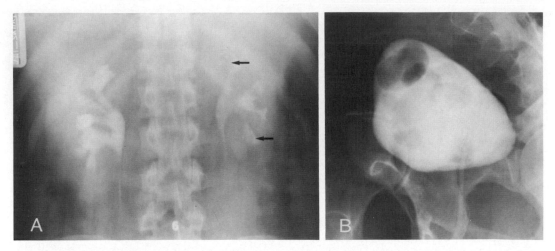

Figure 7.32.   Renal candidiasis. **A,** Excretory urography demonstrates papillary necrosis in the left kidney with multiple small filling defects (*arrows*) representing fungus balls. **B,** Cystogram in the same patient shows multiple large fungus balls.

contrast medium on urography, papillary necrosis, and hydronephrosis. The characteristic finding of candidiasis is the demonstration of multiple filling defects ranging in size from 1 to 4 cm within the collecting system representing fungus balls (Fig. 7.32). Scalloping of the ureters related to submucosal edema, analogous to the changes in the esophagus produced by oral thrush, also has been reported. With diminished renal function, antegrade or retrograde pyelography may be necessary to demonstrate changes in the renal collecting system. On ultrasound, the fungus balls may be recognized as hyperechoic masses within the collecting system with no acoustic shadowing. On CT, low-attenuation lesions represent microabscesses that are best demonstrated after contrast enhancement.

Percutaneous nephrostomy with percutaneous removal of the fungus balls has been reported as an adjunctive therapy.

Other Fungal Infections

Infection with coccidiomycosis occurs as a result of an active focus of infection elsewhere, usually in the lungs. Renal manifestations including papillary necrosis, cavitation, and parenchymal calcification have all been reported. Cryptococcus infection may produce cavitation, papillary necrosis, and multiple parenchymal abscesses.

Brucellosis

Brucellosis of the kidney occurs primarily in meat packers or from the ingestion of unpasteurized milk. The renal infection occurs as a result of hematogenous dissemination of the organism. The renal involvement is radiologically similar to that produced by tuberculosis with extensive calcification, cavitation, and infundibular strictures.

Actinomycosis

Actinomycosis of the kidney usually occurs as a result of infection of the gastrointestinal tract with spread to the kidney through a renoalimentary fistula or by fistulization through the diaphragm from the lung. The causative organism, *Actinomycosis israelii,* while producing mycelial colonies similar to fungi, is actually a bacterium usually sensitive to penicillin. Infection may result in acute pyelonephritis, pyonephrosis, or a granulomatous renal abscess.

Hydatid Disease

Renal hydatid disease is caused by infestation by a tapeworm, usually *Echinococcus granulosis.* Dogs or other canines constitute the primary host for the disease. The eggs of the worm are swallowed, hatch in the gastrointestinal tract, and then enter the portal circulation, where the oncospheres lodge in multiple organs, mainly the liver and lungs. Renal hydatid disease occurs in only approximately 2 to 3% of patients, and may be primary or secondary. In primary hydatid disease, the worms reach the kidney through the arterial circulation; in secondary renal infestation, the worms spread to the urinary tract as a result of involvement of an adjacent organ, such as the liver.

Within the kidney, the worms form a characteristic three-layered hydatid cyst that may grow rapidly and destroy the kidney or may progress very slowly, producing minimal clinical symptoms. One or more daughter cysts may form from the mother cyst. Symptoms of renal involvement are nonspecific, but include flank pain, renal colic, and eosinophilia. At the time of presentation, the average hydatid cyst is approximately 8 cm in diameter.

Radiologic manifestations include a well-defined soft tissue mass in the renal fossa on plain films. Curvilinear calcification is present in the wall of the cyst in approximately one third of the cases. On urography, distortion of the renal pelvis or calyces may be evident (the "crescent sign"). Communication between the cyst and the collecting system results in a characteristic appearance, especially when filling of the daughter cysts (the "bunch of grapes" sign) is present. Extensive renal destruction may result in a nonfunctioning kidney.

On sonography, hydatid cysts appear as round, homogeneous, echo-free masses. The presence of daughter cysts may be readily identified. Dependent echoes within the cyst secondary to hydatid sand (hooks, scoleices, and brood capsules of the worms) may be present. When the patient is moved or changes position, movement of these echoes produces the "falling snowflake" sign, said to be pathognomonic of the disease.

The advisability of diagnostic cyst puncture in hydatid disease has been debated for many years. While such a procedure is diagnostic, concern that the puncture will cause spread of the disease to uninfected areas has been raised. In addition, venous intravasation of the cystic fluid has been reported to cause acute anaphylaxis.

RENAL MANIFESTATIONS OF AIDS

A wide variety of abnormalities (Table 7.2) may be found in the kidneys of patients with acquired immune deficiency syndrome (AIDS). Nonspecific imaging findings including nephromegaly, increased or decreased echogenicity, parenchymal calcification, hydronephrosis, infarction, and acute pyelonephritis have been reported.

Table 7.2.
Renal Manifestations of AIDS

Immunologic
   Hemolytic-uremic syndrome
   HIV nephropathy/nephrotic syndrome
   Vasculitis
Infections
   Candidiasis
   Cryptococcosis
   Cytomegalovirus
   Mucorrmycosis
   Pyogenic infection
   Pneumocystis carinii infection
   Tuberculosis
Miscellaneous
   Interstitial nephritis/drug toxicity
   Amyloidosis
Neoplasms
   Kaposi sarcoma
   Lymphoma
   Renal adenocarcinoma
Vascular
   Cortical necrosis
   Renal infarction

Studies have suggested that patients with AIDS as a result of intravenous drug abuse are more likely to have renal abnormalities than patients with sexually transmitted forms of AIDS. Human immunodeficiency virus (HIV) nephropathy, the most common form of renal dysfunction associated with AIDS, is discussed in Chapter 10.

Opportunistic Infections

HIV infection results in an increased susceptibility to both opportunistic and pyogenic renal infections as a result of depletion of T-helper lymphocytes. Among the opportunistic infections, *Pneumocystis carinii,* although usually thought of primarily as a pulmonary disease, is becoming more common in extrapulmonary sites because of the widespread use of pentamidine inhalers for prophylaxis. The disease may spread by hematogenous and lymphogenous dissemination to a variety of organs, including the kidneys. Punctate renal calcifications (Fig. 7.33) are characteristic of renal involvement, but have

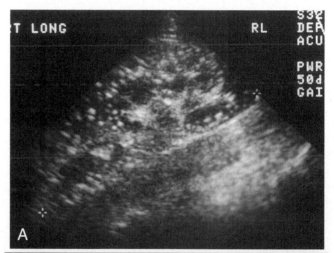

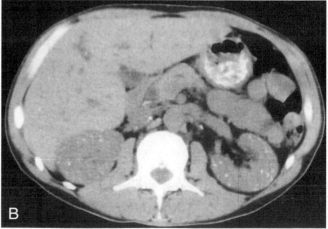

Figure 7.33. *Pneumocystitis carinii* infection. **A,** Longitudinal ultrasound of the right kidney shows multiple focal areas of increased echogenicity. **B,** The presence of punctate bilateral renal calcification is confirmed by computed tomography. (Courtesy of Alec J. Megibow, M.D.)

been reported in *Mycobacterium avium-intracellulare* (MAI) and cytomegalovirus infection as well. The calcification, unlike tuberculosis or candidiasis, may be present in both active and inactive disease. MAI infection is reported in approximately 5.5% of patients with AIDS. The symptoms of MAI are nonspecific and include fever, generalized lymphadenopathy, and anorexia. Focal echogenic lesions in the kidneys on sonography, as well as the development of frank renal abscesses, are reported. Disseminated candidiasis may result in acute pyelonephritis, parenchymal microabscesses, and the development of fungus balls. Other opportunistic infections in patients with AIDS include tuberculosis, mucorrmycosis, and cryptococcosis.

Renal Neoplasms

Renal lymphomas associated with HIV infection are usually of the highly aggressive non-Hodgkin's type and have a poor prognosis. The most common manifestation is bilateral discrete parenchymal masses, ranging in size from 1 to 3 cm. Generalized adenopathy with or without ureteral obstruction is generally present. In a review of 110 patients with untreated AIDS-related lymphoma, Radin and associates found renal involvement in 11% of the patients. Renal involvement with Kaposi sarcoma, although the most common neoplasm associated with HIV infection, is generally microscopic, and therefore, is seldom demonstrated on imaging studies. Bulky retroperitoneal lymphadenopathy and/or diffuse tumor infiltration in the retroperitoneum may, however, be associated with ureteral obstruction.

SUGGESTED READING

General References/Pathophysiology

Benson M, Li Puma JP, Resnick MI: The role of imaging studies in urinary tract infection. *Urol Clin North Am* 13(4):605, 1986.

Corriere JN Jr, Sandler CM: The diagnosis and immediate therapy of acute renal and perirenal infections. *Urol Clin North Am* 9(2):219, 1982.

Ditchfield MR, deCampo JF, Nolan TM, et al.: Risk factors in the development of early renal cortical defects in children with urinary tract infection. *AJR* 162:1394, 1994.

Gold RP, McClennan BL, Rottenberg RR: CT appearance of acute inflammatory disease of the renal interstitium. *AJR* 141:343, 1983.

Hoddick W, Jeffrey RB, Goldberg HI, et al.: CT and sonography of severe renal and perirenal infections. *AJR* 140:517, 1983.

Majd M, Rushton GH, Jantausch B, Weidermann BL: Relationship among vesicoureteral reflux. P-fimbriated Escherichia coli, and acute pyelonephritis in children with febrile urinary tract infection. *J Pediatr* 119(4):578, 1991.

Morehouse HT, Weiner SN, Hoffman JC: Imaging in inflammatory disease of the kidney. *AJR* 143:135, 1984.

Parsons CL: Pathogenesis of urinary tract infections. Bacterial adherence, bladder defense mechanisms. *Urol Clin North Am* 13(4):563, 1986.

Rauschkolb EN, Sandler CM, Patel S, et al.: Computed tomography of renal inflammatory disease. *J Comput Assist Tomogr* 6(3):502, 1982.

Roberts JA: Pyelonephritis, cortical abscess, and perinephric abscess. *Urol Clin North Am* 13(4):637, 1986.

Soulen MC, Fishman EK, Goldman SM, Gatewood OMB: Bacterial renal infection: role of CT. *Radiology* 171:703, 1989.

Talner LB, Davidson AJ, Lebowitz RL, Dalla Palma L, Goldman SM: Acute pyelonephritis: can we agree on terminology? *Radiology* 192:297–305, 1994.

Wan YL, Le TY, Bullard MJ, et al: Acute gas-producing bacterial renal infection: correlation between imaging findings and clinical outcome. *Radiology* 198:433, 1996.

Wicks JD, Thornbury JR: Acute renal infections in adults. *Radiol Clin North Am* 115(2):245, 1979.

Acute Pyelonephritis

Davidson AJ, Talner LB: Late sequelae of adult-onset acute bacterial nephritis. *Radiology* 127:367, 1978.

Dinkle E, Orth S, Dittrich M, et al.: Renal sonography in the differentiation of upper from lower urinary tract infection. *AJR* 146:775, 1986.

Ditchfield MR, De Campo JF, Cook DK, et al.: Vesicoureteral reflux: an accurate predictor of acute pyelonephritis in childhood urinary tract infection? *Radiology* 190(2):413, 1994.

Edell SL, Bonavita JA: The sonographic appearance of acute pyelonephritis. *Radiology* 132:683, 1979.

Goldman SM, Fishman EK: Upper urinary tract infection: the current role of CT, ultrasound and MRI. *Semin Ultrasound CT MR* 12(4):335, 1991.

Harrison RB, Shaffer HA: The roentgenographic findings in acute pyelonephritis. *JAMA* 241(16):1718, 1979.

Ishikawa I, Saito Y, Onouchi Z, et al.: Delayed contrast enhancement in acute focal bacterial nephritis: CT features. *J Comput Assist Tomogr* 9(5):894, 1985.

June CH, Browning MD, Smith LP, et al.: Ultrasonography and computed tomography in severe urinary tract infection. *Arch Intern Med* 145:841, 1985.

Kanel KT, Kroboth FJ, Schwentker FN, Lecky JW: Intravenous pyelogram in acute pyelonephritis. *Arch Intern Med* 148(10): 2144, 1988.

Kass EJ, Fink-Bennett D, Cacciarelli AA, Balon H. Pavlock S: The sensitivity of renal scintigraphy and sonography in detecting nonobstructive acute pyelonephritis. *J Urol* 148:606, 1993.

Lillienfeld RM, Lande A: Acute adult onset bacterial nephritis: long term urographic and angiographic follow-up. *J Urol* 114:14, 1975.

Majd M, Rushton HG: Renal cortical scintigraphy in the diagnosis of acute pyelonephritis. *Semin Nucl Med* 22(2):98, 1992.

McDonough WD, Sandler CM, Benson GS: Acute focal bacterial nephritis: focal pyelonephritis that may simulate renal abscess. *J Urol* 126:670, 1981.

Rosenfield AT, Glickman MG, Taylor KJW, et al.: Acute focal bacterial nephritis (acute lobar nephronia). *Radiology* 132:553, 1979.

Senn E, Zaunbauer W, Bandhauer K, et al.: Computed tomography in acute pyelonephritis. *Br J Urol* 59:118, 1987.

Silver TM, Kass EJ, Thornbury JR, et al.: The radiological spectrum of acute pyelonephritis in adults and adolescents. *Radiology* 118:65, 1976.

Tsugaya M, Hirao N, Sakagami H, et al.: Renal cortical scarring in acute pyelonephritis. *Br J Urol* 69(3):245, 1992.

Zaontz MR, Pahira JJ, Wolfman M, et al.: Acute focal bacterial nephritis: a systematic approach to diagnosis and treatment. *J Urol* 133:752, 1985.

Renal and Perirenal Abscesses

Gerzof SH, Gale ME: Computed tomography and ultrasonography for diagnosis and treatment of renal and retroperitoneal abscesses. *Urol Clin North Am* 9:185, 1982.

Morgan WR, Nyberg LM Jr: Perinephric and intrarenal abscesses. *Urology* 26(6):529, 1985.

Percutaneous Drainage of Renal and Perinephric Abscesses

Bernardino ME, Baumgartner BR: Percutaneous abscess drainage in the genitourinary tract. *Radiol Clin North Am* 24:539, 1986.

Gobien RP, Stanley JH, Schabel SI, et al.: The effect of drainage tube size on adequacy of percutaneous abscess drainage. *Cardiovasc Intervent Radiol* 8:100, 1985.

Lowe LH, Zagoria RJ, Baumgartner BR, Dyer RB: Role of imaging and intervention in complex infections of the urinary tract. *AJR* 163:363, 1994.

Sacks D, Banner MP, Meranze SG, et al.: Renal and related retroperitoneal abscesses: percutaneous drainage. *Radiology* 167:447, 1988.

Pyonephrosis

Jeffrey RB, Laing FC, Wing VW, et al.: Sensitivity of sonography in pyonephrosis: a reevaluation. *AJR* 144:71, 1985.

Subramanyam BR, Raghavendra BN, Bosniak MA, et al.: Sonography of pyonephrosis: a prospective study. *AJR* 140:991, 1983.

Yoder IC, Pfister RC, Lindfors KK, et al.: Pyonephrosis: imaging and intervention. *AJR* 141:735, 1983.

Gas-forming Renal Infections

Evanoff GV, Thompson CS, Foley R, et al.: Spectrum of gas within the kidney. Emphysematous pyelonephritis and emphysematous pyelitis. *Am J Med* 83:149, 1987.

Gervais DA, Whitman GJ: Emphysematous pyelonephritis. *AJR* 162(2):348, 1994.

Lautin EM, Gordon PM, Friedman AC, et al.: Emphysematous pyelonephritis: optimal diagnosis and treatment. *Urol Radiol* 1:93, 1979.

Wan YL, Lee TY, Tsai CC, et al.: Acute gas-producing bacterial renal infections: correlation between imaging findings and clinical outcome. *Radiology* 198:433–438, 1996.

Zweig GJ, Li YP, Srinantaswarny S, Chandramouli S, et al.: Gas-forming infections of the abdomen: plain film findings. *Appl Radiol* 19:37, 1990.

Xanthogranulomatous Pyelonephritis

Eastham J, Ahlering T, Skinner E: Xanthogranulomatous pyelonephritis: clinical findings and surgical considerations. *Urology* 43(3):295, 1994.

Goldman SM, Hartman DS, Fishman EK, et al.: CT of xanthogranulomatous pyelonephritis: radiologic-pathologic correlation. *AJR* 141:963, 1984.

Hayes WS, Hartman DS, Sesterbenn IA: From the Archives of the AFIP: xanthogranulomatous pyelonephritis. *RadioGraphics* 11(3): 485, 1991.

Parker MD, Clark RL: Evolving concepts in the diagnosis of xanthogranulomatous pyelonephritis. *Urol Radiol* 11:7, 1989.

Sandler CM, Foucar E, Toombs BD: Xanthogranulomatous pyelonephritis with air containing intrarenal abscesses. *Urol Radiol* 2:113, 1980.

Subramanyam BR, Megibow AJ, Raghavendra BN, et al.: Diffuse xanthogranulomatous pyelonephritis: analysis by computed tomography and sonography. *Urol Radiol* 4:5, 1982.

Van Kirk OC, Go RT, Wedel VJ: Sonographic features of xanthogranulomatous pyelonephritis. *AJR* 134:1035, 1980.

Zafaranloo S, Gerard PS, Bryk D: Xanthogranulomatous pyelonephritis in children: analysis by diagnostic modalities. *Urol Radiol* 12:18, 1990.

Malacoplakia

Arap S, Denes FT, Silva J, et al.: Malcoplakia of the urinary tract. *Eur Urol* 12:113, 1986.

Hartman DS, Davis DJ Jr, Lichtenstein JE, et al.: Renal parenchymal malacoplakia. *Radiology* 136:33, 1980.

Long JP Jr, Althausen AF: Malacoplakia: A 25-year experience with a review of the literature. *J Urol* 141:1328, 1989.

Miller OS, Finck FM: Malacoplakia of the kidney: the great impersonator. *J Urol* 103:712, 1970.

Chronic Pyelonephritis

Hodson CJ: Reflux nephropathy: a personal historical review. *AJR* 137:451, 1981.

Kay CJ, Rosenfield AT, Taylor KJW, et al.: Ultrasonic characteristics of chronic atrophic pyelonephritis. *AJR* 132:47, 1979.

Ransley PG, Risdon RA: Reflux and renal scarring. *Br J Radiol* (14 suppl):1, 1978.

Renal Tuberculosis

Cohen MC: Granulomatous nephritis. *Urol Clin North Am* 13(4): 647, 1986.

Kollins SA, Hartman GW, Carr DT, et al.: Roentgenographic findings in urinary tract tuberculosis: a 10 year review. *AJR* 121(3):487, 1974.

Roylance J, Penry JB, Davies ER, et al.: The radiology of tuberculosis of the urinary tract. *Clin Radiol* 21:163, 1970.

Fungal Infections

Clark RE, Minagi H, Palubinskas AJ: Renal candidiasis. *Radiology* 101:567, 1971.

Dembner AG, Pfister RC: Fungal infection of the urinary tract: demonstration by antegrade pyelography and drainage by percutaneous nephrostomy. *AJR* 129:415, 1977.

Fisher J, Mayhall G, Duma R, et al.: Fungus balls of the urinary tract. *South Med J* 72(10):1281, 1979.

Gerle RD: Roentgenographic features of primary renal candidiasis. *AJR* 119:731, 1973.

Irby PB, Stoller ML, McAninch JW: Fungal bezoars of the upper urinary tract. *J Urol* 143:447, 1990.

Michigan S: Genitourinary fungal infections. *J Urol* 116:390, 1976.

Shirkhoda A: CT findings in hepatosplenic and renal candidiasis. *J Comput Assist Tomogr* 11(5):795, 1987.

Stuck KJ, Silver TM, Jaffe MH, et al.: Sonographic demonstration of renal fungus balls. *Radiology* 142:473, 1981.

Zirinsky K, Auh YH, Hartman BJ, et al.: Computed tomography of renal aspergillosis. *J Comput Assist Tomogr* 11:177, 1987.

Hydatid Disease

Aragona F, DiCandio G, Serretta V, et al.: Renal hydatid disease: report of 9 cases and discussion of urologic diagnostic procedures. *Urol Radiol* 6:182, 1984.

Saint Martin G, Chiesa JC: "Falling snowflakes", an ultrasound sign of hydatid sand. *J Ultrasound Med* 3:257 1984.

Renal Manifestations of AIDS

Glassock RJ, Cohen AH, Danovitch G, Parsa P: Human immunodeficiency virus (HIV) infection and the kidney. *Ann Intern Med* 112:35, 1990.

Kay CJ: Renal diseases in patients with AIDS: sonographic findings. *AJR* 159:551, 1992.

Kuhlman JE, Browne D, Shermak M, et al.: Retroperitoneal and pelvic CT of patients with AIDS: primary and secondary involvement of the genitourinary tract. *RadioGraphics* 11(3):473, 1993.

Miles BJ, Nelser M, Farah R, Markowitz N, Fisher E: The urological manifestations of the acquired immunodeficiency syndrome. *J Urol* 142(3):771, 1989.

Miller FH, Parikh S, Gore RM, et al.: Renal manifestations of AIDS. *RadioGraphics* 13:587, 1993.

Radin DR, Esplin JA, Levine AM, Ralls PW: AIDS-related non-Hodgkin's lymphoma: abdominal CT findings in 112 patients. *AJR* 160(5):1133, 1993.

Wachsberg RH, Obolevich AT, Lasker N: Pelvocalyceal thickening in HIV-associated nephropathy. *Abdom Imaging* 20:371, 1995.

8

Vascular Diseases

ANATOMY

Arterial

The renal arteries branch from the aorta near the level of the L1–L2 interspace. The right renal artery usually arises from the lateral or anterolateral aspect of the aorta and slightly lower than the left renal artery, which arises from the lateral or posterolateral aspect of the aorta. Thus, aortography should be performed in the anteroposterior or slight right posterior oblique projections to demonstrate the origin of the renal arteries to best advantage.

In as many as 40% of patients, one or both kidneys are supplied by more than one renal artery. Accessory renal arteries arise from the aorta and are usually inferior to the main renal artery (Fig. 8.1). Occasionally an accessory renal artery supplies the upper pole of the kidney, and rarely an accessory renal artery may arise from the celiac, hepatic, or mesenteric arteries. Anomalous kidneys, such as a horseshoe or pelvic kidney, almost always have multiple renal arteries that arise from the aorta or iliac arteries near the kidneys.

The inferior adrenal artery and arteries supplying the renal capsule, renal pelvis, and ureter arise from the main renal artery. Occasionally, the gonadal, middle adrenal, or inferior phrenic arteries also may arise from the renal artery.

The main renal artery divides into dorsal and ventral rami that run posterior and anterior to the renal pelvis. The larger ventral division supplies the anterior and superior aspects of the kidney, whereas the dorsal division supplies the posterior and inferior portions of the kidney. The junction of these ventral and dorsal divisions creates a relatively avascular plane (Brodel's line), which is the preferred track for placing percutaneous nephrostomies.

Segmental branches arise from the dorsal and ventral rami and run along the infundibulae before dividing into interlobar arteries. These interlobar arteries course between the pyramids and the cortical columns parallel to the outer surface of the kidneys before branching into arcuate arteries, which run along the bases of the medullary pyramids.

Collateral pathways that provide arterial supply to the kidney when the main renal artery is compromised include the inferior adrenal, capsular, ureteric, gonadal, intercostal, lumbar, and pelvic arteries. The upper three lumbar arteries allow blood from the aorta to communicate with pelvic, ureteral, or capsular arteries, which anastomose with renal branch arteries. When the ureteral artery serves as a major collateral, the dilation and tortuosity resulting from increased blood flow may cause the artery to impinge on the ureter, causing notching (Fig. 8.2).

Although the intrarenal arteries have been considered end arteries, some intrarenal collateral pathways exist. Trueta described small coiled arteries that lie near the calyces. They arise from the interlobar arteries and communicate with vessels in the pelvic mucosa, as well as with adjacent interlobar arteries. Perforating arteries also provide communication between renal arcuate or interlobular arteries and capsular vessels. These intrarenal collateral arteries are not sufficient to prevent renal infarction, but may minimize the effects of ischemia by helping to preserve renal parenchyma.

Venous

In general, the venous anatomy parallels the arterial circulation. Accessory renal veins are less frequent than

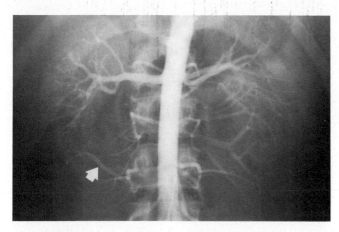

Figure 8.1.   Accessory renal artery. An abdominal aortogram demonstrates an accessory renal artery (*arrow*) supplying the lower pole of the right kidney.

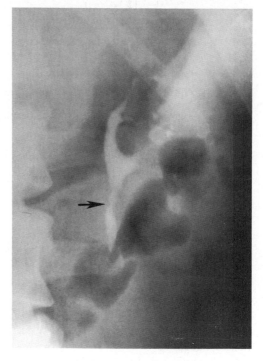

Figure 8.2.   Ureteral notching. Collateral arteries create extrinsic compression (*arrow*) on the proximal ureter in this patient with renal artery stenosis.

accessory arteries and occur more commonly on the right. However, the left renal vein may bifurcate to encircle the aorta and become a circumaortic renal vein. This anomaly is caused by the persistence of the posteriorly located left supracardinal vein and a midline supracardinal anastomosis between right and left vessels. It is a relatively common anomaly, reported in 2 to 16% of patients, according to anatomic and angiographic studies. Using computed tomography (CT), Reed and colleagues found a circumaortic left renal vein in 19 (4.4%) of 433 patients (Fig. 8.3). The posterior portion of this venous collar typically runs inferiorly before crossing behind the aorta to reach the inferior vena cava (IVC).

Patients with a circumaortic left renal vein are asymptomatic, although one case with hematuria and proteinuria has been reported. Knowledge of this anomaly is important when surgery is contemplated or during collection of renal or adrenal vein samples. The ventral vein usually drains the ventral and inferior portions of the kidney, whereas the dorsal component drains the dorsal and superior segments.

A circumaortic left renal vein also can be seen during angiography. Late films from a selective left renal arteriogram may demonstrate ventral and dorsal components. During venography, care must be taken not to overlook the more inferior entrance of the dorsal vein into the IVC. Both left renal veins also may be seen during inferior vena cavography.

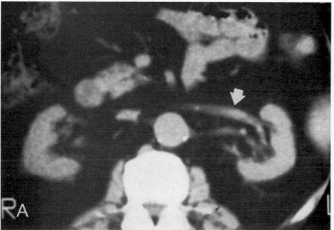

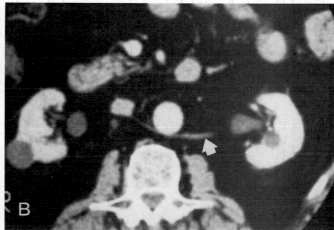

Figure 8.3.   Circumaortic left renal vein. **A,** The anterior portion (*arrow*) of a circumaortic left renal vein is in its normal location. **B,** The posterior portion (*arrow*) runs behind the aorta.

Another common anomaly, the retroaortic left renal vein, is seen less frequently. In the same series of CT examinations reported by Reed and colleagues, 8 of 433 (1.8%) patients had a single retroaortic renal vein (Fig. 8.4). Both of these anomalies can be recognized by CT, and venography is seldom necessary for confirmation. Patients are asymptomatic, but recognition is important if surgery involving this region is planned.

The left renal vein receives the inferior phrenic, capsular, ureteric, adrenal, and gonadal veins. In addition, rich collateral vessels usually anastomose with branches of the hemiazygos and ascending lumbar veins. These vessels are particularly important, because they may preserve the kidney should venous thrombosis occur. In patients with a left-sided IVC, the left common iliac vein continues cephalad as the left IVC and drains into the inferior aspect of the left renal vein.

The right renal vein is shorter than the left, and has a more oblique course to the IVC. It receives capsular and ureteric veins as well as some retroperitoneal collaterals, but the right inferior phrenic and gonadal veins enter directly into the IVC.

Valves may occur in the renal veins. There is a marked variation in the reported incidence of renal vein valves in anatomic studies, ranging from 28 to 70% on the right and from 4 to 36% on the left. Not surprisingly, valves are demonstrated less frequently on venography. Their significance lies in surgical planning, but they also can cause difficulty to the angiographer by inhibiting reflux of contrast medium or passage of a catheter during venography or venous sampling (Fig. 8.5).

Renal vein varices may be idiopathic or may result from renal vein thrombosis or portal hypertension. Varices are believed to cause hematuria in some patients, although this causal relationship is difficult to prove.

Renal vein varices, like varicoceles, are more common on the left than on the right. Thus, an anatomic eti-

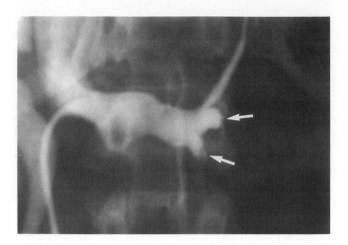

Figure 8.5.   Renal vein valves. Contrast is prevented from reaching the intrarenal veins by valves (*arrow*).

ology is postulated. Compression of the left renal vein between the superior mesenteric artery and the aorta ("nut-cracker" phenomenon) may result in left renal vein hypertension, hematuria, and varix formation. Abnormal branching of the superior mesenteric artery from the aorta has been demonstrated by magnetic resonance (MR) in some patients.

Collateral pathways exist for venous drainage of blood from the kidney in case of occlusion of the main renal vein. Inferior phrenic or adrenal, gonadal, and ureteric veins commonly enter the left renal vein, whereas only the ureteric vein enters the right renal vein. Any of these vessels, as well as a variety of small retroperitoneal veins that enter the renal veins, may function as collateral vessels. The right adrenal, inferior phrenic, and gonadal veins enter directly into the IVC.

In renal vein thrombosis, the clot usually propagates along the entire renal vein and these collateral vessels also are occluded. A local occlusion, such as surgical ligation, however, may allow these collaterals to take over drainage of the kidney. This occurs much more readily with occlusion of the left renal vein, because it receives more potential collateral vessels than the right renal vein.

Circumcaval (Retrocaval) Ureter

Venous anomalies may affect the ureter. Persistence of the right subcardinal vein traps the ureter behind the IVC. The ureter crosses posterior to the IVC and then passes around the medial border anteriorly to partially encircle the cava. This anomaly, which occurs in approximately 1 in 1100 patients, has been termed a retrocaval or circumcaval ureter. The term circumcaval ureter is preferred, because it is possible for the ureter to lie behind the vena cava without encircling it. A circumcaval ureter is more common in men than women.

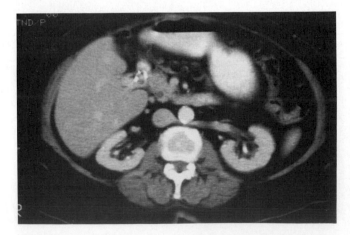

Figure 8.4.   Retroaortic left renal vein. The left renal vein passes behind the aorta to enter the inferior vena cava.

A circumcaval ureter is usually an incidental finding. Most patients are asymptomatic, although right flank pain may be sufficient to bring this anomaly to attention.

The most common complication is obstruction, caused by constriction of the retrocaval segment of the ureter by the IVC. In a few cases, fibrous bands or adhesions of this segment of the ureter have been reported. The hydronephrosis and stasis predispose to stone formation and infection.

Two radiographic patterns of circumcaval ureter have been recognized by Bateson and Atkinson. The more common form has an S-shaped deformity of the midureter as it courses around the IVC. The narrowing of the ureter occurs at the lateral border of the psoas muscle, suggesting that the obstruction is not caused by compression by the IVC. The second type has less severe hydronephrosis, but the point of obstruction is at the lateral wall of the IVC. However, ureteral obstruction is not necessarily present in a circumcaval ureter.

When the classic (type I) appearance is seen in urography, the diagnosis of circumcaval ureter can be suggested (Fig. 8.6). However, an inferior vena cavogram or CT is needed for confirmation. In the less severe form (type II), medial deviation must be distinguished from other etiologies, such as retroperitoneal fibrosis or a retroperitoneal mass.

Circumcaval ureter can be recognized on CT by following the opacified ureter around the IVC. Computed tomography also demonstrates the more lateral location

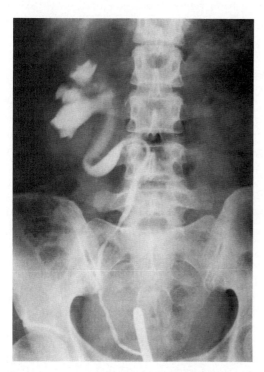

Figure 8.6. Circumcaval ureter. Failure of regression of the postcardinal vein traps the ureter behind the inferior vena cava.

of the cava which usually lies lateral to the right pedicle of the third lumbar vertebral body.

Lymphatic

There is an extensive lymphatic system within the kidney that provides an accessory drainage route for excess fluid. In normal states, approximately one fourth of lymphatic flow from the kidney occurs through small lymphatic vessels that permeate the capsule and communicate with lymph vessels in the perinephric space. The remainder of the renal lymph fluid is drained into large lymph vessels in the renal hilum. The renal lymphatics are not directly imaged, but enlarged vessels may be detected by CT.

DISEASES OF INTRARENAL ARTERIES

A variety of entities affect intrarenal arteries. Although the etiology and clinical course may be different, the radiographic manifestations are similar. Because the disease process is usually generalized, both kidneys are affected and are reduced in size. Small infarcts result in a slightly irregular contour. Renal function may be markedly impaired, but if imaged by urography or retrograde pyelography, the renal collecting system will be normal. The most characteristic findings of diseases affecting intrarenal arteries are the multiple microaneurysms seen with renal arteriography.

Collagen Vascular Diseases

The vasculitides affect the glomeruli and other renal vessels. They may be classified as primarily involving medium and large renal arteries or small vessels and capillaries. Although any of the systemic vasculitides may involve the kidneys, this discussion will concentrate on those that do so commonly.

Polyarteritis Nodosa

Renal involvement occurs in 90% of patients with polyarteritis nodosa (PAN). Patients with PAN often present clinically with hematuria; other abnormalities such as proteinuria are detected on urinalysis. Renal ischemia occurs as a result of involvement of medium vessels, and renin-mediated hypertension is common. The small aneurysms seen in PAN may occasionally rupture and produce an intraparenchymal or perinephric hematoma.

With the exception of arteriography, radiographic imaging studies demonstrate nonspecific findings. Parenchymal scarring may be seen with urography, ultrasound, or CT. Areas of hemorrhage due to aneurysm rupture are best defined by CT (Fig. 8.7), but, if large, also can be detected by urography or ultrasonography. The most definitive radiographic examination is arteriography, where small aneurysms occur at the bifurcation of interlobular or arcuate arteries (Fig. 8.7). These aneurysms are not

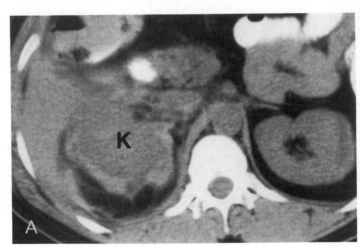

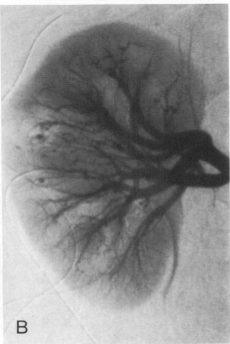

Figure 8.7. Polyarteritis nodosa. **A,** A computed tomography scan demonstrates high-density fluid surrounding the right kidney (*K*), indicating an acute perinephric and subcapsular hematoma. **B,** An arteriogram reveals multiple small aneurysms of the small intrarenal arteries.

limited to the kidneys, because arteries in the liver, spleen, pancreas, muscle, and gastrointestinal tract often are involved.

Although these small aneurysms are typical of PAN, they are not pathognomonic. Similar aneurysms may be seen in patients with systemic lupus erythematosus, Wegener's granulomatosis, intravenous drug abuse, and renal metastases.

Wegener's Granulomatosis

Patients with Wegener's granulomatosis have necrotizing granulomas of the respiratory tract, a focal necrotizing angiitis involving small arteries and veins, and a focal necrotizing glomerulitis that leads to fibrin thrombi and local necrosis of individual glomerular tufts. It occurs most commonly in the fourth and fifth decades and has a slight male preponderance.

Symptoms of upper airway involvement, including sinusitis, otitis media, pharyngitis, and epistaxis, dominate the clinical presentation. Although nodular, infiltrative, or cavitary lung lesions are commonly seen, the pulmonary involvement is generally asymptomatic.

Renal disease may be absent in the limited form of Wegener's granulomatosis, but a rapidly progressive glomerulonephritis is life-threatening in the full syndrome. The most common manifestations of renal disease are hematuria and proteinuria. Hypertension is uncommon.

The radiographic manifestations in the kidneys are nonspecific and reflect the degree of renal failure. Microaneurysms, parenchymal scarring, and areas of hemorrhage may be seen. The findings are indistinguishable from those of PAN.

Systemic Lupus Erythematosus

Most patients with systemic lupus erythematosus have renal involvement, and many die of renal failure. The larger renal vessels are usually unaffected, but interlobular arteries may be affected by inflammatory changes and may be narrowed. The predominant renal changes consist of a focal glomerulonephritis with thickening of the basement membrane resulting in the "wire loop" appearance on histologic preparations.

The radiographic appearance depends on the stage of involvement. Before the onset of renal failure, the kidneys appear normal. Microaneurysms, similar to those seen in PAN, may occasionally be seen on angiography. Although renal infarcts are common (Fig. 8.8), they are usually too small to be seen without selective magnification arteriography.

Intravenous Drug Abuse

The vasculitis associated with intravenous drug abuse has clinical and pathologic features similar to polyarteritis nodosa. Although methamphetamine is a common drug used by patients in whom a vasculitis develops,

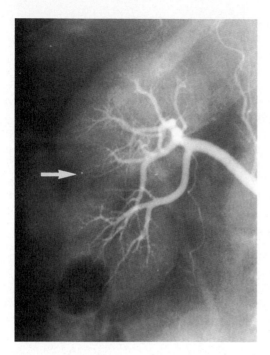

Figure 8.8. Systemic lupus erythematosus. A renal infarct can be appreciated by the cortical scar (*arrow*).

they are usually exposed to multiple drugs. Circulating hepatitis antigen-antibody complexes or drug contaminants also may be responsible for vascular injury. The radiographic appearance of multiple aneurysms 1 to 5 mm in diameter occurring at bifurcations, vascular stenoses, and complete vascular occlusion with infarction is indistinguishable from other vasculitides.

Scleroderma

Progressive systemic sclerosis is a generalized disorder manifested by vascular and connective tissue fibrosis. Narrowing of the interlobular arteries due to intimal thickening may be present, as may fibrinoid necrosis of the afferent arterioles.

Scleroderma occurs most commonly in the fourth and fifth decades, and shows a significant female preponderance. The incidence of renal involvement is variously reported, but the kidneys may be affected in up to 80% of patients. Renal failure often is the cause of death.

The radiographic manifestations are nonspecific. Before the onset of renal failure, the kidneys may appear normal. Hypertension is common, such that the vascular changes seen on angiography may be due to either nephrosclerosis or scleroderma. However, the microaneurysms seen with the vasculitides are not seen with scleroderma.

Radiation Nephritis

Radiation nephritis may be acute or chronic, may cause hypertension, or may result merely in proteinuria. It is a degenerative process that affects the tubules and glomeruli. The vascular changes that consist of fibrinoid necrosis occur late in the course and involve primarily arcuate and interlobar arteries. As little as 1000 rads may induce radiation nephritis, and microscopic changes can be seen with lower doses. Typically, however, doses of at least 2000 to 2500 rads within a 5-week period are needed to cause significant renal damage.

Acute radiation nephritis is manifested by proteinuria and hypertension after a latent period of 6 to 13 months. Uremia, malignant hypertension, and congestive heart failure follow. The prognosis of these patients is poor, with a mortality of approximately 50%.

Patients who develop chronic radiation nephritis may or may not have been affected by acute radiation nephritis. Chronic radiation nephritis has an insidious onset of mild proteinuria, anemia, and azotemia, beginning 18 months to several years after radiation exposure. Although the clinical course is more protracted, the mortality of 50% is similar to acute radiation nephritis.

The radiographic appearance of radiation nephritis depends on the radiation dose and the time between the radiation exposure and the imaging study. In the acute phase, diminished renal function may be manifested only by decreased concentration of excreted contrast medium. In the chronic phase, an area of diminished enhancement is seen. In a patient studied at 3 months, Moore and colleagues (1986) described a normal initial CT scan with an increased persistent nephrogram on scans obtained 2 hours later. This finding may be caused by tubular stasis of contrast with continued water re-absorption and increasing concentration of contrast in the renal tubules.

Arteriolar Nephrosclerosis

Systemic hypertension affects the vascular tree of the kidney more consistently and more extensively than any other region of the body. The degree of change is largely a function of the severity and duration of the hypertension.

Benign Nephrosclerosis

The vascular sclerotic process is accelerated by hypertension. Arteriolar vasospasm with intramural edema is followed by muscular hypertrophy, and later, by intramural arteriolar fibrosis and hyaline degeneration. Glomerular and tubular changes are the result of ischemia. The kidneys are small because of irregular cortical thinning.

The clinical symptoms of patients with benign nephrosclerosis are usually limited to those of hypertension, and the physical examination reveals primarily cardiac and retinal changes. Mild proteinuria may be present.

Malignant Nephrosclerosis

The walls of the arterioles are markedly thickened by an eosinophilic granular material. An endothelial prolif-

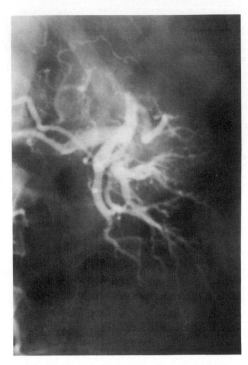

Figure 8.9. Arteriolar nephrosclerosis. A selective left renal arteriogram demonstrates tortuosity and rapid tapering of intrarenal arteries in this man with long-standing hypertension.

eration with concentric layers of collagen occurs in the afferent arterioles and intralobular arteries.

Men develop malignant hypertension more often than women, and most patients have a long history of benign hypertension. Patients with malignant hypertension have a diastolic blood pressure greater than 130 mm Hg and have papilledema. Neurologic symptoms and renal failure are common.

Laboratory tests reveal proteinuria in almost all patients. Elevated plasma renin and aldosterone along with hypokalemia are manifestations of secondary aldosteronism. Untreated malignant hypertension has a poor prognosis, and renal failure is the most common cause of death in these patients.

The radiographic findings reflect the degree of involvement of the kidneys. Unless there is a renal artery stenosis to protect one of the kidneys, involvement is systemic.

On excretory urography, the kidneys appear normal to small. The calyces remain normal, even in areas of marked cortical thinning.

Increased tortuosity and more rapid tapering of intrarenal arteries is seen with angiography (Fig. 8.9). More severe changes include filling defects and loss of cortical vessels.

EMBOLISM AND INFARCTION

The most common source of renal artery emboli is a diseased heart. Patients with atrial enlargement secondary to valvular heart disease or a dyskinetic left ventricle after myocardial infarction provide the source of mural thrombi that may dislodge and become renal artery emboli. Smaller emboli may arise from an ectatic or aneurysmal aorta, or even from cholesterol plaques in a patient with severe atherosclerosis.

Unlike arterial stenoses that are slowly progressive and may cause atrophy or collateralization, emboli produce acute ischemia that may result in infarction. The typical clinical features include the sudden onset of flank pain, hematuria, proteinuria, fever, and leukocytosis. However, the presentation is variable, and the diagnosis often is missed. Despite documented unilateral involvement, a decrease in renal function is seen in many patients.

The radiographic appearance of renal embolism depends on the size of the embolus and location of the arterial occlusion. Excretory urography demonstrates an absence of enhancement of the affected segment of the

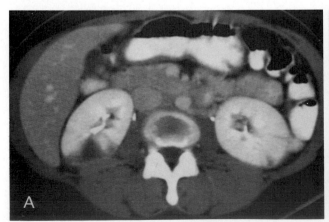
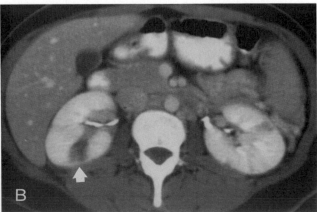

Figure 8.10. Renal infarction. **A,** Several wedge-shaped unenhancing areas indicate infarction due to emboli from subacute bacterial endocarditis. **B,** Capsular vessels preserve a thin peripheral rim (*arrow*).

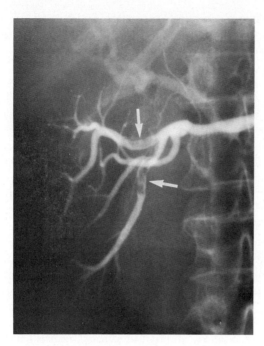

Figure 8.11. Renal embolus. Emboli are seen (*arrows*) as filling defects within the contrast-filled arteries.

kidney, reflecting lack of vascular perfusion. If the main renal artery is occluded, there is no renal function in the affected kidney. A swollen, edematous kidney is seen on ultrasound as an enlarged kidney with decreased echogenicity.

Retrograde pyelography reveals a normal collecting system with sharply cupped calyces. If there is much swelling, there may be attenuation of the intrarenal collecting system.

The absence of contrast enhancement in the affected renal tissue is best demonstrated by CT. Smaller infarcts are seen as wedge-shaped, low density areas within an

otherwise normal-appearing kidney (Fig. 8.10). If the entire kidney is affected, the increase in size due to edema can be identified by the large size and more rounded configuration. Even if the entire renal artery is occluded, capsular branches remain patent and enhance the outer rim of the kidney. The preservation of this outer 2 to 4 mm of cortex has been described on excretory urography, but it is best seen on CT (Fig. 8.10).

Radionuclide renography may suggest the diagnosis by demonstrating an area devoid of radionuclide activity. However, arteriography is needed for a definitive diagnosis. Sharp vessel cut off will be seen if the embolus completely occludes arterial flow. Incompletely occluding emboli appear as a filling defect within a contrast-filled artery (Fig. 8.11).

After the acute phase of renal infarction, atrophy begins. The infarcted tissue contracts, leaving a cortical scar (Fig. 8.12). The parenchymal loss reflects the distribution of the affected artery. If the main renal artery is occluded, the entire kidney will be affected. The kidney atrophies uniformly. There is no appreciable renal function, but renin may be elaborated and may cause hypertension.

Treatment of renal artery embolism depends on the patient's underlying medical condition and the status of the contralateral kidney. Attempts at revascularization can be made with lytic therapy delivered directly into the renal artery through an arterial catheter. Although this is not rewarding as often as lysis of clot that forms behind an arterial stenosis, excellent results have been reported. Many patients are treated with anticoagulant therapy, although surgical revascularization may be attempted in selected cases.

Arterial Thrombosis

Thrombosis of the renal artery occurs most commonly as a complication of severe atherosclerosis. In such cases,

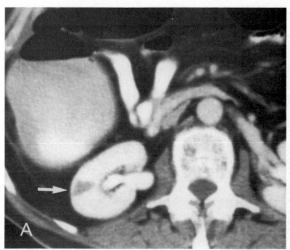
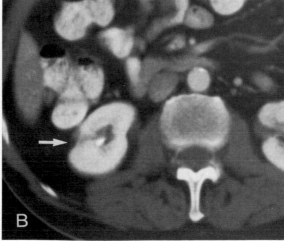

Figure 8.12. Chronic infarction. **A,** An acute infarction is seen as a wedge-shaped unenhanced area with preservation of the periphery by capsular vessels (*arrow*). **B,** Six months, later a cortical scar is present (*arrow*).

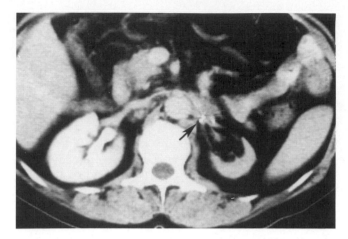

Figure 8.13.   Chronic infarction. The left renal artery was removed during retroperitoneal tumor resection. Surgical clips (*arrow*) are seen on the renal artery. The kidney is atrophic and does not enhance.

atherosclerosis usually involves a variety of other arteries, including coronary and carotid arteries, which dominate the clinical picture. This gradual occlusion of the renal artery that finally results in thrombosis is usually clinically silent and results in ipsilateral renal atrophy.

Acute thrombosis of the renal artery may occur after trauma. It usually follows blunt abdominal trauma in which the forces of acceleration or deceleration produce intimal tears, with resulting dissection of the renal artery and thrombosis. Renal artery thrombosis also may

result from subintimal dissection of the renal artery during arteriography. This is more likely to occur during an attempted transluminal angioplasty than during a diagnostic renal arteriogram.

With acute renal artery thrombosis, the kidney remains normal in size. Unless extensive renal artery collaterals have developed, there is no renal function, and intravascular contrast medium will not be excreted. Retrograde pyelography demonstrates a normal collecting system.

Color flow Doppler ultrasound also may be used in the diagnosis of renal artery thrombosis. The most common finding is absence of an intrarenal arterial signal. If there is incomplete occlusion or collateral vessels are present, a severe tardus-parvus abnormality is detected. In some patients, ultrasound may demonstrate a proximal renal artery stump.

Computed tomography reveals lack of enhancement, although a thin peripheral rim often remains viable because of collateral circulation through capsular arteries. Because collateral blood flow also may come from ureteric, gonadal, lumbar, or adrenal arteries, additional portions of the kidney, such as the medulla also may be preserved. Arteriography may be used to confirm the diagnosis of an occluded main renal artery.

With gradual occlusion, the kidney usually diminishes in size over time and a small kidney remains (Fig. 8.13). If collateral vessels are present, there may be a small amount of renal function preserved. The renal contour is smooth, unless small infarcts have already occurred. The calyces remain normal if visualized by retrograde pye-

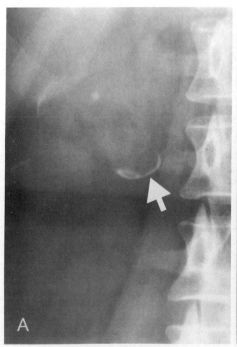

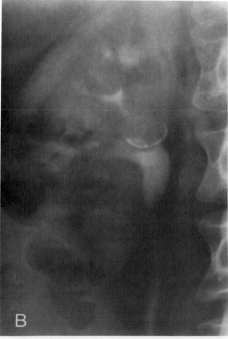

Figure 8.14.   Renal artery aneurysm. **A,** Curvilinear calcification (*arrow*) in the region of the renal hilum indicates a renal artery aneurysm. **B,** Excretory urography confirms that it is extrinsic to the collecting system.

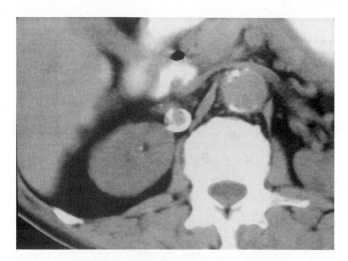

Figure 8.15.   Renal artery aneurysm. A densely calcified left renal artery aneurysm (*arrow*) is clearly visible on this unenhanced computed tomography examination.

lography or if there is sufficient function remaining to image the collecting system during urography.

ANEURYSM

Aneurysms of the renal arteries are uncommon. They are rare in autopsy series, but may be seen during angiography. The most common etiology is atherosclerosis, but a dissecting aneurysm also may involve the renal artery. Mycotic aneurysms usually involve the aorta, but may occasionally affect the renal artery.

Most patients are asymptomatic, and the aneurysm often is discovered incidentally during abdominal arteriography. Because hypertensive patients often undergo angiography to identify a renovascular etiology, it is not surprising that many patients found to have a renal artery aneurysm are hypertensive. In some patients, surgical resection of the aneurysm results in cure of the hypertension. However, these patients usually have an associated renal artery stenosis and lateralizing renal vein renin levels.

Renal artery aneurysms often contain clot and may give rise to renal emboli with or without infarction. The risk of rupture is small, but is more likely in hypertensive or pregnant patients. Calcified aneurysms rarely rupture.

If calcified, a renal artery aneurysm can be recognized on the plain abdominal radiograph (Fig. 8.14). However, the appearance of a curvilinear calcification could be caused by a tortuous or wandering splenic artery, or even a nonvascular etiology.

An aneurysm is seen as a hypoechoic mass along the course of the renal artery. The Doppler signal arising from the aneurysm depends on the amount of thrombus and the size of the neck of the aneurysm.

Renal artery aneurysms also may be demonstrated by CT. Calcification along the wall of the aneurysm is readily detected on unenhanced images (Fig. 8.15). After contrast administration, variable enhancement is found, depending on the amount of thrombus within the aneurysm.

Arteriography is required for a definitive diagnosis (Fig. 8.16), and even small, noncalcified aneurysms are easily identified unless thrombosed. The aneurysm may be partially or completely filled with thrombus, which prevents its opacification. Thus, thrombosed uncalcified aneurysms may be missed by arteriography.

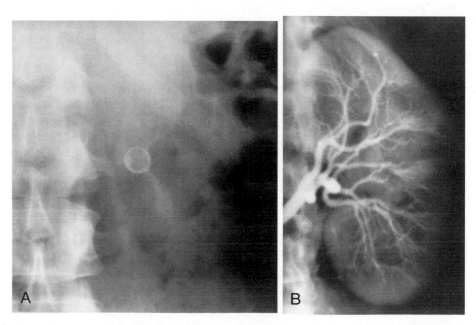

Figure 8.16.   Renal artery aneurysm. **A,** A ring of calcium in the region of the left renal artery is identified on an abdominal radiograph. **B,** A selective left renal arteriogram reveals a renal artery aneurysm (*arrow*).

Surgical treatment for a renal artery aneurysm is usually not necessary. If renin-dependent hypertension can be demonstrated, resection is indicated. However, the presence of symptoms including flank pain or hematuria may be coincidental with, but not caused by the aneurysm, and surgery should be undertaken with caution.

Mycotic Aneurysm

A mycotic aneurysm is one that arises as a result of an infectious process in the arterial wall. They may occur as a result of septic emboli, often from bacterial endocarditis, but also are seen in intravenous drug abusers. Septic emboli tend to lodge at a branch point, a site of rapid vessel tapering, or a sharp bend in the artery. Mycotic aneurysms also may result from direct spread from a contiguous infection or from bacteria lodging in the vasa vasora or in the diseased intima.

Once established, the infection weakens the arterial wall and has a high incidence of rupture. Identification of a mycotic aneurysm also may be the first clue to an underlying bacterial endocarditis. Because the aneurysm may harbor bacteria despite antibiotic therapy, surgery may be needed to eradicate the site of infection.

ARTERIOVENOUS FISTULA

An arteriovenous fistula is an abnormal communication between the arterial and venous circulation that bypasses the capillary bed. Congenital fistulae or arteriovenous malformations (AVMs), also known as angiomas or angiodysplasias, are uncommon.

Congenital

Congenital AVMs often are asymptomatic and may not be detected in patients until they are well into adult life. They are found more often in women than men, and hematuria is the most common presenting complaint. If large enough, an AVM may decrease perfusion to the renal parenchyma, resulting in renal ischemia and renin-mediated hypertension.

The findings on excretory urography are dependent on the size and location of the lesion. Large AVMs located near the collecting system may create extrinsic compression on the renal pelvis. If there is hematuria, blood clots may be seen.

Color flow Doppler ultrasound has become the best noninvasive modality to evaluate AVMs and arteriovenous fistulae. Malformations are seen as focal flow areas with a mixing of Doppler shift frequencies. However, this technique is insensitive to AVMs with minimal flow.

Arteriography may be needed for a definite diagnosis, and many small AVMs can only be detected with selective-magnification renal arteriography. Arteriovenous malformations often are classified as cirsoid or aneurysmal. Cirsoid AVMs have multiple small arteriovenous

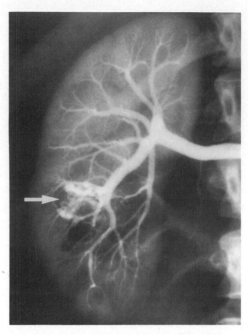

Figure 8.17. Congenital arteriovenous malformation. A tangle of vessels is seen in the right kidney (*arrow*).

communications (Fig. 8.17), whereas aneurysmal AVMs have only a solitary communication. The cirsoid variety tends to be located adjacent to the collecting system and often causes hematuria. The aneurysmal AVM is more likely to cause an abdominal bruit and hypertension.

Acquired

Acquired arteriovenous fistulae do not have the female preponderance seen with congenital AVMs. Because trauma due to a penetrating injury or biopsy is the most common etiology, they often are seen in men.

Idiopathic

Arteriovenous fistulae that appear to be acquired rather than congenital, but do not have an identifiable etiology are classified as idiopathic. They may arise by erosion of a renal artery aneurysm into the adjacent vein.

The physiologic effect of an arteriovenous fistula depends on the size of the fistula and its specific location. The artery supplying the fistula enlarges, and collateral vessels may develop if the fistula is larger than the artery feeding it. In some cases, retrograde flow may occur in the artery distal to the fistula. The draining veins are dilated, and their walls are thickened. This venous arterialization may even be associated with the development of atherosclerotic plaques.

The most common clinical manifestation of renal arteriovenous fistulae is an abdominal bruit. Approximately half of symptomatic patients have cardiomegaly and congestive heart failure. Hematuria also is common.

Hypertension, which is usually diastolic, is renin mediated. The renal artery blood pressure and flow distal to the shunt are diminished. This relative renal ischemia stimulates renin secretion.

The most frequent etiology of an acquired arteriovenous fistula (Fig. 8.18) is renal biopsy. Many more acquired arteriovenous fistulae occur than are probably diagnosed, because imaging is performed only in those patients symptomatic enough to suggest a large fistula. Arteriovenous fistulae also may be seen as a complication of selective renal arteriography, especially during percutaneous transluminal angioplasty. In such cases, a stiff guidewire often is needed to lead the angioplasty catheter through the site of the renal artery stenosis. If the guidewire is passed out too far into the kidney, it will penetrate the renal artery and may enter an adjacent vein.

Acquired arteriovenous fistulae may be easier to detect with ultrasound than congenital AVMs. Increased flow velocity is found in the feeding artery and the draining vein. The flow at the shunt site is highly turbulent. The resistive index in the feeding artery is markedly reduced.

Small arteriovenous fistulae may heal spontaneously. Thus, many patients who develop a fistula after renal biopsy or angiography are not treated unless symptoms develop. Some of these fistulae may enlarge and require treatment.

Significant arteriovenous fistulae may be treated with transcatheter occlusion. It is critical to assess the size of

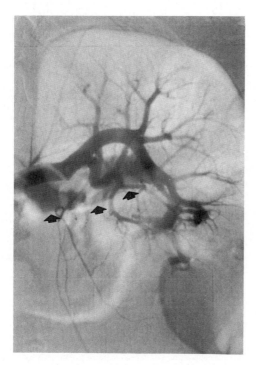

Figure 8.18. Acquired arteriovenous fistula. An arteriogram demonstrates rapid filling of the renal vein (*arrows*) after renal biopsy. Both the supplying artery and draining vein are enlarged.

the communication and be sure that any embolic material will be captured in the fistula and not pass through to become a pulmonary embolus. The most common indications for treatment are persistent hematuria or hypertension that can be localized to the kidney containing the fistula. If all the communicating branches can be occluded, percutaneous therapy should be successful. If transcatheter occlusion cannot be performed, surgery may be needed.

Postnephrectomy

Although uncommon, a fistula may develop between the stump of the renal artery and the stump of the renal vein or vena cava after nephrectomy. Postoperative infection or excessive bleeding requiring packing during surgery contribute to their development. These fistulae tend to be large and may be hemodynamically significant.

RENAL VEIN THROMBOSIS

Thrombosis of the renal vein is usually caused by an underlying abnormality of hydration, the clotting system, or the kidney itself. Occasionally extrinsic compression may occlude the IVC or the renal vein and may cause clot formation due to absent or slow flow. Renal or left adrenal tumors may grow along the veins, resulting in tumor thrombus in the renal vein. Renal vein thrombosis is more common on the left side, presumably reflecting the longer left renal vein as opposed to the right.

The clinical manifestations of renal vein thrombosis depend on the age of the patient, the specific disease process, and the speed with which it occurs. In infants, renal vein thrombosis often is an acute event incited by dehydration due to a volume-depleting illness such as severe diarrhea. The kidney swells and renal function deteriorates. If the venous occlusion is not relieved, the kidney will infarct and atrophy.

In adults, the most common underlying abnormality is membranous glomerulonephritis. Approximately 50% of patients with membranous glomerulonephritis have renal vein thrombosis. Thrombosis occurs less frequently in lipoid nephrosis, immunoglobulin A (IgA) nephropathy, or minimal change disease. Although patients with renal vein thrombosis often present with the nephrotic syndrome, the protein loss is caused by the underlying renal disease rather than the venous thrombosis. In patients with no renal disease and renal vein thrombosis, little or no proteinuria is seen.

Masses that produce extrinsic compression on the renal vein also may induce renal vein thrombosis. Retroperitoneal fibrosis, a tumor mass, acute pancreatitis, trauma, and retroperitoneal surgery may each incite renal vein thrombosis. Thrombocytosis, elevated clotting factors, or dehydration also may induce renal vein thrombosis. When thrombosis is gradual in onset, symptoms may be mild. If sufficient collateral vessels exist, renal function may be unaffected. If thrombosis occurs more acutely, collateral vessels are less likely to develop and clinical symptoms such as back pain are common. Laboratory abnormalities are nonspecific; the marked proteinuria seen in these patients is caused by the underlying nephrotic syndrome rather than by the renal vein thrombosis. Pulmonary embolism is a common associated problem.

The radiographic findings also depend on the underlying disease process and the extent of collateral venous flow. If collateral veins are unable to drain the kidney adequately, the kidney will be enlarged. A persistent nephrogram is seen on excretory urography, and the collecting system is attenuated. However, because renal function is impaired, retrograde pyelography may be required to exclude obstruction. However, sharp calyces are usually seen well enough on an excretory urogram to exclude obstruction.

Ultrasound often is used to exclude ureteral obstruction, but also may demonstrate an enlarged, relatively hypoechoic kidney. In some cases, renal vein thrombosis can be imaged. With Doppler ultrasound, an arterial wave form is detected proximal to the venous clot. There is a shift in the antegrade systolic frequency and reversal of flow during diastole. However, these findings are not specific for renal vein thrombosis, because they also may be seen with acute tubular necrosis or transplant rejection.

Computed tomography may be used to exclude a renal mass such as a carcinoma growing into the renal vein. Renal enlargement with diminished opacification reflecting impaired function is seen. Edema in the renal sinus space and venous collaterals may be identified. (Fig. 8.19) Intravenous contrast should opacify the renal veins; absence of enhancement of a kidney that has arterial flow implies venous thrombosis (Fig. 8.20). With current generation scanners, CT is highly sensitive in detecting renal vein thrombosis.

Magnetic resonance imaging is proving to be even more accurate than CT for vascular imaging, because it does not rely on good cardiac function to propel a bolus of contrast medium to the renal veins and because it is less susceptible to motion artifact. It often is used to detect and delineate venous extension of renal adenocarcinoma, but can also be applied to renal vein or caval thrombosis. Rapidly acquired gradient-recalled echo images can be obtained without intravascular contrast media. This is especially valuable in patients with a contraindication to iodinated contrast media (Fig. 8.21).

Although renal venography is still the most definitive test, it is seldom needed because of the high accuracy of CT and MR. The normal renal vein should be visual-

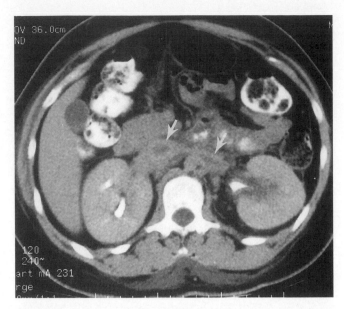

Figure 8.19. Renal vein thrombosis. Thrombus is seen in the inferior vena cava and left renal vein (*arrows*) on an enhanced CT scan in this patient with systemic lupus erythematosus. Edema is present in the renal sinus space, and collateral vessels can be seen in the perinephric space.

ized during the venous phase of a renal arteriogram. Absence of venous opacification implies obstruction. Direct renal venography also may be used to demonstrate venous thrombosis, but it is seldom necessary.

Anticoagulation is the standard therapy for renal vein thrombosis. This prevents clot propagation, while endemic enzyme systems lyse or recanalize the thrombosed vessel. Pulmonary embolism is a common complication of renal vein thrombosis. Lytic therapy may be used in patients in whom the thrombosis is more acute and in whom the clinical manifestations are more severe.

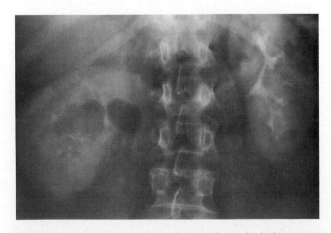

Figure 8.20. Renal vein thrombosis. The right kidney is enlarged and functions poorly. A small amount of contrast medium opacifies the intrarenal collecting system, which is attenuated but shows no evidence of obstruction.

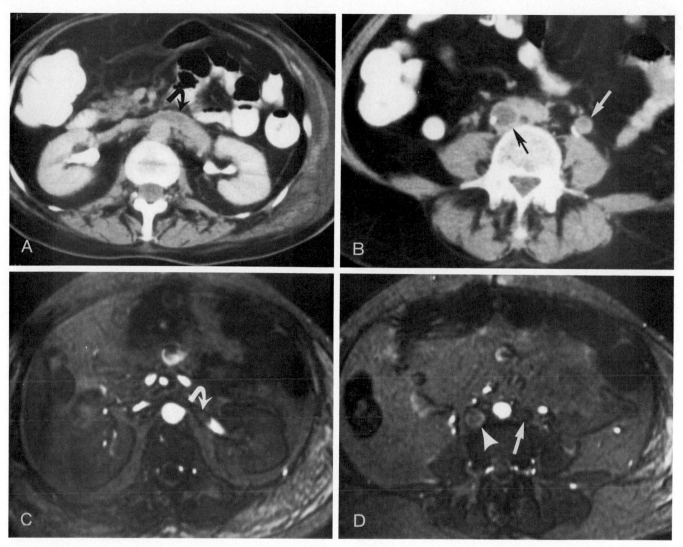

Figure 8.21.   Renal vein thrombosis. **A,** A computed tomography scan through the level of the left renal vein demonstrates thrombosis (*arrow*) by the absence of enhancement. **B,** Below the kidneys, thrombosis of the inferior vena cava (*black arrow*) and left gonadal vein (*white arrow*) can be seen. **C,** A magnetic resonance image using a gradient-recalled echo technique confirms the renal vein thrombosis by the absence of signal (*arrow*). **D,** At a lower level, thrombosis of the inferior vena cava (*arrowhead*) and left gonadal vein (*arrow*) also are seen.

GONADAL VEIN THROMBOSIS

Thrombosis of the gonadal veins unrelated to tumor thrombus is seen most commonly in women during the postpartum period. Stasis of blood, increased levels of circulating clotting factors, and damage to the vessel wall are contributing factors. Ovarian vein thrombosis also may be seen as a consequence of gynecological surgery or pelvic inflammatory disease. Postpartum ovarian vein thrombosis is more common on the right; the left side may be spared by reflux of blood into the gonadal vein.

Abdominal radiographs and excretory urography are unrevealing, although hydronephrosis of pregnancy may be evident. Gray-scale and Doppler ultrasound may demonstrate an echogenic thrombus in an enlarged ovarian vein. However, much of the ovarian vein may be hidden by overlying bowel gas, and CT is usually the preferred imaging modality. A low-density thrombus is easily detected on an enhanced abdominal CT examination (Fig. 8.22). Magnetic resonance imaging also may be used to detect ovarian vein thrombus (Fig. 8.21).

Patients with gonadal vein thrombosis often are treated with antibiotics and anticoagulation.

RENAL LYMPHANGIOMATOSIS

Renal lymphangiomatosis is a rare disorder in which lymphatic tissue fails to develop a normal communication with the rest of the lymphatic system. Cystic masses

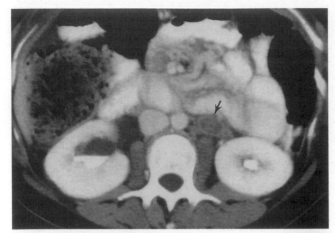

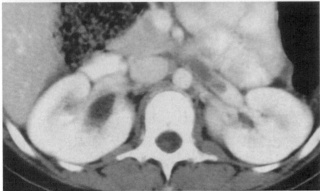

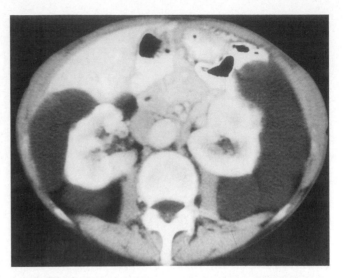

Figure 8.23. Lymphangiomatosis. Multiple, bilateral, thin-walled cysts are seen in the perinephric space.

Figure 8.22. Ovarian vein thrombosis. **A,** Thrombosis of the left ovarian vein (*arrow*) is demonstrated on this enhanced computed tomography scan. **B,** More cephalad images demonstrate thrombus extension into the left renal vein. Incidentally, note the hydronephrosis of pregnancy involving the right kidney in this recently postpartum female.

cysts, whereas the cysts are perinephric in lymphangiomatosis.

Because lymphangiomatosis is benign and most patients are asymptomatic, there is no treatment.

develop, usually in the perinephric space immediately adjacent to the kidney, as a result of obstruction of larger lymphatics that drain through the renal pelvis.

Patients may present with a palpable abdominal mass, or perinephric cystic masses may be found incidentally on cross-sectional imaging studies. The condition is usually bilateral and may be hereditary. Pregnancy may exacerbate the condition. Renal function is normal.

Abdominal radiographs and excretory urography will likely appear normal. Multiple cystic masses are seen with sonography. In some cases, debris from previous hemorrhage may be seen. Multiple thin-walled cystic masses are seen on CT (Fig. 8.23). The density of the cystic masses approximates that of water, unless hemorrhaging has occurred, in which case the density is elevated.

Renal lymphangiomatosis must be distinguished from autosomal dominant polycystic kidney disease (ADPKD). Patients with ADPKD have innumerable parenchymal

SUGGESTED READING

Anatomy

Bateson EM, Atkinson D: Circumcaval ureter: a new classification. *Clin Radiol* 20:173, 1969.

Beckmann CF, Abrams HL: Renal vein valves: incidence and significance. *Radiology* 127:351, 1978.

Beckmann CF, Abrams HL: Circumaortic venous ring: incidence and significance. *AJR* 132:561, 1979.

Beckmann CF, Abrams HL: Idiopathic renal vein varices: incidence and significance. *Radiology* 143:649, 1982.

Beinart C, Sniderman KW, Weiner M, et al.: Left renal vein hypertension: a cause of occult hematuria. *Radiology* 145:647, 1982.

Crosse JEW, Soderdahl DW, Teplick SK, Clark RE: Nonobstructive circumcaval (retrocaval) ureter. *Radiology* 116:69, 1975.

Hoeltl W, Hruby W, Aharinejad S: Renal vein anatomy and its implications for retroperitoneal surgery. *J Urol* 143:1108, 1990.

Hohenfellner M, Steinbach F, Schultz-Lampel D, et al.: The nutcracker syndrome: new aspects of pathophysiology, diagnosis and treatment. *J Urol* 146:685, 1991.

Lautin EM, Haramati N, Frager D, et al.: CT diagnosis of circumcaval ureter. *AJR* 150:591, 1988.

Nielsen PB: Retrocaval ureter: report of a case. *Acta Radiol* 51:179, 1959.

Reed MD, Friedman AC, Nealy P: Anomalies of the left renal vein: analysis of 433 CT scans. *J Comput Assist Tomogr* 6(6):1124, 1982.

Sampaio FJB, Aragao AHM: Anatomical relationship between the intrarenal arteries and the kidney collecting system. *J Urol* 143:679, 1990.

Trueta J: *Studies of the Renal Circulation.* Springfield, Illinois, Charles C Thomas, 1947.

Collagen Vascular Diseases

Anderson R: Arteriography in polyarteritis nodosa. *Br J Urol* 40(5):556, 1968.

Easterbrook JS: Renal and hepatic microaneurysms: report of a new entity simulating polyarteritis nodosa. *Radiology* 137:629, 1980.

Fauci AS, Haynes BF, Katz P, Wolff SM: Wegener's granulomatosis: prospective clinical and therapeutic experience with 85 patients for 21 years. *Ann Intern Med* 98:76, 1983.

Halpern M, Citron BP: Necrotizing angiitis associated with drug abuse. *AJR* 3:663, 1971.

Litvak AS, Lucas BA, McRoberts JW: Urologic manifestations of polyarteritis nodosa. *J Urol* 115:572, 1976.

Longmaid HE, Rider E, Tymmkiw J: Lupus nephritis: new sonographic findings. *J Ultrasound Med* 6:75, 1987.

Radiation Nephritis

Jongejan HTM, van der Kogel AJ, Provoost AP, Molenaar JC: Radiation nephropathy in young and adult rats. *Int J Radiat Oncol Biol Phys* 13:225, 1987.

Moore L, Curry NS, Jenrette JM: Computed tomography of acute radiation nephritis. *Urol Radiol* 8:89, 1986.

Willett CG, Tepper JE, Orlow EL, Shipley WU: Renal complications secondary to radiation treatment of upper abdominal malignancies. *Int J Radiat Oncol Biol Phys* 12:1601, 1986.

Renal Embolism and Infarction

Gasparini M, Hofmann R, Stoller M: Renal artery embolism: Clinical features and therapeutic options. *J Urol* 147:567, 1992.

Hann L, Plister RC: Renal subcapsular rim sign: new etiologies and pathogenesis. *AJR* 138:51, 1982.

Hélénon O, Rody FE, Correas J, Melki P, Chauveau D, Chrétien Y, Moreau J: Color Doppler US of renovascular disease in native kidneys. *RadioGraphics* 15:833–854, 1995.

Lessman RK, Johnson SF, Coburn JW: Renal artery embolism—clinical features and long term follow up of 17 cases. *Ann Intern Med* 89(4):477, 1978.

Malmed AS, Love L, Jeffrey RB: Medullary CT enhancement in acute renal artery occlusion. *J Comput Assist Tomogr* 16:107, 1992.

Renal Artery Aneurysm

DuBrow RA, Patel SK: Mycotic aneurysm of the renal artery. *Radiology* 138:577, 1981.

Tham G, Ekelund L, Herrlin K, et al.: Renal artery aneurysms: natural history and prognosis. *Ann Surg* 197(3):348, 1983.

Arteriovenous Fistulae

Chew QT, Madayag MA: Post-nephrectomy arteriovenous fistula. *J Urol* 109:546, 1973.

Crotty KL, Orihuela E, Warren MM: Recent advances in the diagnosis and treatment of renal arteriovenous malformations and fistulas. *J Urol* 150:1355, 1993.

Ekelund L, Gothlin J: Renal hemangiomas: an analysis of 13 cases diagnosed by angiography. *AJR* 125:788, 1975.

Takaha M, Matsumoto A, Ochi K, et al.: Intrarenal arteriovenous malformation. *J Urol* 124:315, 1980.

Takebayashi S, Aida N, Matsui K: Arteriovenous malformations of the kidneys: Diagnosis and follow-up with color Doppler sonography in six patients. *AJR* 157:991, 1991.

Renal Vein Thrombosis

Bradley WG, Jacobs RP, Trew PA, et al.: Renal vein thrombosis: occurrence in membranous glomerulonephropathy and lupus nephritis. *Radiology* 139:571, 1981.

Brennan RE, Curtis JA, Koolpe HA, et al.: Left renal vein obstruction associated with nonrenal malignancy. *Urology* 19(3):329, 1982.

Clark RA, Wyatt GM, Colley DP: Renal vein thrombosis: an underdiagnosed complication of multiple renal abnormalities. *Radiology* 132:43, 1979.

Duckett T, Bretan PN, Cochran ST, Rajfer J, Rosenthal JT: Noninvasive radiological diagnosis of renal rein thrombosis in renal transplantation. *J Urol* 146:403–406, 1991.

Gatewood OMB, Fishman EK, Burrow CR, et al.: Renal vein thrombosis in patients with nephrotic syndrome: CT diagnosis. *Radiology* 159:117, 1986.

Grant TH, Schoettle BW, Buchsbaum MS: Post partum ovarian vein thrombosis: diagnosis by clot protrusion into the IVC at sonography. *AJR* 160:551, 1993.

Jacoby WT, Cohan RH, Baker ME, et al.: Ovarian vein thrombosis in oncology patients: CT detection and clinical significance. *AJR* 155:291, 1990.

Keating MA, Althausen AF: The clinical spectrum of renal vein thrombosis. *J Urol* 133:938, 1985.

Tempany CMC, Morton RA, Marshall FF: MRI of the renal veins: Assessment of nonneoplastic venous thrombosis. *J Comput Assist Tomogr* 16:929, 1992.

Wei LQ, Rong ZK, Gui L, Shan RD: CT diagnosis of renal vein thrombosis in nephrotic syndrome. *J Comput Assist Tomogr* 15:454, 1991.

Winfield AC, Gerlock AJ, Shaff MI: Perirenal cobwebs: a CT sign of renal vein thrombosis. *J Comput Assist Tomogr* 5(5):705, 1981.

Witz M, Kantarovsky A, Morag B, Shifrin EG: Renal vein occlusion: a review. *J Urol* 155:1173, 1996.

Renal Lymphangiomatosis

Leder RA, Frederick MG, Hall BP, Elenberger CD: Genitourinary case of the day. *AJR* 165:197–200, 1995.

Meredith WT, Levine E, Ahlstrom NG, Grantham JJ: Exacerbation of familial renal lymphangiomatosis during pregnancy. *AJR* 151:965–966, 1988.

9

Renal Hypertension

Hypertension is a common medical problem that affects as many as one third of the population at some time. It is defined as a diastolic pressure of 90 mm Hg or more and is graded as mild, moderate, severe, or malignant. Unfortunately, most cases of hypertension are idiopathic. No etiology can be found, and the patient must be treated with antihypertensive medication. In a minority of patients, however, a specific etiology can be identified. In many of these patients, appropriate therapy results in cure.

The major etiologic categories of hypertension are renovascular, renal, endocrine, and neurologic. Renal parenchymal and renovascular hypertension are discussed in this chapter. Adrenal etiologies are addressed in Chapter 15.

ETIOLOGIES

Renal Parenchymal

A large number of parenchymal abnormalities have been associated with hypertension including pyelonephritis, glomerulopathies, ureteral obstruction, and renal mass lesions. Although many of these entities are common, they are seldom causally related to hypertension. However, documentation of a causal role has been shown in some cases, with relief of hypertension when the parenchymal abnormality has been alleviated.

Hydronephrosis

Unilateral ureteral obstruction may cause hypertension by activating the renin-angiotensin system. Acute ureteral occlusion has been shown to result in unilateral renin secretion and the development of hypertension in dogs. Human data confirm this increased renin secretion in patients with acute ureteral obstruction, but not in patients with chronic ureteral obstruction. Surgical intervention should cure those patients with lateralizing renin levels.

Renal Cyst

Renal cysts, as well as other masses, may rarely cause renin mediated hypertension. This may be due to compression of the main renal artery or of a branch renal artery that is causing ischemia. The resultant increased serum renin level leads to hypertension. Decompression of the cyst relieves the pressure on the renal artery and cures the hypertension. Cystic drainage can be performed percutaneously, but sclerosis may be needed to prevent recurrence. If this cannot be done, surgery may be required.

Chronic Pyelonephritis

Chronic pyelonephritis is another curable etiology of hypertension, although hypertension in most patients with chronic pyelonephritis is idiopathic. Patients more likely to become normotensive after nephrectomy for chronic pyelonephritis are younger, have a more recent onset of hypertension, have a more severely involved ipsilateral kidney, and have a nearly normal contralateral kidney. Lateralizing renal-vein renin levels may be used to predict patients likely to respond to surgery.

Renal Carcinoma

Both renal adenocarcinoma and Wilms' tumor may cause hypertension in several different ways. The mass may cause extrinsic compression on the renal artery, resulting in ischemia and increased renin secretion. Very vascular tumors may cause hypertension due to arteriovenous shunting. Rarely, a renal carcinoma or Wilms' tumor may produce renin. In some patients, hypertension may be the presenting finding, and the renal tumor may be detected during the hypertension work-up. Arteriography performed in these patients must include both main renal arteries to exclude a significant renal artery stenosis (RAS) and possible renovascular hypertension in the contralateral kidney.

Juxtaglomerular Tumors

A renin-secreting tumor of the juxtaglomerular cells is a rare cause of hypertension. Patients with a juxtaglomerular tumor, or reninoma, tend to be young and often are younger than 20 years of age. The most frequent symptoms are related to the hypertension and include headache, polydipsia, polyuria, and neuromuscular complaints resulting from hypokalemia. Hypertension in these patients is usually moderate to severe.

The tumor is usually small and confined to the kidney, although a large (6.5-cm) tumor and a reninoma arising in the perinephric space have been reported. Juxtaglomerular tumors are usually sharply marginated and may be separated from the normal renal parenchyma by a pseudocapsule.

Detection of a renal mass by excretory urography depends on the size and location of the tumor. Calcification is not seen. Ultrasound is most frequently useful in demonstrating that the mass seen at urography is solid rather than cystic. The juxtaglomerular tumor is relatively echogenic due to the numerous interfaces caused by the small vascular channels in the tumor.

Although computed tomography (CT) is quite sensitive in detecting these tumors, their appearance is nonspecific. Contrast enhancement is needed, because the tumor may be isodense with normal renal parenchyma on unenhanced scans.

Reninomas may be detected at arteriography during an evaluation for possible renovascular hypertension. The tumor is typically hypovascular, even on selective renal arteriography. It is detected by displacement of small intrarenal arteries (Fig. 9.1).

Renal-vein renin sampling will demonstrate elevated renin levels arising from the tumor. However, selective sampling from branch renal veins may be needed to confirm the abnormal renin secretion.

Although few juxtaglomerular tumors have been reported, they appear to be benign. Thus, simple tumorectomy or partial nephrectomy is curative.

Ask-Upmark Kidney

Segmental hypoplasia has been recognized as a cause of hypertension since Ask-Upmark reported findings regarding six patients in 1929. The affected kidney is small and has few pyramids and a deep cortical groove overlying an abnormal calyx or recess extending from the renal pelvis. Hyperplasia of juxtaglomerular cells has been reported, and excess renin secretion has been documented in some cases. The process may be unilateral or bilateral.

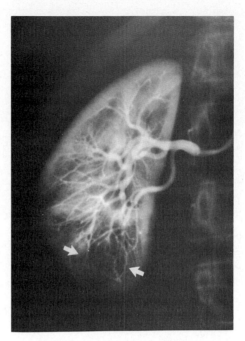

Figure 9.1. Juxtaglomerular tumor. A small hypovascular mass (*arrows*) is seen in the lower pole.

An Ask-Upmark kidney may be seen in children and adults. Most children with an Ask-Upmark kidney are hypertensive, and often the hypertension is severe. The condition is more common in female patients and is highly associated with vesicoureteral reflux and urinary tract infection.

Because many patients have vesicoureteral reflux, there is some controversy over the etiology. The renal abnormalities are similar, and it may be impossible to distinguish the changes due to vesicoureteral reflux from an Ask-Upmark kidney radiographically.

On excretory urography, the affected kidney is small and contains one or more deep cortical scars. The contralateral kidney often demonstrates compensatory hypertrophy. The calyx underlying the cortical scar is dilated and clubbed. Hypertrophy of adjacent renal tissue may splay the infundibulum, creating a mass effect.

Arteriography demonstrates a normal renal artery. The size of the renal artery is proportional to the size of the kidney, which often is small. The size of the orifice of the renal artery also is proportional to the size of the vessel, indicating its congenital etiology (Fig. 9.2).

Trauma

Trauma may cause hypertension by causing injury to the renal artery or hypertension may be due to the compressive effect of a subcapsular hematoma. Traumatic injury may create an intimal hematoma or partial tear of the renal artery that results in renal ischemia. Selective renal arteriography is needed to detect the arterial le-

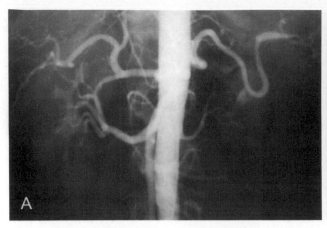

Figure 9.2. Ask-Upmark kidney. **A,** Aortography demonstrates a small left renal artery, but no focal stenosis. **B,** A focal parenchymal scar (*arrow*) is seen on later-phase films. Elevated renins were measured from the left renal vein.

sion, which may affect the main renal artery or a branch vessel. Those patients with partial renal damage may be treated medically, because the hypertension may resolve spontaneously. If the kidney is threatened, however, urgent repair is required.

Another mechanism of trauma-induced hypertension is the development of a subcapsular hematoma that compresses the renal parenchyma, creating local ischemia and resulting in increased renin secretion. This phenomenon was first demonstrated by Page in 1939, when he produced arterial hypertension in laboratory animals by wrapping one kidney in cellophane. This induced a proliferative reaction that formed a fibrocollagenous shell, compressing the renal parenchyma. The hypertension results from excess renin secretion due to ischemia caused by the mass effect of the hematoma compressed against the kidney by the renal capsule.

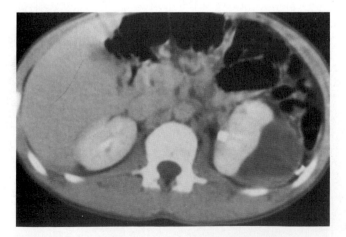

Figure 9.3. Subcapsular hematoma. Compression of the renal parenchyma indicates the subcapsular location. The compression creates local ischemia resulting in increased renin secretion.

The development of hypertension is not acute, but may take months or even years after the trauma.

A subcapsular hematoma is easily seen on CT (Fig. 9.3). If hypertension develops subsequently, renal-vein renin levels should be measured. These will usually lateralize to the affected kidney. Arteriography shows no arterial injury, but the renal distortion by the subcapsular mass is seen. Evacuation of the hematoma should result in cure.

Renovascular Hypertension

Only a small minority of hypertensive patients have a renovascular etiology; the vast majority of patients have essential hypertension. Estimates vary, but the prevalence of renovascular hypertension among all hypertensive patients is only approximately 1 to 4%. It is difficult to predict on a clinical basis which patients have renovascular hypertension, but some characteristics make it more likely.

Renovascular hypertension is more common among patients at either age extreme. Patients younger than 20 years of age or older than 50 years of age are more likely to have a renovascular etiology, whereas patients with essential hypertension are usually between 30 and 50 years of age at onset. However, fibromuscular dysplasia, the second most common cause of renovascular hypertension, typically affects women between 30 and 55 years of age. Rapid acceleration or severe hypertension is another indication of a renovascular etiology, as is a severe hypertensive retinopathy. A flank bruit found on physical examination also suggests a renovascular etiology; it is especially common in patients with fibromuscular dysplasia. A family history of hypertension, more often is found in patients with essential hypertension.

Renovascular hypertension is renin mediated and occurs as a response to renal ischemia. Renin is an enzyme produced in the juxtaglomerular apparatus of the kidney. It acts on the circulating serum protein angiotensinogen to produce the inactive hormone angiotensin I which, in turn, is converted to the active hormone angiotensin II. Angiotensin II has several properties that increase blood pressure. It stimulates aldosterone secretion from the adrenal cortex, causes arteriolar vasoconstriction, and exerts antidiuretic and antinatriuretic effects on the proximal renal tubule by promoting sodium reabsorption.

The most important factor governing renin release is the afferent arteriole, which acts as a baroreceptor. The transmural pressure across this arteriole may decrease as a result of a reduction in perfusion pressure or decreased compliance of the arteriole.

In patients with renovascular hypertension, the hypertension is dependent on the high circulating levels of angiotensin II. Thus, either saralasin, an angiotensin II antagonist, or the converting enzyme inhibitor captopril may be used to control the hypertension.

Although many different processes may cause stenosis of the main renal artery, the most common are atherosclerosis and fibromuscular dysplasia. Rarely, renal artery stenoses may be congenital, may be caused by Takayasu's aortitis or by the middle aortic syndrome, irradiation, or may be associated with neurofibromatosis.

Atherosclerosis

Atherosclerosis accounts for approximately two thirds of cases of significant narrowing of the main renal artery. The lesions usually occur at the origin of the renal artery or within the first 2 cm (Fig. 9.4). They often are circumferential, but may be eccentric. Because atherosclerosis is a generalized process, both renal arteries are frequently affected. If atherosclerosis is present at the renal ostia, it may not be possible to determine whether the plaque is renal or aortic in location.

Atherosclerosis begins as a proliferation of smooth muscle cells in the intima and creates a mound that protrudes into the lumen. Lipid deposition follows with inflammation, necrosis, and formation of atherosclerotic plaque.

Atherosclerosis is more common in men than women, and is accelerated by smoking. The age at which patients present with hypertension is considerably older than in those with fibromuscular dysplasia.

Fibromuscular Dysplasia

Fibromuscular dysplasia (FMD) has only been recognized for the past 30 years, but it accounts for almost one third of cases of renovascular hypertension. It may involve any layer of the renal artery and is classified as intimal, medial, or adventitial. The medial variety can be subdivided into several more categories.

Intimal fibroplasia consists of a concentric accumulation of collagen beneath the internal elastic membrane. This creates a smooth stenosis, usually in the midportion of the renal artery. It is more common among children and is progressive.

Medial dysplasia is the most common type and accounts for approximately 95% of cases. The subcategories reflect involvement of the inner or outer media, and the presence of collagenous infiltration, smooth muscle hypertrophy, or medial dissection.

Medial fibroplasia is the most common subtype of dysplasia. There is replacement of smooth muscle by collagen that forms thick ridges. These alternate with areas of small aneurysm formation and result in the classic "string of beads" appearance seen with arteriography (Fig. 9.5). This type of medial dysplasia is most commonly seen in women 20 to 50 years of age. Although it is progressive, it is usually responsive to percutaneous transluminal angioplasty.

Collagen infiltrates the outer layer of the media in perimedial fibroplasia. A beaded appearance similar to

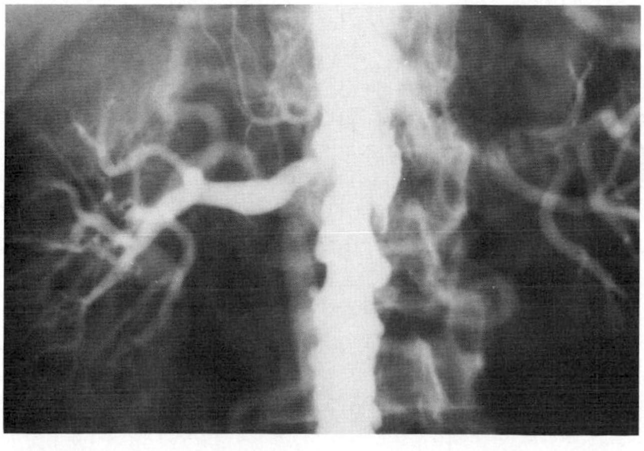

Figure 9.4. Atherosclerosis. Diffuse atherosclerotic changes are seen in the abdominal aorta as well as the right renal artery.

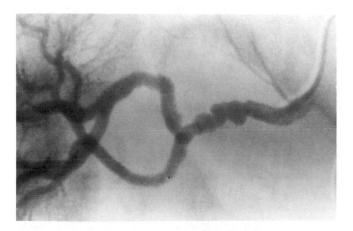

Figure 9.5. Fibromuscular dysplasia. Thick ridges of collagen alternate with aneurysms to create a "string of beads" appearance typical of medial fibroplasia.

that seen in medial fibroplasia is present in the renal arteries, but is less dramatic because true aneurysms do not develop.

True medial hyperplasia is an uncommon form of medial dysplasia and consists of hyperplastic smooth muscle and fibrous tissue. Focal stenoses are seen, but aneurysm formation is not present (Fig. 9.6).

Medial dissection also is uncommon and may be histologically indistinguishable from other forms of medial dysplasia. In this form, a new channel is formed in the outer third of the media.

In adventitial dysplasia, a collagenous infiltrate surrounds the adventitia. Either discrete focal or longer tubular stenoses may be produced.

Fibromuscular dysplasia is not limited to the renal arteries, but also is seen in cephalic, visceral, and peripheral arteries. Fibromuscular dysplasia involves the carotid and vertebral arteries, but tends to spare the intracranial vessels. Transient ischemic attacks may be due to involvement of cephalic vessels by FMD.

Most patients are asymptomatic when the visceral arteries are affected by FMD. Symptoms of intestinal angina have been reported due to lesions in the superior mesenteric artery. The hepatic artery also may be involved, but seldom causes symptoms.

Peripheral arteries are seldom affected, but reports have confirmed involvement of most medium and large muscular arteries. Claudication may result if arterial flow is compromised.

Takayasu's Aortitis

Takayasu's disease is a granulomatous arteritis that commonly involves the aorta and its major branches. It

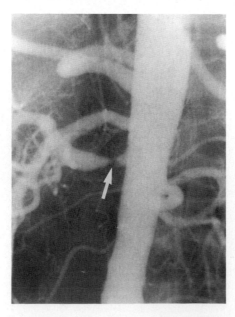

Figure 9.6. Fibromuscular dysplasia. The focal stenosis (*arrow*) suggests medial hyperplasia.

has a marked female preponderance and is usually seen in patients younger than 35 years of age. Although primarily seen in Asians, cases are being reported with increasing frequency in western civilizations. Temporal arteritis is histologically similar, but is confined to small vessels and is typically found in older patients.

Because major branches of the abdominal aorta often are affected, hypertension is a common complication of Takayasu's disease. The hypertension may be caused by coarctation of the aorta or main RAS.

Symptoms of Takayasu's aortitis are nonspecific and often are not recognized until the disease is well advanced. Takayasu's disease is classified into four types.

Arteriography demonstrates vascular narrowing of the aortic arch or great vessels arising from the arch (type 1); descending thoracic and upper abdominal aorta (type 2); aortic arch vessels, abdominal aorta, and major branches (type 3); or pulmonary arteries (type 4). Typically, there is a smooth tapered narrowing of the affected artery. Skip areas may occur, and multiple vessels are commonly involved. The disease may progress to complete occlusion. Treatment is usually surgical, but successful transluminal angioplasty has been reported.

Middle Aortic Syndrome

This rare syndrome of diffuse narrowing of the abdominal aorta often affects the visceral and renal arteries. It occurs in young patients, most often in the second decade of life. Hypertension is typically severe. An abdominal bruit and diminished femoral pulses in a young patient may suggest the diagnosis. The prognosis is poor; the patients often die from cerebral hemorrhage, hypertensive encephalopathy, stroke, and congestive heart failure.

The middle aortic syndrome is distinct from aortic coarctation, which is a congenital lesion. Multiple etiologies are responsible for the middle aortic syndrome and include a chronic inflammatory aortitis, atherosclerosis, and cystic medial necrosis. The disease is progressive and does not respond well to transluminal angioplasty. Thus, treatment consists of surgical revascularization. Although surgery is best performed after the patient is fully grown, the severity of disease may mandate an earlier aggressive surgical approach.

The radiographic manifestations depend on the specific vessels involved. Stenosis of a renal artery may result in a small kidney with delayed excretion of contrast medium on urography.

Arteriography is required to define the vascular involvement. A smooth tapering of the distal thoracic or abdominal aorta is seen. Narrowing often is severe and is usually most marked in the infrarenal aorta. The renal arteries are commonly affected with long stenoses (Fig. 9.7). Lateral views may demonstrate narrowing of the celiac or superior mesenteric arteries in as many as 90% of patients.

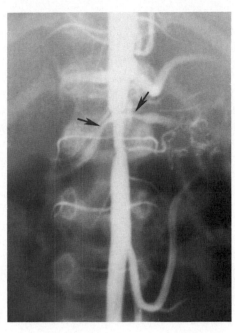

Figure 9.7.   Middle aortic syndrome. Tubular narrowing of the mid-aorta has resulted in bilateral right renal artery stenoses (*arrows*).

The middle aortic syndrome must be distinguished from Takayasu's disease. Patients with Takayasu's disease are usually slightly older and have other manifestations of arteritis, such as fever and an elevated sedimentation rate. The great vessels of the chest often are involved in Takayasu's disease, but not in the middle aortic syndrome.

Renal Transplantation

Approximately 50% of patients develop hypertension after receiving a renal allograft. In the early period after transplantation, acute rejection is the most common cause of hypertension. High-dose glucocorticoid therapy contributes to hypertension, but this can be reduced by using an alternate-day regimen for long-term therapy. Stenosis of the transplant renal artery is another possible cause of hypertension (Fig. 9.8). This stenosis may be caused by acute angulation or extrinsic compression of the artery, ischemic injury during vascular clamping, or intimal fibrosis due to rejection.

The incidence of hypertension is higher if the native kidneys are left in place than if they are removed. This is most likely due to activation of the renin-angiotensin system, because elevated renin levels can be measured in the native renal veins.

Renal Artery Aneurysm

There is an association between renal artery aneurysms and hypertension. However, it is not clear how often the hypertension is caused by the aneurysm.

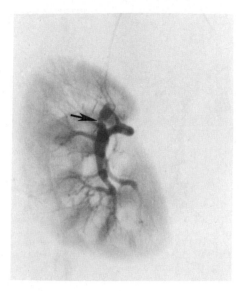

Figure 9.8.   Renal transplant. A focal transplant renal artery stenosis (*arrow*) is seen on this selective arteriogram.

Renin-mediated hypertension may be produced by extrinsic compression of the main renal artery or an intrarenal branch artery by the aneurysm, or by thrombus formation and occlusion of a branch artery.

Vaughan and colleagues reported on 41 hypertensive patients with renal artery aneurysms, but without associated renal or renal artery lesions. Narrowed vessels with delayed flow of contrast and a segmental decreased nephrogram distal to the aneurysm was interpreted as evidence of ischemia. Seven of eight (88%) patients followed for at least one year who underwent ipsilateral nephrectomy were cured. Other investigators, however, have found additional renal artery stenoses that were likely responsible for the hypertension.

SCREENING

Because it is extremely difficult to predict on a clinical basis which patients have renovascular hypertension, a radiographic screening test is needed. However, the prevalence of renovascular hypertension is less than 5% of all hypertensive patients, so it is impractical to apply these tests to all hypertensive patients. Thus, a group of patients at increased risk for renovascular hypertension is selected to undergo radiographic screening for renovascular hypertension. The following criteria often are used to select patients for radiographic screening:

1. Age extreme, usually younger than 20 or older than 50 years;
2. Recent onset of hypertension (less than 1 year);
3. Rapid acceleration of hypertension;
4. Malignant hypertension; and
5. A flank bruit.

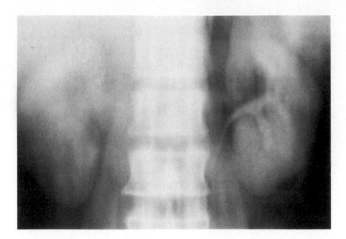

Figure 9.9. Hypertensive urogram. Delayed excretion from the right kidney indicates right renal artery stenosis.

A variety of radiographic screening tests have been used, and there is no consensus as to which is best. The choices may reflect local institutional bias, equipment available, physician interest or expertise, and the characteristics of the patient population.

Hypertensive Urography

Hypertensive urography is performed by rapidly injecting a bolus of contrast medium into a peripheral arm vein and obtaining sequential radiographs of the kidneys at 1-minute intervals for 5 minutes. Additional films also are obtained to examine the kidneys and the remainder of the urinary tract for other pathology.

Findings that suggest renovascular hypertension include a small kidney with delayed excretion (Fig. 9.9) and a delayed intense pyelogram. Extrinsic impression from collateral vessels also may be seen on the ureter or renal pelvis. The most reliable findings are delayed contrast excretion and a small kidney.

Earlier reports on hypertensive urography, including the 1972 publication of a multiinstitutional cooperative study by Bookstein and associates, recommended the use of hypertensive urography to screen patients suspected of renovascular hypertension. Those patients with a positive urogram were recommended for arteriography. However, further analysis has not supported this approach, and the false-negative (22%) and false-positive (13%) rates were too high for use as a screening test. Improvements in competing modalities combined with the insensitivity of the hypertensive urogram have resulted in its abandonment for this purpose.

Radionuclide Renography

Radionuclide renography has been used to detect renovascular hypertension, but results with iodine-131-labeled Hippuran have suffered from disappointingly high false-positive and false-negative rates. However,

the development of quantitative gamma camera renography and the use of technetium-99m diethylenetriaminepentaacetic acid (^{99m}Tc-DTPA) has improved the radionuclide results (Fig. 9.10).

During the past 5 years, radionuclide renography coupled with the administration of the angiotensin-converting enzyme (ACE) inhibitor, captopril, has emerged as the best radiologic method of screening for suspected renovascular hypertension in patients with normal renal function. The strength of the captopril renogram lies not only in a relatively high sensitivity (~90%) and specificity (~95%), but also in its ability to accurately predict which patients are likely to benefit from angioplasty or surgical revascularization. The examination is usually performed as a radionuclide renal perfusion study using ^{99m}Tc-DTPA; the study is then repeated after the oral administration of 50 mg of captopril. A positive study will demonstrate a profound decrease in the perfusion of the kidney when a significant RAS is present (Fig. 9.11).

This technique is effective because captopril does not

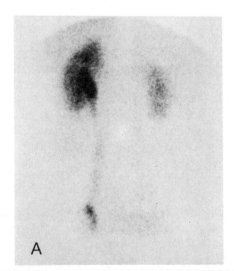

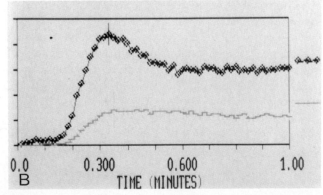

Figure 9.10. Radionuclide renogram. **A,** Posterior image of ^{99m}Tc-DTPA renogram demonstrates a small right kidney with impaired function. **B,** Time-activity curves during bolus injection. The left kidney is normal, but perfusion to the right kidney is markedly reduced.

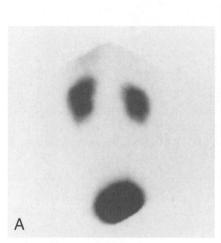
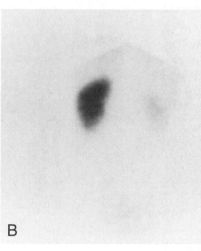
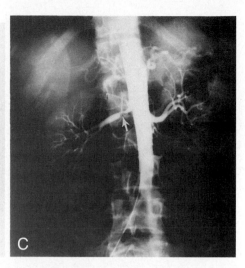

Figure 9.11. Captopril renogram. **A,** A posterior image demonstrates two kidneys of approximately equal size. **B,** A posterior view after 50 mg of an angiotensin-converting enzyme inhibitor (captopril) demonstrates markedly reduced perfusion to the right kidney indicating a hemodynamically significant renal artery stenosis. **C,** A right renal artery stenosis (*arrow*) is confirmed on conventional arteriography.

affect the glomerular filtration rate (GFR) in patients with normal renal arteries or those with essential hypertension. In patients with hemodynamically significant RAS, however, the conversion of angiotensin I to angiotensin II is blocked by the action of captopril; this produces efferent arterial vasodilatation and a corresponding decrease in renal perfusion pressure. This results in a decrease in GFR and a decrease in the accumulation of the tracer in the kidney with RAS.

Acceptance of captopril renography as the primary screening method has been hindered by the lack of a standardized protocol for the performance of the examination, which makes comparison of data from the published series difficult. There are differing opinions regarding whether imaging studies with and without captopril should be performed on separate days and whether a baseline study without captopril is even necessary. Some investigators prefer the use of ^{99m}Tc-DTPA, while others favor technetium-99m-mercaptoacetyltriglycine (^{99m}Tc-MAG$_3$) or even ^{131}I-labeled Hippuran.

Some difficulties and limitations with captopril renography have been reported. When there is significant impairment of renal function, the change in renal accumulation of the radiotracer may be difficult to appreciate. Occasionally, a profound decrease in blood pressure occurs, particularly in patients who are salt- or volume-depleted before the study. A false-positive result may be produced under such circumstances.

Doppler Ultrasound

The velocity of blood flow can be measured with Doppler ultrasound. If the peak velocity in the renal artery exceeds 100 cm/sec or the ratio of the peak renal artery to the peak aortic velocity is greater than 3.5, it is likely that a significant renal artery stenosis exists. However, there are numerous limitations to the use of this technique. The main renal arteries are more difficult to examine than the distal renal artery or its segmental branches. There may be more than one renal artery and the examination is time-consuming. More recently, attention has focused on Doppler study of intraparenchymal arteries to find the Doppler equivalents of the pulsus tardus. Although prolonged systolic acceleration times ($\geq$.07 sec) and reduced acceleration indices (<3.0 m/sec^2) have been reported with severe stenosis, the value for screening remains controversial.

Magnetic Resonance Angiography

Magnetic resonance angiography (MRA) is a noninvasive method of evaluating the renal arteries. As opposed to conventional angiography, which images a vessel lumen, MRA images blood flow. A vascular stenosis creates a flow disturbance that is larger than the anatomic abnormality. For this reason, MRA tends to overestimate the severity of stenosis. High-grade stenosis has the appearance of complete occlusion.

With current techniques, the sensitivity of MRA in detecting a significant stenosis of the main renal artery is approximately 90%. The clarity of the image, however, with current technology often is not sufficient to accurately grade the severity of a stenosis. (Fig. 9.12) In addition, the distal renal artery segmental branches are not seen well enough to be evaluated. This is a major disadvantage in patients suspected of having fibromuscular dysplasia. Accessory renal arteries are usually detected, but the aorta must be carefully scrutinized for polar vessels.

The major advantage of MRA as a screening examination for renal artery stenosis is that it is noninvasive

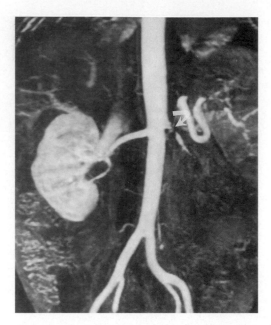

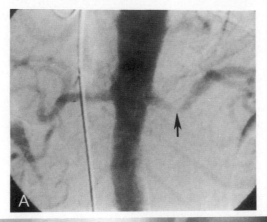

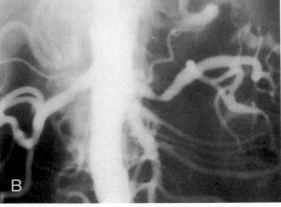

Figure 9.12. Magnetic resonance angiography. A high-grade left renal artery stenosis (*arrow*) is clearly demonstrated on this gadolinium-enhanced magnetic resonance angiogram. (From Prince MR, Narasimham DL, Stanley JC, et al: Breath-hold three-dimensional gadolinium-enhanced MR angiography: developments for imaging the abdominal aorta and its major branches. *Radiology* 197:785, 1995.)

Figure 9.13. Intravenous digital subtraction angiography. **A,** A left renal artery stenosis (*arrow*) is identified. **B,** The lesion is confirmed on a conventional aortogram.

and does not require iodinated intravenous contrast medium. Thus, MRA may be used in patients with compromised renal function without fear of contrast nephropathy. Its merit relative to radionuclide renography and Doppler sonography has not yet been clarified. Thus, in most centers, renal artery stenoses are further evaluated by conventional arteriography before surgical revascularization, unless there are contraindications to iodinated contrast media.

Digital Subtraction Arteriography

Digital subtraction angiography refers to manipulation of angiographic images by a digital computer. These techniques have slightly decreased spatial resolution, but have much better contrast sensitivity than conventional film–screen angiography. When performed with arterial contrast injections, much less contrast medium is required than with conventional arteriography. However, because of the excellent contrast sensitivity, diagnostic arterial images can be obtained after intravenous contrast injections (Fig. 9.13).

Dunnick and colleagues demonstrated improved results of intravenous digital subtraction arteriography (DSA) compared with hypertensive urography for detecting patients with renovascular hypertension. Intravenous DSA detects more patients with renal artery stenosis than urography and also can be used to detect patients with bilateral disease or patients with renal artery stenosis in a solitary kidney. However, intravenous DSA studies are seldom employed, because the images are inferior to intraarterial digital subtraction or conventional film–screen arteriograms.

Intraarterial digital subtraction arteriography (IA-DSA) also may be used to evaluate the renal arteries in patients suspected of renovascular hypertension. Because IA-DSA requires an arterial puncture, it is not as convenient for screening patients as intravenous DSA. However, much less contrast medium is used with IA-DSA, so it is useful in patients with azotemia, in whom a much smaller contrast volume is needed to minimize contrast nephropathy (Fig. 9.14). The quality of studies obtained with IA-DSA is excellent, such that conventional arteriography is no longer required to confirm findings on IA-DSA.

Conventional Arteriography

Conventional arteriography remains the gold standard for the detection of renal artery stenosis, because the spatial resolution of radiographic film is superior to digital systems. Once a lesion is detected, conventional

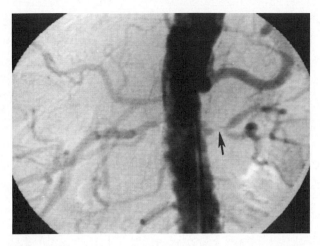

Figure 9.14. Intraarterial digital subtraction angiography. The intraarterial digital technique was used because of azotemia. Generalized atherosclerosis and stenosis of the left renal artery (*arrow*) are present.

arteriography is used to further characterize the stenosis, especially if intervention is contemplated. The etiology of the vascular lesion often can be predicted by its angiographic appearance.

The hemodynamic significance may be assessed by its severity and by the presence or absence of collateral vessels. Lesions must occlude at least 50% of the vessel diameter to be considered significant. However, this measurement is imprecise and does not assess the cross-sectional area or, more importantly, flow. Collateral vessels indicate that the lesion is significant, because alter-

nate pathways to provide flow have developed. Epinephrine may further restrict flow to the kidneys and may make these collaterals more apparent (Fig. 9.15).

The most appropriate treatment often may be determined by the nature and location of the stenosis. A focal stenosis of the main renal artery often responds to percutaneous transluminal angioplasty (PTA), whereas a long stenosis, orifice lesion, or bilateral disease does not do as well. In most centers, percutaneous transluminal angioplasty is the treatment of choice for a renal artery stenosis. However, surgery may be selected for lesions that will be technically difficult for PTA, or for lesions at the renal orifice, which may be caused by atherosclerosis of the aorta, rather than the renal arteries.

Renin Measurement

Because renovascular hypertension is renin mediated, serum renin levels should be elevated. Indeed, peripheral renin levels more often are elevated in patients with renovascular hypertension than in patients with essential hypertension. Sodium depletion has been used to reduce renal blood flow and further stimulate renin secretion.

Selective renal-vein sampling provides a method of measuring the renin level secreted by each kidney. Samples from the main renal veins and inferior vena cava are usually sufficient. If a renin-producing tumor or branch renal artery stenosis is suspected, more selective samples may be needed. The position of the catheter should be monitored fluoroscopically to make sure the catheter is correctly positioned before samples are obtained. Retroperitoneal collateral vessels and the go-

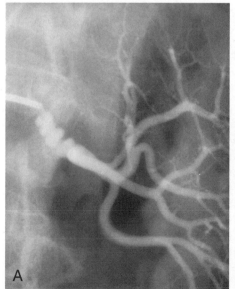
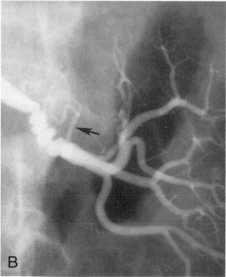

Figure 9.15. Renal artery stenosis with collateral vessels. **A,** A conventional left renal arteriogram demonstrates fibromuscular dysplasia. **B,** Repeat arteriogram after the intraarterial injection of 5 μgm of epinephrine shows collateral vessels (*arrow*) not seen on the initial run.

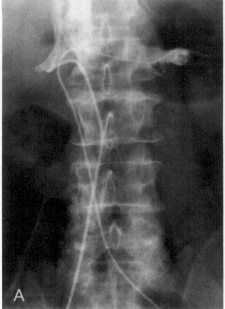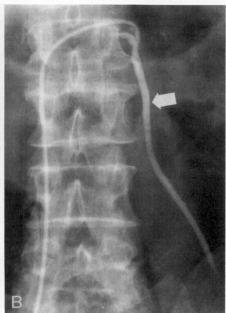

Figure 9.16. Renal vein renin collection. **A,** A catheter lies in each renal artery. **B,** Care must be taken not to draw samples from retroperitoneal or gonadal veins (*arrow*).

nadal veins must be avoided (Fig. 9.16). An ipsilateral/contralateral renal-vein renin ratio of 1.5 or greater is generally considered lateralizing and predictive of renovascular hypertension. Such patients are likely to be cured by correction of the renal artery stenosis.

Multiple studies support the use of this renal-vein renin ratio. A lateralizing ratio predicts a favorable response to correction of the renal artery lesion in more than 90% of patients. However, not all series report such high accuracy. A nonlateralizing result is not nearly as specific, because false-negative rates of greater than 50% are commonly reported. Thus, many physicians prefer to correct the renal artery lesion regardless of the renin measurements.

TREATMENT

Percutaneous Transluminal Angioplasty

Percutaneous transluminal angioplasty was first performed in 1963 and reported in 1964 by Dotter, who inadvertently cannulated an occluded iliac artery. Since then, major advances by Porstmann, Zeitler, and van Andel have contributed to the increasing use and success of the procedure. In 1976, Gruntzig introduced a sophisticated balloon catheter that allowed PTA to be performed on renal and coronary arteries. Since the first report of renal artery PTA in 1978, it has rapidly become accepted as the treatment of choice for many patients with renovascular hypertension.

Mechanism

Transluminal angioplasty procedures are designed to enlarge the lumen of a stenotic artery. Because athero-

matous material is not compressible, it must be fractured and pushed out into the wall of the artery. This requires a dehiscence of the intima of the renal artery. The arterial media also is split and the adventitia is stretched beyond its elastic recoil. The atheromatous plaque is forced into the medial portion of the artery. The adventitia remains intact, the media heals by fibrosis, and there is reendothelialization over the tears in the intima.

A similar process of controlled injury also occurs with nonatherosclerotic stenoses. The intima is disrupted, and the lesions are split or stretched beyond their point of elastic recoil.

Technique

Details of the many techniques and technical maneuvers that may be needed to perform percutaneous transluminal renal angioplasty are beyond the scope of this text; however, some basic principles are reviewed here to facilitate understanding the results and possible complications of the procedure.

The first step in PTA is to cross the stenosis. This is sometimes difficult, especially if the stenosis is tight or if the renal artery makes an acute angle as it arises from the aorta. In some patients, a brachial artery access facilitates crossing the lesion because it results in an obtuse angle of the renal artery rather than the acute angle if approached from below. An angiographic guidewire with a floppy tip is sufficient for most cases. However, steerable guidewires are now available that may be used in difficult cases with very tight stenoses. A platinum-tipped steerable guidewire that is available in 0.014- to 0.038-inch diameter may be used by itself or in coaxial fashion through a catheter.

A difficult stenosis also may be crossed without using a guidewire. A diagnostic catheter may be advanced through the stenosis while contrast is injected through the catheter. The contrast not only demonstrates the path of the catheter, but also tends to keep the tip of the catheter away from the vessel wall.

Once the lesion has been crossed, access should not be surrendered until the procedure is completed. Each time the guidewire is advanced, it has the potential to raise an intimal flap that may lead to further vessel damage and even arterial thrombosis. Thus, the guidewire is left across the lesion and the balloon catheter is passed over the wire until it is centered at the stenosis and ready for inflation.

One of the common problems during catheter and guidewire manipulation is vascular spasm. Arterial vasospasm can be severe enough to cause local ischemia and infarction. Thus, antispasmodic and anticoagulant medications are injected, either after the diagnostic catheter has been inserted or after the stenosis has been crossed. Nifedipine (10 mg orally) is a calcium channel blocker that may be administered 30 minutes before the procedure to prevent spasm. Other calcium channel blockers, such as verapamil hydrochloride, may be injected intraarterially to prevent or reverse arterial spasm. Nitroglycerine (100 μg, intraarterially) also is effective in reversing arterial spasm, especially after a calcium channel blocker has been administered.

The choice of the appropriate balloon angioplasty catheter is critical to the success of the procedure. Low-profile, hydrophilic, high-pressure balloon catheters contribute to a safe and effective dilatation. The size of the balloon depends on the size of the renal artery, not the stenosis. Magnification contributes only a small amount to the perceived vessel size if conventional angiographic films are used. However, magnification may be much greater if digital angiograms are measured. Some catheters now include centimeter markings to facilitate measurement. The diameter of the inflated balloon should be the size of the normal arterial lumen or 1 to 2 mm larger. Slight overdilation is preferable to underdilation. One commonly used method of selecting the appropriate size balloon is to use an angioplasty balloon equal to the size of the renal artery measured on a conventional arteriogram. Because there is slight magnification on the arteriogram, the fully inflated balloon will slightly overdilate the renal artery. In general, a balloon length of 2 cm is sufficient to dilate the renal artery stenosis without causing unnecessary damage to the normal renal artery.

The angioplasty balloon should be inflated with a mixture of contrast medium and saline. This provides sufficient opacity for easy visualization during fluoroscopy, and yet, is a less viscous fluid that will drain easily from the balloon once the dilation is accom-

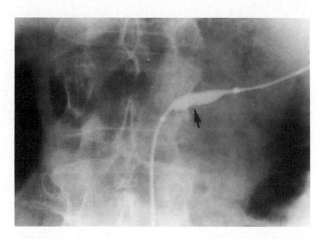

Figure 9.17.   Transluminal angioplasty. Fluoroscopic monitoring confirms proper placement of the angioplasty balloon by demonstration of balloon "waisting" (*arrow*) at the site of stenosis.

plished. Most angiographers dilute the 60% contrast medium used for catheter guidance with an equal amount of saline, resulting in a 30% contrast solution.

Inflation of the balloon should be monitored with a pressure gauge. Currently used polyethylene or Mylar catheters do not expand beyond their predetermined diameter, and too much pressure on injection can lead to balloon rupture. The balloon inflation also should be monitored fluoroscopically, since the stenosis can usually be seen as an indentation on the balloon, and the elimination of this "waist" indicates dilation of the stenosis (Fig. 9.17).

In an alert and cooperative patient, pain also may help monitor the balloon dilation. Some discomfort during dilation is expected. Lack of pain is a sign of underdilation, while severe pain may herald arterial rupture.

The balloon should be left inflated for 30 to 60 seconds, but care must be taken not to move the balloon while inflated. If a fully inflated balloon is moved, it converts the radial force into a shearing force that may completely disrupt the intima.

Results

The overall technical success rate for PTA is generally reported as 80 to 95%. Obviously, the number, type, and location of the lesions contribute significantly to the success or failure of the procedure. Better results can be expected with increased experience, and future reports should demonstrate improvement. Martin and colleagues reported a statistically significant increase in the technical success rate from 93 to 97% when results of the first 100 PTA cases were compared with the second 100 PTA cases. They also noted a concomitant decrease in the total complications from 20 to 13%. A variety of technical innovations also contribute to this improved suc-

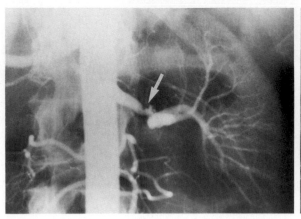
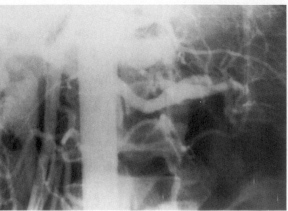

Figure 9.18. Transluminal angioplasty. **A,** A significant left renal artery stenosis (*arrow*) and poststenotic dilation are identified. **B,** After angioplasty, an excellent result is obtained.

cess. Better guidewires, catheters, and vascular sheaths as well as the use of less contrast medium, increased patient hydration, and digital imaging to speed the entire procedure all contribute to these improved results.

Recurrent stenoses occur in 10 to 20% of patients, but are most commonly seen when there is incomplete dilation of the lesion. Thus, it is most important to obtain a good initial result. A restenosis can be approached as a new lesion and attempts at redilating a recurrent stenosis are generally good, but with a slightly decreased success rate.

Some of the problems associated with renal artery angioplasty can be alleviated with a vascular stent. Several different types of stents are available for human use including the Wallstent endoprosthesis (Schneider; Zurich, Switzerland), Nitinol stent (Angiomed; Karlsruhe, Ger-

many), the Strecher stent (Medi-Tech; Watertown, MA), and the Palmaz stent (Johnson & Johnson Interventional Systems; Warren, NJ). Each stent has advantages and disadvantages. In view of the good results reported with balloon angioplasty, stent placement is reserved for patients who have an inadequate dilation, recurrent stenosis, renal artery dissection, or obstructive intimal flaps.

The results of angioplasty vary with the type of lesion responsible for the renal artery stenosis. Thus, the major categories are considered separately.

ATHEROSCLEROSIS. The best results are obtained with short, isolated stenoses in the midportion of the renal artery (Figs. 9.18 and 9.19). If the lesion is located at the origin of the renal artery, it may not be clear whether this is because of atherosclerosis of the renal artery or plaque within the aorta, which merely overhangs the origin of

Figure 9.19. Transluminal angioplasty. **A,** Preliminary arteriogram demonstrates generalized atherosclerotic changes as well as a tight renal artery stenosis (*arrow*). **B,** The lumen is widely patent after percutaneous transluminal angioplasty.

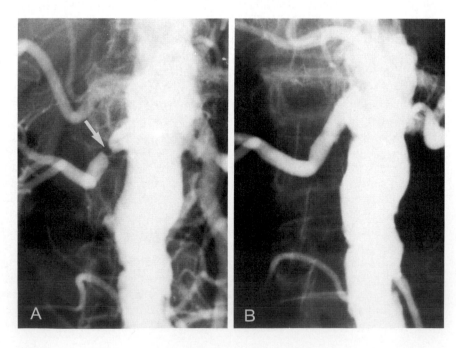

the renal artery. Dilation of atherosclerotic plaque in the proximal portion of the renal artery can be performed with excellent results. However, plaque that arises from the aorta is only displaced during the dilation procedure, and a large residual stenosis often persists.

When patients with atherosclerosis are analyzed, patients with occluded vessels or bilateral stenoses do not do as well as patients with unilateral nonostial lesions. Sos found that two thirds of patients with a unilateral stenosis could be successfully dilated, but only 20% of patients with bilateral stenoses had technical success on both sides. Most patients with a technically successful dilation experience cure or improvement in hypertension. The clinical response in patients with bilateral disease reflects the technical difficulties in obtaining technically successful dilation. If the renal arteries are adequately dilated, a good clinical response often is achieved. However, since there is a high failure rate of one or the other artery, the overall chances of a good clinical response to attempted bilateral renal artery angioplasty are relatively poor.

The likelihood of a successful result for percutaneous dilation of ostial renal artery stenosis has been considered poor. However, Martin and coworkers (1992) found no statistically significant difference in the long-term benefit of percutaneous angioplasty in a group of 110 patients with ostial renal artery stenosis compared with a control group of 94 patients with nonostial stenoses.

The clinical response to PTA cannot be measured immediately or even at discharge from the hospital, because hypertension can recur during the first few months after angioplasty. Thus, at least 3 to 6 months of follow-up are usually required to assess the durability of the clinical response. Lesions do not usually recur after 6 months, although a new lesion may form as the underlying process of plaque formation continues.

When all patients with atherosclerotic plaques are included, approximately 75% have a good clinical response to angioplasty. Approximately 25% of patients are cured (i.e., they become normotensive without medication). Approximately 50% of patients will be improved in that blood pressure is easier to control on fewer medications. Only approximately 25% of patients fail to respond because of the inability to dilate the renal artery stenosis or lack of blood pressure response.

FIBROMUSCULAR DYSPLASIA. Patients with fibromuscular dysplasia almost uniformly have good results from PTA. Since FMD typically occurs in young or middle-aged women, the access vessels are usually free of atherosclerotic plaque and tortuosity. Thus, the lesions are easier to approach. Although tight, web-like stenoses may be present, they seldom prevent guidewire and catheter access. Tegtmeyer, Kellum, and Ayers reported technical success in each of 27 patients with FMD; 10 (37%) were cured and 17 (63%) showed improvement

in hypertension. In 1985, Martin reported similarly excellent results, with 25% of patients cured and 60% improved.

TAKAYASU'S DISEASE. Although experience with PTA of renal artery stenosis secondary to aortoarteritis is not as extensive as with atherosclerosis or FMD, the results have been very good. Scattered reports in the American literature have shown a high rate of technical success and frequently good clinical response. Dong and associates performed PTA on 32 patients with Takayasu's arteritis in Beijing, People's Republic of China. A 6-month follow-up was available on 22 patients, 19 of whom benefited from the procedure. Thirteen patients were cured by PTA, 6 showed improvement, and only 3 failed to respond. All patients with unilateral disease had a good clinical response to PTA, while only 62% of patients with bilateral involvement were cured or improved.

RENAL TRANSPLANTATION. Percutaneous transluminal angioplasty of a renal artery stenosis in a transplanted kidney often is technically difficult. The renal artery may be placed as either an end-to-end anastomosis with the internal iliac artery, or an end-to-side anastomosis with the external iliac artery. Raynaud and colleagues performed PTA on 43 hypertensive renal transplant recipients who had stenosis of the transplant renal artery. In patients with end-to-side anastomoses, an ipsilateral femoral approach was used. In patients with an end-to-end anastomosis, a contralateral femoral approach was used most often, but an axillary approach was occasionally required. The procedure was technically successful in 35 (81%) patients, and 26 (74%) of these achieved clinical success. Most of the technical failures occurred in patients with end-to-end anastomoses.

NEUROFIBROMATOSIS. Renal artery stenosis is a common cause of hypertension in young patients with neurofibromatosis. The renal artery is surrounded by ganglioneuromatous or neurofibromatous tissue. Intimal proliferation, thinning of the media, and fragmentation of the elastic tissue lead to arterial stenosis. Percutaneous transluminal angioplasty of these lesions is extremely difficult and is rarely successful. Baxi and colleagues reported successful PTA of a renal artery stenosis in a 19-year-old woman with neurofibromatosis. They suggested that the lesion in that patient was more likely caused by dysplasia, which also may be seen in neurofibromatosis, but more frequently involves small intrarenal arteries.

Complications

Complications of renal artery PTA may be considered as general complications, such as adverse contrast reactions or problems at the puncture site, or as problems specific to renal artery PTA, such as a rupture, dissection, embolus, or thrombosis of the renal artery. Idio-

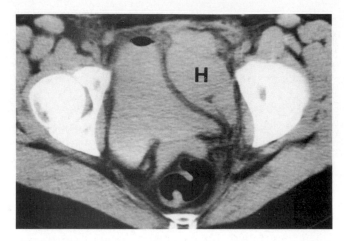

Figure 9.20.   Groin hematoma. A large pelvic hematoma (*H*) is detected by computed tomography after percutaneous transluminal angioplasty.

syncratic reactions to contrast media are rare, but should be treated as a reaction to intravenous contrast injection. Contrast-induced renal failure is a frequent problem, because many of these patients have preexisting azotemia, which is the primary risk factor for contrast nephropathy. Good hydration and judicious use of contrast medium will help to decrease the incidence of contrast-induced renal failure. Intraarterial digital subtraction techniques are particularly helpful in avoiding this problem, because much less contrast medium is required. Problems related to the puncture site at the groin or axilla include bleeding, hematoma (Fig. 9.20),

or false aneurysm formation. The use of a sheath helps to reduce trauma to the vessel at the puncture site and may decrease the incidence of these complications.

Major complications involving the renal artery occur in approximately 5% of patients. Renal artery dissection may result from a subintimal position of the guidewire or may result from the dilation of the renal artery by the angioplasty balloon. The location of the catheter after crossing the stenosis should be tested with a small contrast injection. Even when the PTA proceeds without problem, a renal artery dissection may occur. Gardiner and associates reported three such cases, each of which resolved without surgical intervention.

Thrombosis of the renal artery may be incited by disruption of the arterial intima, the presence of foreign material, or decreased flow due to occlusion of the renal artery by the angioplasty catheter. Vasospasm also may contribute to thrombosis by decreasing arterial flow (Fig. 9.21). Systemic anticoagulation is essential to prevent this problem. Prevention of arterial spasm by premedication supplemented with intraarterial nitroglycerin also is useful.

Renal artery rupture is an acute emergency that must be treated surgically. The rapid blood loss through the renal artery is life-threatening (Fig. 9.22). If rupture occurs, the catheter should be left in the renal artery and the balloon inflated in an attempt to occlude the bleeding vessel. This can be attempted while the patient is in the angiography suite, but does not alleviate the need for immediate surgery.

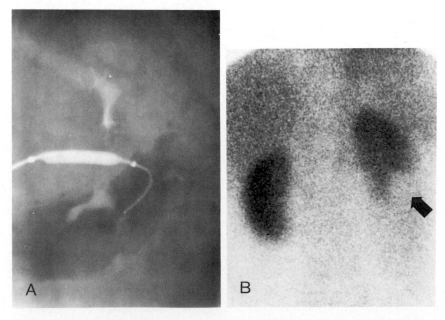

Figure 9.21.   Renal infarct. **A,** During angioplasty the guidewire was passed into a lower-pole vessel, inducing spasm. **B,** A radionuclide scan demonstrates absent perfusion to a portion of the lower pole of the left kidney (*arrow*).

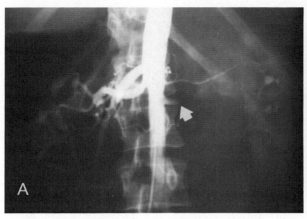 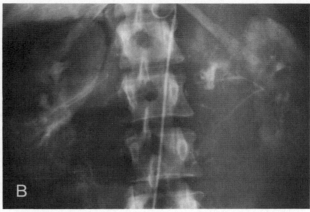

Figure 9.22.   Renal artery rupture. **A,** A sharp cutoff of the left main renal artery is seen (*arrow*). **B,** Contrast extravasation is appreciated on later films. The left kidney is displaced laterally by the retroperitoneal hematoma.

Embolization

Percutaneous transcatheter renal artery embolization may be used in a variety of clinical situations in which renal ablation is desired without surgery.

Patients with end-stage renal disease may have hypertension that is difficult to control. The native kidneys of renal transplant recipients are not routinely removed, as these kidneys may help to excrete water and secrete two important hormones, vitamin D_3 and erythropoetin. These patients are poor surgical risks, and mortality from bilateral nephrectomy ranges from 5 to 10%. The morbidity and mortality of transcatheter renal ablation (as judged by small series and case reports) is lower than surgical nephrectomy.

Renovascular hypertension is occasionally caused by a branch renal artery stenosis that cannot be crossed for PTA. If the feeding branch artery can be cannulated, that segment of the kidney can be infarcted in an attempt to cure the hypertension.

A variety of materials may be used to occlude the main renal artery or branch vessels to infarct renal tissue. Gelatin particles have been used, but recanalization may occur and an additional occluding material, such as a Gianturco coil, is needed. Cyanoacrylate, sodium tetradecol sulfate, and absolute ethanol also have been used successfully. As with embolization procedures for renal malignancy, these agents must be used with care to minimize complications.

RENOVASCULAR HYPERTENSION IN CHILDREN

The incidence of hypertension in children is 1 to 2%, much lower than the incidence in the adult population. The majority of these hypertensive children have a secondary cause.

Acquired renal parenchymal disease is the most common cause of hypertension among children. Other causes include the hemolytic uremic syndrome, renal trauma, nephrotic syndrome, and chronic pyelonephritis. Both acute glomerulonephritis and congenital malformation account for approximately 20% of cases of renal hypertension. In approximately 10%, it is renovascular hypertension. Children with renovascular hypertension tend to be younger and have higher levels of blood pressure than children with essential hypertension. Creatinine and urinalysis are usually normal in both groups.

The most common etiology of renovascular hypertension among children is FMD. Surprisingly, FMD is seen more commonly among boys than in girls. As in adults, the proximal portion of the renal artery is seldom involved, but unlike the adult population, the classic "string of beads" appearance is seldom seen in children.

Renal artery stenosis due to neurofibromatosis is the next most common etiology for renovascular hypertension in children. The proximal renal artery is involved, and an associated hypoplasia of the abdominal aorta may be involved.

The middle aortic syndrome due to nonspecific aortitis was responsible for 4 of the 30 cases of renovascular hypertension reported by Stanley and coworkers. An irregular narrowing of the aorta with stenosis of the proximal renal artery is seen in these patients, and bilateral involvement is usual.

Hypertensive urography is even less sensitive in children than in adults. Radionuclide tests are more promising, but in view of the high incidence of a secondary cause of hypertension, most children with suspected renovascular hypertension, undergo conventional arteriography. Digital techniques may be used, because less contrast medium is needed, and the examination may be performed more quickly than with conventional angiographic filming. However, intraarterial injections often are needed to maintain a good contrast bolus and to obtain optimal images.

Renal vein renin sampling is as useful in children as in adults. A lateralizing result correlates with a good response to intervention. Subselective samples may be required if segmental disease is present. Thus, venous samples are best obtained after angiography.

The treatment of renal artery stenosis causing renovascular hypertension in children has traditionally been surgical. However, PTA has become the treatment of choice in adults, and is being used with increasing frequency in children.

The success rate for PTA in children is lower than in adults for two reasons. The smaller size of the vessel and more frequent arterial vasospasm make children more difficult to angiogram and dilate. The most common etiologies of renal artery stenosis in adults, atherosclerosis and FMD, respond well to PTA, whereas many children have a more fibrotic process that cannot be adequately dilated.

Mali and associates reported the use of PTA in 12 children and adolescents with renovascular hypertension. They subdivided their patients on the basis of the length and location of the renal artery stenosis. Those patients with a short stenosis in the mid- or distal portion of the renal artery responded well to PTA. The patients with a short stenosis near the origin of the renal artery were dilated, but had a poor clinical response. Percutaneous transluminal angioplasty was technically unsuccessful in patients with a long stenosis at or near the origin or the renal artery.

SUGGESTED READING

Renal Parenchymal Hypertension

Amparo EG, Fagan CJ: Page kidney. *J Comp Assist Tomogr* 6(4):839, 1982.

Bonsib SM, Meng RL, Johnson FP Jr: Ask-Upmark kidney with contralateral renal artery fibromuscular dysplasia. *Am J Nephrol* 5:450, 1985.

Dunnick NR, Hartman DS, Ford KK, et al.: The radiology of juxtaglomerular tumors. *Radiology* 147:321, 1983.

Haab F, Duclos JM, Guyenne T, Plouin PF, Corvol P: Renin secreting tumors: diagnosis, conservative surgical approach and long-term results. *J Urol* 153:1781–1784, 1995.

Hattery RR, Hartman GW, Williamson B: Computerized tomography of nonvascular causes of renal hypertension. *Urol Radiol* 3:261, 1982.

Himmelfarb E, Rabinowitz JG, Parvey L, et al.: The Ask-Upmark kidney: roentgenographic and pathological features. *Am J Dis Child* 129:1440, 1975.

Kala R, Fyhrquist F, Halttunen P, et al.: Solitary renal cyst, hypertension and renin. *J Urol* 116:710, 1976.

Lemann J, Taylor AJ, Collier BD, Lipchik EO: Kidney hematoma due to extracorporeal shock wave lithotripsy causing transient renin mediated hypertension. *J Urol* 145:1238, 1991.

Messina LM, Reilly LM, Goldstone J, et al.: Middle aortic syndrome: effectiveness and durability of complex arterial revascularization techniques. *Ann Surg* 204:331, 1986.

Pak K, Kawamura J, Yoshida O: Hypertension with elevated renal vein renin secondary to unilateral hydronephrosis. *Urology* 16:499, 1980.

Schonfeld AD, Jackson JA, Somerville SP, Johnson CF, Anderson

PW: Renin-secreting juxtaglomerular tumor causing severe hypertension: diagnosis by computerized tomography-directed needle biopsy. *J Urol* 146:1607, 1991.

Sonda LP, Konnak JW, Diokno AC: Clinical aspects of nonvascular renal causes of hypertension. *Urol Radiol* 3:257, 1982.

Von Knorring J, Fyhrquist F, Ahonen J: Varying course of hypertension following renal trauma. *J Urol* 126:798, 1981.

Renovascular Hypertension

Berland LL, Koslin DB, Routh WD, Keller FS: Renal artery stenosis: prospective evaluation of diagnosis with color duplex US compared with angiography. *Radiology* 174:421, 1990.

Bude RO, Rubin JM: Detection of renal artery stenosis with Doppler sonography: it is more complicated than originally thought. *Radiology* 196:612, 1995.

Dunnick NR, Sfakianakis GN: Screening for renovascular hypertension. *Radiol Clin North Am* 29:497,1991.

Kaatee R, Beek FJA, Verschuyl EJ, et al: Atherosclerotic renal artery stenosis: ostial or truncal? Radiology 199:637, 1996.

King BF: Diagnostic imaging evaluation of renovascular hypertension. *Abdom Imaging* 20:395, 1995.

Lagneau P, Michel JB: Renovascular hypertension and Takayasu's disease. *J Urol* 134:876, 1985.

Laragh JH: The modern evaluation and treatment of hypertension: the causal role of the kidneys. *J Urol* 147:1469, 1992.

Lewis VD, Meranze SG, McLean GK, et al.: The midaortic syndrome: diagnosis and treatment. *Radiology* 167:111, 1988.

Mann SJ, Pickering TG: Detection of renovascular hypertension. State of the art: 1992. *Ann Intern Med* 117:845, 1992.

Portstmann W, Wierny L: Intravasale rekanalisation inoperabler arterieller obliterationeu. *Zentrabl Chir* 92:1586, 1967.

Silverman JM, Friedman ML, Van Allan RJ: Detection of main renal artery stenosis using phase-contrast cine MR angiography. *AJR* 166:1131, 1996.

Simon N, Franklin SS, Bleifer KH, et al.: Clinical characteristics of renovascular hypertension. *JAMA* 220:1209, 1972.

Spies JB, LeQuite MH, Robison JG, et al.: Renovascular hypertension caused by compression of the renal artery by the diaphragmatic crus. *AJR* 149:1195, 1987.

Wise KL, McCann EL, Dunnick NR, et al.: Renovascular hypertension. *J Urol* 140:911, 1988.

Wylie EJ, Binkley FM, Palubinskas AJ: Extrarenal fibromuscular hyperplasia. *Am J Surg* 112:149, 1966.

Aneurysm

Cummings KR, Lecky JW, Kaufman JJ: Renal artery aneurysms and hypertension. *J Urol* 109:144, 1973.

Vaughan TJ, Barry WF, Jeffords DL, et al.: Renal artery aneurysms and hypertension. *Radiology* 99:287, 1971.

Hypertensive Urography

Bookstein JJ, Abrams HL, Buenger RE, et al.: Radiologic aspects of renovascular hypertension. *JAMA* 220:1225, 1972.

Thornbury JR, Stanley JC, Fryback DG: Hypertensive urogram: a nondiscriminatory test for renovascular hypertension. *AJR* 138:43, 1982.

Radionuclide Renography

Chen CC, Hoffer PB, Vahjen G, et al.: Patients at high risk for RAS: A simple method of renal scintigraphic analysis with Tc^{-99m}DTPA and captopril. *Radiology* 176:365, 1980.

Dondi M, Monetti N, Fanti S, et al.: Use of technetium ^{99m}MAG$_3$ for renal scintigraphy after angiotensin-converting enzyme inhibition. *J Nucl Med* 32:424, 1991.

Postma CT, Van Oijen AHAM, Barantsz JO, et al.: The value of tests predicting renovascular hypertension in patients with RAS treated by angioplasty. *Arch Intern Med* 151:1531, 1991.

Russell CD, Thorstad B, Yester MV, et al.: Comparison of technetium^{-99m} MAG$_3$ with Iodine^{-131} Hippuran by simultaneous dual channel technique. *J Nucl Med* 29:1189, 1988.

Setaro JF, Chen CE, Hoffer PB, et al.: Captopril renography in the diagnosis of RAS and the prediction of improvement with revascularization experience. *Am J Hypertens* 4:698S, 1991.

Sfakianakis GN: Renal scintigraphy following angiotensin converting enzyme inhibition in the diagnosis of renovascular hypertension (captopril scintigraphy). *J Nucl Med Technol* 17(3):160, 1989.

Sfakianakis GN, Bourgoignie JJ, Jaffe D, et al.: Single-dose captopril scintigraphy in the diagnosis of renovascular hypertension. *J Nucl Med* 28:1383, 1987.

Doppler Ultrasound

Berland LL, Koslin DB, Routh WD, et al.: Renal artery stenosis: prospective evaluation of diagnosis with color duplex US compared with angiography. *Radiology* 174:421, 1990.

Hélénon O, Rody FE, Correas JM, et al.: Color Doppler US of renovascular disease in native kidneys. *RadioGraphics* 15:833–854, 1995.

Patriquin HB, Lafortune M, Jequier JC, et al.: Stenosis of the renal artery: assessment of slowed systole in the downstream circulation with Doppler sonography. *Radiology* 184:479, 1992.

Kliewer MA, Tupler RH, Carroll BA, et al.: Renal artery stenosis: analysis of Doppler waveform parameters and tardus-parvus pattern. *Radiology* 189:779, 1993.

Platt JF: Duplex Doppler evaluation of native kidney dysfunction: obstructive and nonobstructive disease. *AJR* 158:1035, 1992.

Magnetic Resonance Angiography

Debatin JF, Spritzer CE, Grist TM, et al.: Imaging of the renal arteries: value of MR angiography. *AJR* 157:981, 1991.

Debatin JF, Ting RH, Wegmüller H, et al.: Renal artery blood flow: quantitation with phase-contrast MR imaging with and without breath holding. *Radiology* 190:371, 1994.

Prince MR: Gadolinium-enhanced MR aortography. *Radiology* 191:155, 1994.

Prince MR, Narasimham DL, Stanley JC, et al.: Breath-hold three-dimensional gadolinium-enhanced MR angiography: developments for imaging the abdominal aorta and its major branches. *Radiology* 197: 785, 1995.

Digital Subtraction Angiography

Dunnick NR, Svetkey LP, Cohan RH, et al.: Intravenous digital subtraction renal angiography: use in screening for renovascular hypertension. *Radiology* 172:219, 1989.

Svetkey LP, Himmelstein SI, Dunnick NR, et al.: Prospective analysis of strategies for diagnosing renovascular hypertension. *Hypertension* 14:247, 1989.

Tonkin IL, Stapleton FB, Roy S, III: Digital subtraction angiography in the evaluation of renal vascular hypertension in children. *Pediatrics* 81:150, 1988.

Wilms GE, Baert AL, Staessen JA, et al.: Renal artery stenosis: evaluation with intravenous digital subtraction angiography. *Radiology* 160:713, 1986.

Renal Vein Renin

Harrington DP, Whelton PK, Mackenzie EJ, et al.: Renal venous renin sampling: prospective study of techniques and methods. *Radiology* 138:571, 1981.

Roubidoux MA, Dunnick NR, Klotman PE, et al.: Renal vein renins: inability to predict response to revascularization in patients with hypertension. *Radiology* 178:819, 1991.

Sos TA, Vaughan ED, Pickering TG, et al.: Diagnosis of renovascular hypertension and evaluation of "surgical" curability. *Urol Radiol* 3:199, 1982.

Thibonnier M, Joseph A, Sassano P, et al.: Improved diagnosis of unilateral renal artery lesions after captopril administration. *JAMA* 251:56, 1984.

Thind GS: Role of renal venous renins in the diagnosis and management of renovascular hypertension. *J Urol* 134:2, 1985.

Percutaneous Transluminal Angioplasty

Baert AL: Renal artery stent placement. *Radiology* 191:619, 1994.

Baxi R, Epstein HY, Abitbol C: Percutaneous transluminal renal artery angioplasty in hypertension associated with neurofibromatosis. *Radiology* 139:583, 1981.

Becker GJ, Katzen BT, Dake MD: Noncoronary angioplasty. *Radiology* 170:921, 1989.

Castaneda-Zuniga WR, Formanek A, Tadavarthy M, et al.: The mechanism of balloon angioplasty. *Radiology* 135:565, 1980.

Dong ZJ, Li S, Lu X: Percutaneous transluminal angioplasty for renovascular hypertension in arteritis: experience in China. *Radiology* 162:477, 1987.

Dotter CT, Judkins MP: Transluminal treatment of arteriosclerotic obstruction: description of a new technique and a preliminary report of its application. *Circulation* 30:654, 1964.

Freiman DB: Transluminal angioplasty of the renal arteries. *Radiol Clin North Am* 24(4):665, 1986.

Gardiner GA, Meyerovitz MF, Stokes KR, et al.: Complications of transluminal angioplasty. *Radiology* 159:201, 1986.

Gruntzig A, Kumpe DA: Technique of percutaneous transluminal angioplasty with the Gruntzig balloon catheter. *AJR* 132:547, 1979.

Gruntzig A, Vetter W, Meier B, et al.: Treatment of renovascular hypertension with percutaneous transluminal dilatation of a renal-artery stenosis. *Lancet* 1:801, 1978.

Harker CP, Steed M, Althaus SJ, Coldwell D: Flash pulmonary edema: an acute and unusual complication of renal angioplasty. *J Vasc Interv Radiol* 6:130–132, 1995.

Hayes JM, Risius B, Novick AC, et al.: Experience with percutaneous transluminal angioplasty for renal artery stenosis at the Cleveland Clinic. *J Urol* 139:488, 1988.

Hennequin LM, Joffre FG, Rousseau HP, et al.: Renal artery stent placement: long-term results with the Wallstent endoprosthesis. *Radiology* 191;713, 1994.

Kim PK, Spriggs DW, Rutecki GW, et al.: Transluminal angioplasty in patients with bilateral renal artery stenosis or renal artery stenosis in a solitary functioning kidney. *AJR* 153:1305, 1989.

Klinge J, Mali WPTM, Puijlaert CBAJ, et al.: Percutaneous transluminal renal angioplasty: initial and long-term results. *Radiology* 171:501, 1989.

Losinno F, Zuccalà A, Busato F, Zucchelli P: Renal artery angioplasty for renovascular hypertension and preservation of renal function: long-term angiographic and clinical follow-up. *AJR* 162;853, 1994.

Martin LG, Casarella WJ, Gaylord GM: Azotemia caused by renal artery stenosis: treatment by percutaneous angioplasty. *AJR* 150:844, 1988.

Martin LG, Cork RD, Kaufman SL: Long-term results of angioplasty in 110 patients with renal artery stenosis. *J Vasc Interv Radiol* 3;619, 1992.

Martin LG, Price TB, Casarella WJ, et al.: Percutaneous angioplasty in clinical management of renovascular hypertension: initial and long-term results. *Radiology* 155:629, 1985.

Matalon TAS, Thompson MJ, Patel SK, et al.: Percutaneous transluminal angioplasty for transplant renal artery stenosis. *J Vasc Interv Radiol* 3;55, 1992.

Miller GA, Ford KK, Braun SD, et al.: Percutaneous transluminal angioplasty vs. surgery for renovascular hypertension. *AJR* 144:447, 1985.

Park JH, Han MC, Kim SH, et al.: Takayasu arteritis: angiographic findings and results of angioplasty. *AJR* 153:1069, 1989.

Raynaud A, Bedrossian J, Remy P, et al. Percutaneous transluminal angioplasty of renal transplant arterial stenoses. *AJR* 146:853, 1986.

Roubidoux MA, Dunnick NR, Knelson M, Debatin JF: Renal revascularization: indications and results. *Urol Radiol* 14;18, 1992.

Sos TA: Angioplasty for the treatment of azotemia and renovascular hypertension in atherosclerotic renal artery disease. *Circulation* 83;Supp I-162, 1991.

Soulen MC: Renal angioplasty: underutilized or overvalued? *Radiology* 193;19, 1994.

Tegtmeyer CJ, Kellum CD, Ayers C: Percutaneous transluminal angioplasty of the renal artery: results and long-term follow-up. *Radiology* 153:77, 1984.

Tegtmeyer CJ, Sos TA: Techniques of renal angioplasty. *Radiology* 161:577, 1986.

van Andel GJ: *Percutaneous Transluminal Angioplasty—The Dotter Procedure*. Amsterdam, Excerpta Medica, 1976.

Zeitler E, Schoop W, Zahnow, W: The treatment of occlusive arterial disease by transluminal catheter angioplasty. *Radiology* 99:19, 1971.

Embolization

Bachman DM, Casarella WJ, Spiegel R, et al.: Selective renal artery embolization: treatment of acute renovascular hypertension. *JAMA* 238:1534, 1977.

Keller FS, Coyle M, Rosch J, et al.: Percutaneous renal ablation in patients with end-stage renal disease: alternative to surgical nephrectomy. *Radiology* 159:447, 1986.

Nanni GS, Hawkins IF, Orak JK: Control of hypertension by ethanol renal ablation. *Radiology* 148:51, 1983.

Reuter SR, Pomeroy PR, Chuang VP, et al.: Embolic control of hypertension caused by segmental renal artery stenosis. *AJR* 127:389, 1976.

Hypertension in Children

Casalini E, Sfondrini MS, Fossali E: Two-year clinical follow-up of children and adolescents after percutaneous transluminal angioplasty for renovascular hypertension. *Invest Radiol* 30:40–43, 1995.

Chevalier RL, Tegtmeyer CJ, Gomez RA: Percutaneous transluminal angioplasty for renovascular hypertension in children. *Pediatr Nephrol* 1:89, 1987.

Mali WPTM, Puijlaert CBAJ, Kouwenberg HJ, et al.: Percutaneous transluminal renal angioplasty in children and adolescents. *Radiology* 165:391, 1987.

Olson DL, Lieberman E: Renal hypertension in children. *Pediatr Clin North Am* 23(4):795, 1976.

Siegel MJ, St. Amour TE, Siegel BA: Imaging techniques in the evaluation of pediatric hypertension. *Pediatr Nephrol* 1:76, 1987.

Stanley P, Gyepes MT, Olson DL, et al.: Renovascular hypertension in children and adolescents. *Radiology* 129:123, 1978.

Stanley P, Hieshima G, Mehringer M: Percutaneous transluminal angioplastic for pediatric renovascular hypertension. *Radiology* 153:101, 1984.

10

Renal Failure and Medical Renal Disease

RENAL FAILURE

There is no clearly defined set of biochemical or clinical criteria that characterize "renal failure." Most authors use this term to describe a patient whose renal function is insufficient to maintain homeostasis. In this fashion, renal failure is distinguished from the term "renal insufficiency," which characterizes a patient whose renal function is abnormal, but capable of sustaining essential bodily functions. Uremia, the clinical syndrome that results from renal dysfunction, may be present in untreated patients with both renal insufficiency and renal failure. Uremia may result in symptoms related to a number of different organ systems including the gastrointestinal tract (nausea, vomiting), the cardiovascular system (hypertension, cardiac arrhythmias, pericarditis), the nervous system (personality changes, seizures, somnolence), and the hematopoietic system (anemia, bleeding diathesis). The term "end-stage renal disease" often is used to describe a patient with chronic renal failure whose renal deterioration is irreversible and requires dialysis or renal transplantation to sustain life.

Acute Renal Failure

Acute renal failure (ARF) is the sudden rapid deterioration in renal function. Classically, the causes of acute renal failure are divided into three broad categories: (*a*) prerenal, (*b*) renal, and (*c*) postrenal.

Prerenal causes are generally associated with volume depletion or renal hypoperfusion and are the most common causes of ARF. Such conditions include congestive heart failure, diuretic use, sepsis, dehydration, burns, hemorrhage, cirrhosis with ascites, and diabetic ketoacidosis.

Renal causes for ARF may result from damage to any portion of the kidney (i.e., the tubules, the glomerulus, the interstitium or the blood supply). *Acute tubular necrosis* (ATN) is among the most common of these causes. *Interstitial* causes for ARF include acute urate nephropathy, multiple myeloma, and acute interstitial nephritis.

Glomerular damage may cause ARF as a result of acute glomerulonephritis, drug toxicity, Goodpasture's syndrome, systemic lupus erythematosus, and other causes. *Vascular* causes for ARF include acute renal vein thrombosis, renal artery occlusion, and scleroderma.

Postrenal causes for ARF refer to the onset of renal failure secondary to acute obstruction. Although postrenal causes of ARF account for only 15% of the cases, this entity is the most commonly sought cause for ARF, because acute obstruction represents the most easily reversed cause of acute renal dysfunction.

Chronic Renal Failure

The gradual progressive loss of renal function characterizes chronic renal failure. The renal dysfunction is attributable to the loss of functioning renal parenchyma and, as such, is irreversible. The causes of chronic renal failure are protean, but may be related to vascular disease (i.e., generalized arteriosclerosis, arterial infarction), intrinsic renal disease (i.e., chronic glomerulonephritis, adult polycystic kidney disease), systemic disease (i.e., diabetes mellitus, hypertension), or may be the result of long-standing obstruction (i.e., neurogenic bladder disease, posterior urethral valves). In most cases, the process of chronic renal failure eventually results in the need for dialysis or renal transplantation.

IMAGING STUDIES IN RENAL FAILURE

Plain Film Radiography

A plain film of the abdomen offers much valuable information about the patient with renal failure. Although the older literature stressed the value of this study for determining renal size, such information is much more reliably obtained with ultrasound. However, the plain film should be used to detect renal parenchymal calcifications, to detect renal calculi or abnormal gas collections in the patient with urosepsis, and to collect valuable information about the bony pelvis, including the detection of unsuspected renal osteodystrophy or metastatic disease.

Excretory Urography

The role of excretory urography in the assessment of patients with renal failure has greatly declined since the advent of cross-sectional imaging techniques. High-dose urography with tomography became the accepted technique for the evaluation of patients with renal failure in the mid-1960s. When doses of contrast material in the range of 600 mg iodine/kg, careful radiographic technique, tomography, and delayed films were used, such studies were reported to have reliably demonstrated the renal outlines and the collecting system in more than 90% of patients with renal failure. In this fashion, it was possible to exclude obstruction as the cause of renal failure and to make an assessment regarding whether the renal failure was acute or chronic. However, aside from nephrogram analysis (*see* below), the availability of cross-sectional imaging techniques and the concern over the use of intravascular contrast media in patients with renal insufficiency have relegated this procedure to one of historical interest.

Nephrographic Analysis

Fry and Cattell first reported that analysis of the pattern of the nephrogram in patients with renal dysfunction could yield information regarding its etiology. They reported three distinct nephrogram patterns: (*a*) the immediate, faint, persistent nephrogram associated with chronic glomerular disease; (*b*) the increasing dense nephrogram or obstructive nephrogram, usually present in acute extrarenal obstruction, but also present with hypotension (Fig. 10.1), renal ischemia, acute glomerular disease, intratubular obstruction, and acute renal vein thrombosis; and (*c*) the immediate, dense, persistent nephrogram characteristically present in ATN (Fig. 10.2) and occasionally in severe renal inflammatory disease.

The immediate, faint, persistent nephrogram reaches

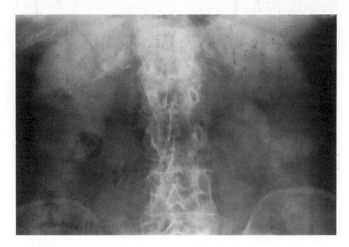

Figure 10.1. A 10-minute film from an excretory urogram demonstrates an increasing dense nephrogram without a pyelogram in a patient who became hypotensive after contrast administration. After fluid resuscitation, the findings resolved.

its maximum intensity shortly after the contrast is injected and persists for several hours. It represents a decrease in the number of functioning nephrons, a decrease in the ability of the kidney to concentrate urine, and an increase in diuresis secondary to azotemia. The pathogenesis of the *obstructive nephrogram* is poorly understood, but probably represents a combination of increasing tubular distention and increased salt and water resorption in the tubule as the result of obstruction. In systemic hypotension, the increasingly dense nephrogram is thought to occur as a result of increased salt and water resorption from the tubules and a reduced rate of clearance of the contrast from the plasma. In a patient suffering an acute hypotensive contrast reaction (*see* Fig. 10.1), the normal nephrogram pattern will be replaced by a dense, persistent nephrogram with a decrease in renal size and the loss of opacification of the collecting

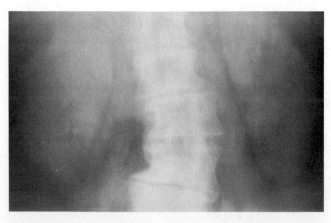

Figure 10.2. A 25-minute film from an excretory urogram in a patient with drug-induced acute tubular necrosis. An unchanging dense nephrogram is present.

system on subsequent radiographs. A variant of the obstructive nephrogram, known as the *striated nephrogram,* occurs when there is prominent visualization of the medullary rays, bundles of cortical nephrons that extend into the medulla. This pattern may be seen in acute extrarenal obstruction, pyelonephritis, and conditions associated with prolonged tubular transit of contrast material. The precise pathophysiology responsible for the immediate dense persistent nephrogram also is poorly understood, but may be related to recirculation of the contrast medium through the venous or lymphatic systems. While these patterns are not always specific, nephrographic analysis is frequently helpful in differential diagnosis.

Ultrasound

Ultrasound is the best available imaging study for the patient with renal failure. Ultrasound does not depend on renal function for the demonstration of renal anatomy; this is in contrast to urography, and to a lesser extent, computed tomography (CT), which depend on the kidney's ability to excrete contrast medium. Therefore, in a patient with renal failure, sonography can easily distinguish a patient with normal-sized kidneys (which generally indicates ARF) from one with small kidneys (which generally indicates chronic renal failure) (Fig. 10.3). Sonography also can readily define the patient with adult polycystic kidney disease and can accurately depict the presence of renal calculi, as a cause of or in association with renal failure.

Ultrasound can screen for renal failure caused by obstruction. Except for patients with bilateral iatrogenic postoperative obstruction, obstructive renal failure is usually chronic in nature and is associated with hydronephrosis; it is therefore readily detectable by ultrasound. Ritchie and colleagues retrospectively evaluated the diagnostic yield of sonography in 394 azotemic patients and found a 29% incidence of obstructive renal failure in a group of patients considered clinically to be at high risk for obstruction (i.e., known pelvic malignancy, known or suspected renal calculus disease, suspected urosepsis, a palpable mass, recent pelvic surgery, or bladder outlet obstruction). In patients without known risk factors, the incidence of obstructive renal failure was 1%. Similar conclusions were reached by Stuck and coworkers in a prospective study.

The accuracy of ultrasound in screening for chronic renal obstruction is discussed in Chapter 16.

Ultrasound also may provide limited information regarding the nature of the underlying renal disease. Normal kidneys have an echogenicity less than that of the liver or spleen. However, using newer ultrasound equipment, some investigators have observed that in many patients with normal kidneys the echogenicity of the renal cortex is equal to that of the liver. Most renal parenchymal diseases result in increased cortical echogenicity (Fig. 10.3). Although such a finding has a high specificity, it has a relatively low sensitivity for detecting renal disease on screening sonography. A small number of renal diseases including lymphoma, acute pyelonephritis, and renal vein thrombosis characteristically result in decreased cortical echoes. Gouty nephropathy, medullary nephrocalcinosis, renal tubular acidosis, and medullary sponge kidney may result in increased medullary echogenicity. Hricak and colleagues compared the ultrasonographic appearance of the kidneys with the results of renal biopsy in 109 patients. Although they found no direct correlation between the ultrasonographic appearance and a specific disease process, they found a significant correlation between increased cortical echogenicity and a decreased level of renal function.

Computed Tomography

Computed tomography should be considered as an imaging study in patients with renal failure when ultrasonography is inconclusive. Even without intravenous contrast medium, CT can detect hydronephrosis, although in some cases differentiation from some forms of renal cystic disease may be difficult. Computed tomography may be useful in delineating the point and nature of an obstruction, as the dilated ureter may be imaged on sequential sections (Fig. 10.4). Computed tomography provides an accurate assessment of renal size and the degree of cortical atrophy that may be present. In some forms of renal cystic disease, CT is the imaging study of choice to detect a complication of the disease process (i.e., hemorrhage complicating adult polycystic

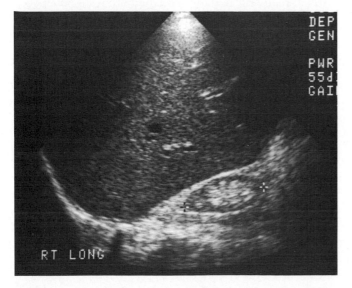

Figure 10.3. Longitudinal sonogram of the right kidney demonstrates a small echogenic kidney characteristic of chronic renal parenchymal disease.

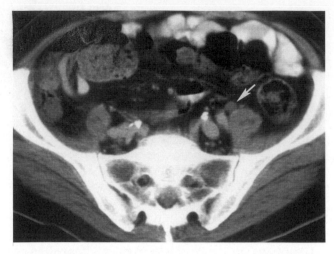

Figure 10.4. Noncontrast computed tomography scan through the pelvis demonstrates a dilated ureter (*arrow*).

disease or the development of a solid renal tumor in patients with acquired cystic disease). Finally, CT is highly sensitive for the detection of renal calculi, even those not demonstrated on conventional radiography.

Radionuclide Studies

Because the excretion of radiopharmaceuticals depends on renal function, they cannot be used to evaluate all patients with renal failure. This is particularly the case with technetium-99m diethylenetriaminepentaacetic acid (^{99m}Tc-DTPA), as it is excreted primarily by glomerular filtration. Iodine 131–labeled Hippuran and technetium-99m-mercaptoacetyltriglycine (^{99m}Tc-MAG$_3$), however, are excreted by tubular secretion, and thus may demonstrate the kidneys even when renal dysfunction is relatively advanced. Because ^{131}I-Hippuran has relatively poor imaging characteristics, its primary use is to produce time-activity curves (*see* Chapter 3) and to evaluate differential renal function when a unilateral process is present. If obstruction is present, a percutaneous nephrostomy tube or a double-J ureteral catheter should be placed before performing a radionuclide scan to estimate residual renal function, because potentially recoverable renal function will likely be overestimated if renography is performed while the kidneys are still obstructed.

Radionuclide determination of the glomerular filtration rate also may be of value in some forms of medical renal disease (*see* Chapter 3).

Other Imaging Studies

The role of *angiography* is extremely limited in the diagnostic evaluation of renal failure. Occasionally the angiographic features of end-stage renal disease will be encountered in patients being evaluated for another purpose. Such features include a pruned, tortuous ap-

pearance of the intrarenal vessels, thinning of the renal cortex, and a slowing of arterial flow within the kidneys. The angiographic nephrogram may have a mottled or lucent appearance. A number of systemic diseases associated with renal failure may demonstrate multiple microaneurysms, including Wegener's granulomatosis, polyarteritis nodosa, and systemic lupus erythematosus (*see* Chapter 8). *Renal venography* is frequently necessary to confirm the diagnosis of renal vein thrombosis.

Magnetic resonance (MR) imaging was initially thought to have great promise for the evaluation of chronic renal failure. This hope was based on reports that loss of the corticomedullary distinction (CMD) was a relatively specific finding in some forms of medical renal disease. It has subsequently been shown, however, that the loss of the CMD is not specific and may be present in normal patients who are well hydrated. There is continued hope, however, that magnetic resonance spectroscopy may provide relatively disease-specific patterns in some forms of renal failure.

Antegrade and *retrograde pyelography* are useful in establishing the diagnosis of ureteral obstruction as a cause for renal failure (*see* Chapter 16).

Small kidneys are found in many conditions that lead to chronic renal failure including chronic glomerulonephritis, diabetic nephrosclerosis, hypertensive nephropathy, generalized renal arteriosclerosis, and analgesic nephropathy.

MEDICAL RENAL DISEASE

Acute Tubular Necrosis

Acute tubular necrosis is the most common form of acute reversible renal failure. It has a wide range of causes including hemolysis, dehydration, hypotension, drugs (contrast media, aminoglycosides, and other antibiotics), heavy metals, and solvent exposure. ATN is commonly seen after cadaveric renal transplantation (*see* Chapter 11). The exact pathogenesis of ATN is poorly understood, but some authorities believe that direct tubular damage is the initiating event and results in filling of the tubular lumen with cellular debris. Others believe that ATN is probably related to a disturbance in the renin–angiotensin axis that results in a global decrease in renal blood flow. Proponents of this theory prefer the term "acute vasomotor nephropathy," because they believe that there is little primary tubular damage and that the renal failure occurs because of a redistribution of blood flow within the kidney.

The renal failure may be oliguric or nonoliguric. During the acute phase, azotemia is present, with blood urea nitrogen and creatinine levels peaking after 10 to 30 days. The return of renal function is typically heralded by the onset of a diuresis and a rapid return of renal function.

The kidneys in patients with ATN are enlarged bilaterally. Urography, although no longer recommended as a diagnostic procedure, characteristically demonstrates a dense persistent nephrogram as discussed above (*see* Fig. 10.2). In a minority of patients, an increasingly dense nephrogram, more characteristic of acute extrarenal obstruction, may be found. The nephrogram may be present for as long as 24 hours after contrast administration. There is typically no opacification of the collecting system.

A variety of sonographic appearances of ATN have been reported. Some authors report an increase in cortical echogenicity with preservation of corticomedullary definition. Others have noted an increase in the echogenicity of the pyramids with a normal cortical appearance, whereas the opposite appearance (i.e., a decrease in the echogenicity and swelling of the pyramids), has been observed by still others. Rosenfield and colleagues have suggested, based on experimentally induced ATN in rats, that the sonographic appearance of ATN depends on its etiology, thus accounting for the variable appearances reported. Platt and coworkers have suggested that an elevated resistive index (RI) on duplex Doppler imaging is present in a majority of patients with renal failure secondary to ATN; they found this elevated RI in only 20% of patients in whom the azotemia was related to prerenal causes.

On CT, nephromegaly with a patchy nephrogram may be found (Fig. 10.5).

Initial enthusiastic reports that MR imaging would be helpful in differentiating renal transplant rejection from ATN have not been borne out. However, a report by Carvlin and colleagues demonstrated that gadolinium-enhanced MR imaging studies show perfusion abnormalities in experimentally induced ATN. Additional work is necessary to confirm the clinical utility of these observations.

Acute Cortical Necrosis

Acute cortical necrosis is a distinct form of ARF that results in ischemic necrosis of the renal cortex, including the columns of Bertin, while the medullary portions of the kidney are relatively spared. The process may occur diffusely throughout both kidneys and may result in complete absence of renal function or may occur in a patchy distribution, resulting in renal insufficiency. In both instances, there is a characteristic sparing of a thin rim of cortical tissue on the outer surface of the kidney because of preservation of the capsular blood supply. A large number of conditions are reported in association with cortical necrosis including burns, sepsis, snake bites, toxins, transfusion of incompatible blood, dehydration, and peritonitis. More than two thirds of the cases, however, are reported to be associated with pregnancy, especially those complicated by placental abruption, septic abortion, or placenta previa. The precise mechanism by which cortical necrosis occurs remains obscure, however, a transient episode of intrarenal vasospasm leading to cortical ischemia is regarded as the probable mechanism by most authors. Other possible explanations include intravascular thrombosis and damage to the glomerular capillary endothelium.

The radiographic findings depend on the stage of the illness. In the early stages of the disease, the kidneys are diffusely enlarged. On urography, there may be faint opacification of the collecting system, particularly if patchy cortical involvement is present. Over the course of several months, there will be smooth renal shrinkage. Characteristically, this will be accompanied by a distinctive form of tram-like calcification throughout the cortex, including the septal cortex (Fig. 10.6 and 12.1A). The appearance of this calcification has been reported as early as 24 days after the onset of the illness, but

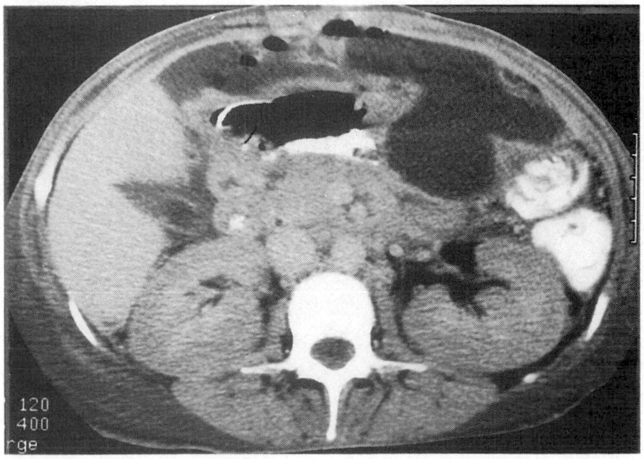

Figure 10.5. Computed tomography scan of the abdomen shows a patchy nephrogram in a patient with acute tubular necrosis secondary to sepsis. Computed tomography was performed in search of an underlying abscess.

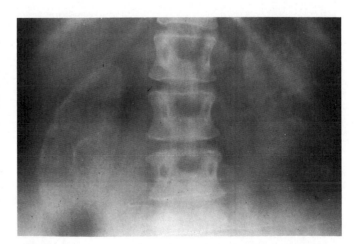

Figure 10.6. Acute cortical necrosis. Bilateral cortical calcifications characteristic of cortical necrosis are present. (From Pollack HM (ed): *Clinical Urography*. Philadelphia, WB Saunders, p. 1771, 1990.)

more characteristically is reported at approximately 2 months. On ultrasonography, the outer cortex is hypoechoic, a finding that has been reported soon after the onset of the disease. On contrast-enhanced CT scans, a zone of absent contrast enhancement at the periphery of the kidneys is said to be characteristic.

Acute Interstitial Nephritis

Acute interstitial nephritis (AIN) is an acute hypersensitivity reaction in the kidney that may result in renal insufficiency or frank renal failure. Three forms of AIN have been described: (*a*) in association with a variety of drugs; (*b*) in association with a number of nonrenal infectious processes (e.g., infectious mononucleosis); and (*c*) in an idiopathic form. Drug-induced AIN is the most common of these. More than 40 compounds, including penicillin, and particularly methicillin, rifampin, sulfonamide derivatives, nonsteroidal antiinflammatory agents, cimetidine, furosemide, and thiazide diuretics, have been associated with AIN.

Cell-mediated immune mechanisms appear to be more important than humorally mediated mechanisms in the pathogenesis of AIN. Histologically, AIN is characterized by an interstitial infiltration of inflammatory cells including eosinophils and mononuclear cells without a significant component of arteritis or glomerulitis. In some forms of AIN, eosinophiluria may be found on clinical examination. Other common clinical signs and symptoms include macroscopic or microscopic hematuria, nonnephrotic range proteinuria, fever, eosinophilia, skin rash, and oliguria. Typically, there is recovery from the renal failure on withdrawal of the drug.

On urography, bilateral nephromegaly with diminished opacification of the collecting system has been reported (Fig. 10.7). On ultrasound, increased cortical echogenicity and renal enlargement may be found. Increased accumulation of gallium-67 (^{67}Ga) citrate in the kidneys also has been reported.

Hematologic Disorders

Sickle Cell Anemia

A variety of morphologic abnormalities, including bilateral renal enlargement, lobar infarction, papillary necrosis (Fig. 10.8), and dilatation of the collecting system have been described in patients with heterozygous and homozygous sickle cell disease. The later abnormality is thought to occur secondary to a decrease in the kidney's ability to concentrate urine. In addition to these structural defects, a number of functional abnormalities including hyposthenuria, hematuria, renal tubular acidosis, and progressive renal insufficiency have been described in patients with sickle cell anemia. This constellation of functional abnormalities is known as *sickle cell nephropathy*.

The older literature suggested that papillary necrosis is uncommon among homozygous patients, whereas it is common in the heterozygous forms, particularly when hemoglobin S is combined with hemoglobin A (SA disease) or hemoglobin C (SC disease). The more recent literature, however, reports that changes of papillary necrosis are present in approximately 25 to 40% of homozygous patients. The appearance of the radiologic abnormalities, however, does not necessarily correlate with the presence of renal functional abnormalities. Papillary necrosis is thought to occur as a result of low oxygen tension in the renal papilla that promotes sickling of the abnormal red blood cells. This, in turn, results in necrosis and ischemia of the papillary tips.

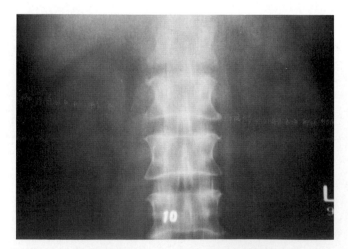

Figure 10.7. Acute interstitial nephritis. Bilateral nephromegaly, a diminished nephrogram, and a faintly opacified collecting system are demonstrated in this patient with drug-induced acute interstitial nephritis.

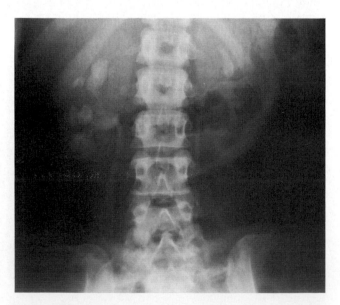

Figure 10.8. Marked calyceal deformity compatible with papillary necrosis is present bilaterally in this patient with known homozygous sickle cell anemia.

Lande and colleagues found that MR imaging in patients with sickle cell disease demonstrates decreased signal from the renal cortex that is especially apparent on T2-weighted images. These authors speculated that the findings were secondary to iron deposition in the renal cortex. Similar findings, however, were not present in a group of patients suffering from β-thalassemia who also were suffering from iron overload.

Recently, a new malignant renal tumor, renal medullary carcinoma, has been described in patients with underlying sickle cell trait (*see* Chapter 6).

Hemophilia

A variety of urographic abnormalities including bilateral renal enlargement, retroperitoneal hemorrhage, and obstructive uropathy secondary to clots within the collecting system or ureter have been described in patients with hemophilia. The most striking feature, bilateral nephromegaly, is of uncertain etiology. Papillary necrosis, thought to be related to concomitant analgesic ingestion, also has been described.

Acute Leukemia

Leukemia is the most common malignant cause of bilateral nephromegaly in children (Fig. 10.9). The renal enlargement is commonly attributed to infiltration of the kidneys by leukemic cells; however, intrarenal hemorrhage and edema also contribute to this appearance. The degree of renal enlargement may be striking, simulating the appearance of polycystic disease. In some cases, the renal enlargement may be asymmetrical, and rarely, it may occur as a focal intrarenal mass (chloroma). The collecting system is generally attenuated, and there may be filling defects in the renal pelvis or calyces secondary to blood clots or uric acid stones.

Multiple Myeloma

Multiple myeloma is one of a group of plasma cell dyscrasias that includes Waldenström's macroglobulinemia, heavy- and light-chain disease, and benign monoclonal gammopathy. The disease results in excess production of immunoglobulins and is characterized by the presence of Bence-Jones proteins in the urine. Renal failure occurs in 30 to 50% of such patients and has been attributed to the abnormal precipitation of myeloma proteins within the renal tubules, dehydration, or superimposed renal infection. Hypercalcemia, as a result of the bone destruction that accompanies the myelomatous lesions in bone, may result in nephrocalcinosis. Because there is excess uric acid production, uric acid calculi also may be found. Amyloidosis develops in approximately 10% of the patients.

Radiologically, the kidneys are enlarged and there may be attenuation of the collecting system as the result of interstitial edema. Poor opacification on urography

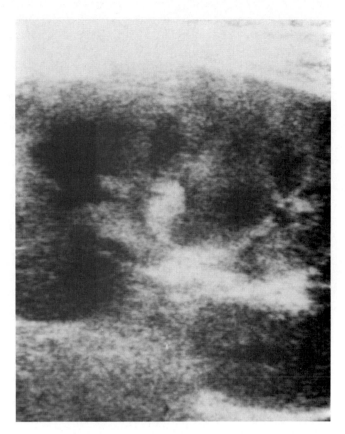

Figure 10.9. Marked nephromegaly is present in this child with proven leukemic infiltration of the kidneys.

typically occurs because of the diminished renal function. On ultrasonography, the kidneys are enlarged with decreased echogenicity that reflects the abnormal fluid accumulation within the kidney.

The administration of intravenous contrast media to patients with multiple myeloma was thought to be contraindicated because of reports that contrast media caused precipitation of the myeloma proteins within the renal tubules, thereby hastening the onset of renal failure. More recent literature, however, suggests that the risks associated with contrast administration in patients with myeloma can be minimized as long as dehydration is avoided.

Amyloidosis

Amyloidosis is characterized by the extracellular deposition of an insoluble fibrillar proteinaceous material with a β-sheet configuration. Although the disease may be localized to one organ, in more than 85% of the cases, a systemic multiorgan form of involvement is present. The disease is known to occur as an idiopathic systemic process (primary amyloidosis); in association with a variety of other chronic diseases including rheumatoid arthritis, tuberculosis, leprosy, chronic osteomyelitis, and some malignancies (*secondary amyloidosis*); in a familial form including that associated with familial Mediterranean fever; in a senile form; or in association with endocrine disorders, including medullary carcinoma of the thyroid and diabetes. Each of these forms is associated with its own characteristic protein subunit. The protein found in patients with primary amyloidosis and those with amyloid disease associated with multiple myeloma are identical and resemble a portion of an immunoglobulin light chain. This fact suggests that the two diseases are different manifestations of a similar underlying blood dyscrasia and most authorities now classify amyloidosis as a blood dyscrasia. A new specific form of amyloidosis has been recognized that results in a multiarticular arthropathy in patients on long-term hemodialysis.

Virtually every organ in the body may be involved; men are affected more commonly than women. The usual age of onset is 55 to 60 years. Most patients experience nonspecific symptoms including weight loss, weakness, and fatigue. Renal involvement occurs in 80% of patients with secondary amyloidosis and 35 to 40% of patients with primary disease. Fifty percent of patients with secondary amyloidosis die of renal failure. Although the kidneys are the most commonly involved organ in the urinary tract, isolated involvement of the renal pelvis, ureter, bladder, urethra, prostate, retroperitoneum, and seminal vesicles has been described. Amyloidosis of the renal pelvis, without renal parenchymal involvement, may be associated with a characteristic pattern of submucosal calcification visible on plain films. Renal vein thrombosis is a well-described complication of renal amyloidosis and may only affect the segmental or interlobar veins as a unique feature. The sudden onset of nephrotic syndrome in a patient with amyloidosis should suggest the development of this complication.

The radiologic findings in renal amyloidosis are nonspecific. Although some patients have normal-sized kidneys, the most consistently described feature is smooth bilateral renal enlargement (Fig. 10.10). As the disease progresses and renal failure ensues, the kidneys decrease in size while retaining their smooth contour. On urography, the nephrogram is typically diminished, and there may be attenuation of the collecting system. On sonography, there is renal enlargement in the acute phase with an increase in cortical echogenicity, presumably related to the abnormal protein deposition. Angiographic features include tortuosity and irregularity of the interlobar arteries, which may be localized to one portion of the kidney. An abnormal accumulation of ^{67}Ga citrate in the kidneys 48 to 72 hours after injection has been described on radionuclide examination.

Rhabdomyolysis/Myoglobinuria

Rhabdomyolysis, an acute disruption of the structural integrity of skeletal muscle cells, is a frequent complication of trauma. Other causes include thermal or ischemic muscle necrosis, drugs (including heroin, amphetamines, and alcohol), and polymyositis. Such injuries result in an increase in the serum concentration of creatine phosphokinase (CPK) and the excretion of an excessive quantity of myoglobin in the urine. Although myoglobin is considered to be nephrotoxic, there is a poor correlation between urine myoglobin levels and the degree of renal failure. In most instances, the renal failure is transient with the eventual return of normal renal function.

Imaging findings have been reported in a few cases. Nephromegaly with an increasingly dense or striated nephrogram on both CT and urography may be found. With more advanced renal failure, severe impairment of contrast excretion may be present (Fig. 10.11).

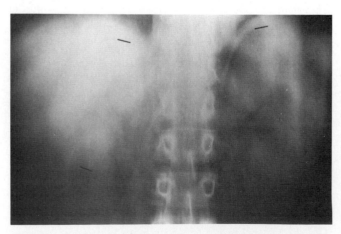

Figure 10.10. Renal amyloidosis. Bilaterally enlarged, poorly functioning kidneys are present on urography in this patient with proven renal amyloidosis. (Courtesy Marco A. Amendola, M.D.)

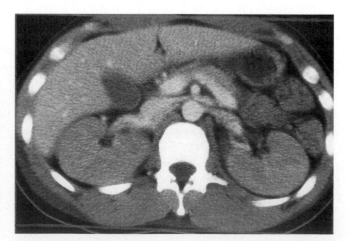

Figure 10.11. Acute renal failure secondary to rhabdomyolysis. The nephrogram is virtually absent despite excellent enhancement of the renal veins, inferior vena cava, and aorta (Courtesy of Akira Kawashima, M.D.).

Acute Urate Nephropathy

Increased nucleoprotein catabolism may occur as a complication of chemotherapy or radiation therapy in patients with leukemia, lymphoma, and other neoplastic disorders. As a consequence, there is a marked increase in plasma uric acid concentration, increased renal tubular secretion, and possibly decreased resorption of the filtered urate load. In such cases, precipitation of urate crystals within the tubules resulting in oliguric renal failure may occur. This form of ARF is termed urate nephropathy.

An increasingly dense nephrogram with enlarged kidneys and an absent or markedly diminished pyelogram has been reported on urography (Fig. 10.12). As contrast medium is a known uricosuric agent, precipitation of acute urate nephropathy in patients with high plasma uric acid concentrations also may theoretically occur after contrast administration.

Increased medullary echogenicity on ultrasonography has been reported in patients with hyperuricemia and clinical evidence of gout.

Diabetic Nephropathy

Diabetic nephropathy is the most common cause of chronic renal failure in the United States. It is believed to occur as a result of glomerular hyperperfusion that results in glomerular hypertension. This results in an increase in transcapillary pressure and protein leakage into the mesangium. This process leads to microalbuminuria and glomerular sclerosis.

The occurrence of diabetic nephropathy is highly correlated with insulin dependence and has recently been correlated with poor glycemic control. Studies have shown that among patients with insulin-dependent diabetes for more than 25 years, the incidence of diabetic nephropathy has declined from more than 25%

during the 1960s to less than 10% during the 1980s, as the importance of glucose control has been recognized. Fully developed nephrotic syndrome generally occurs after 15 to 20 years of insulin dependence, with a resultant decrease in glomerular filtration rate heralding the onset of overt renal failure.

Early in the course of diabetes, imaging studies frequently show generalized nephromegaly. Indeed, diabetes is the most common cause of this finding. In some cases, the nephromegaly may be found before overt glycosuria develops. Although the exact etiology of the renal enlargement is not known, nephron hypertrophy is a possible explanation. Later in the disease process, there is a progressive reduction in renal size and an increase in echogenicity of the renal cortex with preservation of the corticomedullary junction on ultrasonography. With overt renal failure, the kidneys become small, with the echogenicity of the medulla equal to that of the cortex. Platt has suggested that the resistive index (RI) is generally elevated (>0.70) in patients with established diabetic nephropathy, but is normal in diabetics without nephropathy or those with proteinuria but without azotemia.

HIV Nephropathy

Azotemia, with moderate to severe proteinuria, occurs in approximately 10 to 30% of patients with human immunodeficiency virus (HIV) infection. A variety of glomerular lesions, including focal and segmental glomerulosclerosis with mesangial deposits of complement C3, IgM, or IgG, as well as tubular atrophy, have been found on histologic examination. Other forms of glomerulopathy also have been described. The combination of renal insufficiency, nephrotic syndrome, and glomerular changes has been called HIV nephropathy. The disease may result in profound hypoalbuminemia, although hypertension and peripheral edema are characteristically absent. Because renal insufficiency may be the first manifestation of HIV infection, the disorder is properly termed HIV-associated nephropathy rather than acquired immunodeficiency syndrome (AIDS)-associated nephropathy. There is a striking predominance of black male patients. Despite hemodialysis, death usually occurs within 6 months.

On ultrasound examination, approximately 50% of the patients with abnormal renal function will demonstrate normal sonographic findings, while the remainder show increased cortical echogenicity with normal-sized or enlarged kidneys. Hamper and coworkers found there was a correlation between the degree of increased cortical echogenicity and the severity of both the tubular and glomerular changes on histologic examination.

On CT, global renal enlargement with or without hydronephrosis and cortical scarring has been described (Fig. 10.13). On MR imaging, nephromegaly with loss of

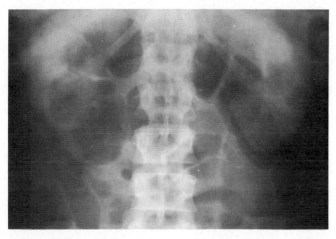

Figure 10.12. Bilateral renal enlargement and an increasing dense nephrogram are present in this patient with acute urate nephropathy.

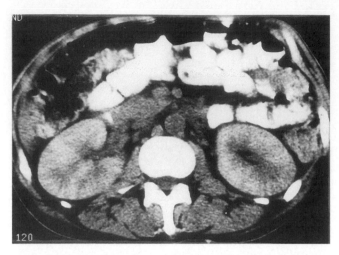

Figure 10.13. HIV nephropathy. Computed tomography scan demonstrates bilateral nephromegaly and a striated persistent nephrogram in this patient with HIV nephropathy. The contrast medium had been administered 24 hours earlier for a computed tomography scan of the head

corticomedullary distinction on T1-weighted images has been found as a nonspecific finding.

Alport's Syndrome

The association of chronic hereditary renal disease, deafness, and ocular abnormalities is known as *Alport's Syndrome.* Although both sexes are affected equally, male patients have a much worse prognosis and usually die of renal failure at an earlier age than do female patients. Clinically, symptoms begin in early childhood and include episodic hematuria, progressive renal failure, and a progressive high-frequency nerve deafness. Ocular abnormalities include congenital cataracts, nystagmus, and myopia. Although there is typically a strong familial history of renal failure, the precise mode of transmission has not been established. On pathologic examination, the kidneys are small but smooth and exhibit a variety of histologic abnormalities including interstitial fibrosis with patchy glomerular involvement. A distinctive histologic feature is the presence of foam cells throughout the renal cortex, but most prominently near the corticomedullary junction.

Small smooth kidneys with impaired excretion of contrast medium are found on radiologic examination. Pruning of the interlobar arteries with an indistinct corticomedullary junction has been reported on angiography.

Miscellaneous Conditions

Nephromegaly has been reported in a variety of other medical conditions including hepatic cirrhosis, diabetes mellitus, infectious mononucleosis, hyperalimentation, paroxysmal nocturnal hemoglobinuria, acute glomerulonephritis, heroin abuse, and Fabry's disease.

SUGGESTED READING

General References and Imaging Studies in Renal Failure

Davidson AJ, Hartman DS: *Radiology of the Kidney and Urinary System, 3rd edition.* Philadelphia, WB Saunders, 1994.

Dawson P, Peters AM: What is the nephrogram? *Br J Radiol* 67(793):21, 1994.

Dyer RB, Munitz HA, Bechtold R, Choplin RH: The abnormal nephrogram. *RadioGraphics* 6(6):1039, 1986.

Evans C: Annotation: renal failure radiology—1987. *Clin Radiol* 38:457, 1987.

Fry IK, Cattell WR: The nephrographic pattern during excretion urography. *Br Med Bull* 28:227, 1972.

Hansen ME, Dunnick NR: Percutaneous intervention in renal failure. *Radiology Rep* 2:137, 1990.

Hricak H, Cruz C, Romanski R, et al.: Renal parenchymal disease: Sonographic-histologic correlation. *Radiology* 144:141, 1982.

Keeton GR, Pillay GP: Diagnostic role of intravenous urography in acute and chronic renal failure. *Urol Radiol* 8:72, 1986.

Mena E, Bookstein JJ, Gikas PW: Angiographic diagnosis of renal parenchymal disease. *Radiology* 108:523, 1973.

Platt JF, Rubin JM, Bowerman RA, et al.: The inability to detect kidney disease on the basis of echogenicity. *AJR* 151:317, 1988.

Ritchie WW, Vick CW, Glocheski SK, et al.: Evaluation of azotemic patients: diagnostic yield of initial US examination. *Radiology* 167:245, 1988.

Schwartz WB, Hurwit A, Ettinger A: Intravenous urography in the patient with renal insufficiency. *N Engl J Med* 269:277, 1963.

Stuck KJ, White GM, Granke DS, et al.: Urinary obstruction in azotemic patient: detection by sonography. *AJR* 149:1191, 1987.

Toyoda K, Miyamoto Y, Ida M, et al.: Hyperechoic medulla of the kidneys. *Radiology* 173:431, 1989.

Acute Tubular Necrosis

Carvlin MJ, Arger PH, Kundel HL, et al.: Acute tubular necrosis: use of gadolinium-DTPA and fast MR imaging to evaluate renal function in the rabbit. *J Comput Assist Tomogr* 11(3):488, 1987.

Love L, Lind JA Jr, Olson MC: Persistent CT nephrogram: significance in the diagnosis of contrast nephropathy. *Radiology* 172:125, 1989.

Nomura G, Kinoshita E, Yamagata Y, et al.: Usefulness of renal ultrasonography for assessment of severity and course of acute tubular necrosis. *J Clin Ultrasound* 12:135, 1984.

Platt JH, Rubin JH, Ellis JH: Acute renal failure: possible role of duplex Doppler US in distinction between acute prerenal failure and acute tubular necrosis. *Radiology* 179(2):419, 1991.

Pozniak MA, Kelcz F, D'Alessandro A, Oberley T, Stratte R: Sonography of renal transplants in dogs: the effect of acute tubular necrosis, cyclosporine nephrotoxicity and acute rejection on resistive index and renal length. *AJR* 158(4):791, 1992.

Rosenfield AT, Zeman RK, Cicchetti DV, et al.: Experimental acute tubular necrosis: US appearance. *Radiology* 157:771, 1985.

Acute Cortical Necrosis

Chugh KS, Jha V, Sakhuja V, Joshi K: Acute renal cortical necrosis: a study of 113 patients. *Renal Failure* 16(1):37, 1994.

Goergen TG, Lindstrom RR, Tan H, et al.: CT appearance of acute renal cortical necrosis. *AJR* 137:176, 1981.

McAlister WH, Nedelman SH: The roentgen manifestations of bilateral renal cortical necrosis. *AJR* 86(1):129, 1961.

Sefczek RJ, Beckman I, Lupetin AR, et al.: Sonography of acute renal cortical necrosis. *AJR* 142:553, 1984.

Acute Interstitial Nephritis

Adler SG, Cogen AH, Border WA: Hypersensitivity phenomena and the kidney: role of drugs and environmental agents. *Am J Kid Dis* 5(2):75, 1985.

Baldwin DS, Levine BB, McCluskey RT, et al.: Renal failure and interstitial nephritis due to penicillin and methicillin. *N Engl J Med* 279(23):1245, 1968.

Ten RM, Torres VE, Milliner DS, et al.: Acute interstitial nephritis: immunologic and clinical aspects. *Mayo Clin Proc* 63:921, 1988.

Hematologic Disorders

Cobby JM, Adler RS, Swartz R, Martel W: Dialysis-related amyloid arthropathy: MR findings in four patients. *AJR* 157:1023, 1991.

Dalinka MK, Lally JF, Rancier LF, et al.: Nephromegaly in hemophilia. *Radiology* 115:337, 1975.

Davidson AJ, Choyke PL, Hartman DS, Davis CJ Jr: Renal medullary carcinoma associated with sickle cell trait: radiologic findings. *Radiology* 195(1):83, 1995.

Davis PS, Barbaria A, March DE, Goldberg RDS: Primary amyloidosis of the ureter and renal pelvis. *Urol Radiol* 9:158, 1987.

Ekelund L: Radiologic findings in renal amyloidosis. *AJR* 129:851, 1977.

Lande IM, Glazer GM, Sarnaik S, et al.: Sickle-cell nephropathy: MR imaging. *Radiology* 158:379, 1986.

Lee VW, Skinner M, Cohen AS, et al.: Renal amyloidosis: evaluation by gallium imaging. *Clin Nucl Med* 11(9):642, 1986.

Mangano FA, Zaontz M, Pahira JJ, et al.: Computed tomography of acute renal failure secondary to rhabdomyolysis. *J Comput Assist Tomogr* 9(4):777, 1985.

Mapp E, Karasick S, Pollack H, et al.: Uroradiological manifestations of S-hemoglobinopathy. *Semin Roentgenol* 22(3):186, 1987.

McCall IW, Moule N, Desai P, et al.: Urographic findings in homozygous sickle cell disease. *Radiology* 126:99, 1978.

McCarthy CS, Becker JA: Multiple myeloma and contrast media. *Radiology* 183:519, 1992.

Odita JC, Ugbodaga CI, Okafor LA, et al.: Urographic changes in homozygous sickle cell disease. *Diagn Imaging* 52:259, 1983.

Pear BL: Other organs and other amyloids. *Semin Roentgenol* 21(2):150, 1986.

Scott PP, Scott WW Jr, Siegelman SS: Amyloidosis: an overview. *Semin Roentgenol* 21(2):103, 1986.

Sueoka BL, Kasales CJ, Harris RD, Heaney JA: MR and CT imaging of perirenal amyloidosis. *Urol Radiol* 11:97, 1989.

Wheeler DC, Feehally J, Burton P, Walls J: The kidney in myeloma. *Br Med J* 292:339, 1986.

Acute Urate Nephropathy

Martin DJ, Jaffe N: Prolonged nephrogram due to hyperuricaemia. *Br J Radiol* 44:806, 1971.

Postlewaite AE, Kelley WM: Uricosuric effect of radiocontrast agents. A study in man of four commonly used preparations. *Ann Intern Med* 74:845, 1971.

Diabetic Nephropathy

Bell DSH: Diabetic nephropathy: Changing concepts of pathogenesis and treatment. *Am J Med Sci* 301(3):195, 1991.

Bojestig M, Arnqvist HJ, Hermansson G, Karlberg BE, Ludvigsson J: Declining incidence of nephropathy in insulin-dependent diabetes mellitus. *N Engl J Med* 330(1):15, 1994.

Platt JF, Rubin JM, Ellis JH: Diabetic nephropathy: evaluation with renal duplex Doppler US. *Radiology* 190:343, 1994.

Rodriguez-de-Velascuez A, Yoder IC, Velasquez RA, Papanicolaou N: Imaging the effects of diabetes on the genitourinary system. *RadioGraphics* 15:1501, 1995.

HIV Nephropathy

Bourgoignie JJ, Pardo V: HIV-associated nephropathies. *N Engl J Med* 327(10):729, 1992.

Bourgoignie JJ, Meneses R, Ortiz C, et al.: The clinical spectrum of renal disease associated with human immunodeficiency virus. *Am J Kidney Dis* 12(2):131, 1988.

Coleburn NH, Scholes JV, Lowe FC: Renal failure in patients with AIDS-related complex. *Urology* 37(6):523, 1991.

Falkof GE, Rigsby CM, Rosenfield AT: Partial, combined cortical and medullary nephrocalcinosis: US and CT patterns in AIDS-associated MAI infection. *Radiology* 162:343, 1987.

Hamper UM, Goldblum LE, Hutchins GM, et al.: Renal involvement in AIDS: Sonographic-pathologic correlation. *AJR* 150:1321, 1988.

Kay CJ: Renal diseases in patients with AIDS: Sonographic findings. *AJR* 159:551, 1992.

Kuhlman JE, Browne D, Shermak M, et al.: Retroperitoneal and pelvic CT of patients with AIDS: Primary and secondary involvement of the genitourinary tract. *RadioGraphics* 11:473, 1991.

Alport's Syndrome

Chuang VP, Reuter SR: Angiographic features of Alport's syndrome. *AJR* 121(3):539, 1974.

11
Renal Transplantation

Renal transplantation is the most desirable treatment for patients with end-stage renal disease, and usually permits homeostasis and a quality of life superior to that achievable by dialysis. Currently, 90 to 95% of transplant recipients survive the first year after surgery, and at least 80% of those transplanted kidneys are functioning. Short-term and long-term survival rates of functioning transplanted kidneys are correlated positively with meticulous immunosuppression, rigid human leukocyte antigen (HLA) matching, experience of the transplant team, and ideal recipient age (between 5 and 50 years). But even in carefully selected and managed patients, it is unusual for functioning kidneys to survive 10 years. Patients may receive subsequent grafts after a first one has failed; duration of function in the first graft is a useful predictor of longevity in the next.

A variety of radiologic procedures are used in the selection of donors and recipients, and in the management and detection of posttransplant complications.

PRETRANSPLANT EVALUATION

Living Donor Evaluation

Most donors are related to recipients. After appropriate HLA matching is performed, the donor undergoes radiologic evaluation to be sure that the kidney considered for donation does not have a morphologic or vascular abnormality that would contraindicate surgery. The remaining kidney must be normal, so that the donor is not at risk for subsequent renal insufficiency. Many prospective donors undergo urography which, if satisfactory, is followed by angiography. In some centers, angiography (usually aortography) is believed to be sufficiently accurate in displaying renal anatomy that urography is omitted. Whether magnetic resonance angiography (MRA) or angiography using spiral computed tomography (CT) will eventually replace standard arteriography remains to be seen.

The ideal transplanted kidney has only one artery. A kidney with two large arteries (Fig. 11.1) often can be successfully transplanted, but the procedure is technically difficult. Tiny accessory arteries that supply only small portions of the kidney may be sacrificed. Because the left renal vein is longer than the right, the left kidney is more desirable for transplantation.

Recipient Evaluation

Radiologic evaluation of the urinary tract in the recipient does not follow a routine path. Virtually all recipients will have had their kidneys imaged in the course of treatment for renal failure; what combination of ultrasound, CT, and radionuclide studies the patients will have undergone depends on the specific renal disease. Sometimes, the specific imaging of the recipient's native kidneys will be necessary during the pretransplant workup. Evaluation for acquired cystic disease and the neoplasm that such kidneys sometimes develop may be performed by CT. Computed tomography may be used to evaluate kidneys in patients with autosomal-dominant polycystic renal disease if extreme enlargement or persistent bleeding makes them candidates for resection. Patients with histories of recurrent urinary tract infections require surgery to treat any vesicoureteral reflux and should have voiding cystourethrography. If symptoms, signs, and cystoscopic or cystometric evaluation of the

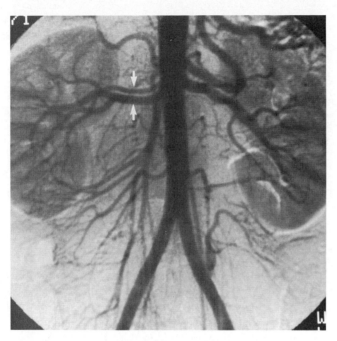

Figure 11.1.   Intravenous digital subtraction angiogram of the abdominal aorta demonstrates two right renal arteries (*arrows*).

bladder suggest problems in the posttransplant period, cystography may be performed. Voiding cystourethrography may be indicated in patients who have been anuric so long that their ability to void normally in the posttransplant period is questioned. Bladders in such patients may have only a small capacity and, when studied by cystography, may demonstrate benign extravasation (Fig. 11.2). This finding does not indicate gross perforation of the bladder, and is not a contraindication to transplantation.

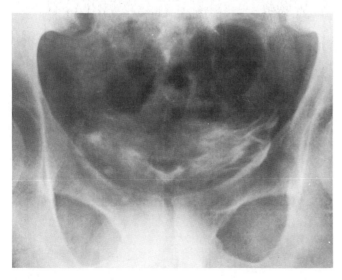

Figure 11.2.   A postvoid film from a voiding cystourethrogram patient with an unused bladder demonstrates benign extraperitoneal extravasation.

TECHNIQUE OF TRANSPLANTATION

The transplanted kidney is usually placed in the left or right iliac fossa extraperitoneally. Most frequently, the artery and vein of the transplanted kidney are anastomosed to the corresponding external iliac artery and vein of the recipient using an end-to-side anastomosis; occasionally, an end-to-end anastomosis between the internal iliac artery of the recipient and the transplant renal artery is performed. In cases of cadaveric donors who have multiple renal arteries, a patch of the aorta containing the renal arterial orifices may be harvested and anastomosed to the common iliac artery. The donor ureter is usually anastomosed to the bladder by a nonrefluxing ureteroneocystostomy.

COMPLICATIONS OF RENAL TRANSPLANTATION

Complications of renal transplantation may be considered as those that affect the renal parenchyma and its small vessels; those that primarily involve the large vessels and their surgery; those that involve the transplanted ureter and its anastomosis; or those that appear as fluid collections in the surgical bed of the recipient. Long-term complications of renal transplantation primarily consist of neoplasms for which recipients are at increased risk.

Renal Complications

Table 11.1 reveals the times during or after transplantation that these complications are most likely to appear. These times, and some of the clinical and radiologic data that can be acquired, frequently permit a reasonably firm diagnosis of the specific complication. However, it often is difficult to establish a specific diagnosis without biopsy of the renal cortex for histologic examination.

Acute Tubular Necrosis

Acute tubular necrosis (ATN) usually occurs in the immediate posttransplant period and is related to ischemia of the transplanted kidney before vascular anastomosis. Such ischemia may occur in cadaveric donors

Table 11.1.
Temporal Sequence of Causes of Parenchymal Complications of Renal Transplants

Acute tubular necrosis	During or immediately after surgery
Hyperacute rejection	During surgery to a few hours afterward
Accelerated acute rejection	First week after surgery
Acute rejection	1–4 weeks after surgery
Chronic rejection	Months to years after surgery
Cyclosporine toxicity	1–3 months after surgery

Modified from Dubovsky EV, Russell CD: Radionuclide evaluation of renal transplants. *Semin Nucl Med* 18:181, 1988.

in the agonal period of the donor and in any donor in the delay between the harvesting of the kidney and completion of vascular anastomosis in the recipient. The duration of the ischemia is directly related to the likelihood of ATN. Most episodes of ATN resolve and appear to have little adverse affect on ultimate graft survival.

Acute tubular necrosis may be manifested as anuria, rising creatinine, and mild enlargement and tenderness of the graft. Graft tenderness and fever are less likely to be prominent signs of ATN than in cases of acute rejection, but the clinical picture usually does not permit firm differentiation of the two conditions.

Acute tubular necrosis usually resolves within a few days to a few weeks of initial onset; however, some cases have persisted for several weeks before recovery.

Cyclosporine Nephrotoxicity

Cyclosporine, together with prednisone, is the mainstay of immunosuppressive therapy. It offers improvement in protection against rejection and is less likely than older drugs to permit opportunistic infection.

Cyclosporine is both nephrotoxic and hepatotoxic. The nephrotoxicity may be acute, subacute, or chronic. Both acute and subacute nephrotoxicity may be treated by lowering the dose; chronic nephrotoxicity is usually not reversible. Acute toxicity appears to potentiate initial graft dysfunction related to ischemia and also may prolong it. Because measurement of blood cyclosporine levels does not always permit distinction of cyclosporine nephrotoxicity from other causes of transplant dysfunction, imaging data may be critical in the differential diagnosis of a failing transplant.

Rejection

Graft rejection continues to represent a significant source of morbidity in the transplant patient. Rejection is currently classified into four categories: (*a*) hyperacute rejection, (*b*) accelerated acute rejection, (*c*) acute rejection, and (*d*) chronic rejection. Virtually every patient experiences some form of rejection in the posttransplant period. Differentiation of graft rejection from other causes of intrinsic renal dysfunction is crucial, because rejection may require increasing the dose of immunosuppressive therapy, whereas cyclosporine nephrotoxicity should be treated in the opposite way.

Hyperacute rejection is mediated by humoral antibodies and often is manifested during surgery; the antigen-antibody reaction causes complement activation, which in turn damages the vascular endothelium, particularly in small vessels. These vessels become filled with fibrin thrombi, thereby making extensive cortical necrosis inevitable. A graft exhibiting hyperacute rejection is usually unsalvageable, and transplant nephrectomy is performed immediately.

Some authors believe that accelerated acute rejection is an antibody-mediated form of rejection identical to hyperacute rejection, but with an onset delayed to 2 or 3 days after surgery. Others believe it is an anamnestic manifestation of cell-mediated immunity. Diagnosis of an accelerated acute rejection usually occurs when a rejection episode occurs in the first week after transplantation. It is frequently, but not always, successfully treated with immunosuppression.

Acute rejection constitutes functional and pathologic changes characterized by a relatively rapid increase in serum creatinine (a rise of 25% or more above the baseline level occurring within 24 to 48 hours), graft swelling and tenderness, and fever. There is usually oliguria. Acute rejection is thought to occur because of a proliferation of C-lymphocytes and to represent a cell-mediated form of immunity. Histologically, it is characterized by a proliferation of mononuclear cells, eosinophils, and plasma cells that infiltrate the interstitium of the kidney. A vascular component also may be present; biopsy specimens in acute rejection are sometimes classified as showing primarily interstitial rejection or both interstitial and vascular abnormalities. A vascular component connotes a poorer prognosis. Acute rejection may occur at any time after transplantation, but most often is encountered during the first through tenth weeks after surgery.

Chronic rejection may appear months to years after surgery, and usually has a more insidious onset than acute rejection. Graft swelling and tenderness, and fever are less prominent features of chronic than acute rejection. Pathologic examination may reveal endothelial swelling, smooth muscle proliferation in small vessels and glomerular changes, along with segmental fibrosis and diffuse infiltration with inflammatory cells. In general, the changes of chronic rejection are irreversible and lead to progressive azotemia and hypertension.

Imaging of Renal Parenchymal Complications

Imaging patients with functional abnormalities of transplanted kidneys is a critical step in the differential diagnosis of the cause of the transplant dysfunction, but imaging findings, considered alone, do not always allow an accurate and specific diagnosis. Sometimes the abnormality is clear, but frequently the clinical or laboratory data must be considered along with the radiologic data to reach a firm diagnosis. Although scintigraphic and Doppler ultrasound findings have been the subjects of considerable investigation, findings that permit accurate distinction among rejection, cyclosporine nephrotoxicity, and ATN in the absence of clinical information have been elusive, and biopsy is frequently necessary.

Hyperacute rejection infrequently leads to an imaging evaluation, because it usually occurs in the operating room. Because renal cortical perfusion is markedly diminished or completely absent, Doppler ultrasound will

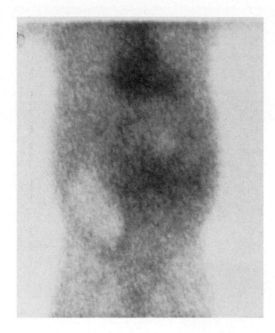

Figure 11.3. Hyperacute rejection. Scintigram obtained 1 day after transplantation shows nearly complete absence of activity in transplanted kidney. (Courtesy of Rashid Fawwaz, M.D.)

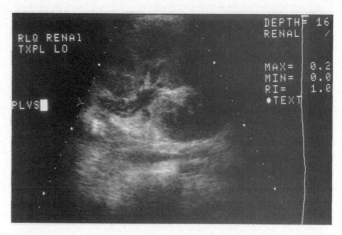

Figure 11.4. Acute rejection. Ultrasound reveals a swollen kidney; the cortex is hypoechoic and the walls of the collecting system are thickened. (Courtesy of Judith Fayter, M.D.)

reveal little or no cortical blood flow, radionuclide examinations will show almost complete absence of perfusion or tubular accumulation (Fig. 11.3), and angiography will reveal total or near-total lack of filling of small vessels.

Accelerated acute rejection demonstrates imaging findings consistent with acute rejection, but occurs within the first week after transplantation. Rare cases of cortical nephrocalcinosis have been described in patients whose transplants underwent severe immediate rejection, but were left in situ for several years.

Acute rejection is most frequently investigated by ultrasound (gray scale, Doppler, and color flow) and radionuclide studies. Gray-scale images (Fig. 11.4) of patients with acute transplant rejection may show an increase in the volume of the kidney, swelling and decreased echogenicity of the renal pyramids, and decreased echogenicity of the cortex. The high echogenicity of the sinus of a normal kidney may be diminished. These findings are thought to reflect edema of the parenchyma and of the renal sinus fat. Edema of the collecting system walls may make them appear thickened. Despite attempts to measure relative volumes of the cortex and medullary pyramids, assessments of echogenicity remain subjective; if the abnormalities are striking, the findings are relatively specific. The sensitivity of these findings to diagnose rejection, however, and the ability to distinguish rejection from cyclosporine nephrotoxicity and ATN when the findings are not clearly present, is poor.

Although there is diminution of total renal blood flow in rejection, cyclosporine nephrotoxicity and ATN, and although there are variations in severity of oligemia among cases of each condition, attempts have been made to use Doppler flow studies to distinguish acute rejection from ATN and cyclosporine nephrotoxicity. In patients with acute rejection—especially those in whom vascular changes predominate in biopsy specimens, as opposed to those in whom the histologic changes are primarily interstitial—the resistive index (RI) often is elevated (Fig. 11.5). The RI (the peak systolic velocity minus the lowest diastolic velocity divided by the peak systolic velocity) is relatively specific for acute rejection when its value is 0.90 or higher, although occasionally elevated RIs may be caused by arterial stenosis, renal vein thrombosis, acute severe ureteral obstruction, severe ATN, acute cyclosporine nephrotoxicity, pyelonephritis, and compression of the kidney by a perirenal fluid collection. With lower RIs, primarily interstitial acute rejection, cyclosporine nephrotoxicity and ATN are possible etiologies. Because rejection and ATN may not affect the entire kidney uniformly, and since resistive indices may vary from observer to observer, the overall accuracy of this method of differential diagnosis is far from ideal. Serial studies, performed by the same examiner, may improve accuracy by reducing interobserver variability and by documenting progression of changes in Doppler spectral patterns (and of renal size and echogenicity changes). In some centers, the pulsatility index (PI) (peak systolic frequency shift − minimal diastolic frequency shift divided by the mean frequency shift) is used as an alternative to measurement of the RI. A PI of 1.5 or greater is generally considered indicative of rejection.

Radionuclide examinations also may assist in distinguishing among the several causes of renal parenchymal dysfunction in transplant patients. In acute rejection associated primarily with vascular changes (Fig. 11.6),

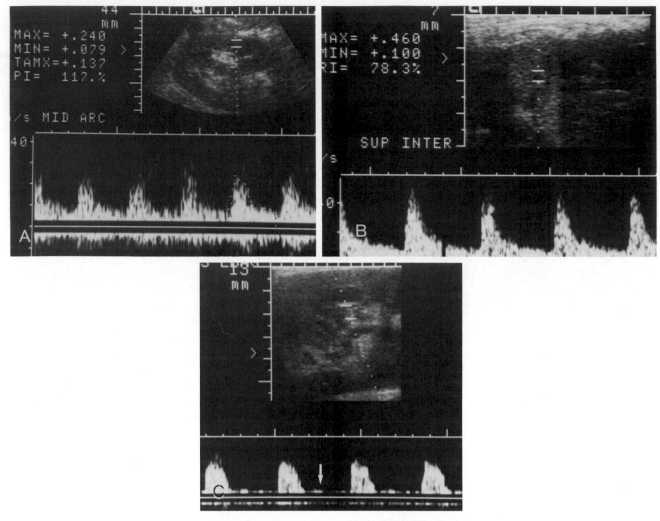

Figure 11.5. Duplex Doppler ultrasonograms. **A,** Normal duplex study with a pulsatility index of 1.17. **B,** Mild rejection; RI = 0.78, PI = 1.7. **C,** Severe rejection with virtually complete absence of diastolic flow (*arrow*).

the rapid increase in activity seen normally is attenuated; the maximum intensity of activity seen in early images is diminished, and the delay between the time of peak activity in the aorta and peak activity in the kidney is prolonged. These findings also may occur in rejection that is primarily of the cellular type, and in ATN and cyclosporine nephrotoxicity, but are less severe in these conditions. The findings may precede clinical evidence of rejection. All parenchymal causes of graft dysfunction exhibit deteriorating tubular function, manifested by diminished activity in later parts of the examination. Once established, ATN and acute rejection may produce scintigraphic findings that are difficult to distinguish. But if the first scans after the operation are abnormal, ATN is likely to be present, whereas if the scans were initially normal but subsequently became abnormal, acute rejection is more likely to be the diagnosis. Acute tubular necrosis followed by acute rejection is difficult to distinguish from ATN without recovery, although the usual course of ATN is a spontaneous return toward normal

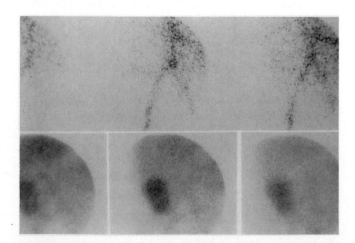

Figure 11.6. Acute vascular rejection. The upper row of scintigrams are dynamic images and reveal diminished renal perfusion as the isotope traverses the iliac arteries. The lower images were obtained 1, 10, and 20 minutes after isotope administration, and reveal persistence of activity in the renal parenchyma. (Courtesy of Rashid Fawwaz, M.D.)

within 1 or 2 weeks of onset. Severe diminution of activity in the kidney, or complete failure of the kidney to accumulate isotope, is a poor prognostic sign.

Indium-111-labeled platelets also have been used to detect acute transplant rejection. The method is relatively sensitive, but does not reliably differentiate rejection from cyclosporine nephrotoxicity, and is expensive. Technetium-99m sulfur colloid and gallium 67 also have been used.

Magnetic resonance imaging (MRI) was initially believed to be promising in differentiating acute rejection from other causes of transplant dysfunction, because the differentiation between cortex and medulla normally visible on T1-dependent images tended to disappear. Subsequently, however, loss of corticomedullary distinction has been found in many causes of renal parenchymal dysfunction, and MRI does not currently play a large role in imaging the parenchyma of renal transplants.

Angiography is not commonly performed to diagnose rejection, but may be indicated for other reasons in transplant patients. With acute rejection, there often is a prolonged arterial phase with poor washout. The nephrogram is diminished, demonstrates patchy opacification, and reveals poor definition of the corticomedullary junction. Arteriovenous shunting may be present. Angiographic findings of acute rejection may be focal.

Chronic rejection produces imaging findings that vary in severity and tend to differ from those of acute processes, but the findings may not permit differentiation of rejection from other chronic conditions affecting a transplanted kidney, such as chronic cyclosporine nephrotoxicity, or the superimposition of diseases such as hypertension or diabetic nephropathy, which may affect transplanted as well as native kidneys.

The kidney often is small. Ultrasound may show increased echogenicity of the cortex; in the rare cases in which mild cortical nephrocalcinosis occurs, cortical echoes may be very strong. The RI value may be normal. A radionuclide scan tends to show relatively rapid uptake and washout; the pattern of poor initial uptake but gradually increasing activity seen with some acute processes is not a feature of chronic rejection (although a bout of acute rejection may be superimposed on a kidney that has been chronically rejecting). Although angiography is not indicated in the diagnosis of chronic rejection, it may be performed on chronically rejecting kidneys when renal artery stenosis is a possibility. The rejection may be manifested as a thinned cortex with a diminished and transient persistent nephrogram; the small vessels are sparse, diminutive, and pruned. Magnetic resonance may reveal absence of corticomedullary distinction on T1-weighted spin-echo images, which is a feature seen in a large number of chronic renal parenchymal diseases. Phosphorus-31 MR spectroscopy has shown phosphate metabolite changes in rejecting kidneys.

Acute tubular necrosis is almost always caused by the ischemia suffered by a kidney from a cadaver donor or ischemia that occurs during a complication of harvesting a kidney from a living donor, and therefore appears within 1 or 2 days after transplantation. Its severity and duration are quite variable, is usually self-limiting, and is usually accompanied by less swelling and tenderness than acute rejection.

Although experimental evidence shows that renal blood flow is lower than normal in cases of ATN, the early phase in a technetium-99m-diethylenetriaminepentaacetic acid (^{99m}Tc-DTPA) renogram (the "perfusion" phase) is relatively well maintained (Fig. 11.7), even though the later phases and the Hippuran or technetium-99m-mercaptoacetyltriglycine (^{99m}Tc-MAG$_3$) curves fail to show rapid parenchymal washout and even show persistent accumulation of the isotope. Sonography—including Doppler—is frequently normal, although occasionally the resistive index may be increased.

Cyclosporine Toxicity. Radionuclide examinations (Fig. 11.8) have been shown to result in a dissociation between the perfusion phase of a ^{99m}Tc-DTPA study (which tends to remain relatively intact) and the clearance phase of a Hippuran or ^{99m}Tc-MAG$_3$ study, which often reveals a prolonged rate of clearance. This is particularly the case in patients with subacute nephrotoxicity. The findings in cyclosporine toxicity are similar to the radionuclide findings produced by ATN or obstruction. The diagnosis of cyclosporine nephrotoxicity, therefore, can only be suggested when serial studies have demonstrated a resolution of the immediately posttransplant ATN; the reappearance of an ascending slope of the Hippuran curve without a new ischemic episode suggests cyclosporine nephrotoxicity. The diagnosis also is based on measure-

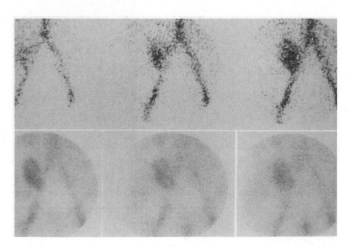

Figure 11.7. Acute tubular necrosis. The top row of dynamic images show rapid early uptake (the "perfusion" phase). The lower row of images, obtained 1, 10, and 20 minutes after administration of isotope, reveal persistence of activity and little excretion into the bladder. (Courtesy of Rashid Fawwaz, M.D.)

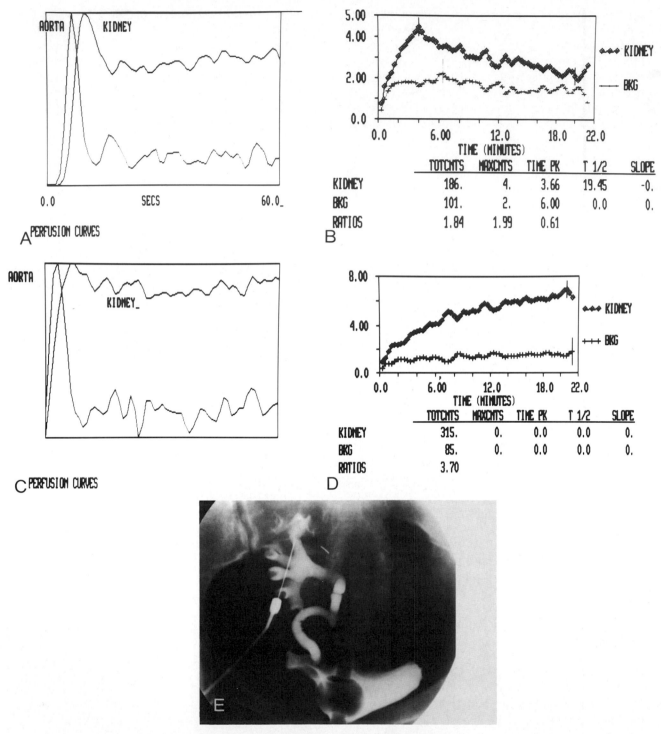

Figure 11.8. Cyclosporine nephrotoxicity. Immediate post-transplant ^{99m}Tc-DTPA perfusion (*A*) and ^{131}I-Hippuran renogram (*B*) curves in a patient who received a living related kidney show good perfusion and excretion. Three days later, the perfusion curve (*C*) remains relatively intact; however, the Hippuran curve (*D*) now demonstrates an ascending slope. An antegrade pyelogram (*E*) shows no evidence of obstruction, thereby confirming that the cause of the transplant dysfunction is cyclosporine nephrotoxicity.

ments of cyclosporine concentration in the blood and by monitoring the effect of dose adjustments.

Graft Infection. Thirty to 60% of patients receiving renal allografts are treated for urinary tract infection within the first 4 months after surgery, and approximately 25% of these patients develop frank sepsis. The incidence and severity of the infection depend on the dose of immunosuppressive therapy, the presence and degree of

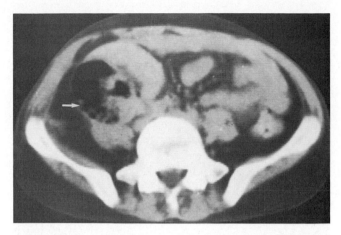

Figure 11.9. Emphysematous pyelonephritis. A computed tomography scan demonstrates air (*arrow*) diffusely infiltrating the transplant kidney in the right iliac fossa.

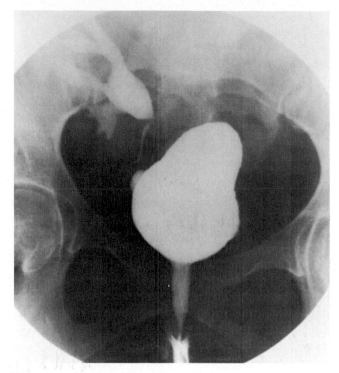

Figure 11.10. A voiding cystourethrogram shows reflux into the transplanted kidney.

control of diabetes mellitus and the coexistence of graft dysfunction.

The organisms responsible are the Gram-negative urinary pathogens commonly found in other patients with urinary infection; graft recipients also may be infected with cytomegalovirus or herpes simplex virus.

Several cases of emphysematous pyelonephritis (Fig. 11.9) have been reported in transplant patients; the diagnosis may be established by demonstrating gas within the renal parenchyma by CT or ultrasound.

There is a relationship between reflux into the transplanted ureter and infection. If a graft recipient suffers multiple infections and if ureteroneocystostomy would be considered if reflux were present and severe, voiding cystography should be performed (Fig. 11.10).

Renal transplant rupture is a dramatic complication that usually occurs within the first 2 weeks of the transplant surgery; it occurs in 3 to 5% of renal allografts. The etiology of rupture is not known with certainty, but it has been speculated that acute rejection, ATN, and vascular occlusion might be predisposing causes. Trauma caused by biopsies also may be contributory.

The imaging findings are some combination of renal parenchymal laceration, intrarenal hematoma, and perirenal hematoma. Ultrasound (Fig. 11.11) may reveal a hypoechoic fluid collection representing a hematoma

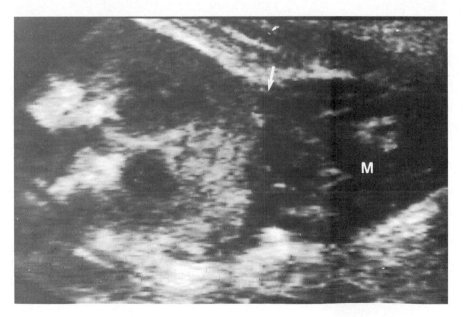

Figure 11.11. Transplant rupture. A longitudinal ultrasound scan demonstrates a hypoechoic mass (*M*) in the inferior portion of the kidney at the site of the rupture (*arrow*).

within the laceration and/or perinephric space, CT may reveal dense clot within the laceration or perinephric space, and radionuclide scans may reveal a focal photopenic region at the site of the laceration.

Vascular Complications

Thrombosis

Thrombosis of the renal artery may occur in the immediate postoperative period; it may be caused by complete or partial occlusion at the anastomotic site or may form as a result of an intimal flap. Renal arterial thrombosis is more common in kidneys that have more than one renal artery and in association with hyperacute rejection. If diminution in renal blood flow is severe or complete, Doppler ultrasound will reveal no evidence of flow within the kidney, radionuclide scintigrams will show no perfusion, and CT with contrast will reveal that the nephrogram is absent. Arteriography will reveal little or no flow to the kidney, and usually demonstrates the thrombus itself. An infarcted kidney, or infarcted portion of kidney, will appear swollen and relatively hypoechoic on gray-scale ultrasound; a hemorrhagic infarct may appear more echogenic.

Renal vein thrombosis in transplanted kidneys is quite rare. The imaging findings are the same as those associated with renal vein thrombosis in native kidneys, including echogenic material and absence of flow in the renal vein and markedly elevated RIs.

Renal Artery Stenosis

Renal artery stenosis is reported to occur in 0.6 to 23% of patients with renal transplants. The real incidence may be higher because asymptomatic patients are not evaluated. Renal artery stenosis may cause diminution in renal function, hypertension, and a bruit.

Stenoses in the host artery proximal to the anastomosis may be related to general arterial sclerosis, especially in patients with diabetes, or may be related to trauma suffered at the time of surgery. Anastomotic stenoses may be related to the surgical technique, to the suture material, or to perfusion injury of the vessels themselves. Postanastomotic stenosis may be related to rejection, abnormal local hemodynamics, or extrinsic compression.

Posttransplant renal artery stenosis requires angiography for accurate evaluation (Fig. 11.12). Because hypertension in transplant recipients is common, a method to determine which of the hypertensive patients have renal artery stenosis noninvasively has been sought. Radionuclide examinations are not sufficiently sensitive to be ideal for this task; Doppler ultrasound of the main renal artery (Fig. 11.13) and of intrarenal vessels has been moderately successful, as has intravenous digital subtraction angiography. Magnetic resonance angiography continues to be evaluated.

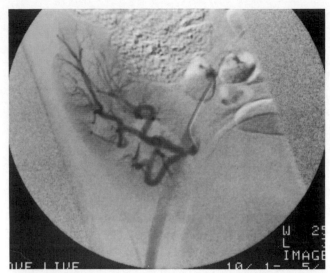

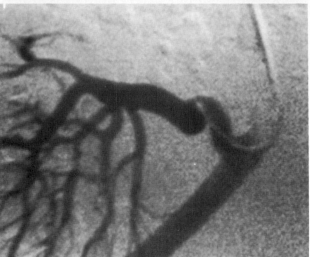

Figure 11.12. A, Renal artery stenosis. An arteriogram shows a stenosis at the site of anastomosis of the renal artery and the internal iliac artery. **B,** A long tubular stenosis is present as a result of kinking of the artery during graft placement.

Percutaneous transluminal angioplasty has become the preferred method by which such stenoses are treated; a large majority of patients have successful outcomes, at least in the short term. The success rates are higher with end-to-side anastomoses than with end-to-end anastomoses. The technique and potential complications are similar to those encountered during percutaneous transluminal angioplasty in native renal arteries.

Renal Arteriovenous Fistula

Because transplanted kidneys frequently undergo biopsy, small postbiopsy arteriovenous fistulae are common. They usually close quickly and spontaneously, but persist in 1 or 2% of patients, and may cause transplant dysfunction or significant arteriovenous shunting. The

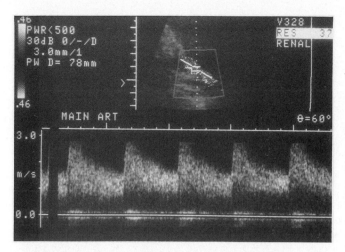

Figure 11.13.   Renal artery stenosis in a transplant. Doppler ultrasound reveals marked spectral broadening produced by turbulence caused by the arterial narrowing. (Courtesy of Judith Fayter, M.D.)

incidence of these persistent symptomatic fistulae appears to be higher in patients treated with cyclosporine than with those treated with azathioprine. Doppler ultrasound (Fig. 11.14) may reveal low-impedance, high-velocity flow through the afferent artery; the draining vein may reveal pulsatile, high-velocity flow. Pseudoaneurysms (Fig. 11.15) are unusual; ultrasound studies reveal them as cystic or complex lesions with Doppler evidence of disorganized flow or alternative patterns of flow toward and away from the transducer.

Angiographic findings (Fig. 11.16) are the same as those encountered in small arteriovenous fistulae or pseudoaneurysms in native kidneys. If they require therapy, they may be amenable to transarterial embolization with coils (Fig. 11.17), Gelfoam (Upjohn, Kalamazoo, MI), or detachable balloons.

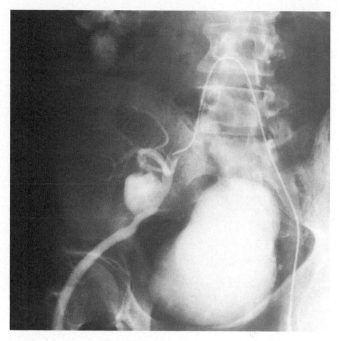

Figure 11.15.   A pseudoaneurysm in the external iliac artery adjacent to the transplant anastomosis is present.

Urologic Complications

Urinary Leak

Urinary leak (Fig. 11.18) most often occurs in the first 3 months after transplantation and is usually discovered within the first few postoperative weeks. Urine may leak from the ureterovesical anastomosis, from a vesicostomy site, or even from injury to the transplanted renal

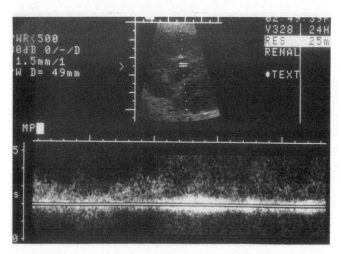

Figure 11.14.   Arteriovenous fistula. Doppler ultrasound reveals continuous flow with marked spectral broadening at the site of the fistula. (Courtesy of Judith Fayter, M.D.)

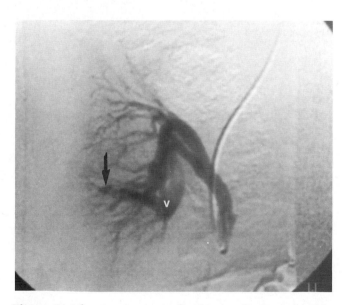

Figure 11.16.   Arteriovenous fistula. A selective transplant arteriogram shows an arteriovenous fistula (*arrow*) with early filling of the renal vein (*v*).

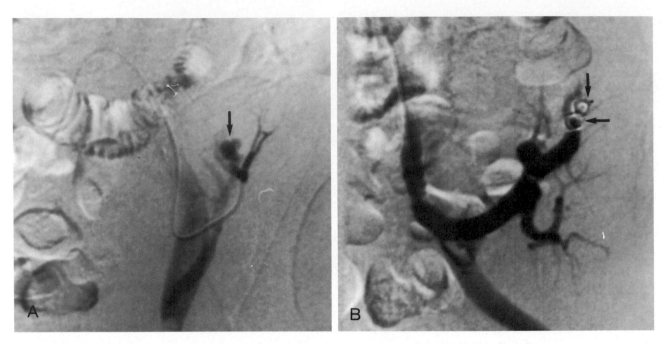

Figure 11.17. A, Subselective renal angiogram shows a large arteriovenous fistula (*arrow*). **B,** After embolization with Gianturco coils (*arrows*), a repeat arteriogram shows closure of the fistula.

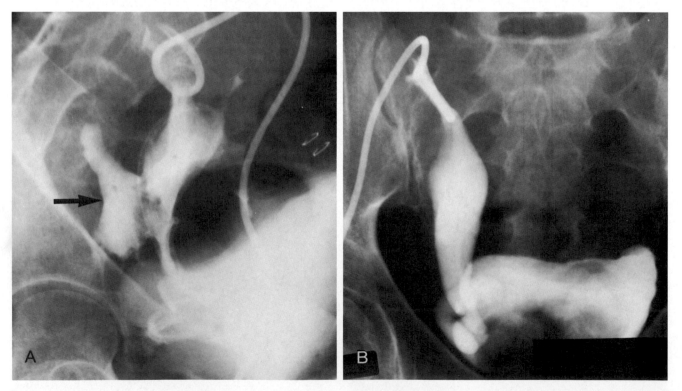

Figure 11.18. A, An oblique view from a nephrostogram demonstrates extravasation from a tear of the renal pelvis. **B,** After removal of the ureteral stent and several weeks of nephrostomy drainage, the leak has completely healed.

pelvis. If the leak is small and transient, the urine is usually resorbed; if it persists, a urinoma frequently forms. Rarely, a ureterocutaneous fistula may develop.

Ureteral Necrosis

Necrosis and sloughing of the distal ureter (Fig. 11.19) is a common urologic complication; it usually causes a urinary leak. It may occur in up to 4% of patients, usually before the 6th postoperative month. It is thought to be caused by ischemia of the distal ureter from interruption of the ureteral arterial blood supply or from a tight submucosal tunnel in the bladder; it also may appear because of rejection.

Ureteral Obstruction

Transient obstruction at the site of the ureteral implantation is common in the immediate postoperative period; it is caused by edema, and usually subsides quickly. Ureteral obstruction that appears months to years after transplantation is more likely to be caused by ureteral ischemic strictures. Rarely, acute obstruction is caused by blood clots, calculi (Fig. 11.20), fungus balls, or sloughed papillae. Stones are reported to occur in approximately 1% of patients with renal allografts; most stone formers are thought to have underlying predisposing conditions. Occasionally, undetected calculi in donor kidneys may cause complications in recipients. Acute ureteral obstruction from a stone may produce pain and graft swelling that simulates acute rejection. The patients may suddenly become oliguric or anuric. Sutures at the site of ureteral implantation or vesicos-

tomies may act as a nidus for the formation of a bladder stone. Any fluid collection may compress the ureter and cause obstruction.

Imaging of Urologic Complications

A variety of radiologic investigations may be helpful in investigating these urologic complications. Plain films may show large urinomas or other fluid collections and also may demonstrate stones. However, because the transplanted kidney and collecting system frequently overlie the iliac bone and sacrum, small or faintly calcified stones may be hard to find.

Excretory urography is only used infrequently because many transplanted patients have compromised renal function, which is a contraindication to intravascular contrast media. Nevertheless, excretory urography is performed occasionally and may demonstrate ureteral obstruction. Urograms may demonstrate accumulation of contrast in a urinoma if there is active large-volume urinary extravasation (Fig. 11.21). Retrograde pyelography is sometimes difficult to perform on transplanted kidneys and ureters, because it is difficult to catheterize a ureter through a ureteroneocystostomy, but contrast may reflux into the transplant ureter during cystography. Cystography may demonstrate a urinary leak when the source is in the wall of the bladder, but may give false-negative results in patients in whom the leak arises from the distal ureter.

Radionuclide examinations often are one of the first studies used to investigate for transplant dysfunction. Patients with urinomas may, in early images, demonstrate a

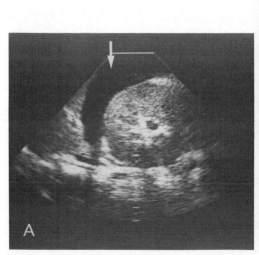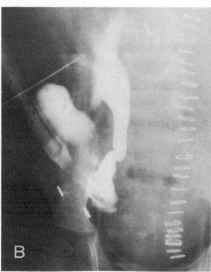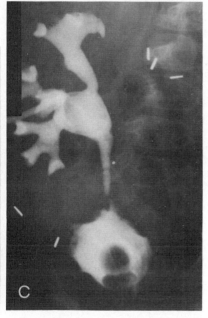

Figure 11.19.   Ureteral necrosis. **A,** An ultrasound examination demonstrates fluid around the transplant kidney (*arrow*). **B,** Antegrade pyelogram shows extravasation from distal ureter as a result of ureteral necrosis. **C,** After percutaneous nephrostomy and stent placement, a nephrostogram shows complete healing.

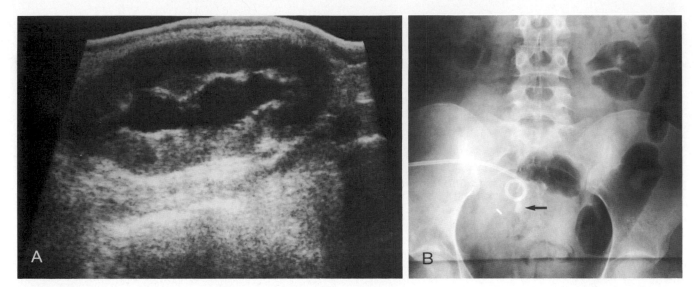

Figure 11.20. A, An ultrasound scan performed to evaluate the sudden onset of oliguria and pain in a transplant patient demonstrates hydronephrosis. **B,** A percutaneous nephrostomy was placed under ultrasound guidance. A follow-up radiograph shows that a stone (*arrow*) lodged in the ureteropelvic junction is the cause of the transplant dysfunction. Percutaneous nephrostolithotomy was subsequently performed.

photopenic region corresponding to the urinoma; the region will gradually accumulate activity in the delayed images if urine is actively excreted into the collection (Fig. 11.22). Ureteral obstruction also may be identified on radionuclide studies. The perfusion phase in a ^{99m}Tc-DTPA examination will be relatively well preserved, and with a Hippuran or ^{99m}Tc-MAG$_3$ examination, there is relatively prompt uptake of the radiopharmaceutical by the transplant kidney. The excretory portion of the study is prolonged, and the renogram curve may have an ascending slope (Fig. 11.23**A**). These findings are similar to those accompanying ATN and cyclosporine nephrotoxicity. Sometimes, direct demonstration of hydronephrosis and hydroureter by scintigraphy, or by other imaging modalities, (Fig. 11.23**B**) makes the diagnosis more specific.

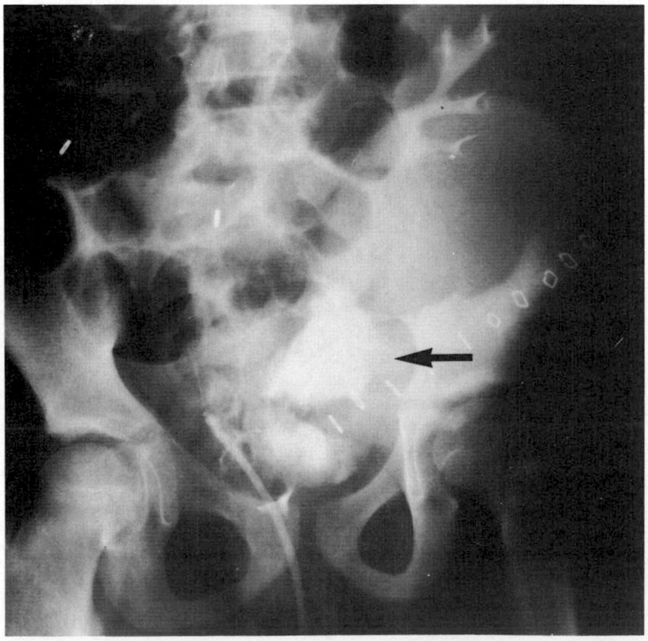

Ultrasound studies also are extremely useful for investigating urologic complications. Ultrasound may show hydronephrosis (Figs. 20**A** and 23**B**) and the degree to which this represents ongoing obstruction may be made clearer by searching for abnormal resistive indices and absent ureteral jets with Doppler. Ultrasound may detect renal or ureteral calculi and peritransplant fluid collections. Hydronephrosis is frequently found in

Figure 11.21. An excretory urogram demonstrating contrast extravasation (*arrow*) as a result of leakage from the ureteroneocystostomy site.

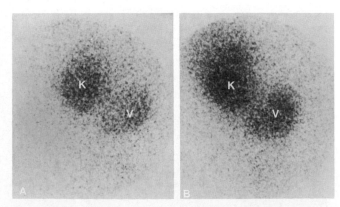

Figure 11.22. A, Initial and **B,** delayed images from ^{131}I-Hippuran radionuclide scan show increasing activity around the transplanted kidney (*K*) as the result of urinary extravasation. Activity also is present in the bladder (*V*).

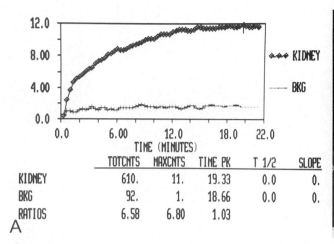

Figure 11.23. Transplant obstruction. **A,** A renogram curve demonstrates an ascending slope compatible with obstruction.

B, Ultrasound examination confirms that transplant hydronephrosis is present.

patients with ureteral sloughing and urinary extravasation. Computed tomography may reveal urinomas or other fluid collections (Fig. 11.24).

Fine-needle antegrade pyelography (Fig. 11.25) is useful in the diagnosis of transplant ureteral obstruction and in detecting and outlining ureteral fistulas. Although it is an invasive technique, and is associated with the risk of hemorrhage and infection, the actual complication rate is quite low. Antegrade pyelography also may be used to perform a Whitaker test, which is most useful in patients who have transplant hydronephrosis but who may not have ureteral obstruction.

Interventional uroradiologic procedures may be used to treat most urologic complications. Percutaneous nephrostomy provides relief of obstruction, and, once inserted, a percutaneous nephrostomy tube may be used for other procedures, such as a Whitaker test.

Some ureteral strictures may be successfully treated with percutaneous balloon dilatation or ureteral stent placement. Although there is a significant rate of short-term failure and long-term restenosis of transplant ureters after balloon dilatation, the technique may provide transient or even permanent relief of obstruction in some patients.

Percutaneous nephrostomy tubes also may be used to treat stones and urinary leaks. The former can be extracted using techniques similar to those employed in the native kidneys. Ureteral or anastomotic leaks may be successfully managed with percutaneous diversion and stent placement.

Peritransplant Fluid Collections

Fluid collections around the transplanted kidney may represent urinomas, hematomas, abscesses, or lymphoceles.

Hematomas

Hematomas usually form in the immediate postoperative period. Ultrasound reveals them as fluid collections; clots or red cell debris may produce regions of echogenicity within them (Fig. 11.26). Clots or layers of debris may appear on unenhanced CT images as denser regions than adjacent solid tissues. Hematomas appear photopenic on the early phases of a radionuclide scintigram, and MRI reveals the same features of hematomas as are seen with extracranial hematomas arising elsewhere.

Urinomas

Urinomas also form relatively early in the posttransplant period, because they are usually caused by acute leaks from the ureteral anastomosis. The fluid in urino-

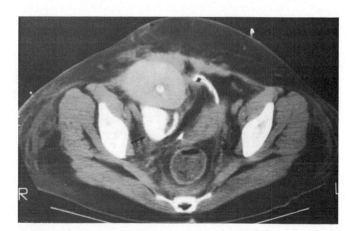

Figure 11.24. Computed tomography demonstrates a collection of extravasated contrast (*arrow*) behind the transplanted kidney.

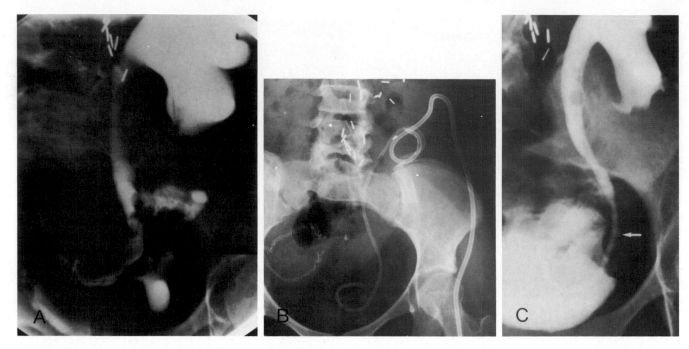

Figure 11.25. A, An antegrade pyelogram shows extravasation from the mid ureter. **B,** A percutaneous nephrostomy and double-J ureteral stent were placed for 6 weeks. **C,** Follow-up nephrostogram shows a small pseudodiverticulum in the distal ureter, (*arrow*) but no further extravasation.

mas appears echo-free on ultrasound, (Fig. 11.19**A**) lucent on CT, and like protein-free fluid (dark on T1-weighted images and bright on T2-weighted images) on MRI. If urine is actively flowing into the urinomas at the time of radionuclide examinations, they may become quite active (Fig. 11.22) if any renally excreted compound is used. Excretory urography is only rarely performed on transplant patients, but it may reveal opacification of a urinoma (Fig. 11.21). Eventually, leaking may cease, and an encapsulated urinoma may not accumulate radionuclide or contrast.

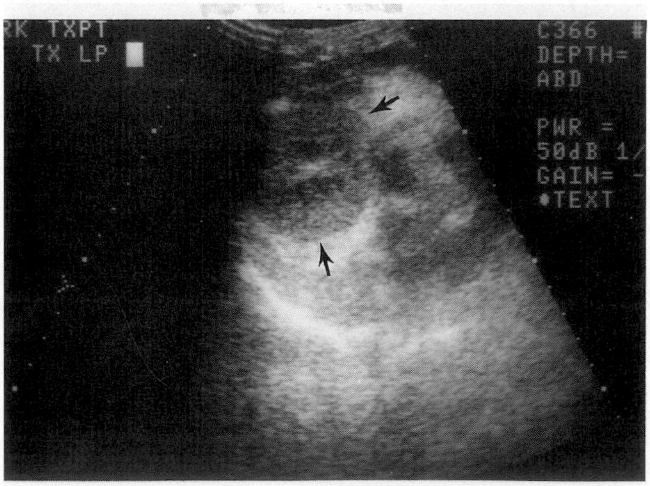

Lymphoceles

Lymphoceles are the most common peritransplant fluid collection; they occur in 1 to 15% of all patients. They usually appear 4 to 6 weeks after transplantation and are frequently associated with previous episodes of rejection. They are believed to be caused by surgical disruption of the recipient's lymphatics at the time of surgery, but there may be a contribution from the transplanted kidney as well.

Lymphoceles are frequently asymptomatic, but, when large, they may compress the collecting system or the ureter and even produce obstruction and impairment of function. They may be palpable and may be associated with pain and ipsilateral leg edema.

Lymphoceles may be detected by a variety of imaging modalities (Fig. 11.27). On radionuclide examinations, they are seen as photopenic areas between the transplanted kidney and the bladder that do not accumulate activity on delayed views. Ultrasound demonstrates fluid-filled structures that often contain fine septations that may be difficult to distinguish from urinomas. They are usually seen at the inferior margin of the transplant between the kidney and the bladder.

On CT scans, lymphoceles are demonstrated as round

Figure 11.26. Perinephric hematoma. The kidney (*arrows*) appears intrinsically normal; the inhomogeneous echogenic region adjacent to it is a clot-containing hematoma. (Courtesy of Judith Fayter, M.D.)

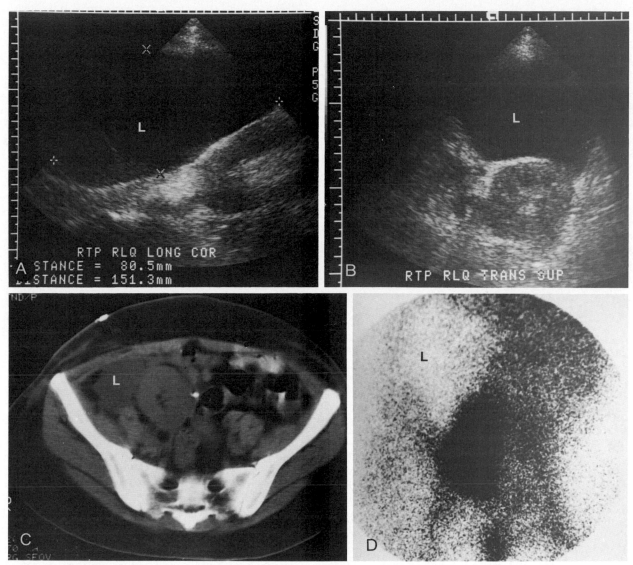

Figure 11.27. Lymphocele (*L*). **A,** Longitudinal ultrasonogram; **B,** transverse ultrasonogram; **C,** computed tomography scan; and **D,** radionuclide scan.

or oval collections with sharp borders and CT values that range from 0 to 20 Hounsfield units (HU). Without contrast, they may be difficult to distinguish from urinomas. After intravenous contrast injection, many, but not all urinomas opacify, whereas lymphoceles do not.

The role of percutaneous drainage of lymphoceles is controversial. Although they may be drained and cured, they recur with sufficient frequency that instillation of a sclerosing agent or surgical therapy may be needed.

The incidence of peritransplant abscess is difficult to estimate from the reported series. Most occur as a complication of pyelonephritis, although abscess as a direct complication of surgery also may occur. Peritransplant fluid collections such as urinomas, hematomas, or lymphoceles may become infected secondarily. Computed tomography and ultrasound are the most helpful imaging modalities in detecting abscesses, but they often are not distinguishable from sterile collections by imaging techniques alone; clinical evidence of infection is usually relied on. Needle aspiration is relatively easy to perform to detect abscesses, and they usually respond to percutaneous catheter drainage.

LONG-TERM COMPLICATIONS OF RENAL TRANSPLANTATION

There is an increased incidence of malignancy in patients treated with immunosuppressive drugs over a long period. Penn classified these patients into five groups, of which three are pertinent to renal transplant recipients: (*a*) there is a 36% incidence of neoplasia in transplant recipients who receive organs from donors with carcinomas; (*b*) the risk of de novo malignancy at some time after transplantation ranges from 6 to 100 times greater than that of the general population in the same age range; (*c*) there is a 53% incidence of recurrence for patients receiving a renal transplant because of a renal cell carcinoma if the interval between treatment of the cancer and transplantation is 1 year or less. Of the organ recipients who develop a de novo malignancy, lymphomas, and Kaposi's sarcoma tumors of the skin, lips, cervix, and rectum are common.

Frick and colleagues have reported the CT appearance of abdominal lymphoma that develops after renal transplantation. The incidence in this series was 1.3% of the transplant population. The lymphomas differed from the usual ones in that they frequently involved extranodal sites, especially in the central nervous system. Computed tomography of posttransplant lymphomas in the abdomen usually reveals bulky masses with inhomogeneous attenuation.

SUGGESTED READINGS

General References

Becker JA, Kutcher R: The renal transplant: rejection and acute tubular necrosis. *Semin Roentgenol* 13(4):352, 1978.

Diethelm AG, Deierhoi MH, Hudson, et al.: Progress in renal transplantation: a single center study of 3359 patients over 25 years. *Ann Surg* 221(5):446, 1995.

Halasz NA, Gambos EA, Ward DM, et al.: Kidney transplantation in the cyclosporine era. *Arch Surg* 122:1001, 1987.

Hanto DW, Simmons RL: Renal transplantation: clinical considerations. *Radiol Clin North Am* 25(2):239, 1987.

Kahan BD, Flechner SM, Lorber MI, et al.: Complications of cyclosporine-prednisone immunosuppression in 402 renal allograft recipients exclusively followed at a single center for from one to five years. *Transplantation* 43(2):197, 1987.

Maklad NF: Ultrasonic evaluation of renal transplants. *Semin Roentgenol* 2(1):88, 1981.

Monaco AP: Clinical kidney transplantation in 1984. *Transplant Proc* 17(1):5; 1985.

Oliver JH III: Clinical indications, recipient evaluation, surgical considerations, and the role of CT and MR in renal transplantation. Radiol Clin North Am 33(3):435, 1995.

Tublin ME, Dodd GF: Sonography of renal transplantation. *Radiol Clin North Am* 33(3):447, 1995.

Donor Evaluation

Flechner SM, Sandler CM, Houston GK, et al.: 100 living-related kidney donor evaluations using digital subtraction angiography. *Transplantation* 40(6):675, 1985.

McElroy J, Novick AC, Streem SB, et al.: A prospective analysis of the accuracy and cost-effectiveness of digital subtraction angiography for living related renal donor evaluation. *Transplantation* 42(1):23, 1986.

Infection

Peterson P, Anderson RC: Infection in renal transplant recipients. Current approaches to diagnosis, therapy and prevention. *Am J Med* 81(suppl 1A):2, 1986.

Potter JL, Sullivan BM, Flournoy JG, et al.: Emphysema in the renal allograft. *Radiology* 155:51, 1985.

Radionuclide Studies

Dubovsky EV, Russell CD, Erbas B: Radionuclide evaluation of renal transplants. *Semin Nucl Med* 25(1):49, 1995.

Kim EE, Pjura G, Lowry P, et al.: Cyclosporin-A nephrotoxicity and acute cellular rejection in renal transplant recipients: correlation between radionuclide and histologic findings. *Radiology* 159:443, 1986.

Kirchner PT, Rosenthall L: Renal transplant evaluation. *Semin Nucl Med* 12(4):370, 1982.

Klintmalm GBG, Klingensmith WC, Iwatsuki S, et al.: TcDTPA and I-131 Hippuran findings in liver transplant recipients treated with cyclosporin A. *Radiology* 142:199, 1982.

Marcos CS, Koyle MA, Darcourt J, et al.: Evaluation of the utility of Indium 111 oxide platelet imaging in renal transplant patients on cyclosporine. *Clin Nucl Med* 11(12):834, 1986.

O'Malley JP, Ziessman HA, Chantarapitak N: Tc-99m MAG3 as an alternative to Tc-99m DTPA and I-131 Hippuran for renal transplant evaluation. *Clin Nucl Med* 18(1):22, 1993.

Shah AN: Radionuclide imaging in organ transplantation. *Radiol Clin North Am* 33(3):447, 1995.

Tisdale PL, Collier BD, Kauffman HM, et al.: Early diagnosis of acute postoperative renal transplant rejection by indium 111 labeled platelet scintigraphy. *J Nucl Med* 27:1266, 1986.

Thomsen HS, Munck O: Use of 99mTc radionuclides to show nephrotoxicity of cyclosporin A in transplanted kidneys. *Acta Radiol* 28:59, 1987.

Acute Rejection: Ultrasound Studies

Fried AM, Woodring JH, Loh FK, et al.: The medullary pyramid index: an objective assessment of prominence in renal transplant rejection. *Radiology* 149:787, 1983.

Griffin JF, Short DC, Lawler W, et al.: Diagnosis of disease in renal allografts: correlation between ultrasound and histology. *Clin Radiol* 37:59, 1986.

Hoddick W, Filly RA, Backman U, et al.: Renal allograft rejection: US evaluation. *Radiology* 161:469, 1986.

Hricak H, Romanski RN, Eyler WR: The renal sinus during allograft rejection: sonographic and histopathologic findings. *Radiology* 142:693, 1982.

Linkowski GD, Warvariv V, Filly RA, et al.: Sonography in the diagnosis of acute renal allograft rejection and cyclosporine nephrotoxicity. *AJR* 148:291, 1987.

Raiss GJ, Bree RL, Schwab RE, et al.: Further observations in the ultrasound evaluation of renal allograft rejection. *J Ultrasound Med* 5:439, 1986.

Acute Rejection: Duplex Sonography

Allen KS, Jorkasky DK, Arger PH, et al.: Renal allografts: prospective analysis of Doppler sonography. *Radiology* 169:371, 1988.

Buckley AR, Cooperberg PL, Reeve CE, et al.: The distinction between acute renal transplant rejection and cyclosporine nephrotoxicity: value of duplex sonography. *AJR* 149:521, 1987.

Murphy AM, Robertson RJ, Dubbins PA: Duplex ultrasound in the assessment of renal transplant complications. *Clin Radiol* 38:229, 1987.

Needleman L, Kurtz AB: Doppler evaluation of the renal transplant. *J Clin Ultrasound* 15:661, 1987.

Posniak MA, Kelcz F, Dodd GF: Renal transplant ultrasound: imaging and Doppler. *Semin Ultrasound CT MR* 12(4):319, 1991.

Rifkin MD, Needleman L, Pasto ME, et al.: Evaluation of renal transplant rejection by duplex Doppler examination: value of resistive index. *AJR* 148:759, 1987.

Rigsby CM, Burns PN, Weltin GG, et al.: Doppler signal quantitation in renal allografts: comparison in normal and rejection transplants, with pathologic correlation. *Radiology* 162:39, 1987.

Rejection-Angiographic Studies

Clark RL, Mandel SR, Webster WR: Microvascular changes in canine renal allograft rejection: a correlative microangiographic and histologic study. *Invest Radiol* 12:62, 1977.

Foley WD, Bookstein JJ, Tweist M, et al.: Arteriography of renal transplants. *Radiology* 116:271, 1975.

Orons PD, Zajko AB: Angiography and interventional aspects of renal transplantation. *Radiol Clin North Am* 33(3):461, 1995.

Magnetic Resonance Imaging

Baumgartner RB, Nelson RC, Ball TI, et al.: MR imaging of renal transplants. *AJR* 147:949, 1986.

Halasz NA: Differential diagnosis of renal transplant rejection: is MR imaging the answer? *AJR* 147:954, 1986.

Hricak H, Terrier F, Demas BE: Renal allografts: evaluation by MR imaging. *Radiology* 159:435, 1986.

Klehr HU, Spannbrucker N, Molitor D, et al.: Magnetic resonance imaging in renal transplants. *Transplant Proc* 19(5):3716, 1987.

Steinberg HV, Nelson RC, Murphy FB, et al.: Renal allograft rejection: evaluation by Doppler US and MR imaging. *Radiology* 163:337, 1987.

Transplant Rupture

Ostrovsky PD, Cart L, Goodman JC, et al.: Ultrasound findings in renal transplant rupture. *J Clin Ultrasound* 13:132, 1985.

Rahatzad M, Henderson SC, Borch GS: Ultrasound appearance of spontaneous rupture of renal transplant. *J Urol* 126:535, 1981.

Computed Tomography

Ehrman KO, Kopecky KK, Wass JL, et al.: Parapelvic lymph cyst in a renal allograft mimicking hydronephrosis: CT diagnosis. *J Comput Assist Tomogr* 11(4):714, 1987.

Letourneau JG, Day DL, Feinberg SB: Ultrasound and computed tomographic evaluation of renal transplantation. *Radiol Clin North Am* 25(2):267, 1987.

Vascular Complications

Flechner SM, Sandler CM, Childs T, et al.: Screening for transplant renal artery stenosis in hypertensive recipients using digital subtraction angiography. *J Urol* 130:440, 1983.

Hohnke C, Abendroth D, Schleibner S, et al.: Vascular complications in 1200 kidney transplantations. *Transplant Proc* 19(5):3691, 1987.

Orons PD, Zajko AB: Angiography and interventional aspects of renal transplantation. *Rad Clin North Am* 33(3):461, 1995.

Raval B, Balsara V, Kim EE: Computed tomography detection of transplant renal artery pseudoaneurysm. CT. *J Comput Tomogr* 9(2):149, 1985.

Raynaud A, Bedrossian J, Remy P, et al.: Percutaneous transluminal angioplasty of renal transplant arterial stenosis. *AJR* 146:853, 1986.

Sniderman KW, Sos TA, Sprayregen S, et al.: Percutaneous transluminal angioplasty in renal transplant arterial stenosis for relief of hypertension. *Radiology* 135:23, 1980.

Sniderman KW, Sprayregen S, Sos TA, et al.: Percutaneous transluminal dilation in renal transplant arterial stenosis. *Transplantation* 30(6):440, 1980.

Taylor KJW, Morse SS, Rigsby CM, et al.: Vascular complications in renal allografts: detection with duplex Doppler US. *Radiology* 162:31, 1987.

Urologic Complications

Becker JA, Kutcher R: Urologic complications of renal transplantation. *Semin Roentgenol* 13(4):341, 1978.

Bennett LN, Voegeli DR, Crummy AB, et al.: Urologic complications following renal transplantation: role of interventional radiologic procedures. *Radiology* 160:531, 1986.

Bushnell DL, Wilson DG, Lieberman LM: Scintigraphic assessment of perivesical urinary extravasation following renal transplantation. *Clin Nucl Med* 9(2):92, 1984.

Curry NS, Cochran S, Barbaric ZL, et al.: Interventional radiologic procedures in the renal transplant. *Radiology* 152:647, 1984.

Glanz S, Gordon DH, Butt K, et al.: Percutaneous transrenal balloon dilatation of the ureter. *Radiology* 149:101, 1983.

Glanz S, Rotter MR, Gordon DH, et al.: Interventional radiologic procedures in the management of the renal transplant patients. *Urol Radiol* 7:97, 1985.

Loughlin KR, Tilney NL, Richie JP: Urologic complications in 718 renal transplant patients. *Surgery* 95:297, 1984.

Schmeller NT, Schuller J, Hofstetter A, et al.: Fine needle antegrade pyelography of transplanted kidneys. *Urol Radiol* 7:19, 1985.

Streem SB, Novick AC, Steinmuller DR, et al.: Percutaneous techniques for the management of urological renal transplant complications. *J Urol* 135:456, 1986.

van Sonnenberg E, Wittich GR, Casola G, et al.: Lymphoceles: imaging characteristics and percutaneous management. *Radiology* 161:593, 1986.

Voegeli DR, Crummy AB, McDermott JC, et al.: Percutaneous management of the urological complications of renal transplantation. *Radiographics* 6(6):1007, 1986.

Long-Term Complications of Renal Transplantation

Frick MP, Salomonowitz E, Hanto DW, et al.: CT of abdominal lymphoma after renal transplantation. *AJR* 142:97, 1984.

Penn I: Malignancies associated with immunosuppressive or cytotoxic therapy. *Surgery* 83(5):492, 1978.

12

••

Nephrocalcinosis and Nephrolithiasis

•••••••••

Intrarenal calcifications may lie in the renal parenchyma (nephrocalcinosis) or in the renal collecting system (nephrolithiasis). Dystrophic calcification is calcification of abnormal tissue such as tumors, cyst walls, inflammatory masses, or vessels. Because dystrophic calcification is caused by the underlying parenchymal abnormality, it is not considered nephrocalcinosis.

Nephrolithiasis is stone formation within the collecting system. Most stones are formed in the pelvocalyceal system and may be passed distally. Occasionally stones may form in a cavity that communicates with the collecting system, such as a calyceal diverticulum, in the bladder, or in a urethral diverticulum. Those conditions that result in nephrocalcinosis often lead to nephrolithiasis.

Because calcification is readily detected on an abdominal radiograph, nephrocalcinosis and nephrolithiasis are routinely evaluated with conventional urography. When supplemented with computed tomography (CT), even relatively lucent stones are easily detected. Furthermore, a variety of interventional techniques are now commonly employed in the treatment of nephrolithiasis and its complications.

NEPHROCALCINOSIS

Calcification of abnormal tissue is termed dystrophic. Dystrophic calcification may occur when the solubility product of calcium and phosphate is exceeded because of a change in pH or may be part of a reparative process. This may occur in a huge variety of lesions, but the most common are tumor, hematoma, an inflammatory mass,

and vascular abnormalities. Dystrophic calcifications will be considered in the discussion of the specific entities.

Calcification of normal renal tissue due to abnormally high levels of calcium is termed metastatic. Metastatic calcification occurs when the solubility product of calcium and phosphate or oxalate in the extracellular fluid is exceeded. Certain diseases have a predilection to calcify specific anatomic areas (Table 12.1). Thus, metastatic nephrocalcinosis may be further subdivided by predominant location.

Cortical Nephrocalcinosis

Cortical nephrocalcinosis is located in the periphery and along the central septa of Bertin. The medullary pyramids are spared. Cortical nephrocalcinosis may be seen on abdominal radiographs as thin peripheral lines of calcification ("tram lines") or as diffuse punctate calcifications representing necrotic cortical tubules. The cortex is echogenic on ultrasound but typically does not have shadowing, and noncontrast CT shows high attenuation of the cortex (Fig. 12.1).

The most common entities to produce cortical nephrocalcinosis are chronic glomerulonephritis and acute cortical necrosis. Cortical nephrocalcinosis also may be seen in Alport's syndrome (hereditary nephropathy and deafness), oxalosis, and in some patients with a rejected renal transplant. Infection with *Pneumocystis carinii*, *Mycobacterium avium intracellulare* (MAI), and cytomegalovirus can result in multiple stippled calcifications in the renal cortex in patients with AIDS (*see* Chapter 7).

Acute cortical necrosis may be caused by ingestion of toxins such as ethylene glycol, exposure to methoxyflurane anesthesia, or an acute vascular insult. Both ethylene glycol and methoxyflurane exposure result in oxalate deposition that causes interstitial fibrosis. Acute hypotension may cause focal tubular necrosis that later calcifies; the typical clinical situation is placenta abruptio with significant hemorrhage.

Hereditary nephritis, or Alport's syndrome, is characterized by glomerulonephritis and interstitial fibrosis, and is frequently associated with nerve deafness. It is inherited as an autosomal dominant trait with variable penetrance. The disease is transmitted to sons and daughters, but it is incompletely expressed in females. Hematuria often begins in childhood and mild protein-

Table 12.1.
Major Causes of Nephrocalcinosis

Cortical Nephrocalcinosis
  Cortical necrosis
  Chronic glomerulonephritis
  Oxalosis
  Alport's syndrome (hereditary nephritis)
Medullary Nephrocalcinosis
  Hypercalcemic states (e.g., hyperparathyroidism)
  Renal tubular acidosis (distal, type I)
  Medullary sponge kidney

uria may be present. Progression to renal failure is slow, with death by the third to fifth decade.

Medullary Nephrocalcinosis

Medullary nephrocalcinosis is central in location, but with peripheral extensions along the medullary pyramids. It is usually a bilateral process with multiple stippled calcifications in the characteristic distribution (Fig.

12.2); the exception is medullary sponge kidney, which may be unilateral or segmental. On ultrasound, the pyramids are echogenic and may or may not have shadowing depending on the size of the calcifications (Fig. 12.3). Computed tomography also clearly shows the high attenuation calcifications in the characteristic medullary distribution (Fig. 12.2).

The most common etiologies to produce medullary nephrocalcinosis are hyperparathyroidism and renal tubular acidosis. Other relatively common causes include tubular ectasia (medullary sponge kidney), the milk-alkali syndrome, and a variety of nephrotoxic drugs such as amphotericin B. Hyperparathyroidism may be caused by a parathyroid adenoma, carcinoma, or hyperplasia of the chief cells. It is most commonly due to a single adenoma. Typically the serum calcium level is high and the phosphate level is low. This helps distinguish primary hyperparathyroidism from secondary hyperparathyroidism resulting from chronic renal disease in which the serum phosphate is elevated.

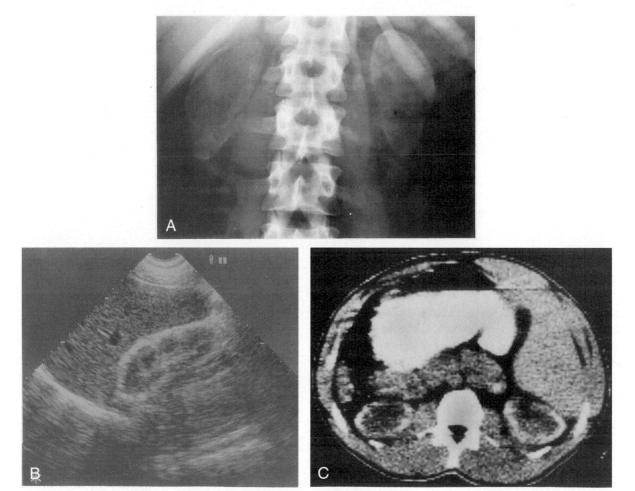

Figure 12.1. Cortical nephrocalcinosis. **A,** Abdominal radiograph shows small kidneys with dense cortical calcification. **B,** Ultrasound of the right kidney shows a very echodense cortex with normal medullary echo pattern. Note that there is no significant shadowing. **C,** Noncontrast Computed tomography scan shows high attenuation renal cortices bilaterally, whereas the medullary regions show normal soft tissue attenuation.

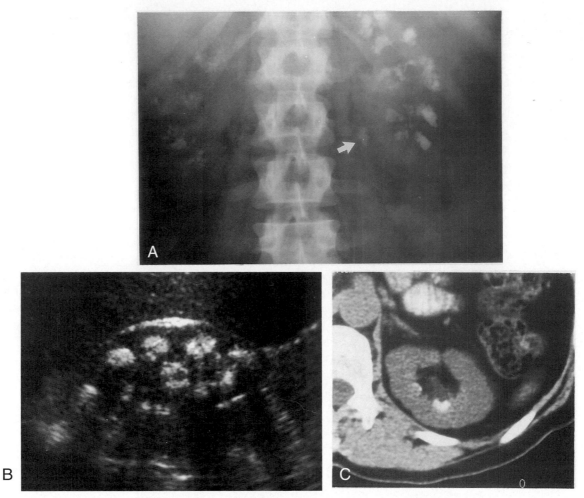

Figure 12.2. Medullary nephrocalcinosis. **A,** Abdominal radiograph reveals dense aggregates of calcifications in the regions of the papillae bilaterally. A stone has passed into the proximal ureter on the left (*arrow*). These dense aggregates are typical of renal tubular acidosis. **B,** Multiple highly echogenic foci in the region of the renal pyramids with shadowing are detected on ultrasound. **C,** Magnified noncontrast computed tomography section through left kidney shows dense calcification in the medulla.

Renal Tubular Acidosis

Patients with renal tubular acidosis (RTA) have a defect in the tubules that prevents the kidney from excreting an acid urine. Thus, the risk of stone formation is increased, as calcium salts are less soluble in alkaline urine than in an acid urine. In adults, primary RTA is caused by an inherited enzymatic defect. The manifestations of urolithiasis, osteomalacia, and hypokalemia can be treated with alkalinizing salts.

A nonhereditary form of primary RTA has been described in children (Lightwood's syndrome). This transient disorder affects infants and lasts several years. However, if treated during the acute period, spontaneous improvement in distal tubular function occurs.

Secondary RTA occurs as a result of a diminished ability of the distal tubule to excrete hydrogen ions. Disease processes that cause secondary RTA by impairing hydrogen ion excretion by the distal tubule include Fanconi's syndrome, Wilson's disease, and amphotericin B toxicity.

Renal tubular acidosis is divided into proximal and distal forms. The proximal variety (type II) of RTA is a result of decreased bicarbonate reabsorption by the proximal tubule. When reabsorption of other substances also is impaired, RTA is known as Fanconi's syndrome. Although biochemically interesting, this proximal form does not have radiographic manifestations.

In the distal (type I) form, the distal renal tubule can no longer secrete hydrogen ions. This results in bicarbonate loss, reduced acid excretion, secondary aldosteronism, and hypokalemia. Nephrocalcinosis occurs in approximately 75% of these patients and commonly appears as clusters of calcifications in the medullary pyramids.

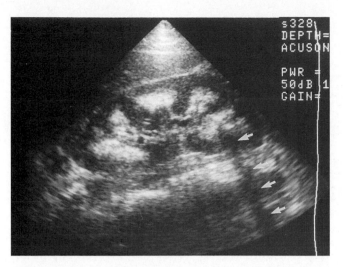

Figure 12.3.   Medullary nephrocalcinosis. Echogenic renal pyramids are seen on an ultrasound examination. Focal shadowing (*arrows*) is caused by a calculus.

Other

Nephrocalcinosis may occur in patients who consume large quantities of antacids and milk for the treatment of peptic ulcer disease. This has been termed the "milk alkali syndrome." Alkaline urine facilitates precipitation of calcium-containing calculi.

The stones found in medullary sponge kidney are cal-

cium phosphate or calcium oxalate. They are usually small, and many more are present than can be detected radiographically. These tiny stones are asymptomatic, but may cause colic if they migrate into the collecting system, enlarge, and begin to pass down the ureter. This condition is caused by cystic dilation of the distal collecting ducts, which causes stasis of urine and stone formation. Because this is an anatomic rather than a metabolic defect, it can occur unilaterally or even segmentally in one or both kidneys. This type of distribution should suggest the diagnosis, as should a linear configuration of medullary calculi (Fig. 12.4). Further evidence is pooling of contrast around the stones in the dilated collecting ducts during excretory urography.

NEPHROLITHIASIS

Nephrolithiasis is a common problem among people from temperate climates. Smith estimates that at least 5% of the female and 12% of the male population will have at least one episode of renal colic due to stone disease by 70 years of age. Interestingly, a low urinary output is believed to aid in urinary tract stone formation, yet people from areas with hot climates such as Africa have a low incidence of stone disease. Perhaps those peoples are genetically less likely to form stones.

In the United States, the southeastern states often are called the "stone belt," because they have the highest incidence of stone disease. Hospital admissions for stone-

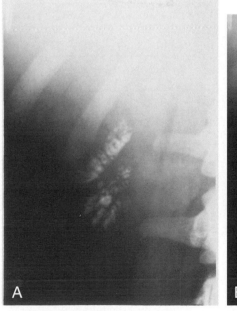
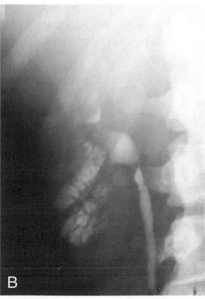

Figure 12.4.   Medullary sponge kidney. **A,** Coned view of the right kidney without contrast shows multiple, somewhat linear calcifications overlying the lower pole. **B,** Excretory urogram reveals the calcifications to involve only the lower-pole calyces. Contrast medium can be seen surrounding the stones. (From Amis ES Jr, Newhouse JH: *Essentials of Uroradiology.* Boston, Little, Brown & Company, 1991.)

related problems are twice as common in the Southeast as the rest of the nation.

There are many etiologies for the production of nephrolithiasis including genetic predisposition, diet, occupation, and lifestyle. A high water intake resulting in an increased urinary output significantly reduces the incidence of stones in patients predisposed to stone formation.

The urine must be supersaturated at least part of the time for stone formation. In addition to solute load, ionic strength complexation, and urine pH affect stone formation. Ionic strength increases the ability of urine to hold ions in solution. Anionic substances, such as citrate phosphate or sulfate may complex calcium, which reduces the free ionic concentration of the crystal components. The urine pH affects complexation and also has a direct effect on the solubility of organic compounds such as uric acid or cystine. Uric acid, for instance, is much more soluble as the pH increases.

Nephrolithiasis is seen 3 times as often in men as in women. The peak age for the onset of renal stone disease is 20 to 30 years, but the tendency for stone formation often is lifelong. Most commonly patients treated for nephrolithiasis are 30 to 60 years of age.

The most common presenting symptom is renal colic, which is usually caused by a ureteral stone. Controversy remains whether or not calyceal stones cause pain. Most calyceal stones are asymptomatic, but occasionally their removal is associated with relief of pain.

Renal colic is abrupt in onset, most frequently begins in the flank, and radiates to the groin. Men may complain of testicular pain, whereas women feel discomfort radiating to the labia majora. Typically, patients suffering renal colic cannot find a comfortable position and continue to move around. Patients with stones in the distal ureter may present with symptoms of bladder irritability.

Hematuria is present in the vast majority of patients with urolithiasis, but may be absent in as many as 15% of patients, particularly if the stone is completely obstructing. Pyuria is uncommon, but a culture should be obtained to detect a urinary tract infection.

The probability of stone passage is related to the size of the stone. Approximately 90% of stones 4 mm or less in diameter pass spontaneously.

Specific Types of Urolithiasis

Calcium Stones

Calcium oxalate and calcium phosphate stones crystallize when the product of the two ions exceeds the solubility product. Thus, both the amount of calcium and the amount of oxalate are important in determining stone formation. A discussion of these factors is beyond the scope of this book, but factors affecting hypercalciuria are presented (Table 12.4).

Hypercalcemia is a common cause of hypercalciuria,

Table 12.2.
Radiolucent Stones

Uric acid
Xanthine
Struvite
Matrix stones

although it is present in a minority of patients, and may result from a variety of metabolic processes. An abnormally large amount of calcium may be absorbed from the digestive tract. This occurs with hypervitaminosis D, sarcoidosis, and the milk-alkali syndrome. Too much calcium may be mobilized from the bony skeleton. This may result from immobilization, extensive bone metastases, or hyperparathyroidism.

Ionized calcium is filtered by the glomerulus, but most of this free calcium is reabsorbed by tubules. However, there is a maximum reabsorption that can occur. If this is exceeded by a high calcium load in patients with hypercalcemia, hypercalciuria will result.

Hypercalciuria also may occur if there is distal renal tubular damage that interferes with hydrogen ion excretion creating RTA. Patients with primary RTA commonly

Table 12.3.
Incidence of Urinary Lithiasis[a]

Calcium oxalate and phosphate, mixed	34
Calcium oxalate, pure	33
Calcium phosphate, pure	6
"Triple phosphate" (struvite + apatite)	15
Uric acid	8
Cystine	3

[a]Percentage of stones analyzed.

Table 12.4.
Causes of Hypercalciuria

Increased absorption
   Hypervitaminosis D
   Milk-alkali syndrome
   Sarcoidosis
   Beryllium poisoning
   Idiopathic hypercalciuria
Increased mobilization from bone
   Hyperparathyroidism
   Immobilization
   Bone metastases
   Multiple myeloma
   Hyperthyroidism
   Cushing's syndrome
Decreased tubular reabsorption
   Renal tubular acidosis
   Fanconi's syndrome
   Wilson's disease
   Amphotericin B toxicity

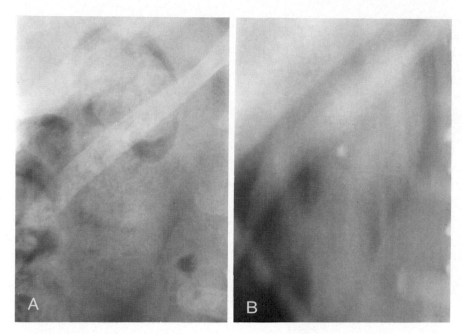

Figure 12.5. Calcium stone. **A,** Overlying bowel gas obscures a right renal stone. **B,** Nephrotomography clearly reveals a 5-mm calcium oxalate stone.

develop nephrocalcinosis, which characteristically involves the medullary pyramids. Secondary RTA may be caused by a variety of diseases including Fanconi's syndrome, Wilson's disease, and amphotericin B toxicity, which also affects the distal renal tubule.

Calcium stones are relatively dense and are usually easily seen on abdominal radiographs. Small stones may be obscured by overlying bowel gas or fecal material, and nephrotomography often is needed for identification and quantification (Fig. 12.5).

Cystine Stones

Patients with cystinuria have a defect in renal tubular reabsorption of the amino acids cystine, ornithine, lysine, and arginine. A positive nitroprusside test is diagnostic, and exchange-column chromatography can identify the amino acids in the urine. The defect is inherited as an autosomal-recessive trait and is present in the intestinal mucosa as well as in the renal tubular cells. Although in some patients a short stature is attributed to lysine deficiency, the only manifestation in most patients is nephrolithiasis. Excess cystine excreted in the urine exceeds its solubility, and cystine stones are produced.

The opacity of cystine stones depends on how much contamination with calcium is present. However, many stones are pure cystine and are still easily seen on abdominal radiographs, although they are not as dense as calcium stones (Fig. 12.6).

Struvite Stones

Magnesium ammonium phosphate (struvite) stones form when the urine pH is more than 7.2. They com-

monly occur in the setting of a urinary tract infection with a urea-splitting Gram-negative enteric organism, often *Proteus mirabilis*. Thus, struvite calculi also are commonly referred to as "infection stones." Because women have more urinary tract infections, struvite stones are seen more frequently in women than in men.

Pure struvite stones are essentially radiolucent and rare. Typically struvite is found mixed with calcium phosphate (apatite), to form the so-called triple phos-

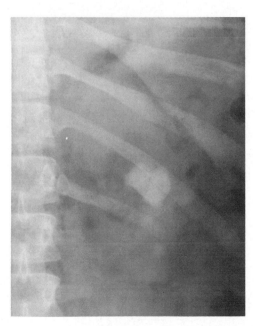

Figure 12.6. Cystine stone. A cystine stone is easily detected on an abdominal radiograph.

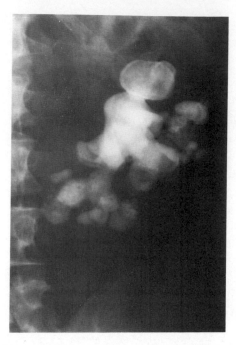

Figure 12.7. Staghorn calculus. A large staghorn calculus is easily seen in the left kidney. The alignment suggests a horseshoe kidney.

phate stones, which are easily seen on plain radiographs. These calcium magnesium ammonium phosphate stones are seen in association with infected urine; to refer to them as struvite alone is a misnomer. They account for approximately 70% of staghorn calculi (Fig. 12.7), the remainder being composed of cystine or uric acid.

Uric Acid Stones

Unlike other mammals, humans lack the enzyme uricase, which converts uric acid into allantoin. In urine, uric acid exists either free or as the much more soluble salt, sodium urate. Acid urine (pH < 5.75) contributes to an increased concentration of the less soluble free uric acid.

Patients with urate calculi have hyperuricosuria, but do not necessarily have hyperuricemia. Idiopathic uric acid lithiasis occurs in patients with normal serum urate levels, but with a persistently low urine pH. This is seen in patients who take medications to acidify their urine, but it also may be present in patients with chronic diarrhea or an ileostomy.

Inborn errors of metabolism may result in hyperuricemia and uric acid lithiasis. Patients with gout or the Lesch-Nyhan syndrome are prone to form uric acid stones. Similarly, an overindulgence in foods high in purine and proteins metabolized to uric acid may lead to hyperuricemia, hyperuricosuria, and uric acid stones. The ingestion of uricosuric drugs such as salicylates and thiazides may increase the urine uric acid concentration sufficiently to allow uric acid stone formation.

In the United States, uric acid stones account for 5 to 10% of renal stones. The reported incidence varies by country; in Israel, approximately 75% of renal stones are uric acid stones.

Uric acid stones are insufficiently radiopaque to be seen on an abdominal radiograph (Fig. 12.8). They account for the majority of "lucent" stones. However, they are still sufficiently dense to be easily seen on CT.

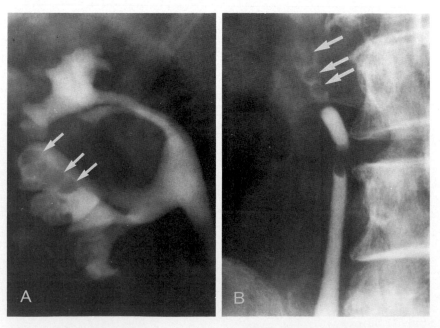

Figure 12.8. Uric acid stones. No stones could be seen on the preliminary radiograph. However, multiple filling defects (*arrows*) representing uric acid stones are identified on **A,** an excretory urogram and **B,** a retrograde pyelogram.

Xanthine Stones

These very rare stones may be seen in patients with hereditary xanthinuria, but also may be present in patients treated with allopurinol, which blocks the conversion of xanthine to uric acid. Xanthine stones are relatively radiolucent, because their density is similar to uric acid stones.

Matrix Stones

Matrix stones are comprised primarily of coagulated mucoids with very little crystalline component. They are found most commonly in patients with urease-producing infections such as *Proteus* species. Matrix stones also are relatively radiolucent (Fig. 12.9) and may be confused with uric acid calculi. However, matrix stones occur in the presence of an alkaline urine, whereas the urine is acidic in patients with uric acid calculi.

Oxalate Stones

Increased excretion of oxalate may be due to an inborn error of metabolism (primary) or may be secondary to other disorders. Hyperoxaluria may cause nephrocalcinosis and may result in calcium oxalate stones. The term *oxalosis* is used to indicate precipitation of oxalate crystals in extrarenal tissues such as the myocardium, lung, spleen, or arterial walls.

The most common cause of secondary oxalosis is small bowel disease, especially after intestinal bypass operations for morbid obesity, but it also may be seen if the distal small bowel is involved in patients with celiac

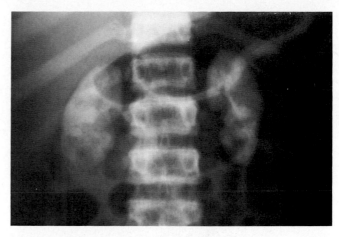

Figure 12.10. Primary oxaluria. Calcium oxalate crystals have precipitated out in the renal parenchyma.

disease or Crohn's disease. These patients have increased absorption of oxalate by the colon because of increased permeability of the colon or increased solubility of oxalate. Other causes of secondary hyperoxaluria include pyridoxine deficiency, methoxyflurane anesthesia, or increased consumption of leafy green vegetables that are high in oxalate.

Primary oxaluria is a rare inborn error of metabolism. There are two biochemical forms, but both result in increased urinary excretion of oxalate salts. Primary oxaluria is inherited as an autosomal recessive trait and shows no sex predilection. Patients present with manifestations of renal stones early in life. Furthermore, dense calcification of the entire kidney (cortex and medulla) can occur (Fig. 12.10).

Calcium oxalate crystals may precipitate out in the renal tubules, which become obstructed and lead to tubular necrosis and atrophy. The crystals may stimulate an immune response in the kidney, causing an interstitial nephritis. This results in progressive atrophy and renal failure.

Patients with hyperoxaluria may present with calcium oxalate stones (Fig. 12.11). However, most patients with such stones do not have a detectable abnormality of oxalate metabolism or increased levels of oxalate excretion.

Stone Disease in Children

In developing countries, bladder calculi are common in children. They most often are uric acid stones and are unrelated to obstruction or infection. In industrialized countries, urinary tract calculi are found much more frequently in the upper urinary tract, as in adults.

The male preponderance of stones seen in adults does not occur in children; boys and girls are equally affected. Black children are affected much less commonly than are white children. Hematuria is the most common

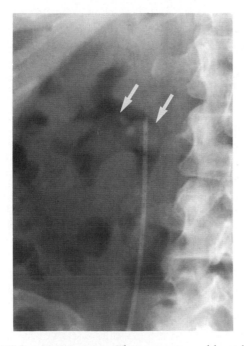

Figure 12.9. Matrix stones. These stones could not be seen on the abdominal radiograph. An air pyelogram demonstrated two large matrix stones (*arrows*).

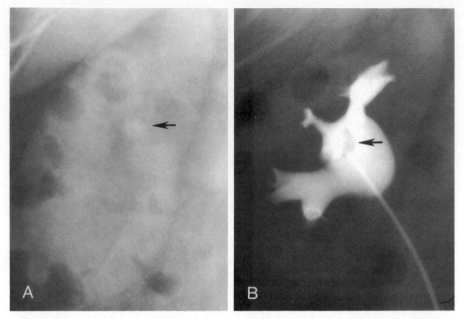

Figure 12.11. Oxalate stone. **A,** A faintly opaque oxalate stone (*arrow*) is appreciated on the preliminary film. **B,** It is seen as a filling defect (*arrow*) in the retrograde pyelogram.

presenting symptom. Rather than the severe pain of ureteral colic seen in adults, children often complain of a more diffuse abdominal pain. The vast majority of pediatric patients have an underlying predisposing factor. Thus, children must be carefully evaluated for metabolic, anatomic, or infectious causes.

In a recent study of stone disease in the pediatric population, Nimkin and colleagues reported that 30% of cases were related to myelodysplasia (76% of these patients had an ileal conduit), 26% had some other type of anatomic urinary tract problem, 17% had known metabolic disease, and the remainder had other miscellaneous conditions or the stones were considered idiopathic.

Nephrolithiasis is rare in very young children, but has been reported in premature babies after furosemide therapy for bronchopulmonary dysplasia. Because urinary calcium excretion varies directly with urinary sodium excretion, furosemide, which increases sodium excretion, also results in hypercalciuria. This is especially marked in preterm babies, because the marked increase in volume of amniotic fluid during the last trimester of pregnancy results from an increased excretion of sodium and water by the fetal kidney. Thus, premature babies have a higher urinary calcium level at birth and are more prone to nephrocalcinosis than full-term children. This nephrocalcinosis is typically medullary, resulting in echogenic renal pyramids. Another cause of this finding is treatment with vitamin D for hypophosphatemic rickets or hypophosphatemic bone disease. Pyramidal hyperechogenicity in a pattern mimicking nephrocalcinosis also can occur in some children with autosomal recessive polycystic kidney disease.

Radiology Diagnosis

Plain Radiograph

Because approximately 90% of urinary tract calculi are radiopaque, the plain abdominal radiograph is the most useful examination in evaluating patients suspected of urolithiasis. Large stones are readily detected on a single film, but small calculi may be obscured by bowel gas or fecal material within the colon. If there are confusing overlying shadows, oblique films or nephrotomograms may be needed. With stones less than approximately 5 mm in diameter, nephrotomograms are usually more effective than oblique films, because the small opacity may be difficult to find on both the anteroposterior and oblique projections. Routine plain nephrotomography also is valuable in following patients with nephrolithiasis, because tomography provides more precise delineation of the extent of the stone burden, especially when small calculi are present.

In addition to overlying bowel contents, the ribs, transverse processes, and sacrum may obscure urinary tract calculi. The lateral edge of the transverse process can be especially confusing, since the cortical margin may mimic a ureteral stone.

Many common calcifications in the abdomen must be distinguished from urinary tract stones. Hepatic or splenic calcifications are seldom a problem, since they often do not overlie the kidneys. However, gallstones may lie over the right renal collecting system. In most cases, gallstones are larger with a characteristic ovoid shape and are easily distinguished from renal stones.

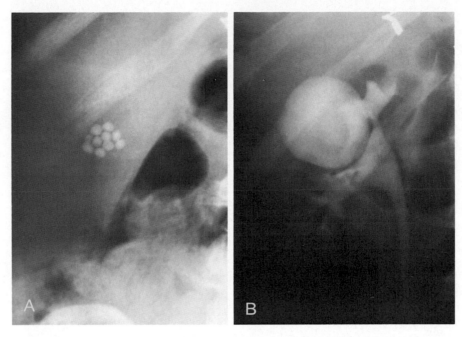

Figure 12.12. Stones in a calyceal diverticulum. **A,** Multiple stones in a spherical configuration in the right upper quadrant suggest gallstones. **B,** An excretory urogram demonstrates their location in a calyceal diverticulum.

However, renal calculi in an obstructed portion of the collecting system or within a calyceal diverticulum (Fig. 12.12) may precisely mimic gallstones. On an oblique radiograph, gallstones should rotate anteriorly, whereas renal stones remain in a more posterior location.

Pancreatic calcification is most frequently seen in chronic pancreatitis. The involvement of the entire gland helps to distinguish these calcifications from renal stones.

Calcification of the costal cartilage of the lower thoracic ribs and arterial calcifications are usually linear, which helps to separate them from renal stones. Furthermore, arterial and rib calcifications lie in predictable locations.

The calcifications most often confused with urinary tract calculi are phleboliths (Fig. 12.13) and calcified mesenteric lymph nodes. Typically phleboliths are rounded, have a central lucency, and are seen in the true pelvis, often below the distal ureter. However, phleboliths are extremely common and are occasionally impossible to distinguish from ureteral stones without opacification of the ureter. Mesenteric lymph nodes typically have a mottled calcification, and oblique films may show them anterior to the retroperitoneum.

In these or other confusing cases, the most valuable maneuver often is comparison with old radiographs. The presence of a pelvic phlebolith that predates renal colic may be sufficient to identify a confusing calcification. In other cases, however, opacification of the col-

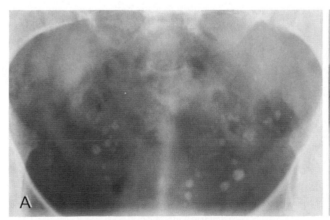
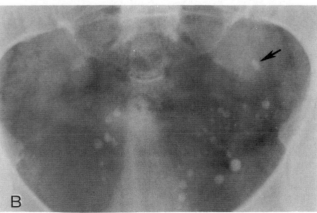

Figure 12.13. Distal ureteral stone. **A,** Multiple pelvic phleboliths are present. **B,** One week later, a distal left ureteral stone (*arrow*) can be detected by comparison with the previous film.

lecting system is needed to separate a urinary tract calculus from an adjacent calcified structure. However, once contrast has been introduced, radiopaque stones become much more difficult to locate. Thus, care must be taken to obtain all preliminary films that are needed before proceeding to contrast injection.

Urography

Excretory urography serves two important functions in the evaluation of the patient with suspected stone disease: (*a*) It delineates the relationship of the collecting system to the calcification on the preliminary film, and (*b*) it demonstrates the degree of obstruction.

Calcifications overlying or within the kidney are seen to be renal stones when their location within the collecting system is demonstrated. Many calcium stones have a density similar to excreted contrast medium, and a careful comparison with the preliminary radiograph is necessary to confirm their location. More lucent stones, such as uric acid calculi, are not seen on the scout film, but are identified as filling defects after the collecting system has been opacified.

The anatomy of the collecting system affects the likelihood of a renal stone to be passed, and the spot where it is likely to stop if it does not pass. Patients with an abnormal collecting system may have focal dilatation due to infundibular stenosis or a calyceal diverticulum, either of which may harbor a stone that is unlikely to pass spontaneously. A ureteropelvic junction obstruction, or even high insertion of the ureter, is likely to keep a stone in the renal pelvis and prevent it from entering the ureter. A ureteral stricture will prevent a stone from passing further.

In patients with an anatomically normal collecting system, a renal stone is most likely to be held up in the renal pelvis, at the point where the ureter crosses over the iliac vessels or at the ureterovesical junction (Fig. 12.14). While 75% of ureteral stones are found distally at the time of diagnosis, stones may hang up at any point along the course of the ureter, and the entire route must be carefully studied in patients with renal colic.

Stones are especially difficult to identify when they overlie the sacrum or ilium. Comparison with old radiographs, if available, is helpful (Fig. 12.13), but in many cases, urography is needed to identify the stone (Fig. 12.15) and site of obstruction.

The anatomy of the collecting system also is pertinent if interventional techniques are planned. Extracorporeal shock wave lithotripsy (ESWL) is best applied to stones in the renal pelvis. If a percutaneous approach will be used, the location of the stone within the collecting system and the relationship of the collecting system to adjacent structures, such as liver, spleen, ribs and diaphragm is critical.

Stones may cause obstruction in a calyx, infundibu-

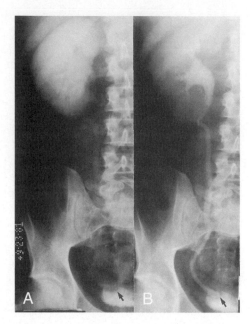

Figure 12.14. Distal ureteral stone. **A,** Thirty-minute film from an excretory urogram reveals an obstructive nephrogram with contrast in the proximal two thirds of the right ureter. A tiny stone can be seen at the ureterovesical junction (*arrow*) with surrounding edema. **B,** Two-hour delayed urogram film reveals contrast columning in the entire right ureter to the previously mentioned stone (*arrow*). (From Amis ES Jr, Newhouse JH: *Essentials of Uroradiology,* Boston, Little, Brown & Co, 1991.)

lum, or at any point along the ureter. When stones remain impacted in an infundibulum for any length of time, there is resultant ballooning of the calyx and thinning of the overlying renal parenchyma, leading to a radiographic pattern that may be indistinguishable from the scarring seen in chronic atrophic pyelonephritis caused by reflux.

The most obvious sign of obstruction is delayed opacification of the collecting system with contrast medium. The nephrogram also is delayed compared with the normal contralateral side, but may have increased intensity with time as contrast is not being excreted from the tubules (Fig. 12.14**A**). The degree of dilation of the collecting system depends on the degree and duration of obstruction. In general, patients with acute ureteral obstruction, either partial or complete, have renal colic severe enough to seek medical attention. Thus, the urogram demonstrates only mild calyceal blunting and mild dilation of the ureter to the point of obstruction. Occasionally a persistent stone or recurrent stone passage may cause greater degrees of dilation of the collecting system (Fig. 12.16). Although these changes are usually quite evident, uncertainty may arise if there has been previous ureteral obstruction after which the collecting system has not returned to normal.

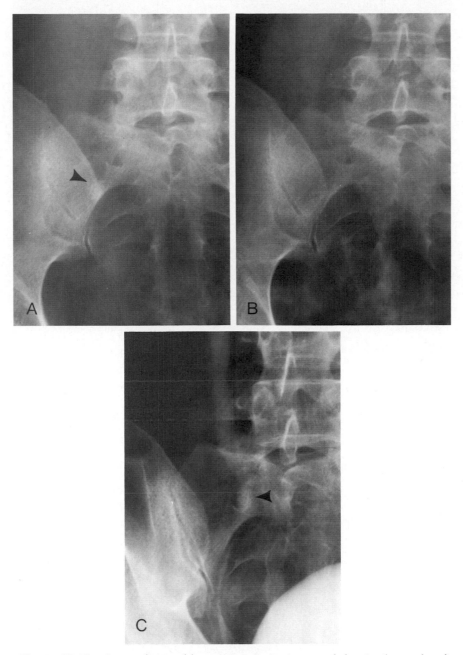

Figure 12.15.   Stone obscured by sacrum. **A,** An increased density (*arrowhead*) blends with the sacrum and ilium. **B,** By comparison with a previous film, it is seen to be recently acquired. **C,** An excretory urogram demonstrates that this density (*arrowhead*) is a partially obstructing ureteral stone.

On occasion, an obstructed collecting system can decompress itself by leakage of urine, typically from one or more calyceal fornices into the renal sinus. This is known as pyelosinus extravasation and can occur with only mild degrees of obstruction. Pyelosinus extravasation is not unusual in patients with ureteral stones and has no clinical significance if the urine is not infected. From the renal sinus, urine may track through the renal hilum and surround the renal pelvis and proximal ureter (Fig. 12.17).

A more subtle change of ureteral obstruction is a persistent full column of contrast medium in the ureter which ends at the stone (Fig. 12.14**B**). Upright films or a film obtained after voiding frequently exaggerates this difference between the mildly obstructed side and the normal side, and helps to facilitate the diagnosis.

Diminished opacity of the ipsilateral ureter is another urographic sign of an obstructing ureteral stone (Fig. 12.18). This sign may be recognized even in the absence of dilation of the collecting system. This presumably oc-

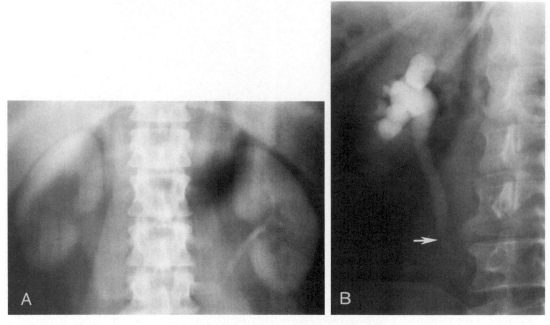

Figure 12.16. Ureteral stone. **A,** Delayed excretion from the right kidney is appreciated on an early nephrotomogram. **B,** On later films ureteropelvocaliectasis ending in the midureter demonstrates the stone location (*arrow*).

curs as a result of decreased concentrating ability of the kidney, but the mechanism is unknown.

Stones that become impacted usually cause edema that may appear as a filling defect within the collecting system. This may have a particularly ominous appearance if a stone impacts at the ureterovesical junction (Fig. 12.14**B**). The halo appearance may suggest a ureterocele or even bladder carcinoma.

Retrograde Pyelography

Retrograde pyelography may be indicated if an excretory urogram is contraindicated, or if there is inadequate excretion of contrast medium into the affected collecting system. Patients with a severe contrast allergy or who are at increased risk for contrast-induced renal failure may be studied with retrograde pyelography. However, there may be slight contrast absorption across the

Figure 12.17. Ureteropelvic junction (UPJ) stone with pyelosinus extravasation. **A,** Coned plain-film view of the left renal fossa shows two calcifications. The lower stone (*arrow*) is in the region of the UPJ. **B,** Thirty-minute film from an excretory urogram reveals mild dilation of the calyces. The renal pelvis (*P*) has not yet opacified and the previously noted stone (*arrow*) is impacted at the UPJ. The other stone noted on the plain film is most likely in the opacified middle calyx, which is ill-defined because of pyelosinus extravasation. Contrast medium can be seen surrounding the not yet opacified renal pelvis and proximal ureter.

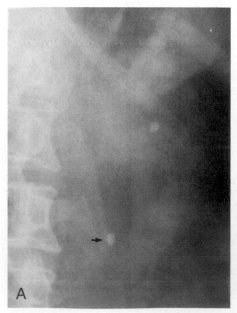

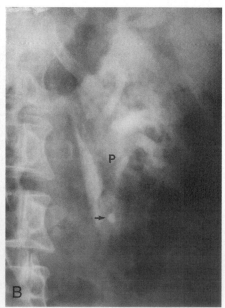

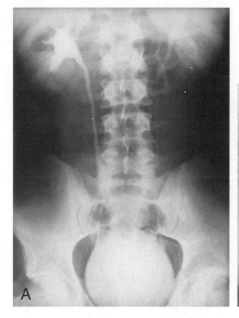

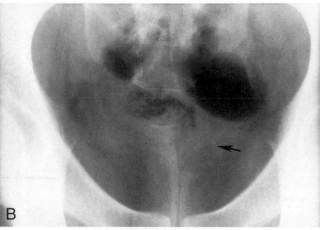

Figure 12.18. Obstructing left ureteral stone. **A,** An excretory urogram demonstrates diminished opacification of the left ureter and renal pelvis. **B,** A small stone (*arrow*) is seen at the ureterovesical junction on the preliminary radiograph.

urothelium, and if extravasation occurs, contrast medium will enter the venous system. Nevertheless, retrograde pyelography is commonly employed in patients with a contraindication to an intravenous contrast injection.

Retrograde pyelography can be particularly useful before interventional techniques. Placing an indwelling ureteral stent catheter allows repeat contrast injection into the ureter, which maximally opacifies the collecting system without the necessity of a large load of intravenous contrast medium. In selected patients, such as those with a severe contrast allergy or a small dense stone, another contrast agent such as air or carbon dioxide may be used (Fig. 12.19).

Antegrade Pyelography

Antegrade pyelography may be used to directly opacify the collecting system if retrograde pyelography is technically unsuccessful. It is also commonly performed in conjunction with pressure flow studies (Whitaker test) or as a prelude to a variety of interventional techniques.

Ultrasound

Both nephrocalcinosis (See Fig. 12.2**B**) and urinary tract calculi (Fig. 12.20) can be identified on ultrasound by the highly echogenic focus and acoustic shadowing of the stone. This can be useful in distinguishing lucent renal stones from other etiologies of a filling defect such as blood clot or tumor. When the kidney is well seen, stones as small as 0.5 mm may be detected sonographically. In the series of 100 patients reported by Middle-

ton and coworkers, ultrasound was 96% sensitive in detecting renal stones compared to abdominal radiography with renal tomography and was more sensitive than an abdominal radiograph alone.

Ultrasound also can be useful in the operating room in detecting small intrarenal calculi. During an open op-

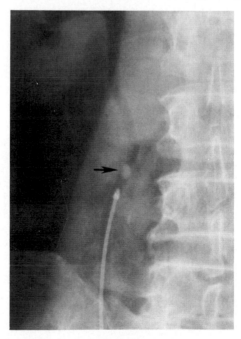

Figure 12.19. Air pyelography. Air was used as the contrast medium to better demonstrate a ureteral stone (*arrow*) during retrograde pyelography.

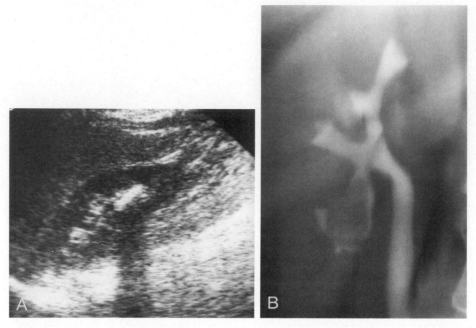

Figure 12.20.   Renal stone. **A,** Ultrasound demonstrates a highly echogenic mass with shadowing in the lower-pole collecting system. **B,** The stone is confirmed on urography.

eration, a balance must be maintained between complete stone removal and minimizing renal damage. Intraoperative radiography, ultrasound, nephroscopy, and plasma coagulum have all been used for this purpose. Ultrasonography is easily applied to the intact kidney and may be used to better define the location of a stone before the initial incision or to look for additional small stones or fragments after the stone is extracted. Ultrasound can be especially helpful if the stone is mobile within the collecting system. However, once the collecting system has been opened, ultrasound is more difficult to interpret, because small amounts of gas create confusing shadows that may mimic or hide a stone.

Ultrasound also is helpful in demonstrating obstruc-

tion of the collecting system (Fig. 12.21). Although the degree of ureteropelvocaliectasis from an acute ureteral obstruction due to a stone is mild, it can usually be distinguished from the normal collecting system in patients who may present with flank pain due to acute bacterial pyelonephritis or a renal infarction. Furthermore, the dilated ureter often can be followed to the point of obstruction and the stone identified (Fig. 12.22). Ultrasonographic evaluation of the ureteral jets also has proved helpful in diagnosing ureteral stones. The frequency and strength of these jets correlates inversely with the degree of ureteral obstruction present; with high degrees of obstruction, there may be no detectable jet or a slow continual dribble of urine from the orifice on the sympto-

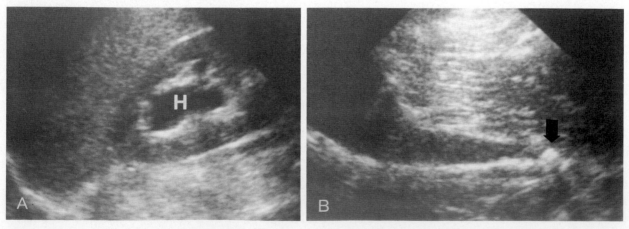

Figure 12.21.   Proximal ureteral stone. **A,** Moderate hydronephrosis (*H*) is seen with ultrasound. **B,** The ureteral dilatation ends at an obstructing ureteral stone (*arrow*).

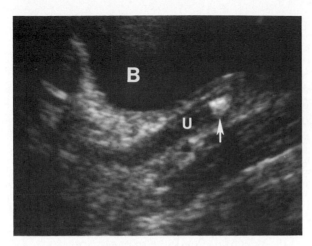

Figure 12.22.   Distal ureteral stone. A dilated ureter (*U*) is seen behind the bladder (*B*). The echogenic focus (*arrow*) is an obstructing distal ureteral stone.

matic side. In fact, the combination of plain abdominal radiography and sonography is reported to be virtually as effective in diagnosing stones as is excretory urography. Furthermore, in females patients, vaginal ultrasound should be considered for evaluation of the distal ureter for calculi, particularly if the transabdominal ultrasound examination is normal or inconclusive.

Computed Tomography

Computed tomography is most valuable in identifying a lucent stone as the etiology of a filling defect within the collecting system. If the defect is small, narrow collimation may be needed to avoid partial volume

artifact. Even lucent stones such as uric acid calculi are easily detected on CT, because their density is far greater than that of normal renal parenchyma, blood clot, or a urothelial tumor (Fig. 12.23). In vitro studies have shown the inability of CT to accurately differentiate among renal stones on the basis of their density because of overlapping values. Calcium oxalate stones are the densest and usually range from 800 to 1000 Hounsfield units (HU). The least dense common stones are uric acid, which range from 150 to 500 HU. There is a greater variation in the density of struvite stones, which may range from 300 to 900 HU, because of their greater range in mineralization. Determination of stone attenuation is more easily performed on stones in the intrarenal collecting system than in the ureter (Fig. 12.24).

Aside from differentiating stones from clot or tumor, CT has recently been advocated for the evaluation of patients with acute flank pain. Noncontrast standard and helical CT studies may demonstrate the cause of flank pain by directly imaging nonopaque stones. Furthermore, CT may identify extraurinary processes not apparent on urography. If the cost differential between urography and CT can be eliminated, it is quite possible that CT, particularly a quick helical scan from kidneys to bladder, could become the modality of choice for evaluating acute flank pain where a ureteral calculus is the suspected cause.

Percutaneous Treatment of Urinary Tract Calculi

Dramatic changes in the treatment of urinary tract calculi have occurred in the last 10 years. Dilation of a

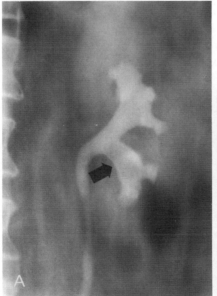
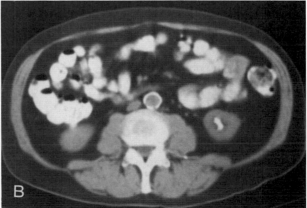

Figure 12.23.   Renal stone. **A,** A filling defect (*arrow*) is present on the excretory urogram. **B,** The high density on an unenhanced computed tomography scan demonstrates that the filling defect is caused by the presence of a stone.

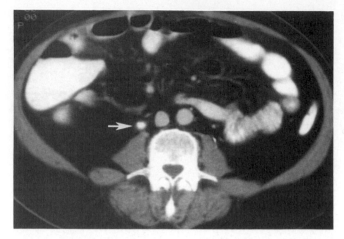

Figure 12.24. Ureteral stone. A stone (*arrow*) is readily identified in the right ureter by computed tomography.

percutaneous nephrostomy (PCN) tract to a size large enough to accommodate an endoscope has provided access to the urinary tract. A variety of catheters, stone baskets, and ultrasonic and electrohydraulic lithotriptors have been used to remove renal and ureteral stones. The success of these techniques has been so great that open surgical procedures are rarely needed. In fact, essentially all stones in either the native or reconstructed urinary tract, regardless of size, location, or hardness, can be managed with extracorporeal shock wave lithotripsy (ESWL) and endourological procedures.

The development of ESWL further advanced these nonoperative techniques. ESWL removes urinary tract calculi by fragmentation and spontaneous passage. This has eliminated the need for a PCN in most patients and has become the primary treatment for symptomatic nephrolithiasis. However, many patients still require percutaneous treatment to supplement ESWL or to treat complications arising from incomplete stone passage.

Expectant Therapy

Because approximately 80% of all urinary tract stones pass spontaneously, intervention may not be needed. More than 90% of stones less than 4 mm in diameter and 50% of stones 4 to 7 mm in diameter pass spontaneously. Rarely can stones 8 mm or larger be passed down the ureter into the bladder. Anatomic abnormalities and the location of the stone affect these rates.

The decision of if and when to intervene depends on the size of the stone, the anatomy of the urinary tract, the condition of the patient, and the presence or absence of other mitigating factors such as urinary tract infection or preexisting renal disease.

Percutaneous Nephrostolithotomy

The cornerstone of percutaneous stone removal is PCN. This determines the tract through which various instruments will be passed to remove the calculi. An ideally placed nephrostomy will avoid violating extrarenal organs (Fig. 12.25), traverse the least vascular plane of the kidney, and yet provide access to all portions of the collecting system that contain stones. The nephrostomy catheter should be sufficiently lateral so that it is not kinked or uncomfortable when the patient is lying supine. The tract also should be straight, so that it can accommodate a rigid nephroscope.

Percutaneous nephrostolithotomy often is more difficult when performed to remove stones, because the collecting system often is not dilated, and frequently a specific entry site is required to reach all of the stones. Furthermore, these access demands may necessitate entry into an upper-pole calyx, which increases the likelihood of puncturing the pleural space. The technique of PCN is discussed in Chapter 3.

In many patients, the renal stone provides an adequate target for placement of the PCN. This is usually true if a solitary calcified stone is to be removed. Multiple stones

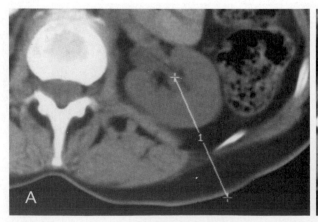
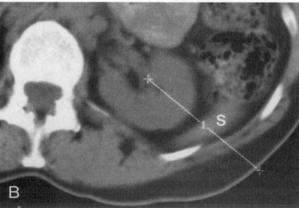

Figure 12.25. Percutaneous nephrostomy route. **A,** A percutaneous nephrostomy should be placed through the least vascular plane of the kidney. **B,** A high or laterally placed nephrostomy increases the risk of injury to the spleen (*S*) or pneumothorax.

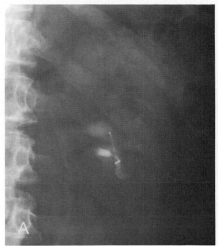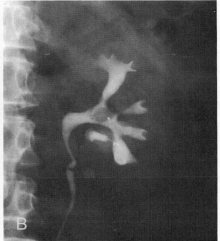

Figure 12.26. Opacification of collecting system. **A,** Faint opacification of the collecting system is seen after intravenous injection of 50 ml of contrast medium. A 3-French dilator has been passed into the renal pelvis. **B,** Injection of contrast medium through the 3-French dilator densely opacifies and mildly distends the collecting system. (From Dunnick NR: Percutaneous approach to urinary tract calculi. In Lang EK (ed): *Percutaneous and Interventional Urology and Radiology.* Berlin, Springer-Verlag, 1986.)

or poorly seen calculi may require opacification of the collecting system before nephrostomy placement.

The collecting system can be opacified from three routes. First, if there is good renal function, intravenous contrast injection will provide adequate visualization. Furthermore, the resultant diuresis provides mild distention of the collecting system. However, optimal opacification is for only a short period, and the patient is subjected to the hazards of intravascular contrast media.

Secondly, retrograde injection of contrast medium through an indwelling catheter provides excellent opacification of the collecting system. Because the contrast medium is not injected intravenously, there is no limit to the volume that can be used. Furthermore, contrast medium can be injected during the puncture, which slightly dilates the collecting system and enlarges the target for the puncture. However, this does require placement of a ureteral catheter by the urologist.

Thirdly, an antegrade pyelogram can be performed with a 22-gauge needle or through a 3-French catheter (Fig. 12.26). This method also avoids intravenous contrast injection and does provide slight dilation of the collecting system. Although ureteral catheterization is not required, an additional puncture of the renal pelvis is needed.

The definitive nephrostomy should be placed at an angle of 30 to 45°. This will allow the tract to pass through the least vascular plane (Brödel's line) of the kidney (Fig. 12.25) unless the kidney is malrotated. The tract should enter the calyx or infundibulum containing the stone. If more than one stone is targeted for removal, the nephrostomy tract should provide access to the locations of the other stones as well.

The nephrostomy tract may be dilated using stainless steel dilators, tapered fascial polyurethane dilators, or a modified angioplasty balloon catheter (Fig. 12.27). In general, the balloon catheter is preferred, because tract dilation is accomplished with less bleeding and presumably less damage to the kidney and other retroperitoneal tissues.

Before catheter manipulation is started, a second or "safety" guidewire should be passed (Fig. 12.28). This second wire can be placed using a larger untapered catheter such as a Ford catheter. Two guidewires provide an extra margin of safety. If the working wire is accidentally dislodged or withdrawn, access can be regained with the safety wire. The most secure position of the working wire is down the ureter. If the tip is in the distal ureter or bladder, it usually provides sufficient stability to permit tract dilation or catheter manipulation.

Once access has been gained and the tract has been dilated to a working size, the stones can be directly extracted, fragmented, and removed in pieces or fragmented and allowed to pass spontaneously. If possible,

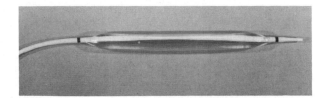

Figure 12.27. Balloon dilating catheter. This polyurethane reinforced catheter can be inflated with pressures as high as 12 atm. (From Carson CC, Dunnick NR: *Endourology.* New York, Churchill Livingstone, 1985.)

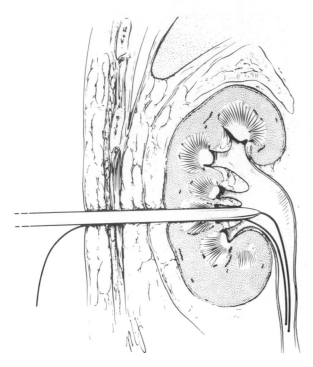

Figure 12.28. Safety wire. A second (safety) guidewire has been passed before dilation with the fascial polyurethane dilators. (From Carson CC, Dunnick NR: *Endourology.* New York, Churchill Livingstone, 1985.)

the stone should be removed intact so that no fragments are left behind to act as a nidus for new stone formation. Furthermore, complete removal of the stone avoids renal colic or hematuria during passage of the fragments.

A large variety of stone baskets are available. Many baskets consist of three, four, six, or eight wires in a helicoid pattern that will fit through a catheter and expand after ex-

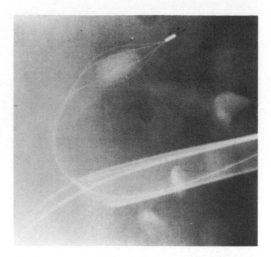

Figure 12.29. Four-wire basket. A helicoid basket has been passed through a Teflon sheath to capture the stone.

iting the catheter tip (Fig. 12.29). Other designs, such as the Hawkins stone basket, use a series of two to four wires along the shaft of the catheter. They have a blunt end that is especially useful in removing calyceal stones.

Forceps also may be used to grasp and extract a renal stone. Flexible forceps with an alligator grasping tip may be introduced through a catheter. Another type of flexible forceps is the three-or four-prong forceps. They may be passed through a catheter and expanded when they exit the distal end within the renal pelvis (Fig. 12.30). These are not widely used, however, because they can exert only a limited pulling force on the stone before losing their grip. Furthermore, the hooks on the grasping end can easily dig into the urothelium and damage the collecting system.

Figure 12.30. Three-prong forceps. The forceps are passed through the nephroscope to remove calculi. **A,** Schematic. **B,** Radiograph. (From Carson CC, Dunnick NR: *Endourology.* New York, Churchill Livingstone, 1985.)

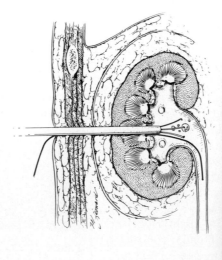

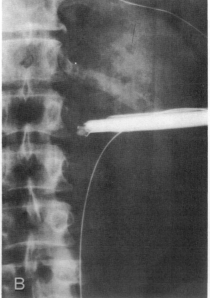

A

B

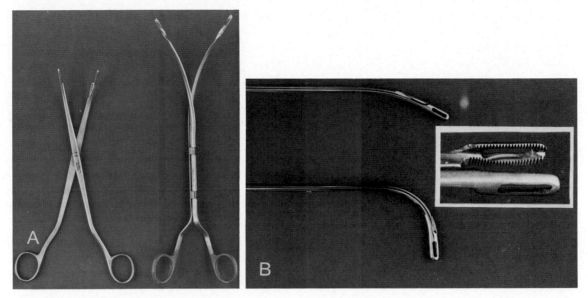

Figure 12.31. Rigid forceps. **A,** The Randall forceps (*left*) open with a conventional scissors action. The Mazzariello-Caprini forceps have a long central fulcrum, which allows better opening when used through a long tract. **B,** A variety of curves are available with either type of forceps. Insert shows the 0.97-mm hole drilled into the grasping end of the forceps, which facilitates its passage over a guide wire. (From Carson CC, Dunnick NR: *Endourology.* New York, Churchill Livingstone, 1985.)

Rigid forceps must be introduced through a straight tract. A Teflon sheath helps to prevent tissue damage during the introduction, manipulation, and withdrawal of the forceps. Three-prong rigid forceps originally designed to be used through a nephroscope are useful in removing renal pelvic or calyceal stones. Randall's forceps open with a scissors-like action (Fig. 12.31). This requires a very short or wide tract to allow the forceps to open sufficiently to engage the stone (Fig. 12.32). The Mazzariello-Caprini forceps open by rotating along the axis (Fig. 12.31). This allows them to be used in a narrower tract. Both Randall and Mazzariello-Caprini forceps should have a groove in the tip, so they can be introduced over a guidewire. Rigid forceps must be used carefully, because they may damage the collecting system. Biplane or C-arm fluoroscopy is helpful to direct the forceps onto the stone.

Ultrasonic Lithotripsy

One of the most effective methods of fragmenting a renal calculus is ultrasonic lithotripsy. The transducer contains a piezoceramic crystal that will resonate at a specific frequency when stimulated by electrical energy (Fig. 12.33). Sound waves of 23,000 to 27,000 Hz are produced and transmitted using an acoustic horn down the hollow steel rod to the stone. The lithotrite probe acts as a drill as it strikes the stone several thousand times per second and gradually fragments the stone to which it is brought into contact. Unfortunately, the lithotrite probe must be a rigid rod, because any articulations would result in significant energy loss.

Electrohydraulic Lithotripsy

Another useful modality for fragmenting renal stones is electrohydraulic lithotripsy. In this technique, a short spark discharge is produced at the tip of the probe. This produces intense heat that vaporizes water and creates a cavitation bubble. The resulting shock wave radiates in all directions. Both this initial shock wave and a second wave that occurs with the collapse of the bubble have an impact on the stone, causing fragmentation.

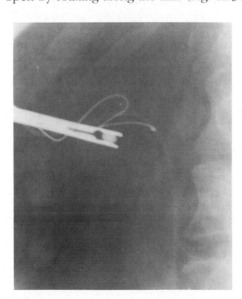

Figure 12.32. Forceps extraction. A renal pelvic stone is grasped by the rigid forceps.

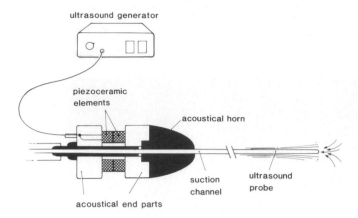

Figure 12.33. Ultrasonic lithotripter. (From Carson CC, Dunnick NR: *Endourology.* New York, Churchill Livingstone, 1985.)

Electrohydraulic lithotripsy is most effective in a one-sixth to one-seventh normal saline solution and is ineffective in normal saline. The heat created at the tip of the probe is easily dispersed in this fluid, but the stone must be free within the collecting system to minimize damage to the urothelium. There is no suction apparatus to remove small stones, so it is desirable to break the stone into pieces just small enough to be removed through the nephrostomy tract.

Chemolysis

Chemolysis can be used as a primary or adjunctive method of removing urinary tract calculi. It is most effective on uric acid stones, but has been successful in treating struvite and cystine stones. However, because of the length of time necessary for stone dissolution and because of the advent of percutaneous lithotripsy techniques and ESWL, chemolysis is now rarely used.

The optimal chemolytic solution depends on the composition of the stone. Triple-phosphate stones contain a mixture of magnesium ammonium phosphate (struvite) and calcium phosphate (apatite). They form in the presence of a urinary tract infection with urease-producing bacteria. Urease splits urea, resulting in a large amount of ammonium ion in an alkaline urine. Thus, triple-phosphate stones can be dissolved with acidifying solutions, such as hemiacidrin or Suby's G solution.

Uric acid and cystine stones can be dissolved with an alkaline solution, such as sodium bicarbonate or tromethamine (THAM). Uric acid stones are the easiest to dissolve and can sometimes be treated with allopurinol, hydration, and oral urinary alkalinization. Raising the urinary pH to 6.8 keeps most of the uric acid in the highly soluble monosodium urate form.

To accomplish stone dissolution effectively, a nephrostomy is needed to bathe the stone directly in a high concentration of the dissolving solution. A large nephrostomy catheter (8–10 French) is needed to pro-

vide good perfusion, and the catheter tip should be placed in close proximity to the stone.

In an unobstructed system, a single catheter is sufficient. The solution is introduced through the catheter; it bathes the stone and is passed down the ureter. The tip of the nephrostomy catheter should be behind the stone, so that the solution introduced through the catheter must wash over the stone before passing down the ureter. If there is ureteral obstruction, a second nephrostomy catheter is required to drain the collecting system. The two catheters should be placed on opposite sides of the stone, so solvent has maximal contact with the stone during irrigation. As an alternative, a double-pigtail ureteral catheter may be used to provide drainage. Infusion rates of 75 to 120 ml/hr are usually sufficient.

Results

In many patients, a variety of percutaneous techniques are used to remove the targeted stones. Thus, the results are reported for percutaneous nephrostolithotomy with the understanding that any or all of these methods may have been employed. For most patients, direct extraction is the technique of choice if the stone is small enough (less than 1 cm) to be removed through the nephrostomy tract. Larger stones must be fragmented, usually with ultrasonic lithotripsy, and the fragments either removed with a basket or forceps, or allowed to pass spontaneously. Chemolysis may be used as the primary therapy in selected patients or as an adjuvant method of eliminating residual fragments. Using various combinations of these techniques, excellent results have been reported.

In 1985, Segura and colleagues reviewed their experience in the percutaneous removal of renal or ureteral stones from 1000 consecutive patients. The targeted stone was successfully removed in 791 of 805 patients (98.3%) with renal stones. The most common reason for failure was inability to provide adequate access to the stone. A similar report by Reddy and associates described their results on 400 consecutive patients after the experience gained from the first 100 patients. As judged by plain abdominal radiographs, they were able to remove all stones from 328 of 332 patients (99%). Two of the four failures were caused by access problems. Lee and colleagues echoed the importance of experience in the analysis of their first 500 patients. Their success rate for the removal of simple pelvicalyceal stones was 98% overall, but was only 89% in the first 100 patients. Furthermore, 14 of the 17 patients requiring open operation after percutaneous nephrostolithotomy failed were among the first 100 patients.

Complications

Percutaneous nephrostolithotomy is a relatively safe and efficacious procedure that has largely replaced

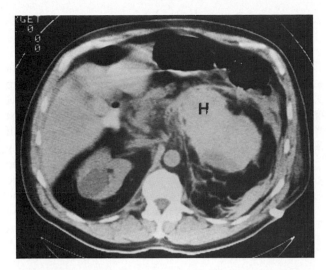

Figure 12.34. Hematoma. A CT scan demonstrates a large left hematoma (H) after percutaneous nephrostolithotomy. (From Dunnick NR, Carson CC, Braun SD, et al.: Complications of percutaneous nephrostolithotomy. *Radiology* 157:51, 1985.)

open surgical procedures for stone removal. However, it is an invasive technique and major complications do occur. In 1985, Dunnick and colleagues reported a 10% complication rate; hemorrhage (Fig. 12.34) and catheter dislodgement were the most common events. They noted that complications decreased with increasing experience, although more difficult cases were accepted in the latter period. In 1987, Lee and colleagues found only a 4% complication rate, with fever and bleeding en-

countered most commonly. Two deaths were reported in this latter series of 582 patients, both in patients with serious underlying medical diseases.

A mail survey tabulating the results of 8595 percutaneous nephrostolithotomy procedures from 62 institutions was reported by Lang. Serious complications declined from a rate of 15% during the first 20 cases to 1.5% afterward. The most common serious complications reported were perirenal abscess (84), hemorrhage requiring transfusion (37), pneumo- or hydrothorax (32), arteriovenous fistula requiring intervention (26) (Fig. 12.35), perforation of the colon (16), and rupture of the renal pelvis or ureteropelvic junction (13). A total of four deaths (0.046%) were reported in this survey. Small perforations of a calyx or the renal pelvis occur frequently, but heal with nephrostomy drainage and should not be considered a significant complication.

Percutaneous stone extraction procedures require frequent radiographic monitoring to access a portion of the collecting system that will allow removal of all the targeted stones. Fluoroscopy also is used to guide tract dilation and stone removal. Because these procedures are frequently difficult and time consuming, relatively high radiation doses may be absorbed by the radiologist and other members of the interventional team. Bush and coworkers examined this problem during 102 procedures for percutaneous removal of renal calculi from the upper collecting system. Fluoroscopy averaged 25 minutes per case, and the average radiation dose to the radiologist at the collar level was 10 mrem per case.

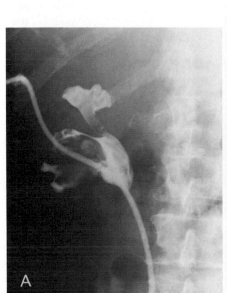

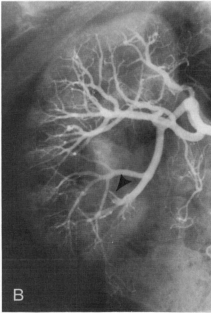

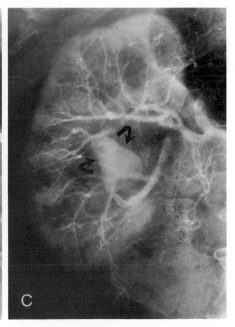

Figure 12.35. False aneurysm. **A,** Filling defect that conforms to the collecting system after nephrostomy tract placement represents a blood clot. **B, C,** Arteriogram obtained after recurrent hematuria from accidental dislodgement of the drainage catheter reveals a false aneurysm (*arrows*) arising from a lower pole branch artery (*arrowhead*). (From Dunnick NR, Carson CC, Braun SD, et al.: Complications of percutaneous nephrostolithotomy. *Radiology* 157:51, 1985.)

To minimize this radiation exposure, members of the interventional team should wear not only a lead apron, but also a thyroid shield and protective leaded glasses. A 0.5-mm lead-equivalent apron allows less than 1% of the x-rays to penetrate while a 0.25-mm lead equivalent apron allows 10% transmission. The glasses should have a side shield as the radiologist often will be facing 90° away from the x-ray beam as he or she looks at the television monitor.

The radiation exposure rate of the fluoroscope should be reduced to the lowest kVp and mA that gives a satisfactory image. Less radiation will reach the operators if the x-ray tube is below the patient rather than overhead. The field of view should be tightly collimated to only the area that must be imaged, and unnecessary fluoroscopy should be eliminated.

Another risk to the interventional team is hearing loss from the high-pitched sound produced by ultrasonic lithotriptors. On the basis of sound level measurements in an acoustic laboratory, Teigland and colleagues estimated that permanent hearing loss could result from 2 hours of continual operation of commercial ultrasonic lithotripsy units if performed on a daily basis. However, ultrasonic lithotripsy is intermittent and is unlikely to exceed 1 hour per patient. Thus, this is not likely to be a problem for most workers. However, people who already have a hearing deficit or who are unusually sensitive may prefer to be more cautious and wear ear plugs during these procedures.

Extracorporeal Shock Wave Lithotripsy

The development and success of ESWL have had a marked impact on radiology. The number of patients undergoing percutaneous nephrostolithotomy has dropped precipitously, and it is now used for difficult or special problem cases. Bush and colleagues found that more than 90% of patients with symptomatic stone disease are now treated with ESWL alone. Percutaneous techniques are used if there is a large stone burden (2%). They also may be applied after ESWL if obstruction occurs or to assist in removal of stone fragments. Others have reported more frequent use of PCN after ESWL. Cochran and coworkers found that 9% of 1456 patients required PCN, with the most common indications being fever and obstruction. Tegtmeyer and associates performed 178 interventional procedures (12%) on 1500 patients treated with ESWL. This trend places even greater demands on the interventional uroradiologist, who is expected to have a high level of technical expertise available for these complicated cases without the benefit of routine cases for training and maintenance of technical skills.

Because ESWL units are large, complex, and expensive pieces of equipment, they have become the central focus of stone treatment centers. They generate a large number of radiographic examinations essential to the treatment of these patients. Cochran and colleagues (1987) reviewed their experience with radiographic procedures for a single year in which 925 patients underwent ESWL. In all, 8478 radiologic studies and procedures were performed pertaining to ESWL. This is approximately 35 radiographic examinations per day. The vast majority of these examinations were abdominal radiographs to follow the progress of stone fragmentation and passage. However, ultrasound, excretory urography, and percutaneous nephrostomies were frequently performed.

Technique

Shock waves are produced by an underwater high-voltage shock discharge of 1-ms duration. This is similar to electrohydraulic lithotripsy, because the discharge causes water vaporization that initiates the shock wave in both techniques. The spark electrodes are located in the focus (F1) of an ellipsoid reflector such that the energy generated is concentrated at a second focal point (F2) outside the ellipsoid (Fig. 12.36). The stone to be fragmented must coincide with this point of highest energy concentration. Biplane fluoroscopy units are used to locate the stone and position the patient over the ellipsoid, so that F2 and the stone coincide.

Since shock waves are much more efficiently propagated through water than air, a path of water is needed between the ellipsoid and the stone. The initial commercial unit (Dornier) used a water bath into which the patient was immersed by a hydraulically controlled sling. Subsequent units, however, have substituted a water bag, eliminating the need for the large cumbersome bath.

Patients are prepared for the treatment with laxatives to reduce bowel gas and fecal material. This helps the fluoroscopic localization of the stones. Either general or epidural anesthesia is administered, and the patient is strapped into the sling and lowered into the water bath. Guided with biplane fluoroscopy, the stone is positioned at the F2 focus of the shock-generating ellipsoid. Approximately 500 to 2000 shock waves are needed to fragment a renal pelvic stone into pieces small enough to be passed down the ureter.

Ureteral obstruction is a contraindication to ESWL, because the stone fragments cannot pass. However, a PCN can be placed and used as the route for stone removal. Similarly, a urinary tract infection is a relative contraindication. Even when the urine clears of infection, a nidus of infection may remain in the calculus material, which can become active when the stone is fragmented. These patients must be treated cautiously, and a nephrostomy catheter may be helpful in preventing obstruction by infected material.

If the stones are poorly calcified, they may be difficult to localize with fluoroscopy. In these patients, a

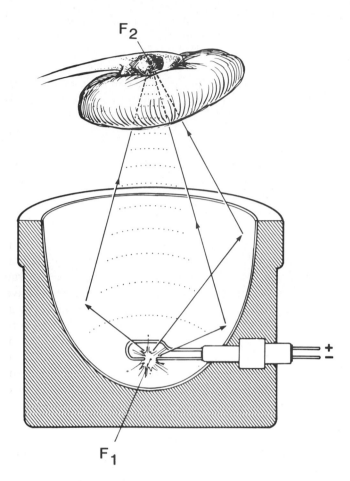

Figure 12.36.   Extracorporeal shock wave lithotripsy. Spark gap electrode and semiellipsoid for focusing shock waves. Electrode is placed at first focus inside ellipsoid with stone placed at second focus. (From Carson CC, Dunnick NR: *Endourology.* New York, Churchill Livingstone, 1985.)

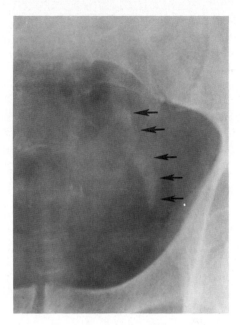

Figure 12.37.   Stone fragments. After ESWL, multiple stone fragments ("steinstrasse") are seen in the distal ureter (*arrows*).

ureteral catheter can be passed and contrast medium can be injected into the collecting system to visualize the stone as a negative filling defect.

Results

The widespread acceptance of ESWL as the primary therapy for urolithiasis attests to its success. However, these shock waves merely disintegrate the stone and the many fragments must still pass through the ureter or a nephrostomy catheter. Thus, it may take days to months to achieve a stone-free status. Radiographs taken within the first few days of ESWL show only fragmentation and partial passage of the stone fragments. If the stone burden was moderate to large, many fragments may accumulate in the distal ureter as "steinstrasse" (Fig. 12.37). A ureteral catheter inserted before ESWL and left in place 3 to 5 days after treatment has been found to facilitate the passage of fragments.

Radiographs obtained 1 to 3 months after ESWL give a more accurate appraisal of the treatment result. Riehle

and coworkers found that 224 of 300 patients (75%) were stone-free as determined by a single abdominal radiograph 3 months after ESWL. Fragments were still present in 70 (23%) patients, and in 6 (2%) patients ESWL showed no appreciable effect. Not surprisingly, patients with solitary stones less than 2 cm in diameter were more often stone-free (87%) than those patients with large or multiple stones (65%).

Graff and colleagues were able to evaluate more than 1000 patients a mean of 19.1 months after ESWL. They found that 72% of these patients remained stone-free. Patients with a stone in the renal pelvis or upper ureter had the best success: 85% and 89%, respectively, were stone-free after follow-up. Patients with multiple stones did not do as well, as only 64% were stone free. Of note, the worst group were those patients with a stone in a lower-pole calyx. Only 58% of these patients were stone-free on follow-up examinations.

The success of ESWL also depends on the composition of the stone. The best results in the Graff series were obtained in patients with calcium oxalate or uric acid calculi. Patients with apatite and cystine stones had the lowest stone-free rates after follow-up.

In a comparison of ESWL with percutaneous nephrostolithotomy, Lingeman and colleagues found similar success rates. Percutaneous nephrostolithotomy was slightly more efficacious in removing the targeted stone (98%) as compared with ESWL (95%), and was significantly better in leaving fewer fragments (7% vs. 24% for ESWL). However, patient morbidity as defined by pain, blood loss, fever, and length of hospital stay was much less in patients treated with ESWL. The significance of these retained stone fragments is unclear, however, because long-term studies have not yet shown whether or not these fragments act as a nidus for new stone formation and increase the recurrence rate.

Complications

The major advantage of ESWL is that open surgery and PCN are avoided. Thus, complications related to these invasive procedures are precluded. The stones are pulverized by shock waves focused on the stone. However, the kidney and adjacent soft tissues also are subject to some of this trauma. Intrarenal, subcapsular, and perinephric hematomas have all been seen and the incidence depends on the imaging modality used for detection, averaging between 15 and 30% on post-ESWL CT and MRI studies.

A decrease in effective renal plasma flow (ERPF) to the kidney treated with ESWL has been demonstrated in some patients. These patients also had increases in both systolic and diastolic blood pressure. Although the mechanism of the development of hypertension after ESWL is not clear, it may be caused by the compressive effect of an intrarenal or subcapsular hematoma, causing decreased perfusion and compensatory renin release (Page kidney). However, not all studies have substantiated this phenomenon, indicating that further experience is needed before it can be confirmed as a significant long-term complication.

Treatment of Staghorn Calculi

Staghorn calculi represent a special treatment problem. Not only is the stone burden great, but the collecting system often is effectively obstructed. Many of these patients have an underlying urinary tract infection that may not be completely eradicated, and there is more likely to be renal damage than in patients with a smaller stone burden.

Anatrophic nephrolithotomy has been the standard surgical procedure for the removal of staghorn calculi. Although the operation is designed to minimize parenchymal damage, a decrease in renal function may be seen, and the convalescent time is long. Since many of these stones recur, repeat operations, which become increasingly difficult, may be required.

Percutaneous nephrostolithotomy also may be a difficult procedure on patients with a staghorn calculus. The stone must be fragmented before removal and long, often repeated sessions with ultrasonic lithotripsy are required (Fig. 12.38). The complication rate is higher than with patients with a smaller stone burden, and more than one percutaneous access is frequently needed. Furthermore, it is difficult to render these patients completely stone-free, and these residual fragments may act as a nidus for more stone formation.

Snyder and Smith compared percutaneous nephros-

tolithotomy with anatrophic nephrolithotomy in a series of 100 patients with staghorn calculi. They found that both techniques were effective in removing the calculus. However, the shorter procedure time and decreased need for blood transfusions and narcotics favored the percutaneous technique. Furthermore, the far more rapid return to work (14.3 vs 54.5 days after discharge from the hospital) was a very strong argument for percutaneous therapy. Although fewer retained stone fragments were seen with open surgery, percutaneous nephrostolithotomy was more amenable to a repeat procedure than anatrophic surgery.

A series of 120 patients with staghorn calculi who underwent percutaneous removal was reported by Lee and colleagues. Most patients (73%) required two or more access routes, and many (24%) underwent multistage procedures. Bleeding was sufficient to require transfusion in 57% of patients, and 27% of patients developed a urinary tract infection. Nevertheless, symptomatic staghorn calculi were successfully removed from 85% of the patients, and the average convalescence time after discharge was only 15 days. A combination of percutaneous nephrostolithotomy and ESWL is probably the best approach to removal of staghorn calculi.

Treatment of Ureteral Calculi

Ureteral calculi present several problems for removal. They often are small and difficult to identify under fluoroscopy. They cannot be reached with a rigid instrument, the spine and bony pelvis limit the application of ESWL, and they may become embedded in the ureteral mucosa. Nevertheless, the variety of instruments that can be used on these stones results in successful removal for most patients.

Because approximately 80% of stones that enter the ureter pass spontaneously, it is reasonable to treat patients expectantly with analgesia and hydration while awaiting stone passage. The ureterovesical junction is the narrowest portion of the urinary tract, so that stones that pass into the bladder can usually be evacuated completely with the urinary stream. Patients with bladder outlet obstruction or stasis due to bladder or urethral diverticula may be exceptions.

The likelihood of a ureteral stone passing can be predicted by its size. Stones 4 mm or less in diameter are usually passed spontaneously and stones greater than 8 mm are unlikely to be passed. Stones that range from 4 to 7 mm in diameter lie in a gray area in which a trial of expectant therapy often is appropriate.

Percutaneous extraction techniques may be applied to ureteral as well as intrarenal stones. This often is done if a nephrostomy has already been established. Access to the ureter is usually easier if a middle or upper-pole calyx has been entered, because the angle down the ureter will be less acute than if a lower pole

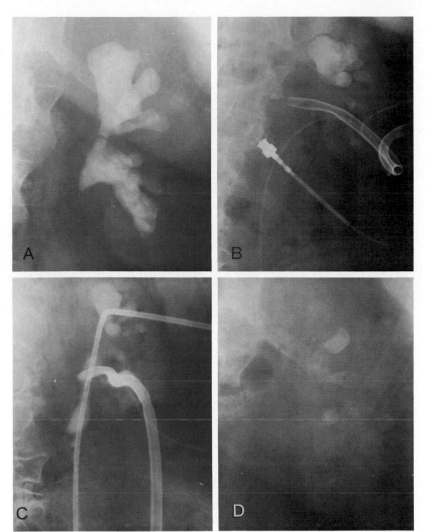

Figure 12.38. Staghorn calculi. **A,** Coned view of preoperative abdominal radiograph. Large staghorn calculus in left kidney. **B,** Retained fragments after first lithotripsy. Council catheter in renal pelvis; Gensini catheter stenting ureter. **C,** Second nephrostomy (Ford straight catheter) placed into upper pole before second lithotripsy. Contrast material in renal pelvis and ureter. **D,** Follow-up radiograph. Multiple retained fragments lodged in peripheral calyces. (From Adams GW, Oke EJ, Dunnick NR, Carson CC: Percutaneous lithotripsy of staghorn calculi. *AJR* 145:803, 1985.)

calyx was entered with the nephrostomy. The four-wire basket with a filiform tip is most useful in the ureter (Fig. 12.39). It is passed through the catheter beyond the stone and then opened. The stone is engaged as the basket is pulled back into the renal pelvis and then out the nephrostomy tract.

If the stone is embedded in the ureteral mucosa, it may not be possible to capture it in the stone basket. Modifications of the four-wire basket, such as the Johnson basket, may be more successful by forcing the edematous mucosa to retract from the stone (Fig. 12.40). Balloon catheters passed distal to the stone and then inflated also have been used to pull the stone back into the renal pelvis, where it can be removed with a stone basket or forceps.

Ureteroscopy has been shown to be effective in reaching and removing stones from a retrograde approach. The ureter must be dilated to accommodate the ureteroscope. If a large stone is encountered, ultrasonic lithotripsy can be employed to fragment it before extraction.

In general, an antegrade approach through a PCN is used for stones in the proximal ureter, whereas a retrograde approach via the bladder is selected when the stone lies in the distal ureter. Dilation of the collecting system above the stone also favors the antegrade approach. Furthermore, if large stones are pulled into the bladder, they may damage the ureterovesical junction. Thus, stones greater than 8 mm in diameter are approached in an antegrade fashion or are fragmented before being extracted.

Using a combination of these techniques as well as chemolysis for known soluble stones, Kahn was able to remove 114 of 120 (95%) ureteral stones. Two patients required surgery for ureteral avulsion, and seven patients had ureteral perforation treated with a double-J ureteral stent.

ESWL can be used on ureteral stones if they lie above the iliac crest. However, the results have not been as good as when the stone lies in the renal pelvis. However, if the ureteral stone is pushed back into the renal pelvis, the results of ESWL are excellent.

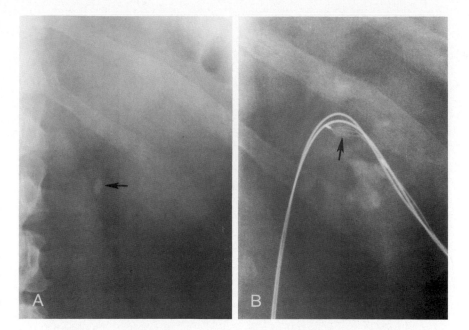

Figure 12.39. Ureteral stone. **A,** A proximal ureteral stone (*arrow*) is identified. **B,** A four-wire basket is used to extract the stone (*arrow*).

Coptcoat and associates reviewed their experience with 100 consecutive patients who required treatment for ureteral stones. Most patients (63) had their stones removed by ESWL after retrograde manipulation. Ureteroscopic techniques were used to remove stones from 29 patients, 26 of whom had distal ureteral stones. Other techniques included percutaneous nephrostolithotomy and cystoscopic removal. Only two patients had open ureterolithotomy, although four patients required surgery for complications of ureteroscopy or stricture.

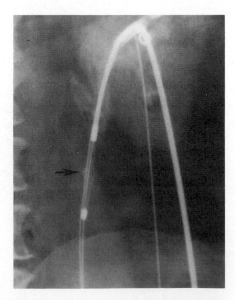

Figure 12.40. Ureteral stone. The four-wire basket was not successful in engaging this stone. The stiff wires of the Johnson basket displaced the edematous mucosa, so the stone (*arrow*) could be captured.

SUGGESTED READING

Nephrocalcinosis and Nephrolithiasis

Burge HJ, Middleton WD, McClennan BE, et al.: Ureteral jets in healthy subjects and in patients with unilateral ureteral calculi: comparison with color Doppler US. *Radiology* 180:437, 1991.

Drach GW: Surgical overview of urolithiasis. *J Urol* 141(Pt II):711, 1989.

Gilsanz V, Fernal W, Reid BS, et al.: Nephrolithiasis in premature infants. *Radiology* 154:107, 1985.

Gleeson MJ, Griffith DP: Struvite calculi. *Br J Urol* 71:503, 1993.

Glowacki LS, Beecroft ML, Cook RJ, et al.: The natural history of asymptomatic urolithiasis. *J Urol* 147:319, 1992.

Goldwasser B, Cohan RH, Dunnick NR, et al.: Role of linear tomography in evaluation of patients with nephrolithiasis. *Urology* 33(3):253, 1989.

Haddad MC, Sharif HS, Shahed MS, et al.: Renal colic: diagnosis and outcome. *Radiology* 184:83, 1992.

Herman TE, Siegel MJ: Pyramidal hyperechogenicity in autosomal recessive polycystic kidney disease resembling medullary nephrocalcinosis. *Pediatr Radiol* 121:270, 1991.

Hewitt MJ, Older RA: Calyceal calculi simulating gallstones. *AJR* 134:507, 1980.

Hillman BJ, Drach DW, Tracey P, et al.: Computed tomographic analysis of renal calculi. *AJR* 142:549, 1984.

Jequier S, Kaplan BS: Echogenic renal pyramids in children. *J Clin Ultrasound* 19:85, 1991.

Katz ME, Karlowicz MG, Adelman RD, et al.: Nephrocalcinosis in very low birth weight neonates: sonographic patterns, histologic characteristics, and clinical risk factors. *J Ultrasound Med* 13:777, 1994.

Kim SH, Lee SE, Park IA: CT and US features of renal matrix stones with calcified center. *J Comput Assist Tomogr* 20:404, 1996.

Korobkin M, Jacobs RP, Clark RE, Minagi H: Diminished radiopacity of contrast material: a urographic sign of ureteral calculus. *Am J Roentgenol* 131:847, 1978.

Laing FC, Benson CB, DiSalvo DN, et al.: Distal ureteral calculi: detection with vaginal US. *Radiology* 192:545, 1994.

Lalli AF: Renal parenchyma calcifications. *Semin Roentgenol* 17:101, 1982.

McLeod RS, Churchill DN: Urolithiasis complicating inflammatory bowel disease. *J Urol* 148:974, 1992.

Middleton WD, Dodds WJ, Lawson TL, et al.: Renal calculi: sensitivity for detection with US. *Radiology* 167:239, 1988.

Miller FH, Parikh S, Gore RM, et al.: Renal manifestations of AIDS. *RadioGraphics* 13:587, 1993.

Mokulis JA, Arndt WF, Downey JR, Caballero RL, Thompson IM: Should renal ultrasound be performed in the patient with microscopic hematuria and a normal excretory urogram? *J Urol* 154:1300, 1995.

Newhouse JH, Amis ES Jr: The relationship between renal scarring and stone disease. *AJR* 151:1153, 1988.

Newhouse JH, Prien EL, Amis ES Jr, et al.: Computed tomographic analysis of urinary calculi. *AJR* 142:545, 1984.

Nimkin K, Lebowitz RL, Share JC, et al.: Urolithiasis in a Children's Hospital: 1985–1990. *Urol Radiol* 14:139, 1992.

Parienty RA, Ducellier R, Pradel J, et al.: Diagnostic value of CT numbers in pelvocalyceal filling defects. *Radiology* 145:743, 1982.

Prien EL: The analysis of urinary calculi. *Urol Clin North Am* 1:229, 1974.

Smith LH: The medical aspects of urolithiasis: an overview. *J Urol* 141:707, 1981.

Smith RC, Rosenfield AT, Choe KA, et al. Acute flank pain: comparison of non-contrast-enhanced CT and intravenous urography. *Radiology* 1995;194:789–794.

Smith RC, Verga M, McCarthy S, Rosenfield AT: Diagnosis of acute flank pain: value of unenhanced helical CT. *AJR* 166:97, 1996.

Sommer FG, Jeffrey RB Jr, Rubin GD, et al. Detection of ureteral calculi in patients with suspected renal colic: value of reformatted noncontrast helical CT. *AJR* 1995;165:509–513.

Percutaneous Nephrostolithotomy

Bush WH, Jones D, Brannen GE: Radiation doses to personnel during percutaneous renal calculus removal. *AJR* 145:1261, 1985.

Carson CC, Dunnick NR: *Endourology.* New York, Churchill Livingstone, 1985.

Dunnick NR: Percutaneous approach to urinary tract calculi. In Lang EK (ed.): *Percutaneous and Interventional Urology and Radiology.* Berlin, Springer-Verlag, 1986.

Dunnick NR, Carson CC, Braun SD, et al.: Complications of percutaneous nephrostolithotomy. *Radiology* 157:51, 1985.

Lang EK: Percutaneous nephrostolithotomy and lithotripsy: a multiinstitutional survey of complications. *Radiology* 162:25, 1987.

Lee WJ, Smith AD, Cubelli V, et al.: Complications of percutaneous nephrolithotomy. *AJR* 148:177, 1987.

Lee WJ, Smith AD, Cubelli V, et al.: Percutaneous nephrolithotomy: analysis of 500 consecutive cases. *Urol Radiol* 8:61, 1986.

Pfister RC, Dretler SP: Percutaneous chemolysis of renal calculi. *Urol Radiol* 6:138, 1984.

Reddy PK, Hulbert JC, Lange PH, et al.: Percutaneous removal of renal and ureteral calculi: experience with 400 cases. *Urology* 134:662, 1985.

Rodman JS, Williams JJ, Peterson CM: State of the art dissolution of uric acid calculi. *Urology* 131:1039, 1984.

Segura JW, Patterson DE, LeRoy AJ, et al.: Percutaneous removal of kidney stones: review of 1,000 cases. *Urology* 134:1077, 1985.

Teigland CM, Clayman RV, Winfield HN, et al.: Ultrasonic lithotripsy: the risk of hearing loss. *Urology* 135:728, 1986.

Extracorporeal Shock Wave Lithotripsy

Barloon TJ, Brown RC, Berbaum KS: Current status of adult uroradiology: a survey of members of the Society of Uroradiology. *AJR* 154:301, 1990.

Baumgartner BR, Dickey KW, Ambrose SS, et al.: Kidney changes after extracorporeal shock-wave lithotripsy: appearance on MR imaging. *Radiology* 163:531, 1987.

Bush WH, Gibbons RP, Lewis GP, et al.: Impact of extracorporeal shock-wave lithotripsy on percutaneous stone procedures. *AJR* 147:89, 1986.

Chaussy C, Schmiedt E, Jocham D, et al.: First clinical experience with extracorporeally induced destruction of kidney stones by shock-waves. *Urology* 127:417, 1982.

Cochran ST, Barbaric ZL, Mindell HJ, et al.: Extracorporeal shock-wave lithotripsy: impact on the radiology department of a stone treatment center. *Radiology* 163:655, 1987.

Cochran ST, Liu E, Barbaric ZL: Percutaneous nephrostomy in conjunction with ESWL in treatment of nephrolithiasis. *AJR* 151:103, 1988.

Fuchs GJ: Interventional urinary stone management [editorial]. *J Urol* 151:668, 1994.

Graff J, Diederichs W, Schulze H: Long-term followup in 1,003 extracorporeal shock-wave lithotripsy patients. *Urology* 140:479, 1988.

Krysiewicz S: Complications of renal extracorporeal shock wave lithotripsy reviewed. *Urol Radiol* 13:139, 1992.

LeRoy AJ: Diagnosis and treatment of nephrolithiasis: current perspectives. *AJR* 163:1309, 1994.

Lingeman E, Coury TA, Newman DM, et al.: Comparison of results and morbidity of percutaneous nephrostolithotomy and extracorporeal shock-wave lithotripsy. *Urology* 138:485, 1987.

Riehle RA, Naslund EB, Fair W, et al.: Impact of shock-wave lithotripsy on upper urinary tract calculi. *Urology* 28:261, 1986.

Tegtmeyer CJ, Kellum CD, Jenkins A, et al.: Extracorporeal shock-wave lithotripsy: interventional radiologic solutions to associated problems. *Radiology* 161:587, 1986.

Williams CM, Kaude JV, Newman RC, et al.: Extracorporeal shock-wave lithotripsy: long-term complications. *AJR* 150:311, 1988.

Yu CC, Lee YH, Huang JK, Chen MT, et al.: Long-term stone regrowth and recurrence rates after extracorporeal shock wave lithotripsy. *Brit J Urol* 72:688, 1993.

Staghorn Calculi

Adams GW, Oke EJ, Dunnick NR, et al.: Percutaneous lithotripsy of staghorn calculi. *AJR* 145:803, 1985.

Lee WJ, Snyder JA, Smith AD: Staghorn calculi: endourologic management in 120 patients. *Radiology* 165:85, 1987.

Snyder JA, Smith AD: Staghorn calculi: percutaneous extraction versus anatrophic nephrolithotomy. *J Urol* 136:351, 1986.

Ureteral Calculi

Banner MP, VanArsdalen KN, Pollack HM: Extracorporeal shock wave lithotripsy of ureteral calculi. *Radiology* 174:12, 1990.

Barr JD, Tegtmeyer CJ, Jenkins AD: In situ lithotripsy of ureteral calculi: review of 261 cases. *Radiology* 174:103, 1990.

Coptcoat MJ, Webb DR, Kellett MJ, et al.: The treatment of 100 consecutive patients with ureteral calculi in a British stone center. *J Urol* 137:1122, 1987.

Kahn I: Endourological treatment of ureteral calculi. *J Urol* 135:239, 1986.

LeRoy AJ, Williams HJ Jr, Bender CE, et al.: Percutaneous removal of small ureteral calculi. *AJR* 145:109, 1985.

Morse RM, Resnick MI: Ureteral calculi: natural history and treatment in an era of advanced technology. *J Urol* 145:263, 1991.

13
Pelvicalyceal System

PAPILLARY NECROSIS

Papillary necrosis (necrotizing papillitis) is a clinical pathologic entity found in association with several diseases that affect the kidney. Each disease is thought to involve renal medullary ischemia, which causes necrosis and sloughing of papillary tissue, which in turn produce radiologic findings and also may be associated with renal functional abnormalities and symptoms. Kidneys that have papillary necrosis also tend to have interstitial nephritis.

Papillary necrosis varies greatly in severity and rate of progression. It may be part of a condition that produces severe acute renal abnormalities with massive sloughing of most papillary tissue, with hematuria and colic, or may follow an indolent course, with only the mildest of nonprogressing radiographic abnormalities and no clinical symptoms at all. The diagnosis may be established by imaging studies (usually urography), by histologic examination of papillary fragments found in the urine, or by pathologic examination of the entire kidney.

The possible etiologies of papillary necrosis may be recalled using the mnemonic NSAID: nonsteroidal antiinflammatory drugs, sickle-cell hemoglobinopathies, analgesic abuse, infection (such as tuberculosis and pyelonephritis), and diabetes mellitus. The mnemonic NSAID itself is one etiology of papillary necrosis that may be increasing in frequency. However, the most common etiologies are tuberculosis, diabetes mellitus, and sickle cell anemia.

Analgesic Nephropathy

Analgesic nephropathy was first described in 1953 in Sweden, where a number of patients with interstitial nephritis were found to have consumed large amounts of analgesics, which usually consisted of combinations of aspirin and phenacetin. The combination has been found to be nephrotoxic, especially to the renal medulla and papillae, and particularly when consumed in large doses for a long time. Although over-the-counter combinations of aspirin and phenacetin have largely been removed from the market, they have been replaced by combinations of aspirin and acetaminophen. Both in combination and alone, these drugs may, in large doses, also produce renal disease. More recently, similar analgesic nephropathy has been found caused by nonsteroidal antiinflammatory drugs (NSAIDs) such as indomethacin, sulindac, and tolmetin.

The association of high levels of consumption of these analgesics and high rates of renal disease from them is clear; they are particularly prevalent in the section of Belgium around the city of Antwerp, in Australia, Germany, Scandinavia, and Switzerland; Britain and the United States have lower rates of consumption and renal disease.

Aspirin and phenacetin interfere with oxidative phosphorylation, which is a protective mechanism against oxidant toxic injury. They also inhibit prostaglandin synthesis, which may reduce renal blood flow. Over time, these changes cause direct toxicity on the collecting tubules, generalized microangiopathy in the peritubular vessels, endothelial necrosis in the interstitial cells, and platelet aggregation in the vasa recta, all of which result in necrosis of all or part of the renal papillae.

Patients with renal disease due to analgesic abuse also have an increased incidence of transitional cell carcinoma, especially of the upper tract (Fig. 13.2).

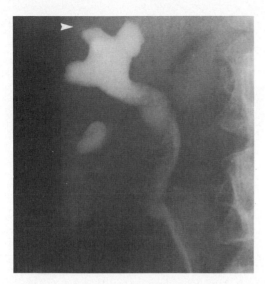

Figure 13.1. Papillary necrosis. Retrograde urogram showing faint calcification in papilla (*arrowhead*) outside the interpapillary line. The filling defect in the renal pelvis is transitional cell carcinoma.

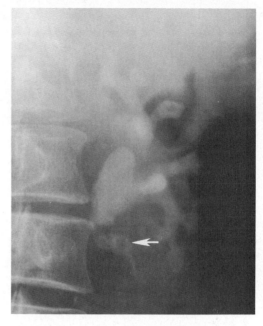

Figure 13.2. Excretory urogram in a patient with analgesic abuse. Ring shadows are seen in the papillary region due to contrast medium surrounding sloughed papillae. A sloughed papilla in the proximal ureter (*arrow*) is seen as a radiolucent filling defect.

Sickle Cell Disease

Sickle cell disease is the result of the homozygous hemoglobin S gene, which is present in approximately 10% of the black Americans and in approximately 30% of black Africans. The gene alters the solubility of hemoglobin, which results in the classic sickle cell shape of erythrocytes; these cells are less malleable than normal, and tend to aggregate in and occlude capillaries, producing regions of ischemia and infarction in the renal medullae and papillae. Up to 50% of patients with sickle cell disease develop renal papillary necrosis. Papillary necrosis also may occur in patients with sickle cell trait.

Infection

The association of pyelonephritis and papillary necrosis is sometimes confusing, in part because of inconsistent meanings for the word "pyelonephritis." There have been published cases of fulminant pyelonephritis in patients with severe diabetic ketoacidosis in whom acute sloughing of renal papillae has clearly occurred; the individual contribution of each disease to the ultimate papillary necrosis, however, is not entirely clear. Also, the term chronic pyelonephritis often is applied to patients who have the nephropathy associated with vesicoureteral reflux (who very often have recurrent bouts of urinary infection as well) in whom focal scarring leads to retraction and disappearance of the papillae. In both conditions, the papillary tissue disappears and the radiologic findings are consistent with papillary necrosis.

When the kidneys are infected by tuberculosis, the bacilli initially lodge in the cortex and move down the nephrons to the medulla, where they cause focal caseating granulomata, which then slough portions of tissue and produce papillary necrosis. A particular "feathery" appearance of the papillae, caused by loss of very small portions of tissue, is one of the patterns that may be produced when tuberculosis is the etiology (*see* Chapter 7).

Diabetes Mellitus

This disease produces a variety of renal abnormalities. Ischemia caused by small-vessel disease can cause papillary necrosis, but the abnormalities are not limited to this region. Diabetic nephrosclerosis affects the entire kidney and may ultimately lead to severe renal failure.

Radiology

The plain film is commonly normal; rarely, a sloughed but retained papilla may develop a ring of calcification on its surface and become visible (Fig. 13.1). If the whole papilla is necrotic, the calcifications may be 5 to 6 mm in diameter. More commonly, only part of the papilla is necrotic and produces a 2- to 3-mm irregularly shaped calcification.

The plain films also may provide other diagnostic clues. Advanced arthritic changes in the hips or spine may be clues to chronic pain that has led to excess analgesic ingestion. Premature vascular calcification, especially in medium to small-diameter vessels, and calcifica-

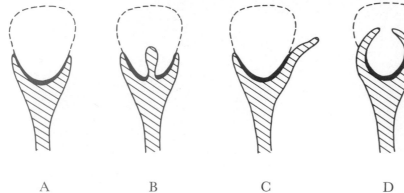

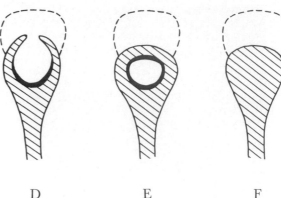

A   B   C   D   E   F

Figure 13.3. Patterns of papillary necrosis. **A,** Normal calyx and papilla. **B,** Central erosion of papilla (medullary type). **C,** Streaky erosion extending from calyceal fornix. **D,** "Lobster claw" deformity resulting from bilateral forniceal erosions into the medullary pyramid above the papilla. **E,** Necrotic papilla retained in calyx after sloughing. If retained long enough, rim-

like calcification of the papilla can occur. **F,** Rounded calyx after passage of sloughed papilla. While this is radiographically similar to the clubbed calyx found in chronic atrophic pyelonephritis, there is usually no adjacent parenchymal scarring. (From Amis ES Jr, Newhouse JH: *Essentials of Uroradiology,* Boston, Little, Brown & Co, 1991.)

tion in the vas deferens may indicate diabetes mellitus. Ischemic necrosis of the femoral head may indicate that the patient has sickle cell disease.

The classic radiologic features of renal papillary necrosis are best shown by excretory or retrograde pyelography (Fig. 13.3). Kidney size may be normal or diminished. There are several patterns of calyceal changes. Small collections of contrast medium may be seen in the papillary region (Fig. 13.4) and may be round, elongated, or irregular in shape. They may extend from the calyceal fornices or directly into the tip of the papillae. The collections usually extend outside the interpapillary line. Central erosion of the papilla is known as the medullary type of papillary necrosis. Alternatively, the entire papilla may become necrotic and slough; this is known as the papillary type of papillary necrosis. If the sloughed tissue has disappeared from the calyx and has been passed down the ureter, urography may reveal a blunted calyceal outline with no remnant of the papilla at all. Alternatively, the entire papilla or large pieces of it may be retained, and may form circular or irregular filling defects (Fig. 13.5); these defects may be calcified on their peripheries. Rarely, urography may be performed while a large papilla that produces ureteral obstruction is being passed. Loss of papillae may be the only abnormalities seen at urography; alternatively, the loss may be followed by more generalized diminution in parenchymal volume with focal or generalized loss in cortical thickness.

Papillary necrosis should not be confused with papillary stones. These papillary stones account for 25% of passed kidney stones, are formed in the interstitium of the papillae, and are 1 to 4 mm in size. They have a particular microscopic appearance with a characteristic

shape; they are convex on one side and concave on the other. Randall's plaques form on the concave side of more than 70% of these stones. The concavity is produced by formation of the stones in the interstitium against the cribriform plate. Papillary stones and Randall's plaques are extratubular and do not affect the collecting ducts, which function normally. There is no alteration in renal function.

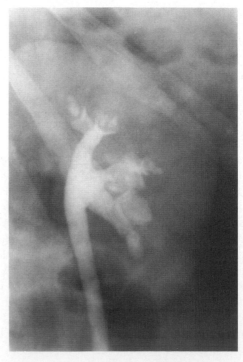

Figure 13.4. Papillary necrosis. Collections of contrast medium of varying sizes are present in the papillary regions adjacent to normal calyces.

MEDULLARY SPONGE KIDNEY

Medullary sponge kidney (MSK) is a condition characterized by dilatation of the renal collecting ducts (ducts of Bellini). The dilatation may be cylindrical or saccular, and may slightly enlarge the affected calyces. The kidney is usually normal in size, but is occasionally enlarged. In approximately 15% of cases, small calcifications are seen within the dilated portions of the collecting ducts. Although the orifices of the ducts in the cribriform plate are normal, the calcifications occasionally erode through the plate and are passed as small stones.

Most patients are asymptomatic. Occasionally, there may be mild hematuria, and the patients who pass calcifications may have episodes of renal colic. There may be a slight association with pyelonephritis. The renal function often is normal; there may be a mild reduction in urinary concentrating capacity and there may be mild hypercalcemia. There are reported associations with ipsilateral hemihypertrophy, cortical renal cysts, calyceal diverticuli, medullary cystic disease, horseshoe kidney, renal ectopia, Ehlers-Danlos syndrome, autosomal-dominant polycystic disease, distal renal tubular acidosis, and hyperparathyroidism with parathyroid adenoma. Some of these associations may be fortuitous or due to an incorrect diagnosis (renal calcification and small cysts may be seen in conditions other than medullary sponge kidney). The disease is rare in children.

Radiology

The plain film is usually normal, but small calcifications may be seen (Fig. 13.6). These calcifications are present in the region of the renal medullary pyramids, may involve both kidneys or only one, may be seen in multiple papillae or one papilla, and may appear as clusters or isolated small stones. Cortical nephrocalcinosis is not part of this condition. On excretory urography, MSK appears as streaks of contrast medium that extend from the surface of the papillae (Fig. 13.7). These streaks often are parallel to each other, perpendicular to the periphery of the kidney, and may appear irregular in outline and of varying caliber. These striations represent fusiform dilatation of the collecting ducts; saccular dilatations also may cause small circular collections of contrast medium to appear. The papillae may be enlarged (Fig. 13.8). The nephrogram features often are not visible on computed tomography (CT); the calcifications may be detected by CT without intravenous contrast and by ultrasound.

The differential diagnosis of this disease is sometimes difficult. A uniform nonstriated papillary blush may be normal; this is especially likely to appear in patients who undergo ureteral compression during urography and may disappear when the compression is removed. The normal papillary blush is not clearly striated, and does not contain cystic collections of contrast medium. A striated nephrogram may be seen in patients with autosomal-recessive polycystic kidney disease. In this condition, however, the striations usually extend farther toward the periphery of the kidney, and the kidneys may be enlarged. The patients are usually younger, and evidence of periportal hepatic fibrosis and portal hypertension may be seen. Papillary and medullary nephrocalcinosis may be caused by a number of conditions other than medullary sponge kidney; with the other causes of nephrocalcinosis, however,

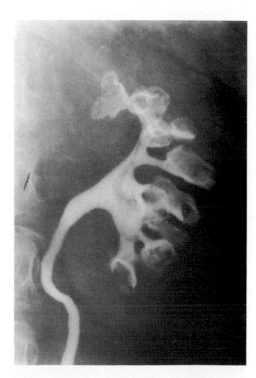

Figure 13.5. Papillary necrosis. The papillae have sloughed but remain in the papillary region. They are seen as filling defects surrounded by contrast medium.

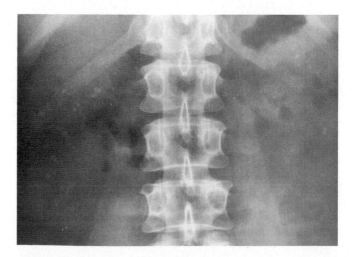

Figure 13.6. The plain film in a patient with known medullary sponge kidney. Multiple punctate calcifications are seen in both kidneys.

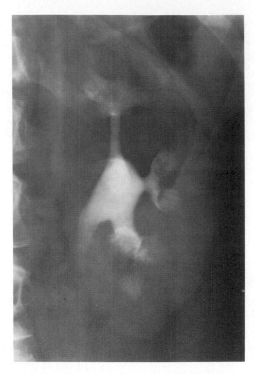

Figure 13.7. Medullary sponge kidney. Contrast medium is seen in several dilated collecting tubules in all calyceal regions. The rays are outside the interpapillary line.

cystic or fusiform dilation of the collecting tubules are not seen. Medullary nephrocalcinosis from medullary sponge kidney and medullary neprocalcinosis from other causes cannot be distinguished by ultrasound.

Benign tubular ectasia is a phrase frequently applied to patients with milder cases of MSK: the striations are usually finer (and more difficult to distinguish from the normal papillary blush), and cystic dilatation or calcifications are not encountered. There has been no convincing demonstration that benign tubular ectasia progresses to more severe cases of MSK.

CALYCEAL DIVERTICULUM

A calyceal diverticulum is a lesion consisting of an outpouching of a portion of the collecting system into the corticomedullary region. It can arise from any part of the collecting system from the renal pelvis to a fornix; it is most commonly seen extending from the fornix of the upper or lower pole calyx. It is sometimes known as a pyelogenic cyst, especially if it arises from the pelvis. These lesions can range in size from a few millimeters to several centimeters in diameter; their necks are virtually always narrow. They may develop calcified stones; characteristically, a cluster of relatively uniformly sized stones may be seen within large diverticuli. They often are asymptomatic, but may appear clinically by producing microhematuria or by association with urinary tract infection. The stones that form within them may pass and cause ureteral colic, but are usually confined to the diverticulum by the narrow neck.

On excretory or retrograde urography, a calyceal diverticulum classically appears as a spherical collection of contrast medium adjacent to a papilla (Fig. 13.9). Oc-

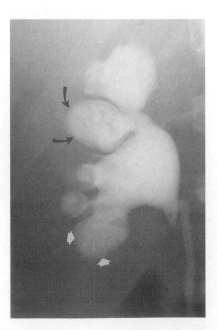

Figure 13.8. Medullary sponge kidney. Excretory urography reveals dense striations and enlargement of several papillae (*arrows*).

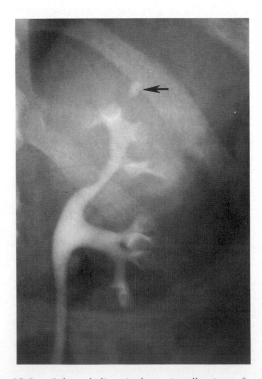

Figure 13.9. Calyceal diverticulum. A collection of contrast material (*arrow*) is seen outside the collecting system. The thin stalk connecting it to the fornix of the calyx cannot be seen.

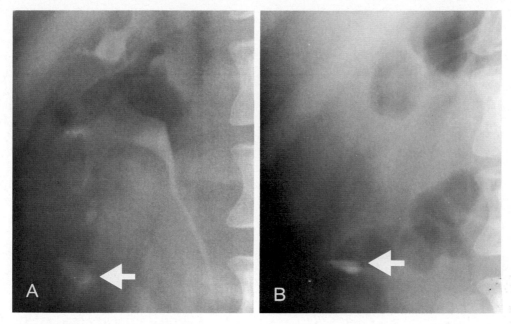

Figure 13.10.   A, Supine film of excretory urogram showing a calyceal diverticulum from the lower pole calyx. **B,** Postvoid upright film shows layering of contrast medium and urine producing a fluid level within the calyceal diverticulum.

casionally, the narrow connecting channel may be visualized, but often the neck is too small to see. In an upright film, if the contrast medium has not completely mixed with urine, a contrast-urine layer may be seen; a similar appearance may occur if multiple small stones layer in the dependent portion when the patient is upright (Fig. 13.10). If the diverticulum is large and arises from the pelvis, it is more likely to cause infundibular or calyceal compression and displacement (Fig. 13.11). The fluid-filled cavity comprising a calyceal diverticulum, together with any stones it contains, may be seen on CT or ultrasound. However, with these modalities, it may be hard to distinguish a diverticulum from a single obstructed hydrocalyx or renal cyst.

RENAL TUBERCULOSIS

Papillary necrosis due to tuberculosis may look similar to that of other etiologies; occasionally, the finely irregular surface of tuberculous papillary necrosis may provide a clue to its cause, as may other renal manifestations of the disease. The adjacent parenchyma may be scarred and calcified.

The epithelial lining of the calyces, infundibuli, pelvis, and ureter may become inflamed and ulcerated from tuberculous infection. After this phase resolves, reactive fibrosis may cause strictures at any of these levels and may produce obstruction. Fibrosis in and around the superior part of the renal pelvis may result in narrowing of the pelvis, with superior retraction producing a sharp pelvic angle known as a "purse-string stricture."

Fibrosis of an infundibulum (Fig. 13.12) can result in an amputated (that is, completely obstructed and nonopacified) calyx. Fibrosis at the ureteropelvic junction may result in caseous pyonephrosis, which may calcify and produce the classic appearance of tuberculous autonephrectomy.

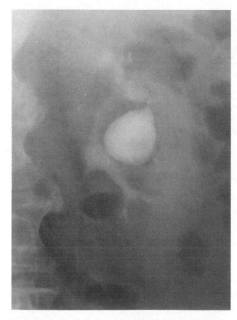

Figure 13.11.   Large calyceal diverticulum. Excretory urography reveals the diverticulum to indent the adjacent renal pelvis; innumerable tiny calcified stones cause it to be quite dense.

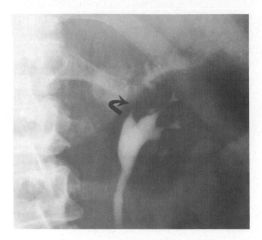

Figure 13.12.   Tuberculosis. Late film from an excretory urogram showing dilated, partially obstructed calyx in the upper pole due to upper pole infundibular stricture. An irregular collection of contrast medium is also seen in the papilla of an adjacent calyx.

The differential diagnosis of benign strictures in the renal collecting system is short. A vessel crossing and compressing an upper pole infundibulum may mimic a stricture, but usually can be distinguished because it is

a solitary finding, because it has the classic configuration of external compression of the infundibulum caused by an adjacent cylindrical structure, and because of the absence of other findings of tuberculosis. Transitional cell carcinoma may obstruct part of the collecting system, but usually a mass or an irregular tumor surface can be detected. Extrinsic infundibular compression due to parapelvic cysts or fat rarely causes obstruction, and cysts usually cause sufficient displacement that the abnormality is clearly due to a space-occupying lesion, rather than an intrinsic stricture. Rarely, brucellosis can mimic tuberculosis, and retroperitoneal fibrosis may occasionally invade the renal sinus and mimic intrinsic pyelocalyceal strictures.

DIFFERENTIAL DIAGNOSIS OF EXTRACALYCEAL CONTRAST MEDIUM

Papillary necrosis, MSK, and tuberculosis may all cause contrast medium to be seen in the papillae outside the interpapillary line (Fig. 13.13), and differentiating among them may be difficult. Both papillary necrosis and MSK are more common in women. Patients with papillary necrosis may have a history of one of the etiologic conditions. Both papillary necrosis and tubercu-

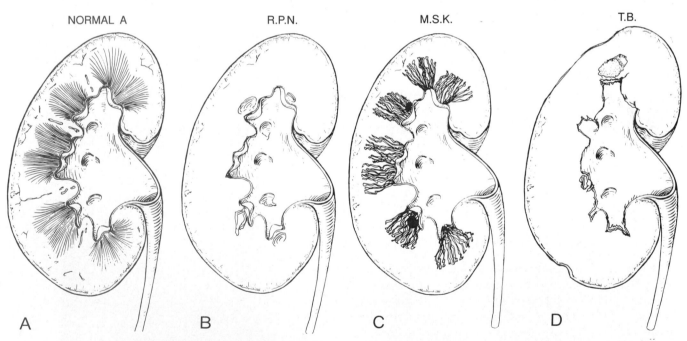

Figure 13.13.   A, Normal. Diagrammatic representation of contrast medium seen in normal collecting tubules after the application of compression in excretory urography. The rays of contrast medium in collecting tubules are outside the interpapillary line. **B,** Papillary necrosis. Diagrammatic representation of necrotic papillae in papillary necrosis. The papilla may be completely (papillary type) or partially (medullary type) necrotic. The calyces are normally cupped unless the necrotic papilla has sloughed and passed into the collecting system in which case the calyx will appear to be blunt. **C,** Medullary sponge kidney. Diagrammatic representation of dilated collecting ducts, some containing small calcifications. The collecting ducts are irregular in outline. The calyx is either normal or flattened. This is the classic appearance of medullary sponge kidney. **D,** Tuberculosis. Diagrammatic representation of intermediate renal tuberculosis. Contrast medium is seen in cavities in the papilla. These collections are irregular and extend toward the cortex. There may be associated scarring opposite the affected papilla. The associated calyx has a motheaten, ragged appearance.

losis may cause pyuria, which most patients with MSK do not have. Urine culture for tuberculosis bacilli makes the critical distinction.

Medullary sponge kidney and benign tubular ectasia usually demonstrate tiny parallel streaks of extracalyceal contrast; this brush-like appearance is occasionally obvious only with a magnifying glass. Calyceal diverticuli, when small, may be difficult to distinguish from single calyces whose papillae have completely sloughed, but calyceal diverticuli usually have extremely thin necks, are eccentric rather than central to the calyx, and may contain a characteristic cluster of small stones. If a series of films has been obtained immediately after contrast injection (1-minute nephrotomograms), the calyceal diverticulum can be seen to opacify after the calyx opacifies, as contrast medium is excreted through the tubules into the calyx and then out to the diverticulum.

RENAL SINUS FAT

The normal renal sinus contains fat that surrounds the pelvicalyceal and vascular structures. This fat is so sparse in infancy and childhood as to be invisible by clinical imaging. But with advancing age, this fat increases in volume and becomes detectable. In anatomically normal patients, this change probably reflects the inexorable loss of renal parenchymal volume that occurs with age. In patients who are obese, who have excess truncal fat from exogenous steroids or Cushing's syndrome, or whose renal parenchymal volume has been reduced by disease, the amount of sinus fat may be considerable. In a few patients in whom the renal parenchyma has been almost completely destroyed, usually by pyelocalyceal stones, the sinus fat can become quite voluminous; this condition is known as replacement lipomatosis, or replacement fibrolipomatosis.

Urography, especially nephrotomography, reveals renal sinus lipomatosis as a region of central renal lucency that surrounds the infundibulae. The infundibulae may look very attenuated, or thinned, or even slightly bowed, but infundibular obstruction is not a feature of this condition. Sinus fat may be indistinguishable from multiple renal sinus cysts during urography.

Ultrasound reveals the fat to be echogenic. Enlargement of the echogenic central renal echo complex is seen, a finding that permits distinction of fat from cysts; the parenchyma may be thinned. Computed tomography directly reveals the sinus fat, which is usually of the same density as other retroperitoneal fat. When extreme thinning of the renal parenchyma causes replacement lipomatosis, the renal sinus fat may be so exuberant as to resemble a central renal fatty mass. In these cases, collecting system calculi may be found and there may be sufficient renal parenchymal damage that the kidney may not function.

VASCULAR IMPRESSIONS

The renal artery and vein and their major branches are in close association with the collecting system, and both normal and abnormal vessels may cause impressions on the pelvis and infundibulae. These impressions are virtually always urographic findings and, although they can usually be specifically diagnosed, they may occasionally require workup with other imaging techniques.

The most common manifestation of pelvicalyceal vascular impression is a band-like or cylindrical lucency that may involve any part of the collecting system, but that is most frequently seen in the upper pole infundibulum or

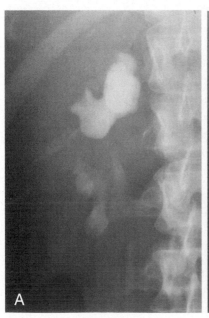 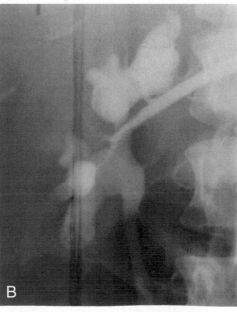

A   B

Figure 13.14. Renal artery partially obstructing upper pole infundibulum. **A,** Excretory urography reveals dilated upper pole calyces. **B,** Renal arteriography shows a branch of the renal artery compressing upper pole infundibulum.

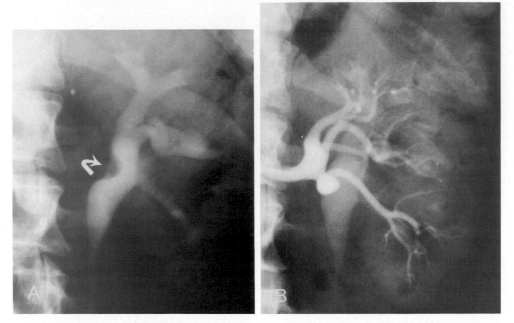

Figure 13.15. **A,** Renal artery aneurysm. Excretory urogram showing renal pelvic defect (*arrow*). **B,** Selective renal arteriography shows a renal artery aneurysm in the exact position of the renal pelvic defect.

on the superior surface of the renal pelvis. The lucency can be made to shrink or disappear if calyceal pressure is increased, either by the application of ureteral compression or the performance of a retrograde pyelogram. If the diagnosis is still not certain, dynamic CT or Doppler ultrasound may demonstrate that the structure producing the lucency is a vessel.

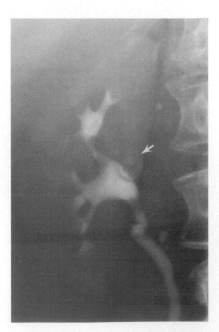

Figure 13.16. Ring-like calcification of renal artery aneurysm (*arrow*) indenting superior aspect of renal pelvis.

Very rarely, a renal artery branch may compress an upper pole infundibulum to the point which the associated calyx may become obstructed and ectatic (Fig. 13.14), a condition referred to as Fraley's syndrome. Surgery may be required to address the associated symptoms or the complications of local hydronephrosis.

Renal artery aneurysms (Fig. 13.15) and arteriovenous malformations that protrude into the renal sinus may indent the collecting system and produce urographic lucencies. Ring-like calcifications in aneurysms (Fig. 13.16) may be clues to the etiology of impressions on the collecting system.

RENAL SINUS HEMORRHAGE

Hemorrhage into the renal sinus or collecting system may occur in a variety of clinical circumstances including benign or malignant renal tumors, arteritis, aneurysms, arteriovenous malformations, trauma, coagulation disorders, or other bleeding diatheses. In the central portion of the kidney, bleeding may occur into the renal sinus or the wall or lumen of the collecting system.

The radiologic appearance depends on the compartment into which bleeding has occurred. Hemorrhage into the collecting system may produce intraluminal clots that appear as filling defects. These filling defects are usually well defined and conform to the configuration of the collecting system. Large blood clots are usually evident and are associated with gross hematuria; small blood clots may be difficult to distinguish from loosened stones or even tumors. Because the kidney produces urokinase, blood clots often dissolve, though they may reform if bleeding persists. Blood clots have moderate echogenicity, less than that of renal sinus fat. They do not produce the acoustic shadowing seen with stones. Computed tomography demonstrates blood clot as an opacity slightly denser than adjacent soft tissues. They can be clearly distinguished from stones, because even "lucent" stones have a CT density of approximately 150 Hounsfield units (HU) or more. Blood clots also may pass down the ureter and may cause ureteral obstruction.

Hemorrhage into the wall of the collecting system is seen most frequently in patients with a bleeding disorder or those receiving anticoagulant medication. Excretory urography reveals an intramural mass that creates a well-defined filling defect that can be linear, circular, or even plaque-like in configuration. (Fig. 13.17) Since the hematomas are usually small, they are difficult to see on CT.

The radiographic appearance of bleeding into the renal sinus includes narrowing of the major infundibula, renal pelvis, or proximal ureter. Although they are often best seen on excretory urography, this narrowing may be large enough to be identified on CT (Fig. 13.18). The density of the hematoma depends on the age of the lesion. Acute thrombus is more dense than unenhanced renal parenchyma. Over time, the clot may liquify to a water density or may be resorbed.

Intraluminal, intramural, and renal sinus hemorrhage may occur independently, in combination, or accompanied by renal parenchymal or perinephric bleeding. The radiographic evaluation should be directed not only at

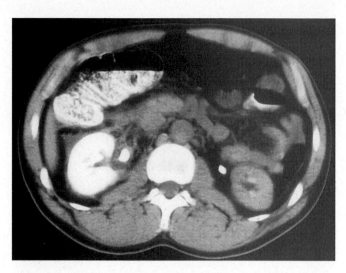

Figure 13.18.   Renal sinus hemorrhage. A persistent right nephrogram is due to ureteral obstruction by a blood clot in this anticoagulated patient. Hemorrhage into the renal sinus is seen surrounding the contrast filled renal pelvis.

diagnosing this hemorrhage, but identifying the underlying etiology. In some cases, extensive bleeding precludes a good CT examination, and a follow-up study may be necessary to exclude a small neoplasm.

BENIGN MASSES

Papillomas

Papillomas are a kind of benign tumor of the transitional epithelium that may appear in the collecting system, ureter, or bladder; they are rare in the upper tract. Some pathologists do not make a clear distinction between papillomas and low-grade transitional-cell carcinomas. Papillomas appear as polypoid filling defects that may have a recognizable stalk. Inverted papillomas are extremely unusual lesions that have a central core composed of transitional epithelium rather than connective tissue and are covered with the normal layer of transitional cell epithelium. They are small and intrinsically benign, but a few patients have been described in whom urothelial malignancy has been found near the inverted papilloma or elsewhere in the urinary tract.

Connective Tissue Tumors

Connective tissue tumors of the collecting system are rare; both malignant and benign tumors originating from muscular, vascular, fibrous, and neural tissues have been described. They present as masses arising from the renal pelvic or calyceal walls. As a group, their surfaces may be less irregular than those of epithelial malignancies, but their specific diagnoses can usually not be established radiologically.

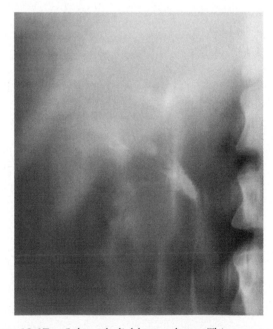

Figure 13.17.   Suburothelial hemorrhage. This tomographic section from an excretory urogram demonstrates an irregular contour to the renal pelvis.

Fibroepithelial Polyps

These are described in greater detail in the chapter on the ureter, but also may appear in the renal pelvis. The pelvic lesions may be more bulky and multilobular than the ureteral lesions, which often are long, thin, and cylindrical.

Leukoplakia (Squamous Metaplasia)

Squamous metaplasia is a rare inflammatory condition, usually associated with chronic infection, which may occur in the collecting system, ureter, or bladder. The term leukoplakia refers to a white patch seen on the surface of an area of squamous metaplasia. Although there is an association between squamous metaplasia and squamous cell carcinoma in the bladder, whether there is such an association in the upper urinary tract is not clear; the malignant potential of the lesion in the renal collecting system is probably low. The lesion may be accompanied by symptoms of urinary tract infection and microhematuria; desquamated flakes of epithelial tissue may appear in the urine.

Retrograde pyelography or excretory urography may reveal the lesion as a flat mass or region of thickening of the renal pelvic wall; the thickening may give a "corduroy" appearance.

Malacoplakia

Malacoplakia is another rare benign inflammatory lesion that is usually accompanied by recurrent bouts of *Escherichia coli* infection. The lesions are usually small; they are rarely larger than 3 mm in diameter, and are commonly multiple. They appear as smooth yellow plaques on gross inspection, which, histologically, contain the typical histiocytes in which Michaelis-Guttmann bodies are seen. Radiographically, they appear as multiple filling defects arising from the wall of the renal pelvis; they usually are flatter than the lesions of pyelitis cystica.

Pyelitis Cystica

These lesions are identical to those sometimes found in the ureter in patients with ureteritis cystica; they are described more fully in Chapter 16. Urography reveals them as multiple, small (2-mm), smooth, hemispherical filling defects protruding into the lumen from the renal pelvic wall.

MALIGNANT TUMORS

Seven to 8% of primary renal malignancies develop in the collecting system. There is a male predilection for urothelial cancer. Most malignancies of the renal collecting system are transitional cell carcinomas; squamous cell carcinomas are unusual and adenocarcinomas are rarer still. The types are usually not distinguishable radiologically. Transitional cell carcinomas have a tendency to be multiple, so that synchronous and metachronous lesions may be seen in a given patient. In general, transitional cell carcinomas of the bladder are much more common than tumors of the upper urinary tract. Up to 40% of patients with transitional cell carcinomas of the collecting system may have carcinomas of the bladder diagnosed within a short time, and patients with a transitional cell carcinoma at any site are at increased risk for developing a subsequent transitional cell carcinoma in the upper urinary tract as well. If transitional cell carcinomas of the upper tract are treated with local resection, the remaining collecting system and ureter are particularly prone to develop another tumor.

A number of predisposing factors seem to place patients at risk for developing upper tract transitional cell carcinoma, including analgesic abuse, exposure to aniline dyes or petroleum derivatives, a long history of heavy smoking, administration of cyclophosphamide, and Balkan nephropathy. Long-standing upper tract stone disease may be a risk factor for squamous cell carcinoma; whether or not leukoplakia or upper urinary tract cholesteatomas increase the risk is debatable.

Any upper urinary tract tumor may present with gross or microscopic hematuria. The patients may have pain, especially if the tumors have caused hydronephrosis, and voided urine may contain exfoliated malignant cells that are detectable on cytologic examination.

Upper urinary tract tumors can be staged by a scheme similar to that used for bladder carcinomas. Stage 0 tumors are limited to the transitional epithelium, stage A lesions have invaded the lamina propria, and stage B tumors have invaded into, but not completely through, the muscularis. The prognosis for these tumors is good; 50% survivals of 5 to 7 years are typical. Stage C tumors have invaded the adjacent fat or renal parenchyma, and stage D tumors have metastasized (nodal and lung metastases are common); the prognosis for these lesions is usually poor, and many patients die of carcinomatosis within 1 year.

Small carcinomas of the collecting system may be best detected initially by excretory or retrograde urography (Fig. 13.19). The images reflect the growth pattern. Tumors may appear as intraluminal filling defects, which may be polypoid or flat; their surface is usually irregular (Figs. 13.20 and 13.21). If the tumor has completely obstructed an infundibulum, the associated calyx may fail to opacify (the "amputated" calyx) and evidence of local hydronephrosis may be visible. If the pelvis or ureteropelvic junction is obstructed, varying degrees of failure to function and hydronephrosis involving the entire kidney may be encountered.

Filling defects may require a differential diagnosis. Lucent stones may need to be excluded by ultrasound, which will show them to have an echogenic surface near the transducer and acoustic shadows deep to them. On

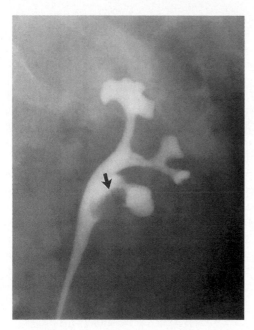

Figure 13.19. Transitional cell carcinoma of the renal pelvis. Retrograde pyelography reveals a solitary renal pelvic filling defect (*arrow*).

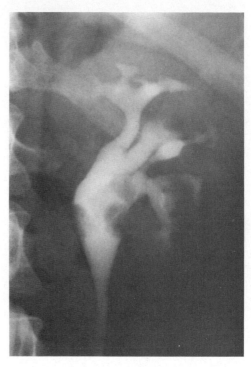

Figure 13.20. Transitional cell carcinoma. Multiple irregular filling defects in renal pelvis and calyces are most consistent with transitional cell carcinoma.

CT, lucent stones show Hounsfield units higher than that encountered in soft tissue. Blood clots may produce filling defects; this diagnosis may be excluded if there is no gross hematuria or may be confirmed if the CT density is consistent with clots or if subsequent examinations prove

them to lyse and disappear. A sloughed papilla may sometimes look like a polypoid tumor, but is usually associated with a blunted calyx at the site from which the

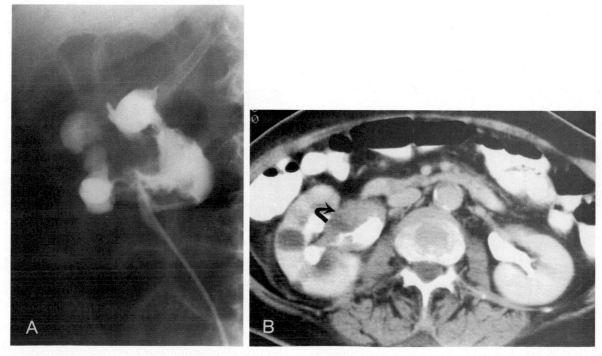

Figure 13.21. A, Transitional cell carcinoma. Retrograde pyelography demonstrates a large irregular filling defect in the renal pelvis. **B,** The soft tissue mass component is shown on this enhanced computed tomography examination.

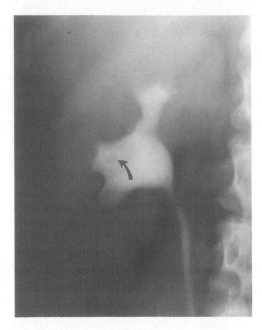

Figure 13.22. Normal papilla causing lucent filling defect in renal pelvis. Note dense ring (*arrow*) caused by contrast in the papilla's fornix.

papilla detached. Fungus balls may be diagnosed by finding hyphae in the urine. Rarely, cholesteatomas may mimic tumors. A normal papilla may protrude into the renal pelvis without an intervening infundibulum; contrast in the papilla's fornix may produce a dense ring around the lucency and provide a clue to the diagnosis (Fig. 13.22). Benign strictures may mimic obstructing tumors; these are usually caused by tuberculosis and may be accompanied by other signs of renal tuberculosis, and sometimes by pyuria and positive urine cultures. Rarely, renal parenchymal tumors may invade the collecting system and mimic transitional cell neoplasms.

Ultrasound and CT are not as sensitive as urography

for detecting small tumors. Ultrasound reveals transitional cell carcinomas to be relatively hypoechoic regions (Fig. 13.23) within the renal sinus, which is normally quite echogenic. Ultrasound also may demonstrate any hydronephrosis that the tumor has produced.

The differential diagnosis of a hypoechoic lesion in the collecting system includes blood clot, fungus ball, and other tumors. Computed tomography reveals the mass directly and also may depict any hydronephrosis. The mass is usually of soft-tissue density and may enhance slightly with intravenous contrast medium. Large tumors may contain low-density necrotic regions that do not enhance. If the tumor appears as a relatively discrete intraluminal mass surrounded by normal-appearing parenchyma, it is likely to be of relatively low (O, A, or B) stage. If the edges of the mass extend into the region of the renal parenchyma and acquire indistinct boundaries (Fig. 13.24), it is likely to be stage C; local lymphadenopathy, which usually indicates stage D disease, also should be sought when the tumors are evaluated with CT.

Arteriography is rarely performed in patients with collecting system tumors. When the tumor is large enough to be visualized, it is usually relatively hypovascular (Fig. 13.25); any visualized tumor neovascularity is likely to appear as tortuous, thread-like vessels rather than as hypertrophied arteries.

VESICOURETERAL REFLUX

Vesicoureteral reflux is dealt with primarily in Chapter 16, and the chronic pyelonephritic changes that it causes in the kidney are described in Chapter 7. However, reflux and chronic pyelonephritis involve changes that appear in the pyelocalyceal system, and are briefly reviewed here.

Low grades of reflux may produce no pyelocalyceal

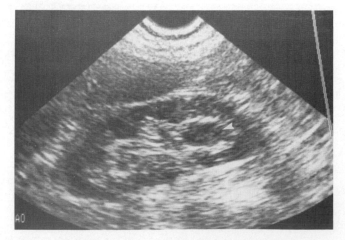

Figure 13.23. Transitional cell carcinoma. Ultrasound examination showing echogenic discrete mass in the lower pole calyceal region.

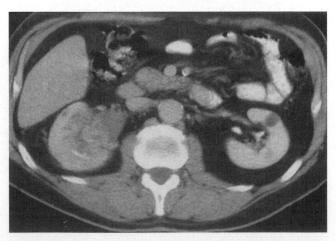

Figure 13.24. Computed tomography of right renal pelvic transitional cell cancer. The tumor occupies the entire renal sinus, has invaded the parenchyma and obstructed the kidney (note diminished nephrogram). There is a simple cyst on the left.

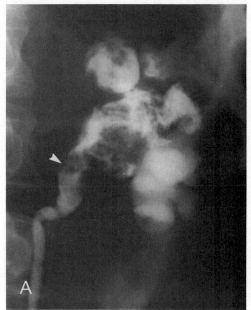
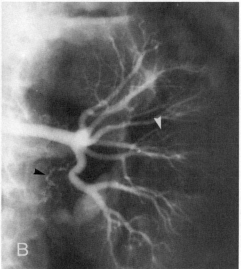

Figure 13.25.   A, Transitional cell carcinoma. Excretory urogram in a patient with invasive transitional cell carcinoma. The tumor has extended into the calyces and through the renal pelvic wall (*arrowhead*). Much of the filling defect represents blood clot. **B,** Selective renal angiography shows small tumor vessels centrally (*white arrowhead*) and tortuous tumor vessels where the tumor has invaded the renal pelvis (*black arrowhead*). Tumor vessels are not commonly seen in transitional cell carcinoma.

changes at all. At the instant in which reflux occurs, there may be varying degrees of pyelocalyceal distention, the morphology of which may be indistinguishable from obstructive hydronephrosis. Depending on the duration and severity of the reflux, the distention may or may not persist between episodes of reflux and after the reflux has resolved naturally or been corrected surgically.

Reflux may cause focal renal scarring (Fig. 13.26). This may be unilateral or bilateral, may involve a very small portion of a kidney or nearly the entire organ. The scarring has a predilection to appear in the poles, especially the upper poles. Because the scarring involves focal thinning of the renal parenchyma that extends from the renal capsule into the calyx, inward retraction of the renal margin and outward retraction of the papillary regions appear. The normal surface of the papilla, which produces the concave outer margin of opacified calyx, becomes flattened or even convex (Fig. 13.27). Focal ca-

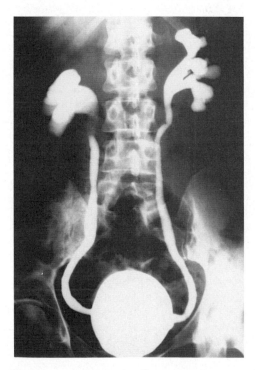

Figure 13.27.   Vesicoureteral reflux. Cystogram in a female patient showing low-pressure grade 4 reflux into dilated pelvicalyceal systems.

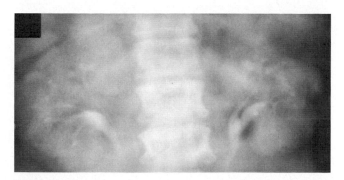

Figure 13.26.   Reflux nephropathy. Excretory urogram with tomography in a 35-year-old woman, showing bilateral parenchymal scarring and blunted calyces in a patient who refluxed in early childhood.

lyceal blunting with associated parenchymal thinning due to reflux is difficult or impossible to distinguish from that which may be caused by calyceal stone disease.

SUGGESTED READING

Papillary Necrosis

Allen RC, Pety RE, Lirenman DS, et al.: Renal papillary necrosis in children with chronic arthritis. *Am J Dis Child* 140:20, 1986.

Andriole GL, Bahnson RR: Computed tomographic diagnosis of ureteral obstruction caused by a sloughed papilla. *Urol Radiol* 9:45, 1987.

Braden GL, Kozinn DR, Hampf FE Jr, et al: Ultrasound diagnosis of early renal papillary necrosis. *J Ultrasound Med* 10(7):401, 1991.

Felatte LC, Minon-Cifuentes JLR, Medina JA: Papillary stones: calcified renal tubules in Randall's plaques. *J Urol* 133:490, 1985.

Gong MB, Davidson AJ: Development and progression of renal papillary necrosis in SA hemoglobinopathy. *Urol Radiol* 2:55, 1980.

Henrich WL: Southwestern Internal Medicine Conference: analgesic nephropathy. *Am J Med Sci,* 295:561, 1988.

Henry MA, Tange JD: Ultrastructural appearances of acute renal papillary lesions induced by aspirin. *J Pathol* 151:11, 1987.

Maher JF: Analgesic nephropathy. Observations, interpretations, and perspectives on the low incidence in America. *Am J Med* 76:345, 1984.

Medullary Sponge Kidney

Gedroyc WMW, Saxton HM: More medullary sponge variants. *Clin Radiol* 39:423, 1988.

Ginalski JM, Portmann L, Jeager P: Does medullary sponge kidney cause nephrolithiasis? *AJR* 155(2):299, 1990.

Zawada ET, Sica DA: Differential diagnosis of medullary sponge kidney. *South Med J* 77:686, 1984.

Leukoplakia and Malacoplakia

Benson RC Jr, Swanson SK, Farrow GM: Relationship of leukoplakia to urothelial malignancy. *J Urol* 131:507, 1984.

Hertle L, Androulakakis P: Keratinizing desquamative squamous metaplasia of the upper urinary tract: leukoplakia-cholesteatoma. *J Urol* 127:631, 1982.

Stanton MJ, Maxted W: Malacoplakia: A study of the literature and current concepts of pathogenesis, diagnosis and treatment. *J Urol* 125:139, 1981.

Tuberculosis

Becker JA: Renal tuberculosis. *Urol Radiol* 10:25, 1988.

Goldman SM, Fishman EK, Hartman DS, et al.: Computed tomography of renal tuberculosis and its pathological correlates. *J Comput Assist Tomogr* 9:77, 1985.

Premkumar A, Lattimer J, Newhouse JH: CT and sonography of advanced urinary tract tuberculosis. *AJR* 148:65, 1987.

Psihramis KE, Donahoe PK: Primary genitourinary tuberculosis: rapid progression and tissue destruction during treatment. *J Urol* 135:1033, 1986.

Renal Sinus Lipomatosis

Faegenburg D, Bosniak M, Evans JA: Renal sinus lipomatosis: its demonstration by nephrotomography. *Radiology* 83:987, 1964.

Subramanyam BR, et al.: Replacement lipomatosis of the kidney: diagnosis by computed tomography and sonography. *Radiology* 148:791, 1983.

Vascular Impressions

Fraley EE: Vascular obstruction of superior infundibulum causing nephralgia. *N Eng J Med* 275:1403, 1966.

Quillin SP, Brink JA, Heiken JP, et al: Helical (spiral) CT angiography for identification of crossing vessels at the ureteropelvic junction. *AJR* 166:1125, 1996.

Renal Sinus Hemorrhage

Fishman MC, Pollack HM, Arger PH, Banner MP: Radiographic manifestations of spontaneous renal sinus hemorrhage. *AJR* 142:1161–1164, 1984

Levitt S, Waisman J, deKernion J: Subepithelial hematoma of the renal pelvis (Antopol-Goldman lesion). *J Urol* 131:939, 1984

Oza KN, Rezvan M, Moser R: Subepithelial hematoma of the renal pelvis (Antopol-Goldman lesion). *Journal of Urology.* 155(3): 1032-1033, 1996

Benign Masses

Irby PB, Stoller ML, MacAninch JW: Fungal bezoars of the upper urinary tract. *J Urol* 143:447, 1990.

Renfer LG, Kelley J, Belville WD: Inverted papilloma of the urinary tract: histogenesis, recurrence and associated malignancy. *J Urol* 140:832, 1988.

Malignant Tumors

Affre J, Michael JR, de Peyronnet R, et al.: Secondary foci of primary tumors of the bladder in the upper urinary tract. *Urol Radiol* 3:7, 1981.

Anselmo G, Rizzotta A, Fielici E, et al.: Multiple simultaneous bilateral urothelial tumors of the renal pelvis. *Br J Urol* 60:312, 1987.

Balfe DM, McClennan BL, AufderHeide JF: Multimodality imaging in evaluation of two cases of adenocarcinoma of the renal pelvis. *Urol Radiol* 3:19, 1981.

Bree RL, Schultz SR, Hayes R: Large infiltrating renal transitional cell carcinomas: CT and ultrasound features. *J Comput Assist Tomogr* 13(3):381, 1990.

Highman WJ: Transitional carcinoma of the upper urinary tract: a histologic and cytopathological study. *J Clin Pathol* 39:297, 1986.

Jarrett TW, Sweetser PM, Weiss GH, et al: Percutaneous management of transitional cell carcinoma of the renal collection system: 9-year experience. *J Urol* 154: 1629, 1995.

Leder RA, Dunnick NR: Transitional cell carcinoma of the kidney and ureter. *AJR* 155:713, 1990.

Marchetto D, Li FP, Henson DE: Familial carcinoma of ureters and other genitourinary organs. *J Urol* 130:772, 1983.

Munechika H, Kushihashi T, Gokan T, et al.: A renal cell carcinoma extending into the renal pelvis simulating transitional cell carcinoma. *Urol Radiol* 12:11, 1990.

Narumi Y, Sato T, Hori S, et al.: Squamous cell carcinoma of the uroepithelium: CT evaluation. *Radiology* 173:853, 1989.

Nyman V, Oldbring J, Aspelin P: CT of carcinoma of the renal pelvis. *Acta Radiol* 33:31, 1992.

Oldbring J. Glifberg I, Mikulowski P, et al.: Carcinoma of the renal pelvis and ureter following bladder carcinoma: frequency of risk factors and clinicopathologic findings. *J Urol* 141:1311, 1989.

Pollack HM: Long-term follow-up of the upper urinary tract for transitional cell carcinoma: how much is enough? *Radiology* 167:871, 1988.

Renfer LG, Kelley J, Belville WD: Inverted papilloma of the urinary tract: histogenesis, recurrence and associated malignancy. *J Urol* 140:832, 1988.

Tasca A, Zattoni F: The case for a percutaneous approach to transitional cell carcinoma of the renal pelvis. *J Urol* 143:902, 1990.

Yousem DM, Gatewood OMB, Goldman SM, et al.: Synchronous and metachronous transitional cell carcinoma of the urinary tract: prevalence, incidence and radiographic detection. *Radiology* 167:613, 1988.

Vesicoureteral Reflux

Hodson CJ: Reflux nephropathy: a personal historical review. *AJR* 137:451, 1981.

Rizzona G, Perale R, Bui F, et al.: Radionuclide voiding cystography in intrarenal reflux detection. *Ann Radiol* 29:415, 1986.

14

Urinary Tract Trauma

RENAL INJURIES

Clinical Features

Hematuria after blunt abdominal injury is common; significant injury to the kidney, however, is relatively uncommon. Hematuria after penetrating injury is virtually always a sign of renal damage that requires evaluation.

The amount of hematuria that should trigger radiologic investigation of the urinary tract after blunt trauma is controversial. Many authorities believe that any amount of hematuria should be investigated, because significant urinary tract injury may be present in patients with little or even no hematuria. Furthermore, there is little correlation between the degree of hematuria and the extent of renal injury present. An oft-cited example is patients suffering from renal pedicle injury in whom hematuria is said to be absent in 25% of the cases.

As a result, screening studies of the urinary tract often are performed in virtually every patient after abdominal trauma. This low threshold for investigation has resulted in a relatively low yield for injury on radiologic screening studies. In a series of patients studied by McDonald and colleagues at a major trauma center, only 18 of 209 urograms performed for blunt trauma in patients with hematuria were considered abnormal (9%). Similar results have been reported from other institutions.

As a result of these statistics, other investigators have sought to refine the criteria that should lead to investigation. Guice and associates found that no significant renal injury would be missed had investigation been limited to those patients with gross or 4+ hematuria on dipstick urinalysis. Fortune and coworkers, in a series encompassing 216 patients, found that in all but 1 of 20 patients with significant urographic abnormalities, hematuria greater than 50 red cells per high-power field was present and that all of the renal injuries present were associated with obvious abdominal injury. Similarly, Nicolaisen and colleagues found that significant renal injury was limited to the group of patients in whom shock and hematuria was present among 306 patients analyzed retrospectively following blunt trauma. There were no significant renal injuries among the 221 patients who had microscopic hematuria, but were not suffering from shock. In patients in the same series who suffered penetrating injuries, however, no such discrimination was possible, and the authors suggest radiologic evaluation be undertaken in all patients suffering penetrating injury and hematuria. These observations have now been confirmed in multiple additional studies both retrospectively and prospectively. Therefore, investigation of hematuria is warranted in those patients suffering penetrating injury, gross hematuria, microscopic hematuria with shock, and those suspected of having major associated intraabdominal injury.

Other clinical findings associated with renal injury include a flank mass or hematoma on physical examination; a soft tissue mass on plain-film studies; a scoliosis of the lumbar spine; and fractures of the lower ribs (Fig. 14.1), lumbar vertebral bodies, or transverse processes. Loss of the psoas shadow is a nonspecific finding on which significant injury cannot be reliably diagnosed or excluded.

Most blunt renal injuries (75%) occur in patients suffering multisystem trauma. In a series from Cass and colleagues (1985), 241 of 831 patients had what were considered to be solitary renal injuries; however, the vast majority (98%) were minor injuries. Only five patients in

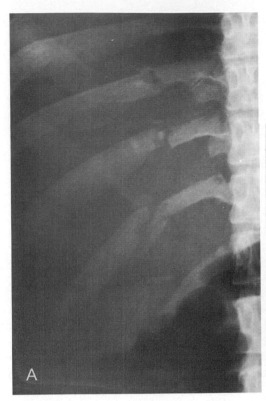

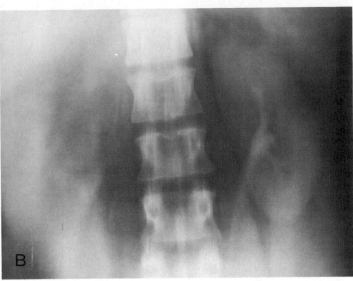

Figure 14.1. **A,** Scout radiograph demonstrates multiple lower right rib fractures. **B,** Tomogram from an IVP demonstrates a poorly defined renal outline, decreased contrast excretion, and poor filling of the collecting system of the right kidney, indicative of a right renal injury.

the entire series suffered significant isolated renal injury. There were 33 significant renal injuries in the group of 590 patients with hematuria who suffered multisystem trauma. Other injuries associated with injury of the kidneys after multisystem blunt trauma include, in order of decreasing frequency: fractures of the extremities, thoracic injury, pelvic fracture, intraabdominal injury, head injuries, and diaphragmatic rupture. The liver and spleen are the abdominal organs most commonly associated with renal injury, followed by the pancreas, the colon, and the small bowel. Studies have shown a strong association between the presence of gross hematuria and nonurologic intraabdominal injury as well following blunt trauma. Knudson and coworkers found that 24% of patients with gross hematuria after blunt trauma had a significant intraabdominal injury; this increased to 65% when shock also was present.

In most series, blunt trauma accounts for 80% of all renal injuries, but the incidence reported depends on the referral pattern of the reporting institution. Approximately three quarters of the reported renal injuries occur in men younger than 50 years of age. Motor vehicle accidents account for about one half of the reported cases; falls, altercations, industrial accidents, and sports injuries comprise the remainder.

Penetrating renal injuries fall into two categories: (*a*)

those related to gunshot wounds and (*b*) those related to stabbings. Limited posterior stab wounds that do not penetrate the renal fossa are managed conservatively by many surgeons. In the remainder, the mere demonstration that the kidney is in the path of the injury or the presence of hematuria is an indication for surgical exploration. More than 80% of gunshot wounds of the kidney are associated with other abdominal injuries, usually of the bowel, the pancreas, the diaphragm, or the liver and spleen.

Anatomy and Mechanism of Injury

The kidney is relatively protected from injury by the rib cage, the vertebral column, and the psoas muscles. The fascial coverings of the kidney and the retroperitoneal fat provide additional protection. Injury of the lower ribs or the vertebra is associated with a higher incidence of renal injury; an injury to the spleen frequently accompanies injury to the left kidney, whereas a liver injury accompanies injury of the right kidney. Bleeding from renal injuries is frequently self-limiting, because Gerota's fascia provides a tamponade effect.

Bleeding within the renal parenchyma results in an intrarenal hematoma. Bleeding that occurs between the renal parenchyma and the renal capsule is a subcapsular hematoma. If the capsule also is torn, hemorrhage confined by Gerota's fascia is termed a perinephric hematoma. Rarely, hemorrhage also may extend beyond Gerota's fascia within the retroperitoneum.

Blunt injuries of the kidney occur as a result of a direct blow to the flank or from deceleration. With a direct blow, the kidney is crushed, causing a laceration or lacerations of the renal parenchyma that result in subcapsular, intrarenal, or perinephric hematomas. With a deceleration injury, acute tension on the renal pedicle may produce a laceration of the renal vein or artery, an intimal tear in the vessel that generally results in secondary thrombosis, or rarely laceration or avulsion of the ureteropelvic junction (UPJ). Penetrating injury usually results in direct injury of the renal parenchyma, the vascular pedicle, or the collecting system.

In patients with a preexisting renal abnormality, relatively minor trauma may cause disproportionate symptomatology that brings the patient to medical attention. Such underlying conditions include calculi, tumors, cystic disease, and some congenital conditions, including UPJ obstruction and horseshoe kidney.

Classification

There is no one uniformly applied classification of renal injuries. As such, comparison of data among published series can be difficult or even misleading. This is a particular problem when one attempts to compare data from one series in which patients are classified according to surgical findings to another series in which the patients have been classified based on radiologic examination. It is preferable, therefore, to use a functional classification in which injuries are grouped according to the severity of the injury and its therapeutic implication rather than by using descriptive terminology, the criteria of which are more subjective in nature. The system most widely used in the radiology literature (Fig. 14.2 and Table 14.1) is described as follows.

Minor injuries (Category I) may be treated expectantly and rarely require surgical intervention. They are the most common form of renal injury, comprising 85% of injuries in most series. In patients suffering isolated renal injuries, minor injuries constitute an even higher percentage of the injuries. In those suffering multisystem trauma, minor injuries still account for 75% of the total. The vast majority of minor renal injuries consist of small to moderate intrarenal hematomas that also are called *renal contusions* (*see* Fig. 14.1). Other injuries included in this group include small subcapsular (Fig. 14.3) or perinephric hematomas, small cortical lacerations, subsegmental renal infarcts, and rarely pyelosinus extravasation associated with blunt injury. In general, these injuries do not involve a break in the renal capsule.

Intermediate injuries (Category II) constitute approximately 10% of cases. They are usually managed conservatively but may, on occasion, require surgical intervention, particularly if clinical deterioration develops.

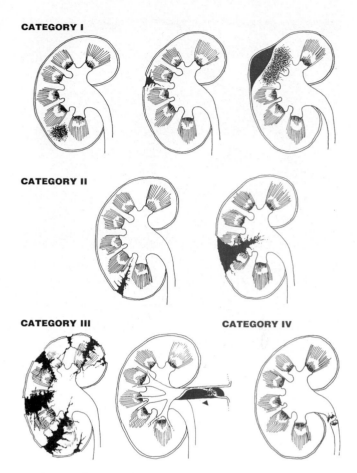

Figure 14.2.   Radiologic classification of renal injuries.

Injuries in this category include major renal lacerations that extend beyond the renal capsule, with or without involvement of the renal collecting system. These lacerations, which when distracted are termed "fractures," may be sufficiently large to be visible radiographically or at the time of surgical exploration. Extensive perirenal hematomas are usually present, and if the laceration involves the collecting system, demonstrate extravasation of contrast medium on radiologic examination (Fig. 14.4). Vascular injuries involving the segmental renal vessels are usually included in this category (*see* Traumatic Renal Infarction).

Table 14.1.
Classification of Renal Injuries

Category	Disease Extent
I	Small intrarenal ("contusions") or subcapsular hematomas, lacerations, small cortical infarcts
II	Deep cortical lacerations with or without involvement of the collecting system
III	Catastrophic renal injuries including multiple lacerations, shattered kidney or vascular injuries involving the renal pedicle
IV	Avulsion of the ureteropelvic junction

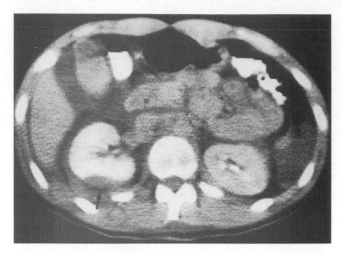

Figure 14.3.   A small subcapsular hematoma is present on the posterior surface of the right kidney (*arrow*).

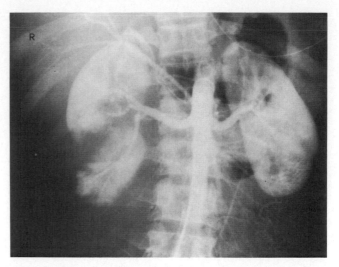

Figure 14.5.   Abdominal aortogram demonstrates multiple right renal lacerations (renal rupture) in a patient who suffered a direct blow to the flank.

Major injuries (Category III), which account for approximately 5% of all renal injuries, virtually always require surgical exploration, because of a threat to the viability of the kidney itself or because of life-threatening hemorrhage. In such situations, immediate surgical exploration and nephrectomy is frequently necessary. Major renal injuries include multiple renal lacerations (Fig. 14.5) or injury of the renal pedicle including avulsion of one or more of the renal veins, and thrombosis or laceration of the main renal artery. Large perinephric hematomas are common, and the tamponade effect of the renal fascia may be lost if it also is torn.

Isolated avulsion of the UPJ (Category IV) (Fig. 14.6) is a rare injury that has principally been described in children with a deceleration injury, but is increasingly found in adults as well. In such cases, the vascular supply of the renal pedicle remains intact; however, the UPJ is sheared from its attachment to the renal pelvis, resulting in a urinoma that surrounds the kidney. It more

commonly occurs in children and adolescents, presumably owing to the great elasticity of the child's blood vessels, which allows the renal vascular supply to remain intact at a force sufficient to cause disruption of the ureter. In addition, the smaller amount of retroperitoneal fat in children provides less cushioning during sudden deceleration. Avulsion of the UPJ may be partial or complete; with partial tears, some contrast medium will be present in the ureter below the site of injury (Fig. 14.7). This is a critical distinction; partial injuries may be treated with a ureteral stent, whereas complete disruption always requires open surgery.

On imaging studies, contrast extravasation will be demonstrated from the region of the UPJ. On computed tomography (CT), contrast extravasation into a urinoma that collects predominately in the medial perinephric space is seen (Fig. 14.6). There will be no associated perinephric hematoma unless a coexisting parenchymal laceration is present. The unopacified ureter may be identified within the area of contrast extravasation when the ureter has been completely avulsed.

Traumatic Renal Infarction

Traumatic renal artery thrombosis is reported to occur in approximately 3% of patients suffering renal injuries. The injury occurs as a result of a contrecoup tearing of the intima of the renal artery in patients suffering acute deceleration. The resulting intimal flap causes thrombosis of the renal artery. The injury may involve the main renal artery and result in global renal infarction, or more commonly may involve a segmental branch vessel and result in focal infarction. The injury generally occurs in patients suffering a fall from a height or as a result of an auto-pedestrian accident. While gross or microscopic hematuria often is present, Cass and col-

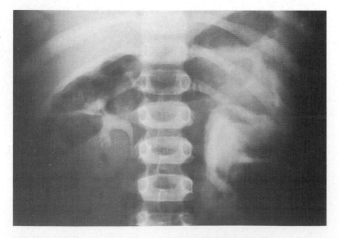

Figure 14.4.   IVP demonstrates obvious contrast medium extravasation from the left kidney. At surgery, a major laceration with involvement of the collecting system was present.

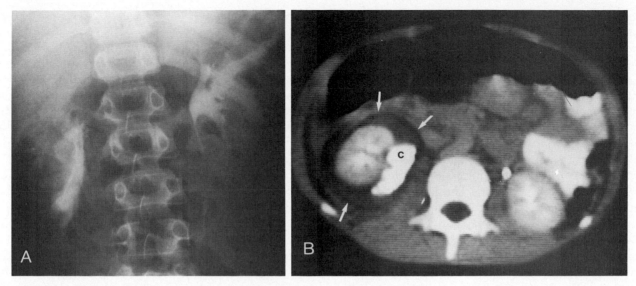

Figure 14.6.   Isolated complete avulsion of the ureteropelvic junction in a child involved in a motor vehicle accident. **A,** IVP demonstrates extravasation of contrast medium from the right kidney. No filling of the right ureter is seen. **B,** Computed to-mography shows no evidence of a renal laceration. A large collection of extravasated contrast (*c*) as well as a perinephric urinoma (*arrows*) are present.

leagues reported the absence of hematuria in as many as 25% of patients.

Traumatic occlusion of a segmental renal vessel is the most common vascular injury of the kidney after blunt renal trauma. Such occlusion results in segmental renal infarction. In the past, when this injury has been diagnosed, some authors have advocated partial nephrectomy or attempted revascularization out of concern that it might result in the subsequent development of hypertension. Bertini and colleagues studied 24 patients with segmental arterial occlusions demonstrated by angiography and found, that while transient hypertension was common initially, none of the 10 patients followed for up to 5 years suffered sustained blood pressure elevation. Similarly, Cass and coworkers studied seven patients who survived renal pedicle injuries for up to 7 years after injury; no sustained hypertension was reported.

The majority of patients suffering global renal infarction eventually develop irreversible loss of renal function and parenchymal atrophy. There are, however, a few isolated reports of spontaneous recovery of some renal function. In such cases, it has been presumed that collateral renal circulation has preserved a small amount of functioning parenchyma.

The management of patients suffering main renal artery occlusion after blunt trauma is controversial and is related to the variable period reported for which the kidney can tolerate warm ischemia. Warm ischemia times for human kidneys has been reported to be as short as 1 to 6 hours by some investigators, while others report successful revascularization after more than

20 hours. Even when revascularization is attempted, reports of successful return of renal function are sporadic; the precise incidence of success is not known, because it is likely that most unsuccessful attempts are not reported. Since the majority of renal pedicle injuries occur in patients suffering multisystem trauma and because the nonrenal injuries are often life threatening, it is not uncommon for several hours of warm ischemia to have

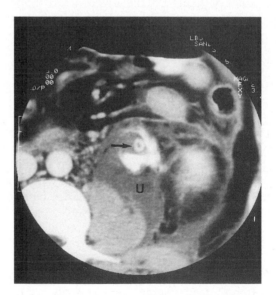

Figure 14.7.   Partial ureteropelvic junction avulsion in an adult. Enhanced computed tomography shows extravasation of contrast/urine adjacent to the psoas muscle with formation of a urinoma (*U*). There is contrast in the ureter surrounding a blood clot (*arrow*). This indicates that the continuity of the ureter remains partially intact.

occurred before consideration of renal-sparing surgery is even possible. In such circumstances, and in view of the absence of a significant incidence of late complications associated with renal infarction, many authorities now believe that attempts at revascularization should be limited to the uncommon patient with bilateral renal artery thrombosis. Therefore, in contrast to previous recommendations that patients found to have unilateral absence of excretion on urography or a cortical rim sign on CT undergo immediate angiography, most investigators now believe that angiography is only necessary in those patients who are being considered for surgery. Routine removal of infarcted kidneys also is deemed unnecessary; in addition, the chance for spontaneous recovery of renal function, albeit small, would be forfeited by such surgery.

Radiologic Examination

Diagnostic Approach to Renal Trauma

There is no single method of imaging evaluation that can be uniformly applied to all patients suspected of suffering urinary tract injury. The exact approach depends not only on the types of injuries the patient has likely suffered, but the philosophy of the attending physicians, local practice, and the type of equipment and support available. Moreover, evaluation of the renal injury can not be carried out isolated from the evaluation of other suspected intraabdominal injuries. A variety of different approaches to a given patient may therefore be acceptable.

As a rule, evaluation of the lower urinary tract should precede evaluation of the upper urinary tract, when both are indicated. In male patients, therefore, urethrography should precede cystography; these examinations should be performed before an evaluation of the kidney. If CT is to be performed for other reasons, CT cystography as described later in this chapter may be used to evaluate possible bladder rupture.

There is great diversity of opinion regarding the value of CT of the abdomen as a screening study for suspected intraabdominal injury. Many trauma surgeons still regard diagnostic peritoneal lavage (DPL) as the method of choice for the detection of intraperitoneal hemorrhage. Diagnostic peritoneal lavage is sensitive, easy to perform, and universally available; however, it does not differentiate inconsequential bleeding from that which requires laparotomy and more importantly, it cannot detect the site of the bleeding. Furthermore, DPL does not detect retroperitoneal injuries and generally is not performed in children (because of the risk of injury to the bladder), those who have had previous laparotomy (because intraabdominal adhesions may cause false-negative results), and in those with retroperitoneal hematomas as

a result of pelvic fractures (because of potential false-positive results).

Computed tomography is much more specific than DPL for both intraperitoneal and retroperitoneal injuries and most importantly can differentiate trivial injuries from those requiring exploration. Computed tomography is, however, not universally available on an immediate basis, is expensive, and is reported to be less sensitive than DPL for the detection of injuries to the bowel or mesentery.

Urography, which has traditionally been used as a screening study for renal injury, is less sensitive and less specific than CT; however, studies have consistently shown that urography yields sufficient information to guide urologic management in the vast majority of patients suffering blunt abdominal injury. Cass and associates found no patients with a renal injury greater than renal contusion among blunt trauma patients with normal urograms. Nicolaisen and colleagues reported similar findings in 214 patients in whom urograms were performed. Bergren and coworkers reported no cases of renal pathology greater than contusion when the results of urography were reported as normal. The preference for the use of urography as a screening study for renal injuries is predicated on the fact that urography is readily available, inexpensive, requires no special equipment and, when normal, except after penetrating injury, obviates the need for further evaluation. Furthermore, clinical signs of renal injury are relatively nonspecific and a large number of patients with hematuria must be screened to demonstrate those with significant renal injuries.

In patients who are hemodynamically unstable, little time is available to study the status of the urinary tract. A single view of the abdomen after a large dose of intravenously administered contrast medium ("one-shot IVP") is generally all that can be obtained; such a study is insufficient to diagnose most renal injuries, but can be used to give information about the gross functional status of the kidney(s). Similarly, most patients suffering from an anterior gunshot wound of the abdomen will require surgical exploration; the goal of imaging in such cases is to establish the presence of gross bilateral renal function. The renal injury will be assessed intraoperatively. Recently, the value of these limited "one-shot" studies in unstable patients has been questioned; a retrospective review of 239 such studies showed that the urographic assessment of contralateral renal function played no role in the management of the renal injury. The authors of this study felt that delaying definitive therapy merely to obtain the urographic study was not justified.

Assessment of the nature and extent of the renal injury is therefore most important in those patients in whom there will be an attempt to avoid exploratory surgery. In hemodynamically stable patients being assessed for wide-impact blunt injury in a major trauma center where CT is available immediately, this goal can be met most efficaciously by abdominal and pelvic CT. In smaller institutions, where there would be a significant delay in obtaining a CT examination, it is perfectly acceptable to use DPL to assess the intraperitoneal viscera and high-dose urography, preferably with tomography, to assess the kidneys.

In patients who have suffered penetrating injury, urography is not sufficiently sensitive to reliably exclude significant injury; therefore, CT should be performed as a first line study. Wilson and Ziegler found renal injuries that required surgery in one third of such patients whose urograms were thought to be normal. In Bergren's series, an alarming 75% of patients (9 of 12) whose urograms were thought to be normal had what the authors called "serious renal pathology" after penetrating injury. However, many of the urograms in this series were performed with a low dose of contrast medium or were limited to a single radiograph. Some urologists will argue that CT is unnecessary, because they believe that all such patients should have renal exploratory surgery. In such cases, the goal of imaging is similar to that in unstable patients (i.e., to exclude an abnormality of the contralateral kidney). In patients with limited posterior stab wounds, however, CT is the method of choice for assessment because exploratory surgery is not mandatory.

The patient with suspected isolated blunt renal injury is perhaps the most controversial. Most such patients do not have evidence of multisystem trauma, but are suspected of renal injury only because of hematuria. Studies have demonstrated that the incidence of significant renal injury in this group of patients is low; therefore, many authorities believe that if imaging is indicated, urography is the study of choice, since a significant injury is unlikely to be overlooked. In all patients in whom urography suggests an abnormality, CT should be performed for further assessment unless hemodynamic instability necessitates immediate surgery.

Excretory Urography

Urography for suspected renal injury should be performed by a thorough but quick routine designed to yield a maximum amount of information. In general, it should be performed with a higher dose of contrast medium than might be used for an elective study to compensate for the large volume of fluid such patients generally receive. A contrast dose of 1 ml/lb generally yields a satisfactory study. Tomography is a valuable adjunct in such patients and should be used whenever feasible. Needless to say, an adequate scout radiograph is absolutely mandatory.

Most commonly, the results of urography are normal in patients suffering from minor renal injuries. In more severe injuries, urographic abnormalities include delayed opacification, incomplete visualization of the renal outlines, displacement of the kidney, poor or incomplete calyceal filling (Fig. 14.1), a diminished nephrogram that might be segmental, as well as nonvisualization of the affected kidney. These findings, however, are generally nonspecific and additional studies often are required to define the specific renal injury that is present.

Some specific urographic findings may be present. A filling defect in the collecting system, in the setting of trauma, usually indicates a blood clot. In some instances, a cleft in the renal parenchyma may be visualized, indicating that there is a renal laceration. Extravasation of contrast medium (Fig. 14.3), indicates a laceration that extends into the renal collecting system, but also may be present with avulsion of the UPJ.

In rare instances, extravasation of contrast medium may be present in less significant injuries. Pyelosinus extravasation may be present from minor injuries or may be demonstrated in patients with preexisting renal calculi. In addition, patients with congenital renal anomalies, such as horseshoe kidney or UPJ obstruction, may demonstrate pyelosinus extravasation when undergoing evaluation for suspected renal trauma. In such instances, CT will demonstrate the extravasation, but will not demonstrate a renal laceration. In most cases of benign extravasation after trauma, urography demonstrates some degree of caliectasis, which suggests the presence of the preexisting condition.

The unilateral absence of excretion on urography (Fig. 14.8) suggests that a renal vascular injury is present. Stables studied 23 patients (20 after blunt trauma) who exhibited unilateral excretion on urography after abdominal injury and found that, in 17 cases, the cause for this finding was traumatic occlusion of the main renal artery. Renal agenesis was found to be responsible in only three patients. Stables concluded that, when such a finding is encountered in a patient who has suffered abdominal injury, a renal artery injury is the most likely etiology. Cass and Luxenberg reported a series of 53 patients (47 after blunt trauma) in whom similar findings were present on urography. In their series, traumatic occlusion of the renal artery was present in 16 patients; the final diagnosis in the remaining patients were parenchymal laceration (12), renal rupture (12), renal contusion (8), branch arterial injury (1), and renal vein laceration (4).

Computed Tomography

Computed tomography for the detection of renal injuries should be performed with 10-mm incrementation and 10-mm collimation or with continuous acquisition technique. A short scan time to minimize respiratory

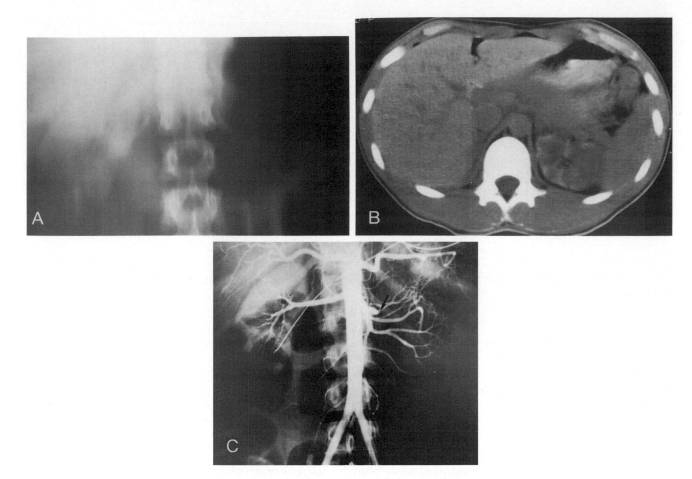

Figure 14.8.   Traumatic occlusion of the renal artery. **A,** IVP demonstrates no visible excretion from the left kidney. **B,** Computed tomography shows only a rim of enhancement of the outer cortex of the left kidney secondary to intact left re- nal capsular vessels. The majority of the renal parenchyma shows no contrast enhancement. **C,** Abdominal aortogram shows the characteristically tapered appearance of traumatic main renal artery occlusion (*arrow*).

motion is desirable. In general, precontrast scans yield too little additional information to be of routine value. If contrast medium has been administered more than 1 hour before the start of the study (i.e., for a preceding urogram), an additional bolus of contrast material should be used. Lang and colleagues have advocated the routine use of dynamic CT to enhance the detection of vascular injuries. With this technique, six to ten CT sections are acquired in rapid sequence after the ad- ministration of a bolus of contrast medium. If a contin- uous acquisition or ultrafast technique is used, a series of delayed scans to visualize the collecting system is necessary unless urography has preceded the CT study.

The accuracy of CT staging of renal injuries has been compared with other imaging studies in several retro- spective series. Cass and Vieira report that CT provided diagnoses in 22 cases of suspected severe renal injuries, while urographic findings were indeterminate in 82% of the cases. Bretan and colleagues studied 85 patients with renal injuries using CT and a variety of other imag- ing techniques. Blunt trauma accounted for 87% of their

cases, while the remainder were secondary to penetrat- ing injury. In 33 patients who subsequently underwent laparotomy, the CT diagnoses were confirmed. In con- trast, the most common finding on urography, dimin- ished opacification, was found to bear no relationship to the severity of the injury found at surgery. In the same series, angiography was found to have appreciably un- derstaged the severity of the injury in 1 of 5 patients in whom this procedure was employed. In addition, CT has a great impact on the management of renal injuries; Erturk and coworkers reported that early CT evaluation allowed confident nonoperative management in 17 of 22 patients with renal injuries. Federle and colleagues have reported equally favorable results using CT in pa- tients suffering penetrating renal injuries.

On contrast-enhanced CT, subcapsular hematomas appear as rounded or elliptical areas of decreased at- tenuation located between the renal cortex and the re- nal capsule (Fig. 14.9). Such hematomas indent the re- nal margins because of their subcapsular location. Intrarenal hematomas (Figs. 14.10 and 14.11) are seen as

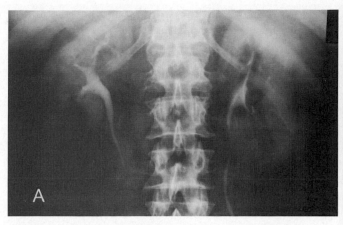

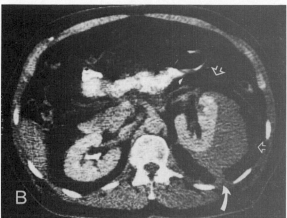

Figure 14.9. Subcapsular hematoma. **A,** IVP shows compression of the calyces of the left kidney and straightening of the lateral renal border. **B,** Computed tomography shows the renal margin to be indented by a large subcapsular hematoma. A small area of extension to the perinephric space is present (*curved arrow*). Gerota's fascia also can be identified (*open arrows*), confirming the subcapsular location of the hematoma.

rounded or ovoid poorly marginated areas of decreased attenuation within the renal parenchyma; in some cases, the small intrarenal lacerations with which they are associated may be visualized extending into the hematoma itself. Perinephric hematomas are located between the renal capsule and Gerota's fascia and are usually associated with an intrarenal hematoma (Fig. 14.12). Perinephric hematomas may be quite large and may extend inferiorly into the true pelvis following the cone of renal fascia, may displace the kidney anteriorly, or occasionally may be quite localized and simulate a subcapsular collection.

The attenuation coefficient of these hematomas depends on their age, with acute hematomas having a higher attenuation value than unenhanced renal parenchyma (Fig. 14.13). With time, their attenuation value decreases

owing to liquefaction of the clot. In addition, the measured attenuation value of these perinephric hematomas may be lower than expected, reflecting their tendency to infiltrate the normal perinephric fat. This tendency also may produce a streaked or bubbled appearance in the retroperitoneum that should not be confused with abscess.

Diagnosis of major lacerations (Fig. 14.14) can be made on CT when a hematoma-filled cleft that extends through the renal capsule is visualized in the renal parenchyma. If the laceration extends into the renal collecting system, extravasation of opacified urine into the perinephric space also will be present (Fig. 14.15). If the lacerated segment has become devitalized, this portion of the kidney will not enhance after contrast administration. Because this segment is surrounded by hematoma

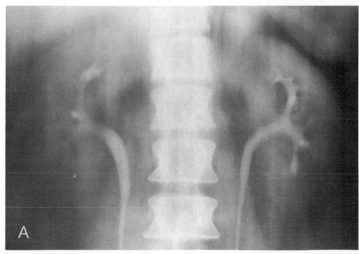

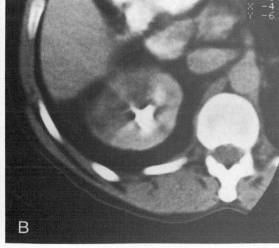

Figure 14.10. Intrarenal hematoma. **A,** IVP shows minimal indistinctness of the right renal outline. **B,** On computed tomography, a poorly marginated area of decreased attenuation in the anterolateral aspect of the right kidney is present.

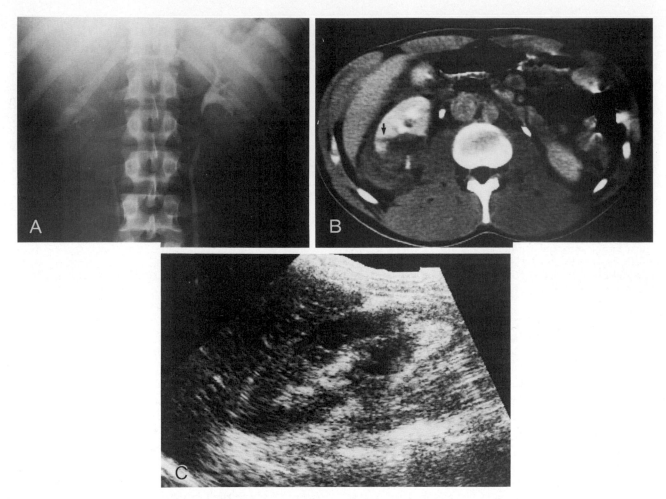

Figure 14.11. Intrarenal hematoma. **A,** IVP shows nonspecific findings including an indistinct right renal outline and poor calyceal filling. **B,** On computed tomography, a large area of decreased density is present in the inferior portion of the right kidney. A small laceration extending into the hematoma is visualized (*arrow*). A small perinephric hematoma is present as well. **C,** Longitudinal ultrasound shows decreased echogenicity in the area of the hematoma and slight anterior displacement of the lower pole of the right kidney.

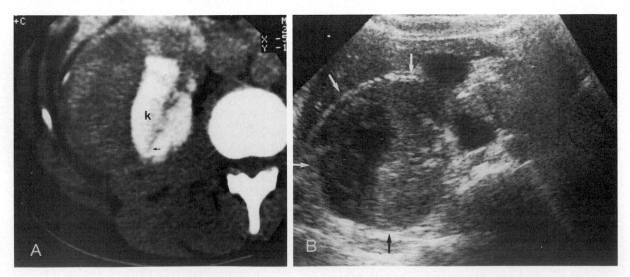

Figure 14.12. Perinephric hematoma. **A,** Computed tomography shows a large perinephric hematoma filling Gerota's fascia. The lateral margin of the right kidney (*k*) is compressed, thereby simulating a subcapsular collection. A small renal laceration also is present (*arrow*). **B,** Transverse sonogram also shows the large perinephric collection (*arrow*).

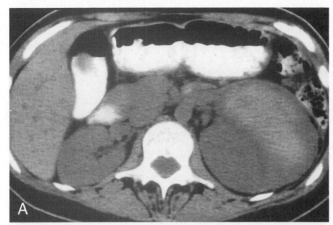

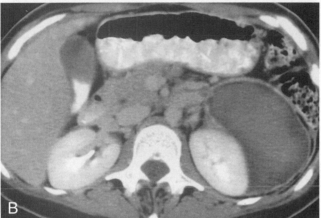

Figure 14.13. Large subcapsular hematoma. **A,** Precontrast scan shows high-density blood adjacent to left kidney, indicating acute hemorrhage. On the postcontrast study, **B,** a relatively thick rind is seen surrounding the hematoma.

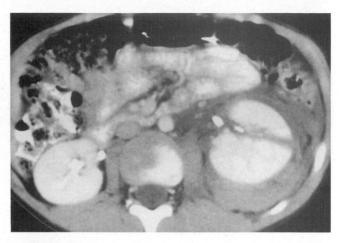

Figure 14.14. Renal laceration. A large renal laceration is present in the left kidney associated with a moderate perinephric hematoma.

and does not enhance, it may be difficult to appreciate as a separate fragment.

Segmental or cortical infarcts are the most common vascular injury after blunt trauma. On CT, infarcts appear as sharply demarcated wedge-shaped areas of diminished or absent contrast enhancement that extend to the renal cortex (Fig. 14.16). If the capsular blood supply remains intact, perfusion of the outer layer of cells results in enhancement of the cortical rim. Most commonly, segmental or cortical infarcts are not associated with a perinephric hematoma, thereby helping to distinguish them from intrarenal hematomas. The sensitivity of CT for the detection of such injuries can be enhanced with the use of dynamic scanning (Fig. 14.17). Indeed, the ability of CT to reliably distinguish these injuries from hematomas depends on the contrast enhancement provided by the bolus of contrast medium. If there has been too long an interval between the contrast administration and the CT study, their sharply marginated appearance will be lost because of collateral circulation.

Thrombosis of the main renal artery results in complete absence of contrast enhancement when studied shortly after injury. In some cases, and especially in those instances where the diagnosis of pedicle injury is delayed, a rim of enhancement in the outer renal cortex may be present owing to circulation from capsular and collateral vessels (Fig. 14.8). Similar findings are frequently present in patients with nontraumatic renal infarction. In the majority of patients with this injury, there will be no evidence of a perinephric or subcapsular hematoma, unless this injury has been caused by a penetrating wound or is associated with injury of another organ. Retrograde opacification of the renal vein of the affected kidney has been reported as a secondary sign of this injury, especially if an infusion technique for contrast enhancement is used.

Angiography

The use of angiography in the evaluation of renal injuries has significantly declined since the advent of CT. In patients in whom angiography is required for another purpose (i.e., the evaluation of a suspected injury of the thoracic aorta), it may be used as a primary imaging technique in the evaluation of suspected renal injuries.

Angiographic assessment of renal injuries may be carried out by a variety of techniques. Film aortography or intraarterial digital subtraction aortography is sufficient for diagnosis of injury of the main renal artery; however, for precise demonstration of intrarenal vascular injuries, selective renal angiography is required.

Angiography is the only method capable of identifying certain traumatic lesions such as arteriovenous fistulae and pseudoaneurysms, and provides definitive diagnosis of traumatic arterial thrombosis and infarcts. The extent of the collateral vascular supply to the injured parenchyma can be directly evaluated. In addition to di-

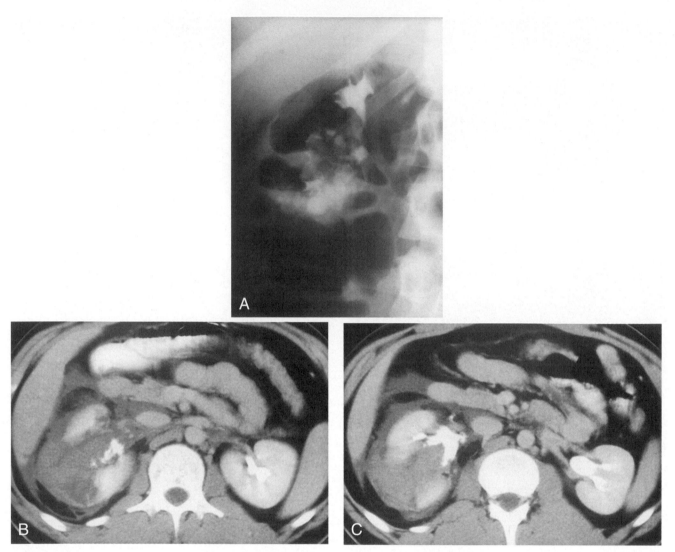

Figure 14.15. Renal laceration with extension into the collecting system. **A,** IVP shows contrast extravasation which obscures lower pole calyces, **B** and **C,** Postcontrast computed tomography shows a distracted renal laceration (fracture) that extends into the collecting system with contrast extravasation into the perinephric space.

agnosis, angiography provides a method by which traumatic renal hemorrhage can be directly diagnosed and treated through transcatheter embolization (Fig. 14.18).

The disadvantages and limitations of angiography must be recognized. The technique is invasive, time-consuming, and expensive, and carries far greater risk of complications than do the noninvasive techniques. Some injuries, particularly perinephric hematomas, either anterior or posterior to the kidney, may be grossly underestimated. Thus, angiographic evaluation of renal injuries is best suited to those situations in which vascular injury is suspected (i.e., a nonvisualized kidney on urography), the evaluation of suspected late complications of renal injury, and those patients in whom transcatheter therapy of renal injury may be necessary.

Angiographic findings in minor renal injuries include

a slowing of arterial flow and evidence of cortical ischemia; these changes produce a striated appearance to the angiographic nephrogram. Intrarenal hematomas demonstrate displacement of the interlobar arteries and a diminished vascular nephrogram. Perirenal hematomas show displacement of the capsular arteries and the pelvic branch vessels. With subcapsular hematomas, there is indentation of the renal margin similar to that seen on urography.

Major renal lacerations (Fig. 14.19) demonstrate a well-defined cleft in the nephrogram on angiographic examination. The degree of displacement of the lacerated segment and its viability can be assessed by an analysis of the nephrogram at the fracture margins. Multiple lacerations are a feature of renal rupture (*see* Fig. 14.5). Traumatic arteriovenous fistulae almost always result from

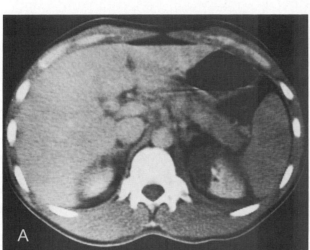
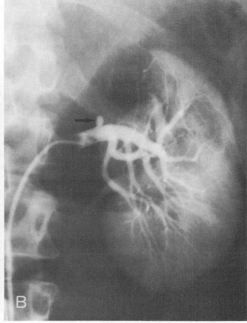

Figure 14.16. Segmental infarct. **A,** Computed tomography demonstrates a sharply marginated area of absent contrast enhancement in the left kidney. There is no associated perinephric hematoma. **B,** Selective left renal angiogram shows an amputated upper segmental artery (*arrow*). (From Sandler CM, Toombs BD: Computed tomographic evaluation of blunt renal injuries. *Radiology* 141:461, 1981.)

penetrating renal injury. The vast majority occur after percutaneous renal biopsy, are not hemodynamically significant, and close spontaneously. Clinically, symptomatic lesions may present with hypertension, evidence of left heart failure, and audible bruit on physical examination. On angiography, opacification of the large draining veins is visible during the arterial phase of the study. The draining vein is usually saccular in appearance; with hemodynamically significant lesions, there may be decreased nephrographic staining and evidence of renal ischemia.

Traumatic arterial pseudoaneurysms are rare injuries that also almost always occur after penetrating trauma. While the diagnosis may be suspected by CT, definitive diagnosis requires angiography.

Segmental renal infarcts are demonstrated as wedge-shaped areas of absent vascular perfusion. The occluded artery responsible for the infarct can usually be identified by its sharply cut-off appearance (Figs. 14.16 and 14.17). Collateral vascular supply through capsular branch vessels also may be identified angiographically.

Occlusion of the main renal artery usually occurs in its proximal one third and has one sharply defined oblique edge (Fig. 14.8**C**) at the point where the intimal injury has occurred. If the occlusion is not acute, collateral supply to the kidney may be visualized on aortography. In kidneys supplied by more than one renal artery, supply through the unaffected vessels may prevent total renal infarction from occurring.

Radionuclide Scanning

Radionuclide scanning of the kidneys after trauma has been used to detect suspected renal injury as an alternative to urography. Such studies may be performed with either technetium-99m diethylenetriaminepentaacetic acid (^{99m}Tc-DTPA), technetium-99m-mercap-

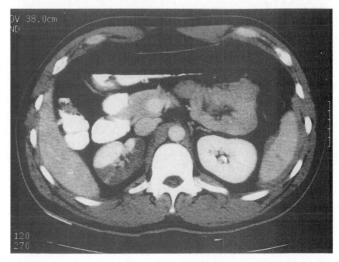

Figure 14.17. Large segmental infarct. Computed tomography shows a large area of absent contrast enhancement corresponding to the posterior segmental branch of the right renal artery. Also noted is a perisplenic hematoma from a small laceration (*not shown*).

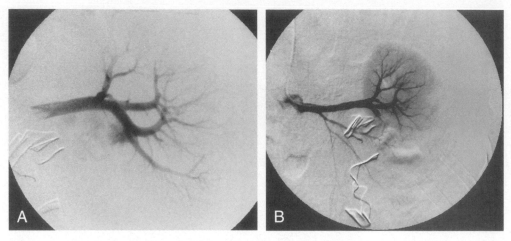

Figure 14.18. Traumatic renal hemorrhage. **A,** Arterial phase study shows frank bleeding from a laceration of a lower segmental artery (*arrow*); **B,** After embolization with Gelfoam (Upjohn, Kalamazoo, MI), the bleeding is controlled.

toacetyltriglycine (^{99m}Tc-MAG$_3$), or ^{99m}Tc-glucoheptonate. For the detection of renal injury, perfusion studies should be acquired by computer for the first 1 minute, followed by immediate static images and a series of delayed static images. Views acquired with a pinhole collimator give the highest spatial resolution and are helpful in detecting major renal lacerations.

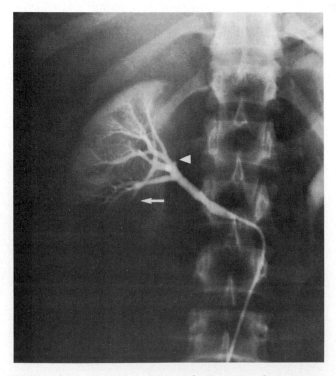

Figure 14.19. Selective right renal angiogram demonstrates a major laceration involving the midportion of the kidney. The lower pole is completely devitalized with traumatic occlusion of the lower pole segmental artery (*arrow*). A segmental infarct involving the upper pole (*arrowhead*) is also seen.

One advantage of radionuclide scanning is the ability to acquire images even in relatively uncooperative patients and children. Radionuclide studies also are of value in patients with known sensitivity to contrast media. Radionuclide scanning should not be used in patients with a nonvisualized kidney on urography, because this study cannot differentiate a congenitally absent kidney from renal artery thrombosis.

Analysis of the radionuclide perfusion curve in patients with renal injuries demonstrate a decrease in the kidney-peak-to-plateau ratio and a delay in the peak activity in the kidney when the renal curve is normalized to that of the aorta. Static imaging reveals diminished uptake and excretion of the radiopharmaceutical in the affected kidney.

Studies reported in the literature have suggested that radionuclide imaging has a higher sensitivity than does urography for the detection of renal injuries. As with urography, the specificity of an abnormal radionuclide study is low.

Renal lacerations may be visualized as photon-deficient areas in the renal parenchyma. A laceration that extends into the collecting system may demonstrate an area of tracer activity outside the kidney, indicating extravasation of urine. Renal infarcts may be diagnosed as photon-deficient areas in the renal parenchyma, but differentiation of this injury from intrarenal hematomas is difficult. Large perinephric hematomas may be visualized as photopenic defects adjacent to the kidney. Urinomas also are present as photopenic areas; however, on delayed images, such areas accumulate activity indicating their uriniferous nature.

Occlusion of the renal artery is suggested by the absence of perfusion to one kidney. In such cases, a photopenic defect may be present in the renal fossa. Large perinephric hematomas that displace the kidney anteriorly may simulate this finding; in this instance, an anterior image of the abdomen usually demonstrates the displaced kidney.

URETERAL INJURIES

Ureteral Injuries Secondary to External Violence

Aside from UPJ avulsion, traumatic injuries of the ureter virtually always occur secondary to penetrating trauma. As such, nearly all ureteral injuries are associated with injuries of other organs including the small bowel, liver, spleen, or a major blood vessel. Ureteral injuries include partial or complete laceration and ureteral contusion, an injury of the ureter that produces ureteral wall damage, but not a frank laceration. Ureteral contusion is generally considered to result from the blast effect of the missile on the ureter (Fig. 14.20). A significant percentage of patients with ureteral injuries do not have hematuria.

The diagnosis of ureteral injury may be established by urography when extravasation of contrast medium is present. The accuracy of urography in establishing this diagnosis is uncertain, because most of the published series are small, and because of the nature of the associated injuries, many of the patients are taken to surgery before urography. Steers and associates report that the urogram was diagnostic in 7 of 8 patients with penetrating ureteral injury in whom this study was performed. In cases when radiologic studies are not performed before surgical exploration, the diagnosis may be established with the aid of intraoperative vital dyes that usually demonstrate the point of injury.

Iatrogenic Ureteral Injury

Surgical injury of the ureter may result from a variety of abdominal, pelvic, urologic, and gynecologic procedures. The risk of surgical injury varies with the type of operation, with the highest risk occurring as a consequence of gynecologic procedures. More than 25% of the ureteral injuries that occur from gynecologic procedures occur during laparoscopy. With radical hysterectomy, ureteral injury may occur in as many as 10 to 30% of patients. The reported incidence of ureteral injury as a complication of abdominal hysterectomy varies between 1.5 and 2.5%, and it may occur even less commonly during other pelvic operations, including vaginal hysterectomy and cesarean section.

Ureteral injury generally occurs when there is inadvertent ligation of the ureter. With radical hysterectomy, injury also may occur when the blood supply of the distal ureters is stripped during dissection of periureteral lymphatics. Patients with this complication have ureteral necrosis and the formation of a urinoma, or the later development of a long ureteral stricture.

Ureteral injury may complicate a number of urologic procedures including ureteroscopy, ureteral stone basketing (Fig. 14.21), retrograde pyelography, and ureterolithotomy. Ureteroscopy is the highest risk procedure, accounting for approximately 70% of urologic injuries. In most of these cases, the injury is a result of ureteral perforation. Ligation of the ureter also may occur during vesicourethral suspension.

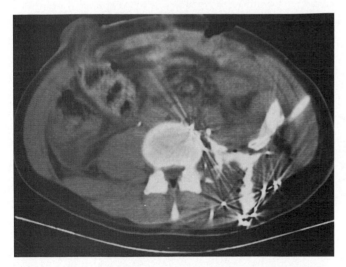

Figure 14.20. Ureteral contusion with subsequent necrosis. Computed tomography demonstrates frank contrast medium extravasation from the left ureter in a patient who suffered a shotgun wound of the left flank. No laceration had been identified at the time of exploratory surgery. However, after several days urine was noted emanating from a surgically placed Penrose drain, prompting computed tomography investigation.

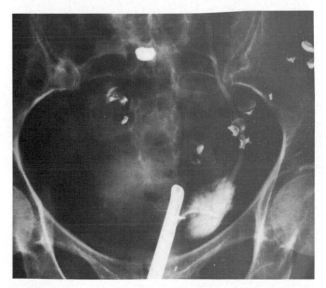

Figure 14.21. Retrograde pyelogram showing extravasation of contrast medium after a traumatic ureteral stone basketing procedure.

Injury of the ureter may complicate other surgical procedures including abdominoperineal resection, enterolysis, resection of abdominal aortic aneurysm, and lumbar laminectomy. In such cases, the injuries consist of ureteral perforation, transection, ligation, or a crush injury associated with inadvertent clamping of the ureter.

Bilateral ureteral injuries are generally recognized in the immediate postoperative period because of anuria. Unilateral injury may be recognized at the time of the original surgery, but more commonly it is not recognized until 10 to 30 days after surgery. Fever and ipsilateral flank pain are the most common symptoms. A significant number of cases go unrecognized until the development of a ureterovaginal (Fig. 14.22) or ureterocutaneous fistula. Dowling and colleagues reported this presentation in 9 of 23 patients (39%) in whom there was delayed recognition of the ureteral injury. In all cases, the diagnosis of ureteral injury was established by urography.

Interventional uroradiologic procedures play an important role in the management of iatrogenic ureteral injury. Harshman and associates reported three patients with ureteral injury after gynecologic surgery who were successfully treated with percutaneous nephrostomy drainage alone. They postulated that the ureteral injury in these patients was secondary to suture ligation or entrapment of the ureter and that with time, there was resorption of the suture material allowing resolution of the

ureteral obstruction. In Dowling's series, 11 of 15 ureteral injuries, including 6 of 7 cases that were believed to have resulted from ureteral ligation, were successfully treated with percutaneous nephrostomy alone or with nephrostomy combined with antegrade ureteral stenting. Lang reported successful management of 15 ureteral fistulas with a combination of nephrostomy and stent placement for periods ranging between 30 and 45 days.

BLADDER INJURIES

Injury of the bladder may occur as a result of blunt, penetrating, or iatrogenic trauma. The susceptibility of the bladder to injury varies with its degree of filling at the time of the accident; a collapsed or nearly empty bladder is much less vulnerable to injury than is a distended organ.

Clinical Features

Signs of bladder injury are relatively nonspecific. Suprapubic tenderness is usually present; however, the etiology of this discomfort may be manifold. Hematuria inevitably accompanies bladder rupture; in some of the reported series, gross hematuria was present in 95% of cases. The urge to void may be absent or normal; in some forms of bladder rupture, the organ may still act as a reservoir and thus a normal urge to void may be present.

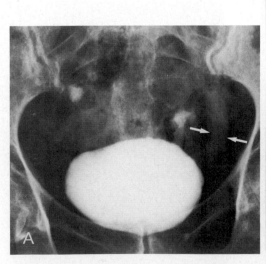
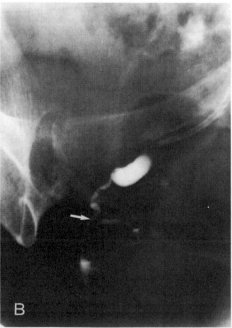

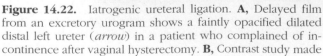

Figure 14.22. Iatrogenic ureteral ligation. **A,** Delayed film from an excretory urogram shows a faintly opacified dilated distal left ureter (*arrow*) in a patient who complained of incontinence after vaginal hysterectomy. **B,** Contrast study made after advancing an end-hole nephrostomy catheter down the ureter demonstrates complete occlusion of the distal ureter and ureterovaginal fistula.

Radiologic Examination

Cystography is the examination of choice for the diagnosis of bladder rupture. Although it is preferably performed with fluoroscopic guidance, it may be performed with fixed radiographic or even portable equipment when the clinical situation demands it. The method by which cystography is performed has been discussed in Chapter 3; however, some modification of the procedure may be necessary in the trauma patient. A minimum of 300 ml of diluted (30%) contrast medium must be used to achieve adequate bladder distention. The use of 14 × 17-inch films that cover the upper abdomen facilitates the diagnosis of intraperitoneal bladder rupture, and therefore should be used for at least one of the radiographs. When fluoroscopic equipment is not used, an initial radiograph after instillation of approximately 100 ml of contrast medium can be used to check for gross extravasation; if none is present, the remainder of the contrast medium is then infused. The postdrainage radiograph is an essential component of the cystogram made for trauma as the diagnosis of bladder rupture may be established only by this film in approximately 10% of cases (Fig. 14.23).

The accuracy of cystography for the diagnosis of bladder injury varies from 85 to 100% in the reported series. Carroll and McAninch report, however, that the accuracy of cystography would have decreased from 100 to 79% in their series had careful technique not been followed. A false-negative cystogram may occur in patients who have suffered penetrating bladder injury, especially when caused by small-caliber bullets. In such cases, it is assumed that the bladder tear seals with hematoma or by the surrounding mesentery, and thus results in a false-negative study.

While cystography is highly accurate in the diagnosis of bladder injury, the cystographic phase of the excretory urogram cannot be relied on to exclude bladder injury (Fig. 14.24). In the series reported by Carroll and McAninch (1983), cystographically verified bladder injuries were found in only 16% of the cases by urography.

Computed tomographic cystography (Fig. 14.25) may be used in place of conventional cystography, particularly in patients undergoing CT for another reason. To perform CT cystography, the bladder is filled in a retrograde fashion with diluted contrast medium and 10-mm of contiguous sections through the pelvis are obtained. Computed tomographic cystography performed in this fashion has an accuracy comparable with conventional cystography. Assessment of the bladder using CT performed with contrast filling only from excreted contrast medium has been shown to be inaccurate in excluding bladder injury. In a prospective study, Mee and colleagues found conventional cystography superior to contrast-enhanced CT for the diagnosis of bladder rupture, when only excreted contrast material was used for the CT study.

Bladder Injury in Blunt Pelvic Trauma

Major bladder injury occurs in approximately 10% of patients suffering a pelvic fracture. Injury of the bladder following blunt trauma may be classified as follows:

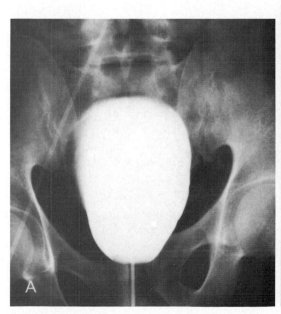
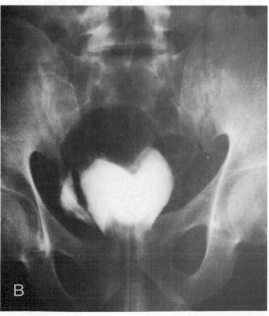

Figure 14.23. A, Filled film from a cystogram demonstrates extrinsic compression of the right side of the bladder, but no evidence of extravasation. Catheter in right femoral artery is from an arteriogram performed immediately before the cystogram. **B,** Postdrainage film shows simple extraperitoneal rupture (type 4a).

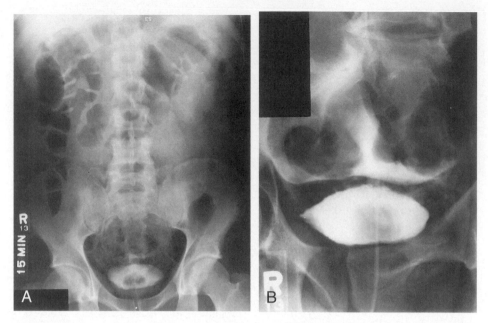

Figure 14.24. **A,** Cystographic phase from an IVP shows a Foley catheter in the bladder, but no evidence of extravasation. **B,** Cystogram performed a few minutes later shows intraperitoneal rupture.

Type 1—Bladder contusion;
Type 2—Intraperitoneal rupture;
Type 3—Interstitial bladder injury;
Type 4—Extraperitoneal rupture
   a. Simple
   b. Complex;
Type 5—Combined bladder injury.

Bladder contusion (type 1) is an incomplete tear of the bladder mucosa after blunt injury that results in an ecchymosis in a localized segment of the bladder wall. Cystography is normal; the diagnosis is usually estab-

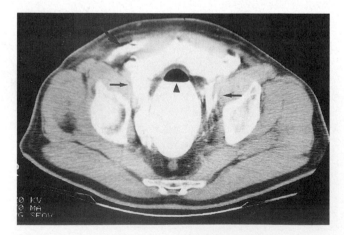

Figure 14.25. Computed tomographic cystogram. Axial section through the bladder shows extraperitoneal bladder rupture (*arrows*). Note small amount of air in bladder from Foley catheter placement (*arrowhead*).

lished by exclusion in patients who have hematuria after pelvic trauma for which no other cause can be found. Cystoscopy is rarely performed for confirmation. Bladder contusion may be present in patients in whom extrinsic compression of the bladder by a pelvic hematoma or hematomas is found.

Bladder contusion is generally regarded as the most common form of bladder trauma; however, it is not a major injury.

Intraperitoneal bladder rupture (type 2) accounts for approximately one third of major bladder injuries. It occurs when there is a sudden increase in intravesical pressure as a result of a blow to the lower abdomen in patients who have a distended bladder. This injury results in rupture of the weakest portion of the bladder wall, the dome, where the bladder is in contact with the peritoneal surface. Intraperitoneal rupture commonly occurs as a seatbelt or steering wheel injury. Approximately 25% of the cases occur in patients without a pelvic fracture. On cystography, contrast medium is seen in the paracolic gutters and outlining the abdominal viscera and loops of the small bowel (Fig. 14.26).

Interstitial bladder injury (type 3) occurs as a result of an incomplete perforation of the serosal surface of the bladder. On cystography, a mural defect in the bladder wall representing the site of injury is present, however, there is no extravasation of contrast medium. This injury is rare, but should be considered a major injury.

Extraperitoneal bladder rupture (type 4) is associated with one or more fractures of the pubic rami or diastasis

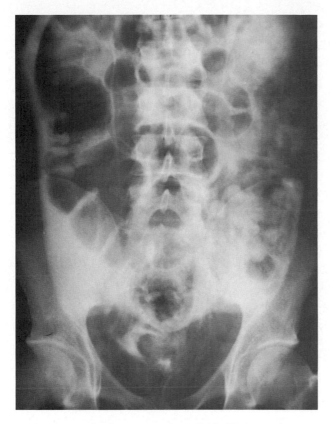

Figure 14.26. Intraperitoneal bladder rupture.

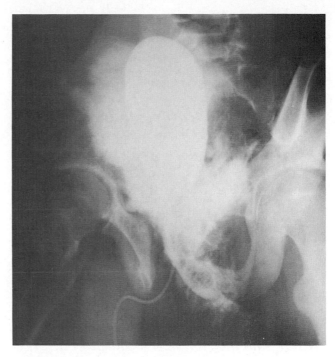

Figure 14.27. Complex extraperitoneal bladder rupture (type 4b). Extravasated contrast medium extends outside the confines of the pelvis into the perineum.

of the symphysis pubis in virtually every case. Classically, the injury occurs when there is a laceration of the extraperitoneal portion of the bladder wall by a bone spicule associated with the fracture. However, recent data have shown that cystograms in such patients often show the site of extravasation to be far removed from the site of pelvic fracture, suggesting that this injury can be caused by other mechanisms. One such explanation is that bladder injury results when stress is applied to the hypogastric wings or to the puboprostatic ligaments, causing the bladder wall to tear. In still other cases, the injury may occur by a mechanism analogous to the intraperitoneal rupture.

In simple extraperitoneal rupture, contrast medium extravasation is limited to the pelvic extraperitoneal space (Fig. 14.23**B**). With complex extraperitoneal rupture, the contrast extravasation extends beyond the perivesical space to the thigh, the scrotum, the penis, or the perineum (Fig. 14.27). Complex extravasation implies that a disruption in the fascial boundaries of the pelvis has occurred as a result of the injury. Thus, extravasation into the perineum may be present with a bladder injury alone; the presence of such extravasation should not be mistaken as evidence of a coexisting urethral injury.

Combined bladder injury (type 5) results in both intraperitoneal and extraperitoneal bladder rupture (Fig. 14.28). In a series by Palmer and associates, this injury

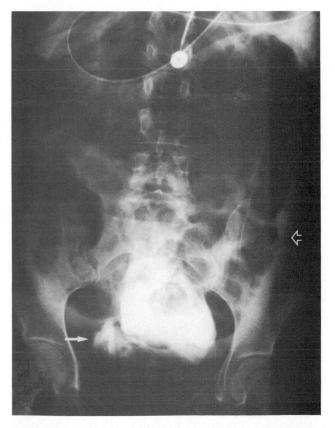

Figure 14.28. Combined bladder injury. The extraperitoneal component (*arrow*) and the intraperitoneal component (*open arrows*) are both demonstrated.

occurred in approximately 0.5% of patients with pelvic fracture and represents approximately 5% of all major bladder injuries. On cystography, both types of extravasation may be demonstrated, however, in some cases only one component is shown.

External Penetrating Bladder Injury

Penetrating injury of the bladder may occur as a result of a bullet wound or as a result of impalement of the bladder by various objects. Penetrating bladder injury may result in intraperitoneal rupture, extraperitoneal rupture, or combined bladder injury.

The diagnosis is usually suggested by cystography and is confirmed at exploration. As in renal injuries, the high association of injury to other viscera mandates surgical exploration in the majority of cases. Vascular injuries are commonly associated with bladder injuries following gunshot wounds; with knife wounds of the bladder, there is a high incidence of associated colon injury.

Iatrogenic and Obstetric Bladder Injury

Injury of the bladder may occur in virtually any type of obstetric, gynecologic, urologic, or pelvic surgery, or as the result of migration of surgically placed devices.

Obstetric bladder injury may result from laceration of the bladder during cesarean birth, injury secondary to trauma from obstetric forceps, or from pressure necrosis of the bladder wall during labor. Vesicouterine fistula is a rare, delayed complication of cesarean section. Such patients may present with menouria (Youseff's syndrome).

Injury to the bladder has been reported during dilatation and curettage of the uterus, laparoscopy, or hysterectomy. Transurethral urologic procedures, especially transurethral biopsy of bladder tumors, occasionally result in bladder injury. Surgically placed instruments that may damage the bladder include intrauterine contraceptive devices, Foley catheters, orthopedic hip nails, Penrose drains, and ventriculoperitoneal shunt catheters.

Spontaneous Bladder Injury

Spontaneous bladder rupture refers to the occurrence of a bladder injury without known antecedent trauma. In most cases, an underlying pathologic condition of the bladder is thought to be responsible. Such conditions include bladder tumors, inflammatory conditions of the bladder, lesions that infiltrate the bladder from outside its walls, and lesions resulting in bladder outlet obstruction.

The term idiopathic bladder rupture is used to refer to the occurrence of bladder rupture when there is no known antecedent trauma and no underlying or adjacent bladder pathology. Most of these cases occur in alcoholics, and it is postulated that the bladder injury results from relatively minor external trauma that the patient is unable to recall.

Table 14.2.
Classification of Injuries of the Male Urethra

Urethral injury in pelvic fracture
   type I
   type II
   type III
Straddle injury
Penetrating injury
Iatrogenic injury

INJURY OF THE MALE URETHRA

Injuries of the male urethra are classified according to their mechanism of injury (Table 14.2).

Urethral Injury in Pelvic Fracture

Clinical Features

Urethral injury in pelvic fracture is a devastating injury because it may be associated with major complications including bulbomembranous urethral stricture, impotence, and urinary incontinence. There is a general correlation between the degree of severity of the urethral injury and the severity of the pelvic ring disruption. However, severe urethral injury may occur with relatively minor pelvic fracture, and urethral rupture has rarely been reported without pelvic fracture. Conversely, severe pelvic fracture may result in relatively minor urethral injury. Patients with urethral injury in pelvic fracture commonly have multisystem injuries. Mortality rates of 9 to 33% are reported in these patients. The reported incidence of urethral injury in pelvic fracture is 4 to 17%. The average age is approximately 30 years, but ranges from 4 to 80 years.

The single most important clinical sign of urethral injury is blood at the external meatus. There may be a high-riding prostate on rectal examination, but in young male patients, it is often difficult to distinguish the prostate from a firm hematoma. The "pie in the sky" (Fig. 14.29) or inverted teardrop bladder on excretory urography is an indication of urethral rupture. Blind urethral catheterization is condemned in suspected urethral injury, although the inability to pass a urethral catheter is considered evidence of urethral rupture. No attempt should be made to pass a catheter until the urethral injury is assessed by dynamic retrograde urethrography.

Mechanism of Injury and Classification

The urogenital diaphragm is attached to the medial surface of the inferior pubic rami. The prostate is attached to the pubis by the puboprostatic ligaments. Pubic ramus fracture with separation or displacement of the symphysis pubis may result in disruption of the urogenital diaphragm and puboprostatic ligaments, causing proximal displacement of the prostate gland.

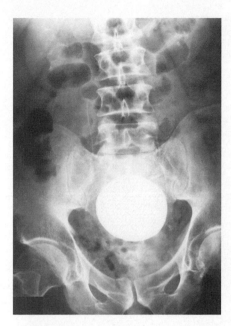

Figure 14.29. "Pie in the sky" bladder.

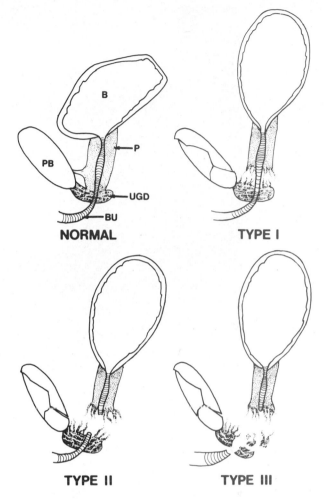

Figure 14.30. Radiologic classification of urethral injury in pelvic fractures. The diagrams describe the types of injury. Type III is the most common.

The classically described urethral injury is separation of the urethra at the junction of the prostatic and membranous urethra produced by a shearing effect at the time of injury. Less severe injury may result in a partial urethral injury, producing a laceration in the urethra at this site. Although membranous urethral tear is still described in the literature as the classic injury, retrograde urethrography has shown that the injury most commonly extends into the proximal bulbous urethra, below the urogenital diaphragm. This is consistent with the anatomy of the region. The apex of the prostate intermingles with fibers of the external sphincter at the urogenital diaphragm, but it is not firmly fixed. When trauma occurs, the prostate readily separates and moves superiorly, taking with it the prostatic and membranous urethras. The membranous urethra has the support of the urogenital diaphragm. The proximal bulbous urethra has no significant support—only fat and loose connective tissue.

In patients with suspected urethral injury, dynamic retrograde urethrography using the Foley catheter method (*see* Chapter 3) is performed. The film is exposed during injection of 10 to 20 ml of contrast medium.

The Colapinto and McCallum radiologic classification of urethral injury is as follows (Fig. 14.30):

- Type I. The urethra remains intact, but may be stretched and narrowed by proximal displacement of the prostate and the accumulation of hematoma elevating the bladder high in the pelvis. The urethra is compressed and may be contused (Fig. 14.31).
- Type II. The urethra is ruptured at the prostatomembranous junction above the urogenital diaphragm. Retrograde injection of contrast medium shows ex-

travasation of contrast medium into the true pelvis above the urogenital diaphragm. No contrast medium extravasates into the perineum (Fig. 14.32).
- Type III. The prostate is dislocated proximally. The urogenital diaphragm is disrupted and the proximal displacement of the prostatomembranous urethra pulls the bulbous urethra proximally. The tear in the urethra occurs below the urogenital diaphragm. Retrograde injection of contrast medium shows extravasation into the perineum and often into the scrotum (Fig. 14.33).

Both the type II and type III urethral injuries may be partial or complete. In partial type II injury, the tear in the urethra is above the urogenital diaphragm. Extravasation occurs into the true pelvis, however, some contrast medium will usually pass into the bladder. In partial type III urethral injury, the tear in the urethra is below the urogenital diaphragm and extravasation is into the perineum, with some contrast medium passing into the bladder. Par-

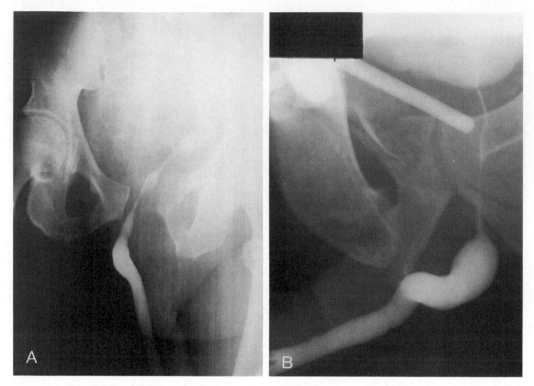

Figure 14.31.   Type I urethral injury. **A,** Dynamic retrograde urethrogram in a patient with pelvic fracture. The study shows an "inverted teardrop" bladder, large pelvic hematoma, intact but stretched urethra, and displacement of the prostate into the pelvis. **B,** Dynamic retrograde urethrogram in a patient with pelvic fracture. The urethra is narrowed and stretched but intact. (**A,** from McCallum RW, Colapinto V: *Urological Radiology of the Adult Male Urinary Tract.* Springfield, IL, Charles C Thomas, 1976.)

tial rupture is reported in 27 to 52% of the cases. Partial ruptures are thought to result in shorter, more readily repaired strictures than do complete ruptures.

Clinical Management

Two schools of thought regarding urethral injuries have existed for many years. Primary repair of the urethral injury involves surgical intervention as soon as possible after the injury. Although this method had fallen out of favor, several recent publications now advocate this approach when the urethral fragments are in relatively close proximity and realignment can be accomplished over a catheter with comparatively small amounts of tissue dissection.

Delayed repair involves only the insertion of a suprapubic catheter for drainage. Because there is no initial at-

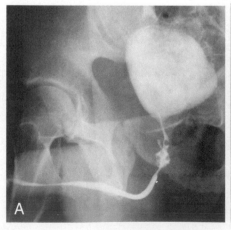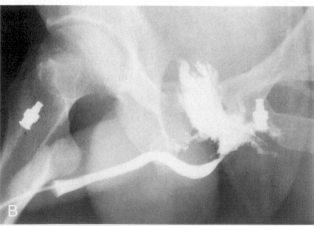

Figure 14.32.   Type II urethral injury. **A,** Partial; contrast medium extravasation is present from the membranous urethra above the urogenital diaphgram. Some contrast medium, however, flows into the bladder indicating a portion of the urethra remains intact. **B,** Complete.

mizes the risk of these complications, since no acute soft tissue dissection is performed. Proponents of immediate repair contend that when a technique that minimizes damage to the neurovascular bundle and the internal urethral sphincter are used, even lower morbidity than is reported with delayed repair are possible.

The initial urethrogram indicates the site of injury and commonly reveals whether the injury is partial or complete. However, a partial injury may appear to be complete if no contrast medium enters the bladder. This appearance in partial rupture is likely due to the presence of a blood clot blocking the urethra. If delayed repair is the chosen method, a urethrogram repeated 7 to 10 days later usually demonstrates that the urethral tear is partial. A second or third urethrogram is necessary in delayed repair immediately before the urethroplasty is performed. In this study, the bladder is filled through the suprapubic cystostomy tube and a retrograde urethrogram is performed at the same time as a voiding study (Fig. 14.34). This examination outlines the full extent of the stricture, provided the patient is able to open the bladder neck. Rarely the bladder neck does not open because the bladder capacity is small, and the bladder neck has not opened for 3 months due to the suprapu-

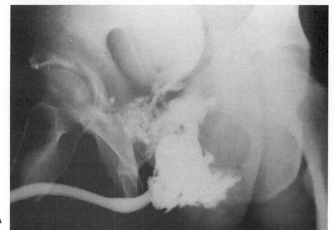
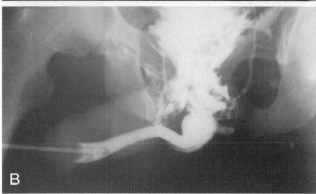

Figure 14.33.   Type III urethral injury. **A,** Partial; contrast medium has extravasated from the urethra into the perineum, but some contrast medium has entered the bladder indicating the urethral injury is partial. **B,** Complete; no contrast medium enters the bladder.

tempt at repair, a urethral stricture occurs in 100% of cases treated by this method. The suprapubic catheter is left in place for approximately 3 months, after which the urethra is repaired by a one- or two-stage urethroplasty. This method of repair is preferable when there is a large amount of soft tissue injury, the urethral fragments are distracted, or extensive associated injuries militate against an immediate approach to the urethral injury. Delayed repair should probably be used whenever the patient is treated in a center where relatively few urethral injuries are seen.

The controversy regarding the best method of treatment of such injuries is related to the high rates of impotence, incontinence, and recurrent stricture disease that are associated with such injuries. The incidence of incontinence has been reported to be as high as 25% and impotence as high as 40% in patients undergoing immediate repair. The high morbidity has been related to the method of repair, because comparable groups undergoing delayed repair have been reported with only 12% incontinence and 2% impotence. The proponents of delayed repair have argued that this method mini-

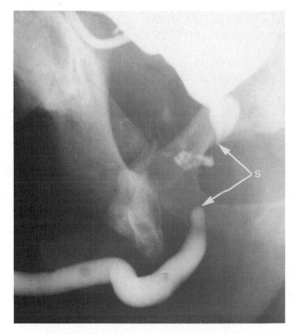

Figure 14.34.   Simultaneous retrograde and voiding urethrogram 3 months after pelvic fracture. A suprapubic catheter was inserted into the bladder at the time of urethral injury. The bladder is filled through the suprapubic cystostomy and the patient attempts to void at the same time as a dynamic retrograde injection is performed. The bladder neck is open, and the proximal prostatic urethra is filled. A small amount of extravasation has occurred. The retrograde injection defines the distal end of the stricture. Between the distal end of the visualized prostatic urethra and the proximal visualized bulbous urethra is hard fibrous scarring (*S*). This is repaired from below by transperineal urethroplasty.

bic drainage. In this instance, the suprapubic catheter should be clamped for 6 to 8 hours before attempting a second voiding study. The combined retrograde and voiding study delineate the length of the stricture. Type III urethral injuries treated by delayed repair have a stricture several centimeters long and extend from the site of the bulbous urethral tear proximally, usually up to the verumontanum. After 3 months, the pelvic hematoma is usually resorbed, and the prostate and bladder neck have returned to a more normal position.

Type II urethral injuries show a much shorter stricture on the preoperative retrograde and voiding study, because resorption of the pelvic hematoma allows the prostate, prostatic urethra, and torn membranous urethra to move back to a normal position with approximation of the torn ends of the urethra.

Type I urethral injuries generally require no surgical intervention. The initial urethrogram showing an intact urethra allows the careful insertion of a small, well-lubricated catheter into the bladder. The bladder can be filled through this catheter and a voiding study is obtained with the patient voiding around the catheter. The bladder is assessed for concomitant bladder tear. If no extravasation occurs from the bladder, the catheter can be removed and the patient allowed to void at will. Repeat retrograde and voiding urethrogram in 3 months demonstrate resorption of the pelvic hematoma and return of the bladder and prostate to a normal position.

Combined Bladder and Urethral Injury

In pelvic fracture, up to 20% of male patients with urethral injury have an associated bladder tear. Type I

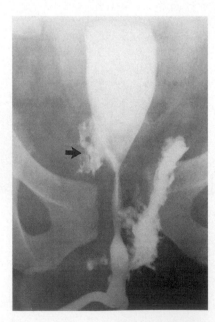

Figure 14.35. Combined urethral and bladder rupture. A retrograde urethrogram demonstrates a partial type III injury associated with an extraperitoneal bladder rupture (*arrow*).

injury, in which the urethra is intact, allows contrast medium to fill the bladder, and the bladder can be assessed for extravasation of contrast medium. Partial type II and type III urethral ruptures allow some contrast medium to enter the bladder, but bladder filling in these cases should not be attempted, because much of the contrast medium injected will extravasate through the tear in the urethra. Occasionally, however, the bladder injury may be shown on the retrograde urethrogram (Fig. 14.35). If delayed repair is to be used, cystography should be performed after placement of the suprapubic catheter. If primary repair is attempted for partial or complete type II or type III injuries, the bladder must be carefully inspected at surgery to exclude bladder tear.

Straddle Injury

Straddle injury most commonly occurs when a male patient falls astride a hard object such as the crossbar of a bicycle, a steel or wooden beam, or the edge of a manhole cover. Kicks to the perineum may also injure the bulbous urethra. The urethra and corpus spongiosum are compressed between the hard object and the inferior aspect of the pubis. This may result in urethral contusion with an intact urethra or partial or complete rupture of the sump of the bulbous urethra. Straddle injury is not generally related to any bony injury.

In minor straddle injury to the urethra, blood is not usually present at the external meatus, although the urethra may be contused. The hematoma is usually confined to Buck's fascia and the tunica albuginea of the corpus spongiosum. More violent straddle injury commonly ruptures Buck's fascia and the hematoma spreads to involve the perineum and scrotum, but is usually well delineated by Colles' fascia bilaterally at its junction with the ischial bones. In such injuries, blood is commonly present at the external meatus.

In minor straddle injury, the retrograde urethrogram may show an intact urethra and the patient can be allowed to void normally. If the urethra is compressed or distorted by hematoma, but intact, and there is no extravasation, a small, well-lubricated catheter may be carefully inserted into the bladder and left for a few days. In more severe straddle injuries, the retrograde urethrogram (Figs. 14.36 and 14.37) generally shows partial or complete rupture. If a partial rupture is present, attempted catheterization may complete the rupture. Suprapubic cystostomy tube insertion is recommended, and repeat urethrography is performed 2 to 3 weeks later. Small partial ruptures may heal without stricture, but the patient should have follow-up urethrography 6 months to 1 year later. Large partial or complete ruptures in the bulbous urethra show extensive extravasation, and if Buck's fascia is lacerated, contrast medium extravasates into the scrotum (Fig. 14.38) and may outline the testicle. Excess injection of contrast

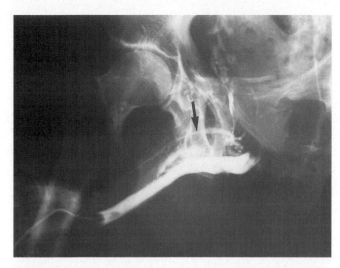

Figure 14.36.   Straddle injury. Typical appearance of straddle injury with extensive venous intravasation. Filling of dorsal vein of the penis is seen (*arrow*).

medium may show contrast medium passing up the anterior abdominal wall beneath Scarpa's fascia. When suprapubic cystostomy is used, large partial and complete rupture results in stricture. These traumatic strictures are usually short (Fig. 14.39), and scarring does not extend to the membranous urethra. Such strictures can be repaired by anterior urethroplasty using a patch or pedicle graft.

Recently, Goldman and colleagues proposed a modification of the Colapinto and McCallum classification which was designed to unify the classification of anterior and posterior urethral injuries into one comprehensive scheme. In this modification, Colapinto/McCallum Type

I, Type II and Type III are unchanged, but three additional categories were added. Type IV injuries are lacerations which extend through the bladder neck into the urethra and which may involve damage to the internal urethral sphincter; it is important that such injuries be recognized because if not properly treated may result in urinary incontinence. Type IVa injuries are injuries of the bladder base which do not actually involve the urethra but simulate true Type IV injuries radiographically and Type V injuries are straddle injuries of the anterior urethra. Types II, III, and V may be either partial or complete.

Penetrating Injuries

Penetrating injuries to the urethra are uncommon. They result from gunshot or knife wounds and more commonly affect the anterior urethra. Penetrating urethral injuries generally require immediate surgical exploration and antibiotic therapy to contain superimposed infection. Knife wounds to the perineum can generally be treated by anastomosis of the cut bulbous urethra. Gunshot wounds may destroy some urethra, and patch or pedicle grafting may be necessary as a one-stage urethroplasty or as the first stage of a two-stage urethroplasty.

Iatrogenic Urethral Injury

This topic is discussed in Chapter 19.

INJURY OF THE FEMALE URETHRA

Clinical Features

Traumatic rupture of the female urethra is rare. It is usually the result of instrumentation, vaginal operation, or obstetric complications. Approximately 1% of ure-

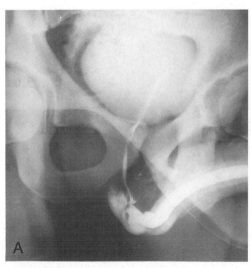

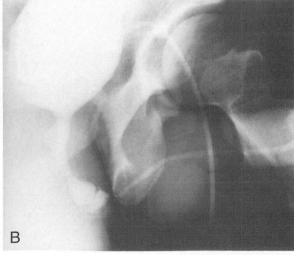

Figure 14.37.   Straddle injury. **A,** retrograde urethrogram shows extravasation from the site of injury in the bulbous urethra; contrast medium, however, flows into the bladder indicating partial injury. **B,** Follow-up voiding cystourethrogram made through a suprapubic catheter shows high-grade focal stricture at the site of the previous injury.

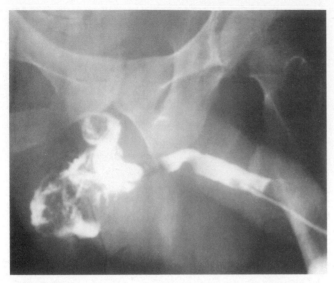

Figure 14.38. Straddle injury with complete urethral disruption. Contrast medium extravasates into the scrotum because of rupture of Buck's fascia.

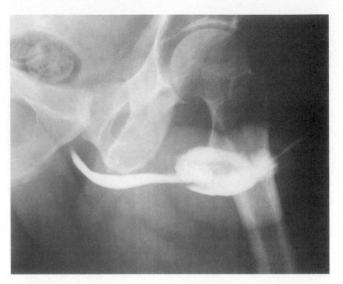

Figure 14.40. Urethral injury in penile fracture. Extensive extravasation of contrast material is present in the penile urethra adjacent to the site of injury of the corpus cavernosum.

thral injuries in females are caused by pelvic fracture. Most reported cases have occurred in female children or young adult females. The rarity of this lesion is likely owing to the shortness of the urethra and to its mobility, because the female urethra is only loosely fixed by the urogenital diaphragm. In pelvic fracture, rupture of the female urethra should be suspected when deep vaginal lacerations are present. There is inability to void or inability to pass a catheter. The urethra may be avulsed at the bladder neck or 1 or 2 cm below the bladder neck. Rupture may be partial or complete. Avulsion

at the bladder neck requires a suprapubic approach with anastomosis of the separated urethral ends over a stenting catheter. More distal urethral rupture may be approached transvaginally with end-to-end urethral anastomosis over a stenting catheter.

The diagnosis of urethral injury in women is generally established on endoscopy.

INJURY OF THE PENIS

Rupture of the corpus cavernosum ("fracture of the penis") is an uncommon injury that generally occurs during strenuous sexual activity. A urethrogram is generally recommended to exclude a concomitant urethral injury (Fig. 14.40). Cavernosography may be useful for the preoperative evaluation of such injuries. In fracture of the erect penis, the tunica albuginea is torn and cavernosography may show the exact site and extent of the tear. This may be useful as the site of a tunica albuginea tear may not be obvious at operation. Urethrocavernous fistula also may occur in the fractured penis and the fistula can be demonstrated on cavernosography.

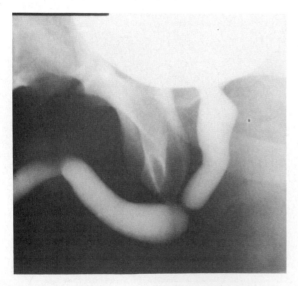

Figure 14.39. Dynamic retrograde and voiding cystourethrogram 3 months after partial rupture from straddle injury. The bladder is filled through a suprapubic cystostomy tube. The stricture is short and well defined.

SUGGESTED READING

General References: Renal Trauma

Bergren CT, Chan FN, Bodzin JH: Intravenous pyelogram results in association with renal pathology and therapy in trauma patients. *J Trauma* 27(5):515, 1987.

Bright TC, White K, Peters TC: Significance of hematuria after trauma. *J Urol* 120:445, 1978.

Boone TB, Gilling PJ, Husmman DA: Ureteropelvic junction disruption following blunt abdominal trauma. *J Urol* 150:33, 1993.

Cass AS, Bubrick M, Luxenberg BE, et al.: Renal trauma found during laparotomy for intra-abdominal injury. *J Trauma* 25(10):997, 1985.

Cass AS, Luxenberg M, Gleich P, et al.: Management of perirenal hematoma found during laparotomy in patients with multiple injuries. *Urology* 26(6):546, 1985.

Cass AS, Luxenberg M, Gleich P, et al.: Type of blunt renal injury rather than associated extravasation should determine treatment. *Urology* 26(3):249, 1985.

Cass AS, Luxenberg M, Gleich P, et al.: Clinical indications for radiographic evaluation of blunt renal trauma. *J Urol* 136:370, 1986.

Eastham JA, Wilson TG, Ahlering TE: Radiographic assessment of blunt renal trauma. *J Urol* 31:1527, 1991.

Eastham JA, Wilson TG, Ahlering TE: Radiographic evaluation of adult patients with blunt renal trauma. *J Urol* 148:266, 1992.

Fortune JB, Brahme J, Mulligan M, et al.: Emergency intravenous pyelography in the trauma patient. *Arch Surg* 120:1056, 1985.

Goldman SM, Wagner LK: Radiologic management of abdominal trauma in pregnancy. *AJR* 166:763, 1996.

Hardeman WS, Husmann DA, Chinn GKW, et al.: Blunt urinary tract trauma: identifying those patients who require radiological diagnostic studies. *J Urol* 138:99, 1987.

Herschorn S, Radomski SB, Shoskes DA, Mahoney J, Hirshberg E, Klotz L: Evaluation and treatment of blunt renal trauma. *J Urol* 274, 1991.

Heyns CF, de Klerk DP, de Kock MLS: Stab wounds associated with hematuria: a review of 67 cases. *J Urol* 130:228, 1983.

Husmann DA and Morris JS: Attempted nonoperative management of blunt renal lacerations extending through the corticomedullary junction: the short-term and long-term sequela. *J Urol* 143:682, 1990.

Husmann DA, Gilling PJ, Perry MO, Morris JS, Boone TB: Major renal lacerations with a devitalized fragment following blunt abdominal trauma: a comparison between nonoperative (expectant) versus surgical management. *J Urol* 150:1774, 1993.

Kisa E, Schenk WG: Indications for emergency intravenous pyelography (IVP) in blunt abdominal trauma: a reappraisal. *J Trauma* 26(12):1086, 1986.

Knudson MM, McAninch JW, Gomez R, Lee P, Stubbs HA: Hematuria as a predictor of abdominal injury after blunt trauma. *Am J Surgery,* 164:482, 1992.

Mee SL, McAninch JW, Robinson AL, et al.: Radiographic assessment of renal trauma. a 10-year prospective study of patient selection. *J Urol* 141:1095, 1989.

Miller KS, McAninch JW: Radiologic assessment of renal trauma: our 15-year experience. *J Urol* 154:352, 1995.

Nicolaisen GS, McAninch JW, Marshall GA, et al.: Renal trauma: reevaluation of the indications for radiographic assessment. *J Urol* 133:183, 1985.

Pollack HM, Wein AJ: Imaging of renal trauma. *Radiology* 172:297, 1989.

Roberts RA, Belitsky P, Lannon SG, et al.: Conservative management of renal lacerations in blunt trauma. *Can J Surg* 30(4):253, 1987.

Sagalowsky AI, McConnell JD, Peters TC: Renal trauma requiring surgery: an analysis of 185 cases. *J Trauma* 23(2):128, 1983.

Stevenson J and Battistella FD: The 'one-shot' intravenous pyelogram: Is it indicated in unstable trauma patients before celiotomy? *J Trauma* 36:828, 1994.

Wilson RF, Ziegler DW: Diagnostic and treatment problems in renal injuries. *Am Surg* 53(7):399, 1987.

Computed Tomography of Renal Trauma

Brennan FJ, Goff WB, II: Seatbelt injury to a pelvic kidney as demonstrated on CT. *J Comput Assist Tomogr* 17(4):1993.

Bretan PN, McAninch JW, Federle MP, et al.: Computerized tomographic staging of renal trauma: 85 consecutive cases. *J Urol* 136:561, 1986.

Cass AS, Vieira J: Comparison of IVP and CT findings in patients with suspected severe renal injury. *Urology* 24(5):484, 1987.

Cates JD, Foley WD, Lawson TL: Retrograde opacification of the renal vein: a CT sign of renal artery avulsion. *Urol Radiol* 8:92, 1986.

Erturk E, Sheinfeld J, DiMarco PL, Cockett TK: Renal trauma: evaluation by computerized tomography. *J Urol* 133:946, 1985.

Fanney DR, Casillas J, Murphy BJ: CT in the diagnosis of renal trauma. *RadioGraphics* 10:29, 1990.

Federle MP, Brown TR, McAninch JW: Penetrating renal trauma: CT evaluation. *J Comput Assist Tomogr* 11(6):1026, 1987.

Federle MP, Kaiser JA, McAninch JW, et al.: The role of computed tomography in renal trauma. *Radiology* 141:455, 1981.

Glazer GM, Francis IR, Brady TM, et al.: Computed tomography of renal infarction: clinical and experimental observations. *AJR* 140:721, 1983.

Lang EK, Sullivan J, Frentz G: Renal trauma: radiological studies. *Radiology* 154:1, 1985.

Lupetin AR, Mainwaring BL, Daffner RH: CT diagnosis of renal artery injury caused by blunt abdominal trauma. *AJR* 153:1065, 1989.

Peitzman AB, Makaroun MS, Slasky BS, et al.: Prospective study of computed tomography in initial management of blunt abdominal trauma. *J Trauma* 26(7):585, 1986.

Rhyner P, Federle MP, Jeffrey RB: CT of trauma to the abnormal kidney. *AJR* 142:747, 1984.

Sandler CM, Toombs BD: Computed tomographic evaluation of blunt renal injuries. *Radiology* 141:461, 1981.

Sclafani SJA, Becker JA: Radiologic diagnosis of renal trauma. *Urol Radiol* 7:192, 1985.

Steinberg DL, Jeffrey RB, Federle MP, et al.: The computerized tomography appearance of renal pedicle injury. *J Urol* 132:1163, 1984.

Yale-Loehr AJ, Kramer SS, Quinlan DM, et al.: CT of severe renal trauma in children: evaluation and course of healing with conservative therapy. *AJR* 152:109, 1989.

Renovascular Injuries

Bertini JE, Flechner SM, Miller P, et al.: The natural history of traumatic branch renal artery injury. *J Urol* 135:228, 1986.

Cass AS, Luxenberg M: Unilateral nonvisualization on excretory urography after external trauma. *J Urol* 132:225, 1984.

Cass AS, Luxenberg M: Traumatic thrombosis of a segmental branch of the renal artery. *J Urol* 137:1115, 1987.

Cass AS, Susset J, Khan A, et al.: Renal pedicle injury in the multiple injured patient. *J Urol* 122:728, 1979.

Halpern M: Angiography in renal trauma. *Surg Clin North Am* 48(6): 1221, 1986.

Heyns CF and Vollenhoven PV: Increasing role of angiography and segmental artery embolization in the management of renal stab wounds. *J Urol* 147:1231, 1992.

Stables DP: Unilateral absence of excretion at urography after abdominal trauma. *Radiology* 121:609, 1976.

Radionuclide Studies

Rosenthall L, Ammann W: Renal trauma. *Semin Nucl Med* 13(3): 238, 1983.

Uthoff LB, Wyffels RL, Adams CS, et al.: A prospective study comparing nuclear scintigraphy and computerized axial tomography in the initial evaluation of the trauma patient. *Ann Surg* 98(5):611, 1983.

Ureteral Injuries

Beamud-Gomez A, Martinez-Verduch M, Estorness-Moragues F, et al.: Rupture of the ureteropelvic junction by nonpenetrating trauma. *J Pediatr Surg* 21(8):702, 1986.

Boone TB, Gilling PJ, Husmann DA: Ureteropelvic junction disruption following blunt abdominal trauma. *J Urol* 150(1):33, 1993.

Bright TC III, Peters PC: Ureteral injuries secondary to operative procedures. *Urology* 11(1):22, 1977.

Cass AS: Blunt renal pelvic and ureteral injury in multiple injured patients. *Urology* 22(3):269, 1983.

Dowling RA, Corriere JN Jr, Sandler CM: Iatrogenic ureteral injury. *J Urol* 135:912, 1986.

Fry DE, Milholen J, Harbrecht PJ: Iatrogenic ureteral injury. *Arch Surg* 118:454, 1983.

Hall SJ, Carpinito GA: Traumatic rupture of a renal pelvis obstructed at the ureteropelvic junction: case report. *J Trauma* 37(5):850, 1994.

Harshman MW, Pollack HM, Banner MP, et al.: Conservative management of ureteral obstruction secondary to suture entrapment. *J Urol* 127:121, 1982.

Kenney PJ, Panicek DM, Witanowski LS: Computed tomography of ureteral disruption. *J Comput Assist Tomogr* 11(3):480, 1987.

Lang EK: Diagnosis and management of ureteral fistulas by percutaneous nephrostomy and antegrade stent catheter. *Radiology* 138:311, 1981.

Sieben DM, Howerton L, Amin H, et al.: The role of ureteral stenting in the management of surgical injury of the ureter. *J Urol* 119:330, 1978.

Selzman AA, Spirnak JP: Iatrogenic ureteral injuries: a 20-year experience in treating 165 injuries. *J Urol* 155:878, 1996.

Spirnak JP, Persky L, Resnick MI: The management of civilian ureteral gunshot wounds: a review of 8 patients. *J Urol* 134:733, 1985.

Steers WD, Corriere JN Jr, Benson GS, et al.: The use of indwelling ureteral stents in managing ureteral injuries due to external violence. *J Trauma* 25(10):1001, 1985.

Bladder Injuries

Carroll PR, McAninch JW: Major bladder trauma: the accuracy of cystography. *J Urol* 130:887, 1983.

Carroll PR, McAninch JW: Major bladder trauma: mechanisms of injury and unified method of diagnosis and repair. *J Urol* 132:254, 1984.

Corriere JN Jr, Sandler CM: Management of the ruptured bladder: seven years experience with 111 cases. *J Trauma* 26(9):830, 1986.

Corriere JN Jr, Sandler CM: Mechanisms of injury, patterns of extravasation and management of extraperitoneal bladder rupture due to blunt trauma. *J Urol* 139:43, 1988.

Eisenkop SM, Richman R, Platt LD, Paul RH: Urinary tract injury during cesarean section. *Obstet Gynecol* 60(5):591, 1982.

Huffman JL, Schraut W, Baley DH: Atraumatic perforation of bladder. *Urology* 22(1):30, 1983.

Lis LE and Cohen AJ: CT cystography in the evaluation of bladder trauma. *J Comput Assist Tomogr* 14(3):386, 1990.

Mee SL, McAninch JW, Federle MP: Computerized tomography in bladder rupture: diagnostic limitations. *J Urol* 137:207, 1987.

Palmer JK, Benson GS, Corriere JN Jr: Diagnosis and initial management of urological injuries associated with 200 consecutive pelvic fractures. *J Urol* 130:712, 1983.

Sandler CM, Hall JT, Rodriguez MB, et al.: Bladder injury in blunt pelvic trauma. *Radiology* 158:633, 1986.

Sandler CM, Phillips JM, Harris JD, et al.: Radiology of the bladder and urethra in blunt pelvic trauma. *Radiol Clin North Am* 19(1):195, 1981.

Shumaker BP, Pontes JE, Pierce JM Jr: Idiopathic rupture of the bladder. *Urology* 15(6):566, 1980.

Urethral Injuries

Casselman RC, Schillinger JF: Fractured pelvis with avulsion of the female urethra. *J Urol* 117:385, 1977.

Colapinto V, McCallum RW: Injury to the male posterior urethra in fractured pelvis: a new classification. *J Urol* 118:575, 1977.

Follis HW, Koch MO, McDougal WS: Immediate management of prostatomembranous urethral disruptions. *J Urol* 147:1259, 1992.

Goldman SM, Sandler CM, Corriere JN, Jr., and McGuire EJ: Blunt urethral trauma: a unified, anatomical-mechanical classification. *J Urol.* (In press)

Herschorn S, Thijssen A, Radomski SB: The value of immediate or early catheterization of the traumatized posterior urethra. *J Urol* 148:1428, 1992.

Netto NR, Ikari O, Zuppo VP: Traumatic rupture of the female urethra. *Urology* 22:601, 1983.

Perry MO and Husmann DA: Urethral injuries in female subjects following pelvic fractures. *J Urol* 147:139, 1992.

Sandler CM, Harris JH, Corriere JN, et al.: Posterior urethral injuries after pelvic fracture. *AJR* 137:1233, 1981.

15

....

The Adrenal Gland

....

ANATOMY

The adrenal glands lie within the perinephric space along with the kidneys. In most patients, there is sufficient perinephric fat that they are easily seen on computed tomography (CT) (Fig. 15.1). The right adrenal gland lies anteromedial to the upper pole of the right kidney and immediately posterior to the inferior vena cava. The left gland is anteromedial to the upper pole of the left kidney and posterior to portions of the splenic vein and artery. The right adrenal gland consistently extends above the upper pole of the kidney, whereas the left adrenal gland more often is found at the level of the left upper pole and may extend to the renal hilus.

Both adrenal glands have an inverted Y configuration, with the tail of the Y pointing anteromedially. The angle between the two arms is more acute in the cephalad portion and widens inferiorly as the gland tends to straddle the upper pole of the kidney (Fig. 15.2). In patients with renal agenesis or ectopy, the ipsilateral adrenal gland has a more linear shape, rather than the inverted Y configuration (Fig. 15.3).

The adrenal glands weigh approximately 5 g each and vary from 3 to 6 mm in width. This small size makes it difficult to distinguish a normal from an atrophic or hyperplastic adrenal gland on the basis of size.

The arterial supply to the adrenal glands is from many small arterial branches from one of three main feeding arteries. This produces a comb-like appearance, with small arteriae comitantes arising from one of three dominant vessels (Fig. 15.4). The arteries supplying the superior portion of the gland come from the superior adrenal artery, which is usually a branch of the inferior phrenic artery. The middle adrenal artery arises directly from the aorta and provides vessels for the midportion of the gland. The inferior aspect of the adrenal gland is supplied by branches of the inferior adrenal artery, which most often branches from the renal artery.

Each adrenal gland is drained by a single central vein. On the right side, the adrenal vein enters directly into the posterior aspect of the inferior vena cava (Fig. 15.5). Occasionally, however, the adrenal vein may join an accessory hepatic vein before entering the inferior vena cava. The left adrenal vein enters the inferior phrenic vein before joining the left renal vein. The right adrenal vein is shorter and has a smaller diameter than the left adrenal vein. This explains the increased difficulty in obtaining a venous sample from the right adrenal vein compared with the left.

FUNCTIONAL DISEASES

The adrenal glands are small, and patients seldom present with pain or a palpable adrenal mass. Because the adrenal gland is an active site of synthesis of a variety of hormones, patients may present with symptoms of hormone excess or, less likely, hormone deficiency.

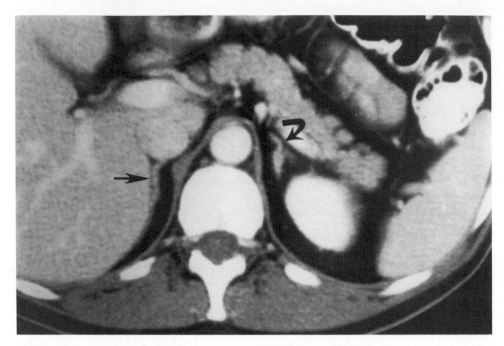

Figure 15.1. Normal adrenal glands. The right adrenal (*arrow*) lies behind the inferior vena cava and medial to the liver. The left adrenal (*curved arrow*) is anteromedial to the upper pole of the left kidney.

Thus, adrenal diseases are discussed as hyperfunctional disorders in which excess hormone is produced, disorders of adrenal insufficiency, and diseases in which adrenal function is normal. Because these hormones can be readily measured, there is seldom doubt as to which category a patient belongs (Table 15.1).

Cushing's Syndrome

Cushing's syndrome is the manifestation of excess glucocorticoids. These steroids may come from exogenous or endogenous sources. Exogenous Cushing's syndrome is seen in patients treated with large doses of steroids. Endogenous Cushing's syndrome is caused by overproduction of cortisol by the adrenal cortex. This can be caused by an autonomous adrenal tumor, benign or malignant, or by adrenal hyperplasia from unregulated corticotropin (ACTH) production.

Cushing's disease refers to bilateral adrenal hyperplasia due to excess ACTH production by a pituitary adenoma. However, the pituitary gland is not always the source of ACTH in patients with adrenal hyperplasia; a variety of other tumors, such as oat cell carcinoma, bronchial adenoma, and tumors of the ovary, pancreas, thymus, and thyroid also may secrete ACTH.

The characteristic appearance of a patient with Cushing's syndrome includes truncal obesity, hirsutism, abdominal striae, and muscle atrophy. Hypertension and glucose intolerance are common findings. The diagnosis of Cushing's syndrome may be confirmed by measuring plasma or urinary 17-hydroxycorticosteroid levels, which are elevated.

The most common etiology of endogenous Cushing's syndrome is bilateral adrenal hyperplasia, which accounts for approximately 70% of cases. Approximately 90% of these patients also have a pituitary adenoma secreting increased amounts of ACTH. Ectopic sources of ACTH cause the other 10% of cases.

A few patients with adrenal hyperplasia have macronodules that can be seen in the adrenal glands on CT examination. These macronodules usually measure less than 3 cm and may be less than 1 cm in diameter. Macronodular hyperplasia is caused by an ACTH-secreting pituitary microadenoma in the majority of cases. A benign but autonomous adrenal cortical adenoma is the etiology of 20% of cases of endogenous Cushing's syndrome, and a primary adrenal cortical carcinoma is responsible for approximately 10% of cases.

Conn's Syndrome

Conn's syndrome, or primary aldosteronism, is the result of excess aldosterone produced by the adrenal glands. As with Cushing's syndrome, it may be caused by adrenal hyperplasia or an adrenal tumor. A benign adenoma secreting an unregulated amount of aldosterone is the most common etiology of primary aldosteronism, being responsible for almost 70% of cases. Bilateral adrenal hyperplasia accounts for 30% of cases.

Adrenal hyperplasia may be further subdivided into idiopathic hyperaldosteronism (IHA) and primary adrenal hyperplasia (PAH). Idiopathic Hyperaldosteronism is far more common than PAH. Bilateral adrenalectomy does not effectively control the hypertension

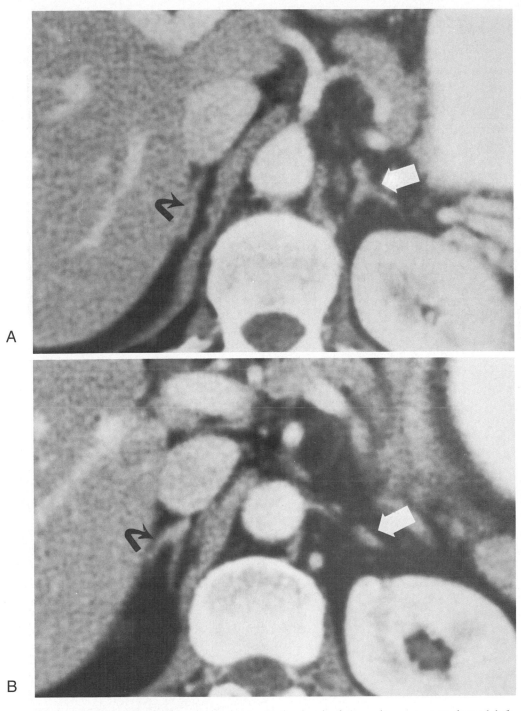

A

B

Figure 15.2.   Normal adrenal glands. **A,** At the level of the celiac axis a Y-shaped left adrenal (*arrow*) is appreciated, but only the anteroposterior limb of the right adrenal (*curved arrow*) is present. **B,** At lower levels the right adrenal (*curved arrow*) becomes Y-shaped, whereas only a portion of the lateral limb of the left adrenal (*arrow*) is identified.

and hypokalemia in patients with IHA, so they are treated medically. Although morphologically PAH resembles IHA, PAH may be unilateral or bilateral, and adrenalectomy is an effective treatment for unilateral cases. Rarely does a primary adrenocortical carcinoma secrete enough aldosterone to cause a recognizable clinical syndrome.

The syndrome Conn described in 1955 includes hypokalemia, hypertension, elevated serum aldosterone, but low serum renin levels. Excess levels of aldosterone cause sodium retention, an increase in the plasma volume, and hypertension. Because potassium is exchanged for sodium in the distal tubule, sodium retention creates hypokalemia.

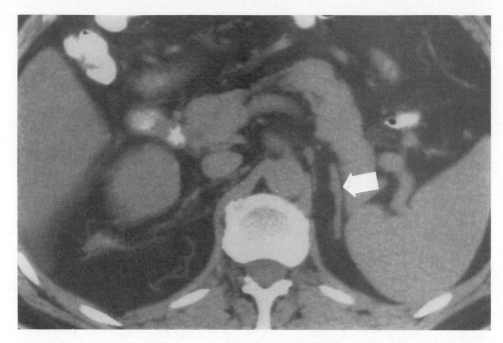

Figure 15.3.   Left renal agenesis. The left adrenal gland (*arrow*) has a linear rather than an inverted Y configuration.

Figure 15.4.   Adrenal arteries. The adrenal gland is supplied by many small arterial branches that arise from the inferior phrenic artery, aorta, and renal artery.

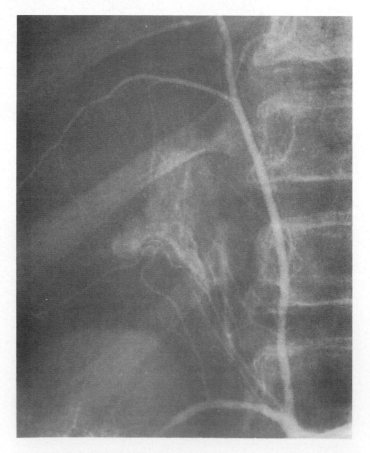

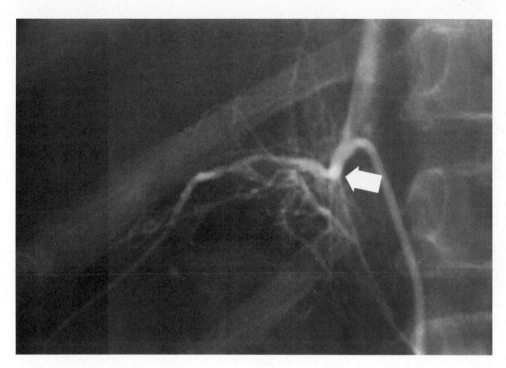

Figure 15.5. Adrenal vein. A single draining right adrenal vein (*arrow*) enters directly into the inferior vena cava.

Aldosteronism also occurs in patients with renovascular hypertension. However, this form of secondary aldosteronism is distinguished from primary aldosteronism by measuring the serum renin level, which is low in Conn's syndrome.

Laboratory tests also can be used to help distinguish between hyperplasia or an adenoma, as the etiology of primary aldosteronism. However, these tests are not entirely accurate and radiographic confirmation is usually obtained. Furthermore, if an adenoma is present, radiographic techniques are needed to localize the tumor.

Adrenogenital Syndromes

These syndromes are the result of an inborn error in the adrenal enzyme system that blocks or impairs the synthesis of cortisol or aldosterone. Low serum levels of cortisol stimulate ACTH secretion by the pituitary gland, while inadequate concentrations of aldosterone lead to increases in renin and angiotensin. Each of the six different enzyme deficiencies results in a different form of congenital adrenal hyperplasia. The clinical manifestations are determined by the degree of deficiency of cortisol or al-

Table 15.1.
Causes of Primary Adrenal Insufficiency

Idiopathic (autoimmune disease)
Bilateral adrenalectomy
Granulomatous disease
Metastases
Lymphoma
Hemorrhage

dosterone and by the biologic properties of the biochemical intermediates that are formed and secreted in excess.

Deficiencies of 21-hydroxylase or 11B-hydroxylase are the most common forms of congenital adrenal hyperplasia. Insufficient 21-hydroxylase impairs production of cortisol and aldosterone. Because androgens do not require 21-hydroxylase for their synthesis, they are overproduced in response to high levels of ACTH. The clinical manifestation depends on the sex of the patient and the age at which the androgen excess appears. Virilization is seen in women, and precocious puberty is found in young boys.

When a deficiency of 11B-hydroxylase exists, cortisol secretion is impaired. This results in an increase in ACTH, and the precursor 11-deoxycortisol is oversecreted. This precursor is a mineralocorticoid that induces hypertension. Because androgens do not require 11B-hydroxylation, virilization or precocious puberty may result.

Virilizing Tumors

Androgen-producing tumors are rare, may be benign or malignant, and occur in either males or females at any age. Patients whose virilization is due to a tumor usually present at a later age than those with congenital adrenal hyperplasia.

The typical clinical manifestations include amenorrhea, hirsutism, enlargement of the clitoris, and deepening of the voice. Elevated testosterone levels also are frequently found in adrenal tumors, so a high testosterone level cannot be used to distinguish a gonadal from an adrenal tumor.

Feminizing Tumors

Feminizing tumors are quite rare. They are usually seen in men, but have been reported in prepubertal girls and postmenopausal women. Gynecomastia is the predominant clinical manifestation.

Adrenal Insufficiency

Adrenal insufficiency may result from inadequate stimulation by ACTH (secondary) or may be caused by tissue destruction of the adrenal glands (primary). Because normal adrenal function depends on ACTH, any disorder that impairs the ability of the pituitary gland to secrete ACTH may lead to adrenal hypofunction. With decreased ACTH activity, cortisol and adrenal androgen secretion diminish, but aldosterone secretion remains relatively intact. Thus, patients with hypopituitarism can tolerate sodium deprivation better than patients with primary adrenal insufficiency. Furthermore, hypopituitary patients do not develop mucocutaneous hyperpigmentation, as this depends on excessive ACTH secretion.

Primary adrenal insufficiency, or Addison's disease, occurs only after at least 90% of the adrenal cortex has been destroyed. Idiopathic adrenal atrophy is the most common cause of Addison's disease in the United States and is most likely an autoimmune disorder. The other common cause of Addison's disease is destruction of the adrenal glands by a granulomatous disease, usually tuberculosis. However, other causes such as infarction, amyloidosis, hemorrhage, or destruction by histoplasmosis, blastomycosis, disseminated fungal infection, lymphoma, and metastatic tumor have been reported.

Histoplasmosis is usually a mild pulmonary infection. Occasionally histoplasma cells disseminate to multiple sites, which usually heal without sequelae. Disseminated histoplasmosis can occur in otherwise healthy individuals, but immunocompromised patients or those at either end of the age spectrum are most susceptible. Organs commonly involved by disseminated histoplasmosis include the liver, spleen, adrenal glands, and lymph nodes. Adrenal insufficiency may occur when both adrenal glands are involved.

With histoplasma infection, the adrenal glands enlarge symmetrically. They maintain a normal configuration, but have low-density centers with peripheral enhancement. Calcification may develop during the healing phase. This appearance may be seen with infection by granulomatous diseases. The diagnosis may be confirmed by percutaneous biopsy, although the pathologist must be alerted to the possibility of histoplasma infection so that special stains are used.

The clinical onset of Addison's disease is usually gradual and may be difficult to recognize. Manifestations are primarily a function of cortisol and aldosterone deficiency. Because cortisol deficiency results in increased pituitary secretion of ACTH and other melanocyte-stimulating hormones, patients with Addison's disease develop a characteristic hyperpigmentation. Treatment includes cortisol and aldosterone replacement, as well as saline to correct extracellular fluid depletion.

The radiographic manifestations of adrenal insufficiency depend on the cause of adrenal dysfunction. The plain abdominal radiograph may reveal adrenal calcification, commonly seen in tuberculosis or histoplasmosis.

The most useful examination is CT, which defines the size and shape of the adrenal glands. In idiopathic Addison's disease, severe cortical atrophy is present, such that the adrenal glands may be difficult to detect.

Granulomatous involvement by tuberculosis or histoplasmosis is usually bilateral. The glands are enlarged, but often maintain a normal configuration. Calcification is common.

If adrenal hemorrhage is acute, it may be recognized by the increased density of the recent hemorrhage. As the density of the hematoma decreases, it becomes indistinguishable from other adrenal masses. Although adrenal metastases are common, adrenal insufficiency rarely occurs. This is because so much of the adrenal cortex must be destroyed before insufficiency ensues.

Radiology

Urography

The plain radiograph is usually unrewarding in patients with hyperfunctioning adrenal cortical disease, although large masses can be recognized. Calcification may be present in an adrenal carcinoma, but this is a nonspecific finding. Excretory urography will be normal unless the adrenal mass displaces the kidney. Because the adrenal glands lie anteromedial to the upper pole of the kidneys, an adrenal mass will push the upper renal pole laterally, creating a more vertical renal axis. If the adrenal lesion is huge, the ipsilateral kidney also will be displaced inferiorly.

Ultrasound

Although the normal adrenal gland may be difficult to image with ultrasound, tumors larger than 2 cm often can be detected (Fig. 15.6). The right adrenal gland is usually easier to study, because the liver provides a good acoustic window. Obese patients are more difficult to image because of the higher sound attenuation of fat.

In patients with hyperfunction of the adrenal glands, ultrasound has two major uses. Large functioning tumors, such as adrenal carcinomas, may be difficult to distinguish from adjacent organs, such as the kidney or liver. The multiple scan projections that can be used with ultrasound may allow a tissue plane to be distinguished that could not be seen with CT. Some adenomas may have sufficient lipid within them to appear as low-density (near-water) masses. Without intravenous contrast administration, CT is

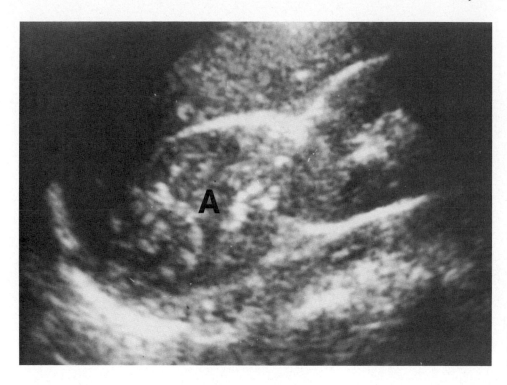

Figure 15.6. Adrenal tumor. Ultrasound demonstrates a solid suprarenal mass (*A*) easily distinguished from an adrenal cyst.

unable to differentiate a small homogeneous adenoma from an adrenal cyst. Ultrasound may be valuable in demonstrating the solid nature of the adenoma.

Computed Tomography

The modality routinely used to evaluate the adrenal glands is CT. The perinephric fat present in most patients allows the adrenal glands to be clearly displayed, and tumors as small as 5 mm in diameter can be identified (Fig. 15.7). The adrenal glands must be carefully examined using contiguous 3- or 5-mm collimated slices. Intravenous contrast medium is not usually needed, but may be used to distinguish an adrenal mass from the upper pole of the kidney.

Figure 15.7. Adrenal adenoma. A small right adrenal adenoma (*arrow*) is detected by computed tomography.

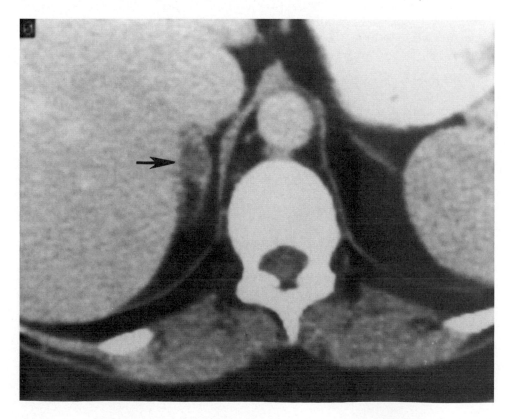

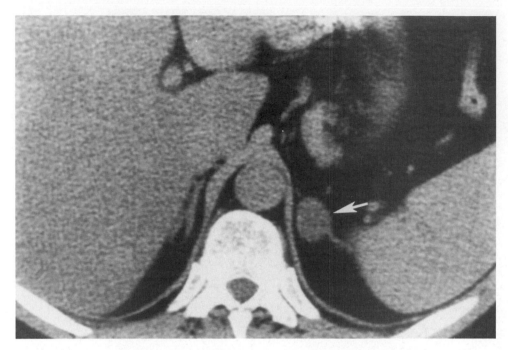

Figure 15.8.   Adrenal adenoma. An aldosterone-secreting adenoma (*arrow*) is seen in the left adrenal gland.

The adenomas in Conn's syndrome are usually the most difficult adrenal tumors to detect because they tend to be the smallest, averaging less than 2 cm in diameter. Careful study of the adrenal gland is required and repeat, narrowly collimated sections may be needed. The left adrenal gland may be particularly troublesome (Fig. 15.8).

Patients with Cushing's syndrome, conversely, are relatively easy to examine by CT. The tumors in these patients are larger than those causing Conn's syndrome, and the adrenal glands are clearly depicted by the abundant retroperitoneal fat (Fig. 15.9). Tumors that are greater than 4 cm in diameter or that demonstrate central necrosis are suspicious for malignancy and may be instances of a primary adrenocortical carcinoma rather than an adenoma.

Figure 15.9.   Adrenal adenoma. Cortisol-secreting adenomas (*A*) are easy to detect because of the abundant retroperitoneal fat.

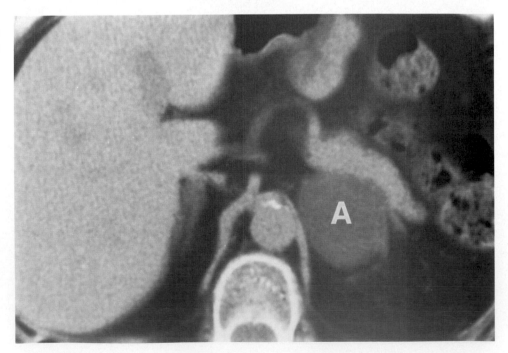

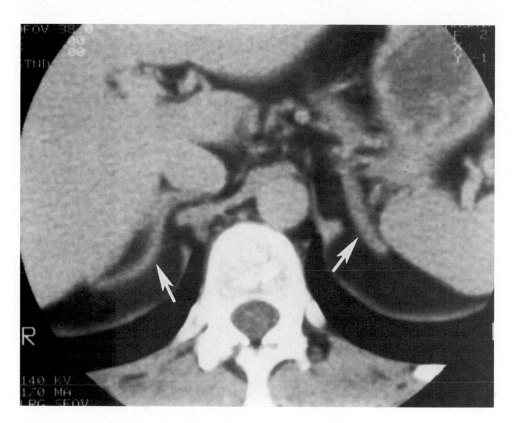

Figure 15.10.   Bilateral adrenal hyperplasia. Both adrenal glands (*arrows*) are thick and elongated in this patient with Cushing's disease.

Bilateral adrenal hyperplasia is seen as enlargement of the entire adrenal gland, but without a focal mass. The limbs of the adrenal gland are thicker and longer, and they are seen over a larger series of CT sections (Fig. 15.10). On the right side, the false impression of a fatty adrenal mass may be created as the horizontal arm is forced posteriorly by the liver. The normal perinephric fat seen between the two arms may be misinterpreted as a myelolipoma.

Enlargement of the adrenal gland is usually more obvious in patients with Cushing's syndrome than in those with Conn's syndrome. However, there is significant overlap with the appearance of normal adrenal glands, and hyperplasia should not be diagnosed by morphology alone. Furthermore, patients with adrenal hyperplasia also may have discrete nodules that cannot be distinguished from an autonomous adrenal adenoma.

Arteriography

Adrenal arteriography is seldom used in the evaluation of functional adrenal diseases. Computed tomography is a superior method of detecting adrenal hyperplasia or an adrenal tumor. Occasionally arteriography is used to identify the tissue of origin of a large upper quadrant mass, because delineation of the vessels supplying the mass defines the organ from which it developed.

Venography

Because each adrenal gland is drained by a central vein, the entire gland can be visualized with a single contrast injection. An adenoma is detected as a focal mass that displaces intraadrenal veins (Fig. 15.11). However, the veins, especially the right, are small and catheterization may be difficult.

Adrenal venography should be performed with hand injections because the vessels are small and because it is easy to cause extravasation. This usually results in back pain that is self-limited and without sequelae. Occasionally this sequence of events may damage the adrenal gland, and adrenal insufficiency has been reported. However, attempts to ablate aldosterone-containing adrenal glands in this manner were unsuccessful, and adrenal venography is generally safe. The few major complications reported are usually caused by clot formation, which can be avoided with heparinization.

Venous Sampling

Although venography can be used to detect an adrenal mass, it is more often employed to provide samples of blood from the adrenal veins for hormone analysis. Venous sampling can be valuable in patients with Conn's syndrome, because the aldosterone-secreting adenoma often is less than 1 cm and may be too small

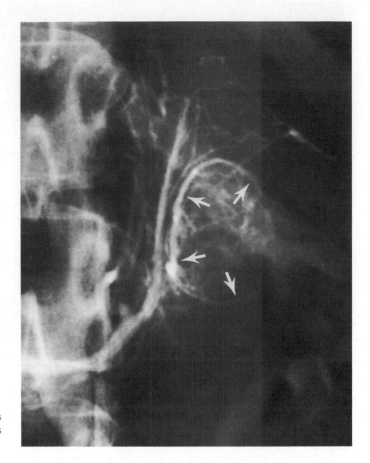

Figure 15.11. Adrenal adenoma. An adrenal adenoma is defined by the displacement of adrenal veins (*arrows*) in this patient with Conn's syndrome.

to be detected by CT. Venous sampling is rarely needed in evaluating patients with Cushing's syndrome, but may be applied to those patients suffering from masculinizing or feminizing tumors.

Bilateral adrenal venous samples are obtained and are compared with each other and with a sample obtained from the inferior vena cava below the renal veins. ACTH may be administered to the patient before drawing the venous samples in an effort to increase hormone output and to make side-to-side differences more pronounced.

Catheterization of the left adrenal vein is relatively easy, and satisfactory adrenal venous samples can reliably be obtained. The right adrenal vein is smaller and more difficult to find. Once the catheter has cannulated this vessel, it is difficult to obtain the 7 to 10 ml of blood required for hormone analysis. The catheter often falls out of the right adrenal vein, and the sample is diluted with blood from the vena cava.

This problem of dilution can be offset by measuring an adrenal hormone that is unaffected by the presence of an adrenal tumor. In the case of Conn's syndrome, measurement of cortisol will demonstrate how "pure" the adrenal vein sample is. Thus, an aldosterone/cortisol ratio is obtained and is compared with similar ratios

from the contralateral adrenal vein and the inferior vena cava.

In experienced vascular laboratories, the technique of adrenal venous sampling is quite accurate and provides tumor localization that may not be obtained with other imaging techniques. However, these syndromes are relatively uncommon, and few laboratories have sufficient experience to maintain a high level of experience.

An additional venous sampling technique is occasionally used in patients with Cushing's syndrome due to bilateral adrenal hyperplasia. In these patients, the source of the ACTH is usually a pituitary adenoma but may be from an ectopic source, such as a lung tumor. In this situation, blood samples are obtained from the right and left petrosal sinuses and ACTH is measured.

Magnetic Resonance Imaging

The perinephric fat provides excellent contrast for magnetic resonance imaging (MRI) as well as CT. The spatial resolution of MRI is similar to that of CT, and the additional parameters available to distinguish benign from malignant lesions may be useful. For most patients with hyperfunction of the adrenal cortex, MRI does not provide additional information after a CT examination.

Radioisotope Scanning

Cortical imaging agents have been developed that can localize hyperfunctioning adrenal cortical tumors, particularly in patients with Cushing's syndrome. The labeling agent iodine-131–19-iodocholesterol is given intravenously, and scans are obtained after a delay of 2 to 14 days. However, the success of CT in localizing these adrenal tumors has made this examination unnecessary in most centers.

ADRENAL MEDULLA

Pheochromocytoma

Pheochromocytomas are tumors comprised of chromaffin cells and are usually located in the adrenal medulla. Extraadrenal pheochromocytomas (paragangliomas) may lie anywhere between the base of the brain and the epididymis, but usually lie along the sympathetic chain in the retroperitoneum. They are rare tumors and account for less than 1% of patients with systemic hypertension.

Patients may complain of episodes of headaches associated with palpitation and diaphoresis. If the pheochromocytoma is located in the bladder wall, micturition may induce a symptomatic episode.

Hypertension is the most common finding and is present in more than 90% of patients. Hypertension from a pheochromocytoma may be difficult to distinguish from renovascular or essential hypertension; however, patients with a pheochromocytoma are more likely to have labile hypertension with discrete paroxysmal attacks. These patients also are prone to hypertensive attacks during anesthesia induction. Manipulation of the gland during surgery, percutaneous adrenal biopsy, or even selective adrenal arteriography also may induce a hypertensive crisis.

Pheochromocytomas are associated with other endocrine tumors. The multiple endocrine neoplasia (MEN) syndrome, type 2A, includes medullary carcinoma of the thyroid and parathyroid hyperplasia as well as pheochromocytoma (Table 15.2). The MEN syndrome, type 2B, comprises pheochromocytoma, medullary carcinoma of the thyroid, and mucocutaneous manifestations of mucosal neuromas, intestinal ganglioneuromatosis, and a marfanoid habitus (Table 15.3). The majority of patients with the MEN 2A or MEN 2B syndromes have pheochromocytomas that are bilateral and almost always intraadrenal. All manifestations of the syndrome may not oc-

Table 15.2.
Multiple Endocrine Neoplasia, Type 2A

Medullary carcinoma of thyroid
Pheochromocytoma (usually bilateral)
Parathyroid adenoma

Table 15.3.
Multiple Endocrine Neoplasia, Type 2B

Medullary carcinoma of thyroid
Pheochromocytoma (usually bilateral)
Mucosal neuromas
Intestinal ganglioneuromatoses
Marfanoid habitus

cur at the same time. Thus, a careful history of a previous endocrine abnormality should be obtained in evaluating patients who may fall into these categories. These syndromes are inherited in an autosomal-dominant fashion.

Pheochromocytoma is associated with neurofibromatosis and the von Hippel-Lindau syndrome (Table 15.4). A syndrome of familial pheochromocytomas not associated with other endocrine tumors has also been noted. In 1977, Carney and colleagues reported the association of a gastric leiomyosarcoma, a pulmonary chondroma, and a functioning extraadrenal pheochromocytoma. This rare combination of neoplasms often is termed Carney's triad.

Although 90% of all pheochromocytomas are located in the adrenal medulla, there is a striking difference between sporadic tumors and those associated with the MEN syndromes. The sporadic pheochromocytomas are located outside the adrenal gland in as many as 25% of cases, while those associated with the MEN 2 syndromes are virtually always intraadrenal. Pheochromocytomas found in patients with MEN 2 syndrome are usually multicentric, and involve both adrenal glands in more than 80% of cases.

The histologic appearance also differs in sporadic and MEN 2–associated cases. In sporadic cases, the tumor is well encased with normal adjacent medulla. In patients with MEN 2 syndrome, the medulla is hyperplastic and the tumor may be multicentric.

If a pheochromocytoma is suspected, the diagnosis can be made by measuring elevated levels of serum or urine catecholamines. Urinary metanephrines or vanillylmandelic acid (VMA) is elevated in more than 90% of patients when measured on 24-hour urine collections. Epinephrine, norepinephrine, and dopamine can be measured by liquid chromatography, which further aids in the diagnosis. Several separate determinations should be made because of the episodic hormone secretion

Table 15.4.
Pheochromocytoma Syndromes

Multiple endocrine neoplasia, type 2A
Multiple endocrine neoplasia, type 2B
von Hippel-Lindau disease
Neurofibromatosis
Carney's triad

found in these patients. Furthermore, patients taking medications such as methyldopa or mandelamine may have falsely high catecholamine levels.

In the past, provocative tests using an adrenal stimulator such as glucagon have been used. Although an occasional patient may still benefit from this procedure, it has largely been abandoned. Because glucagon may induce a hypertensive crisis, it should not be used in patients undergoing an abdominal CT scan to identify a suspected pheochromocytoma. Fortunately, motion artifact from bowel peristalsis is seldom a limiting factor in the currently used scanners.

Pheochromocytomas are usually benign, but approximately 13% demonstrate malignant behavior. Extraadrenal pheochromocytomas are more likely to be malignant than intraadrenal tumors.

The treatment of patients with pheochromocytoma is surgical resection. Biochemical confirmation of the diagnosis and accurate preoperative radiologic localization have made these operations much safer. Nevertheless, patients undergoing surgical resection must still receive adrenergic blockade before the induction of anesthesia as well as careful monitoring during the operation to treat any crises. Both an α-adrenergic blocker (phenoxybenzamine) as well as a β-blocker (propranolol) are advocated, while nitroprusside may be used to treat hypertensive episodes. This same regimen may be used in patients requiring invasive radiologic procedures such as arteriography, venography, or percutaneous biopsy.

Radiology

ULTRASOUND. Ultrasound may be used to localize an intraadrenal pheochromocytoma (Fig. 15.12), but also may identify ectopic tumors lying in the paraaortic area. Pheochromocytomas tend to be more echogenic than normal adrenal tissue, possibly owing to the hypervascularity they usually exhibit. By varying the angle of the transducer, ultrasound may be able to detect a tissue plane not seen with CT and may determine the organ of origin of a large upper quadrant mass. Ultrasound also is often helpful in children, in whom the relative lack of retroperitoneal fat makes CT evaluation difficult.

COMPUTED TOMOGRAPHY. As with tumors of the adrenal cortex, CT is the primary localizing examination in patients with an intraadrenal pheochromocytoma (Fig. 15.12). Most intraadrenal pheochromocytomas are detected, and a sensitivity of 95% can be expected. Care must be taken when examining patients with the MEN syndrome, however, because the tumors in these patients often are smaller (Fig. 15.13). Because most extraadrenal pheochromocytomas (paragangliomas) lie in the paraaortic region, they also are demonstrated on an abdominal CT examination (Fig. 15.14).

MAGNETIC RESONANCE IMAGING. Pheochromocytomas

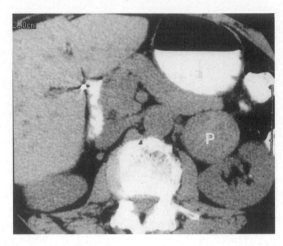

Figure 15.12. Pheochromocytoma. A 4-cm left adrenal pheochromocytoma (*P*) is seen on this unenhanced computed tomography examination.

are both identified and characterized by MRI. T1-weighted sequences are used to identify the mass, while the high signal intensity seen on T2-weighted images helps to characterize it as a pheochromocytoma (Fig. 15.15). This intense T2-weighted signal helps to distinguish a pheochromocytoma from an adrenal adenoma.

Magnetic resonance imaging can identify pheochromocytomas in areas that may be a problem for CT. Tumors in the wall of the urinary bladder or the paracardiac region often are problematic on CT, but are clearly recognized with MRI. Postoperative patients in whom retroperitoneal tissue planes are disrupted may be difficult to examine with CT.

NUCLEAR MEDICINE. Metaiodobenzylguanidine (MIBG) is an analogue of guanethidine that is taken up by adren-

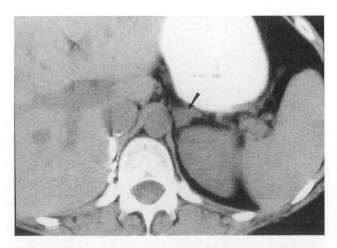

Figure 15.13. Multiple endocrine neoplasia (MEN) syndrome. This patient with a history of medullary carcinoma of the thyroid, had a right pheochromocytoma removed (*surgical clips*) 2 years earlier. A small left adrenal mass (*arrow*) is detected on this unenhanced computed tomography scan.

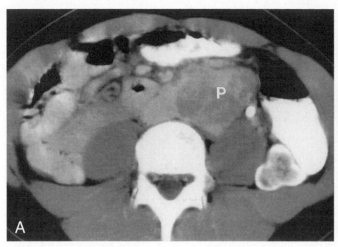

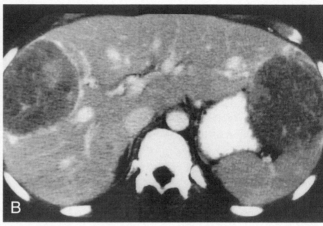

Figure 15.14.   Paraganglioma. **A,** A heterogeneous mass (*P*) in the left paraaortic region on an enhanced computed tomography examination was found to be an extraadrenal pheochromocytoma. **B,** Hepatic metastases demonstrate its malignant nature.

ergic tissue. When MIBG is labeled with a radionuclide, pheochromocytomas can be localized (Fig. 15.16).

The overall accuracy of MIBG is similar to that of CT and MRI; however, scintigraphy has several advantages. With a single injection of radionuclide, the entire body can be scanned. This is particularly helpful for ectopic tumors or for the detection of metastatic deposits. MIBG also can detect medullary hyperplasia, which is seen in patients with MEN syndromes and may be an early manifestation of a developing pheochromocytoma.

However, MIBG is not widely used to detect or localize pheochromocytomas. ^{131}I-MIBG has recently gained approval of the Food and Drug Administration (FDA), but is not universally available. Furthermore, the spatial resolution is poor, and studies require 1 to 3 days to complete.

Neuroblastoma

Neuroblastomas are primitive tumors that arise from sympathetic nervous system tissue (Table 15.5). They may occur in the neck, thorax, abdomen, and pelvis, but no

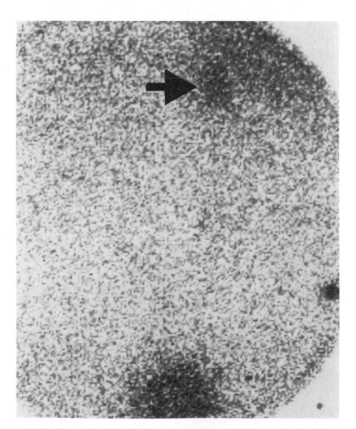

Figure 15.16.   Pheochromocytoma. Increased radionuclide activity in the region of the right adrenal gland (*arrow*) on this metaiodobenzylguanidine (MIBG) scan helps to localize a pheochromocytoma.

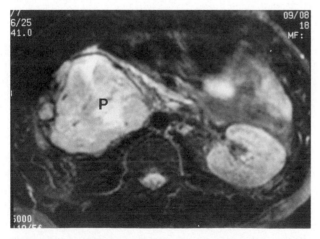

Figure 15.15.   Pheochromocytoma. This fast spin-echo image demonstrates a large mass (*P*) in the right paracaval region. The high signal intensity is typical of pheochromocytomas.

definite primary site can be found in a significant minority of patients. The most common location is the adrenal gland, which accounts for approximately 35% of patients.

Neuroblastomas usually occur in young children. Approximately 25% of cases occur in the first year of life and as many as 60% occur by the age of 2 years.

Although neuroblastoma is the most common extracranial malignant tumor in childhood, its incidence is only 1 to 3 per 100,000 children per year. An increased incidence is seen in neurofibromatosis, and familial associations have been reported.

Some neuroblastomas spontaneously mature into benign ganglioneuromas. Histologically, neuroblastomas contain densely packed small round cells that may be difficult to differentiate from other tumors, such as Ewing's sarcoma, lymphoma, or rhabdomyosarcoma. Other tumors may contain more mature ganglion cells mixed with neuroblasts and are classified as ganglioneuroblastomas. A mature ganglioneuroma is benign, but careful evaluation of the entire tumor is necessary because there may be marked variation in different parts of the tumor.

The most common presentation of a child with a neuroblastoma is with an abdominal mass discovered by a parent. Other presenting symptoms include opsoclonus and myoclonus, paresis due to tumor extension through the neural foramina, Horner's syndrome, or bone pain due to metastatic disease. Most patients have elevated urinary catecholamines when measured as catechol excretion per milligram of creatinine. More than 50% of patients excrete high levels of VMA and up to 90% of patients have an elevation of VMA or homovanillic acid.

The staging system described by Evans and associates in 1971 is still the one most commonly used to stage neuroblastomas. Stage I tumor is confined to the organ of origin. In stage II, the tumor has grown outside the organ of origin but not across the midline. Regional lymph nodes may be involved, but must be on the same side as the tumor. Stage III tumors extend in continuity across the midline. Lymph node involvement may be bi-lateral. Patients with stage IV tumors have widespread disease involving the bony skeleton, distant lymph nodes, and distant organs. A variant of stage IV, stage IV-s is attributed to patients whose primary tumor would be considered stage I or II, but in whom there is limited metastatic disease to the liver, skin, or bone marrow. These patients are usually infants younger than 1 year of age.

Radiology

UROGRAPHY. The plain abdominal radiograph may demonstrate a pattern of stippled calcification that helps distinguish a neuroblastoma from a Wilms' tumor. Evidence of bone metastases or widened neural foramina also may be detected with plain radiographs.

Excretory urography may be useful to distinguish an extraadrenal tumor from an intrarenal Wilms' tumor. The kidney often is displaced inferiorly by an adrenal neuroblastoma. The contralateral kidney must also be evaluated, because the adjacent kidney may be compromised or removed as the neuroblastoma is excised.

Ultrasound

Sonography and CT have replaced urography as the primary modalities for evaluating a patient with a suspected neuroblastoma. Ultrasound is especially valuable in small children, who have a paucity of retroperitoneal fat. A mass of heterogeneous echogenicity is usually seen in the region of the adrenal gland (Fig. 15.17). The margins are poorly defined, and a capsule is not present. A sonographic "lobule" of homogeneous increased echogenicity consisting of an aggregate of cells separated from the surrounding tumor by collagen deposition has been described in a minority of patients. Ultrasound also can be used to detect involvement of adjacent vascular structures, such as the inferior vena cava.

Computed Tomography

Unenhanced CT scans are more sensitive than plain radiographs in detecting the mottled calcification commonly seen in neuroblastoma (Fig. 15.18). Intravenous contrast medium is commonly used to distinguish a renal from an extrarenal mass (Fig. 15.19). Computed tomography may be used to identify neuroblastomas in the abdomen, pelvis, or chest. Involvement of adjacent organs or retroperitoneal lymph nodes can be detected.

Ganglioneuroblastomas and ganglioneuromas are differentiated from neuroblastomas by a greater degree of cellular maturation. Ganglioneuroblastomas are malignant tumors, but may be partially or totally encapsulated. Ganglioneuromas are benign tumors with an intact capsule. They are seen as a well-defined, homogenous retroperitoneal mass (Fig. 15.20).

Table 15.5.
Neuroblastoma Staging

Stage	Disease Extent
I	Confined to organ of origin
II	Contiguous extension beyond organ of origin but not beyond midline. Regional ipsilateral lymph nodes may be involved
III	Contiguous extension beyond midline. Regional lymph nodes may be involved bilaterally
IV	Remote disease involving skeleton, parenchymatous organs, soft tissues, or distant lymph nodes
IVs	Stage I or II disease and remote disease confined to one or more of the following sites: liver, skin, or bone marrow

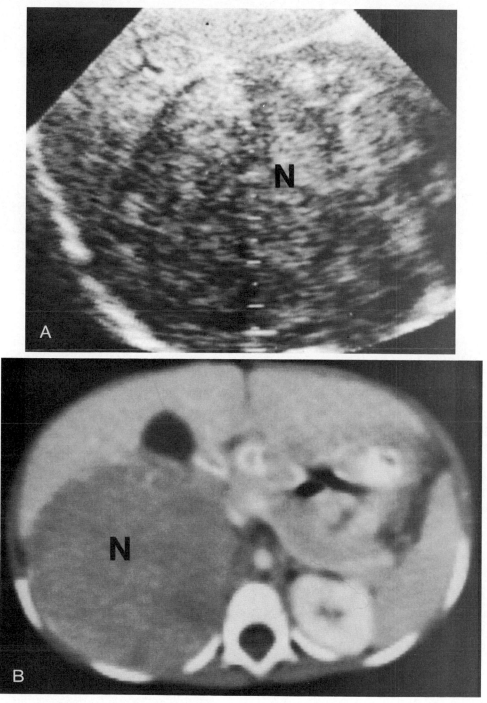

Figure 15.17. Neuroblastoma. **A,** A large neuroblastoma (*N*) with heterogeneous echogenicity is defined by ultrasound. **B,** Although there is very little retroperitoneal fat, the tumor (*N*) is easily detected on computed tomography because of its large size.

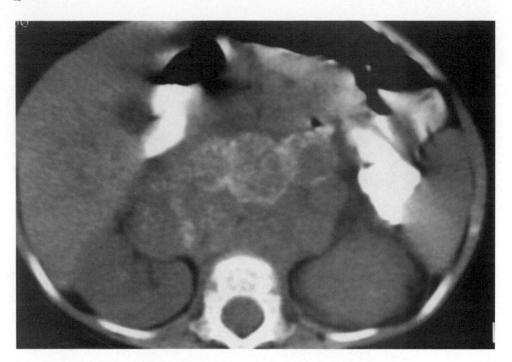

Figure 15.18. Neuroblastoma. Calcification is seen in this malignant tumor involving paraaoric lymph nodes.

Magnetic Resonance Imaging

Magnetic resonance imaging is a useful study in children with neuroblastoma if the child is sedated and motion artifact is reduced or eliminated. The tumor has a signal intensity slightly lower than liver or renal cortex on T1-weighted images. On T2-weighted sequences, the intensity is higher than liver but similar to kidney (Fig. 15.21).

The ability to scan in any plane is especially helpful. Using the coronal plane and T1-weighted sequences, the neuroblastoma can be distinguished from the kidney and liver. T2-weighted images have superior contrast differentiation and are used in differentiating the extent of the tumor from adjacent normal tissue.

Nuclear Medicine

Because neuroblastomas commonly metastasize to bone, radionuclide bone scans are useful. In addition, many primary tumors demonstrate uptake of a skeletal tracer. MIBG is sensitive for the detection of neuroblastomas and may be useful in confirming neuroblastoma as the etiology of an abdominal mass.

Treatment

Surgical excision is indicated in patients with stage I or II disease, as well as stage II disease originating in the mediastinum. In patients with more advanced disease, chemotherapy is used first to reduce the size of the primary tumor and control metastases. Irradiation also may be used in combination with chemotherapy. Unfortunately the overall survival remains less than 50%.

NONFUNCTIONAL DISEASES

Adenoma

Benign, nonhyperfunctioning adrenal adenomas are commonly encountered on abdominal CT examinations. Hedeland and colleagues found adrenal adenomas in 8.7% of 739 consecutive postmortem examinations, whereas Commons and Callaway (1948) found adenomas greater than 3 mm in diameter in 2.86% of 7437 autopsies. Both studies found more adenomas among older patients and those with diabetes or hypertension.

Adenomas consist of cords of clear cells separated by fibrovascular trabeculae. It is often difficult to distinguish a benign adenoma from an adrenal cortical carcinoma. Although carcinomas are more likely to have hemorrhage, necrosis, pleomorphism, and giant cells, these features also may be seen in benign adenomas.

Nonhyperfunctioning adenomas are almost always detected as an incidental finding. Occasionally, they are large enough to cause pain or compress adjacent structures. Rarely does hemorrhage into an adenoma occur.

Radiology

Calcification may rarely be seen on an abdominal radiograph, and large adenomas may displace the ipsilateral kidney. Ultrasound can detect adrenal adenomas when they reach 2 to 3 cm in diameter. Furthermore, ul-

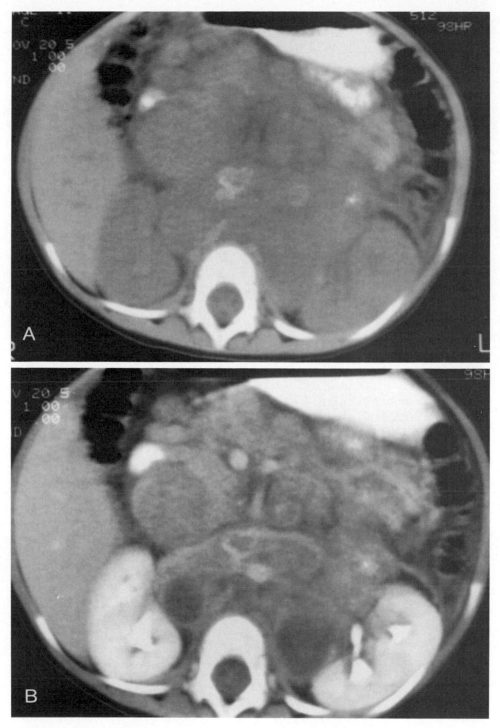

Figure 15.19. Neuroblastoma. **A,** Paraaortic masses are present, but are difficult to distinguish on an unenhanced computed tomography examination. **B,** After contrast injection the kidneys and large retroperitoneal vessels are clearly defined.

trasound may be helpful in distinguishing a solid tumor from a cyst.

Most adenomas are detected during a CT examination of the upper abdomen. Typically, the nonhyperfunctioning adenoma is a well-defined, rounded, homogeneous mass (Fig. 15.22). Calcification is uncommon and central necrosis or hemorrhage is rare. The density of an adrenal adenoma is lower than other soft tissue masses because of the higher lipid content found in these tumors. The presence of lipid can be used to

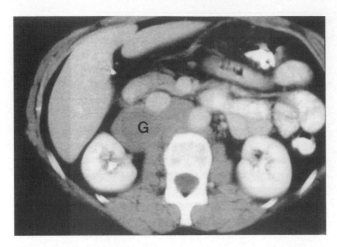

Figure 15.20. Ganglioneuroma. This retroperitoneal mass (*G*) was detected as an incidental finding on an enhanced computed tomography examination.

distinguish benign adenomas from adrenal metastases, because metastases do not contain lipid. In the series reported by Korobkin and colleagues, the mean attenuation for nonhyperfunctioning adrenal adenomas on unenhanced CT scans (3 Hounsfield units [HU]) was significantly lower than for nonadenomas (32 HU). In this series, none of the nonadenomas had an attenuation coefficient less than 18 HU. Other authors have suggested using a threshold of 10 HU to exclude metastases. Lesions with a density below this threshold value could be confidently diagnosed as a benign adenoma, while those whose density is greater must undergo per-

cutaneous biopsy to confirm the presence of metastatic disease.

Magnetic resonance imaging can detect adrenal masses almost as well as CT. Nonhyperfunctioning adenomas seem to be less intense than adenomas secreting aldosterone or cortisol. However, this is seldom a clinical problem, because adrenal hyperfunction can be assessed by measuring serum hormone levels.

Magnetic resonance imaging also may be useful in distinguishing a nonhyperfunctioning adrenal adenoma from metastatic tumor. Metastases typically have a higher signal intensity on T2-weighted sequences (Fig. 15.23). Several methods have been employed to demonstrate this difference. Because the normal adrenal gland is small, it is difficult to measure the signal from normal adrenal cortex. Thus, a ratio of the intensity of the adrenal tumor and adjacent fat, muscle, or liver have been employed. Data from several studies suggest there are cutoff points below which all lesions are adenomas and above which all lesions are metastases. However, this leaves an overlap group which includes 21 to 31% of cases. Others have used calculated T2 values to distinguish benign from malignant masses, but similar overlap has been observed.

Krestin and coworkers have demonstrated that gadolinium enhancement may be used to distinguish adenomas from metastases on fast gradient-recalled echo images. Using dynamic perfusion studies after intravenous administration of gadolinium-DTPA, they demonstrated that metastases enhanced to a significantly higher signal intensity than adenomas. Furthermore, the adenomas had much faster washout of this contrast medium.

Figure 15.21. Neuroblastoma. A large right neuroblastoma (*N*) is easily seen on this T2-weighted (TR = 2000, TE = 35) magnetic resonance image.

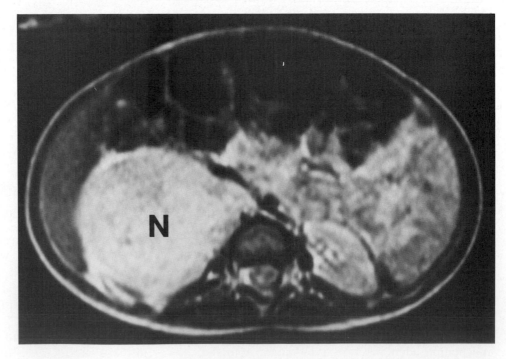

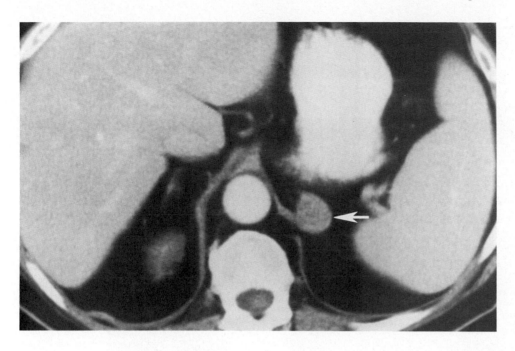

Figure 15.22. Benign adenoma. A left adrenal mass (*arrow*) was found to be a nonhyperfunctioning adenoma at autopsy.

The most accurate of the MR techniques for distinguishing an adenoma from a metastasis is chemical shift imaging. Because protons in water precess at different frequencies than those in triglyceride when exposed to a magnetic field, even small quantities of lipid can be detected (Fig. 15.24). Chemical shift imaging was used to demonstrate the presence of lipid in 26 of 27 adenomas and in none of 12 metastases studied by Mitchell and associates in 1992. These excellent results have been confirmed by several investigators.

Radionuclide imaging with a cortical labeling agent such as NP59 also may be useful. Studies with NP59 show that these nonhyperfunctioning adenomas accumulate the radiopharmaceutical. Thus, radionuclide uptake indicates a benign lesion. Absence of radionuclide activity suggests a metastatic tumor, but also is consistent with an adrenal cyst or hematoma.

Nuclear medicine techniques also can take advantage of differences in metabolic activity. Since malignant cells use more glucose than benign tissue, adrenal metastases would be expected to have increased uptake of the radiotracer 2-[fluorine-18]-fluoro-2-deoxy-D-glucose (FDG) compared with adenomas. Boland and colleagues recently demonstrated that positron emission tomography (PET) with FDG accurately categorized 14 malignant and 10 benign adrenal masses.

Carcinoma

Primary adrenal cortical carcinoma is an uncommon malignancy that occurs with a frequency of approximately 1 case per 1 million population. Men and women are affected equally, but functional tumors are more common among female patients. Although the median age at presentation is the fifth decade, patients ranging from 1 to 80 years of age have been reported.

Adrenal carcinomas occur more commonly in the left gland than in the right, and up to 10% may be bilateral. They are usually quite large at presentation, although a tumor as small as 1 cm has been reported. They have a nodular surface and are incompletely encapsulated. Central tumor necrosis and hemorrhage are common.

The microscopic appearance is variable. Some carcinomas are well differentiated such that differentiation from an adenoma is difficult. In more frankly malignant lesions, highly abnormal cells with giant nuclei, multinucleation, and atypical mitoses are found.

The most common presentation of patients with an adrenal carcinoma is abdominal pain or a palpable mass. Approximately 50% of these tumors are functional and may be detected by the manifestations of excess hormone production. Cushing's syndrome is most frequent, followed by virilization and feminization. Hyperaldosteronism is rarely caused by carcinoma.

Many of the "nonfunctional" carcinomas may produce hormones that do not cause a clinical syndrome. This can be demonstrated by measurement of urinary 17-ketosteroid levels.

Surgical excision is the only effective therapy. Chemotherapy with ortho para DDD (OP' DDD) and radiation therapy may be given for palliation, but they do not improve survival.

Radiology

A large upper abdominal mass may be detected on plain abdominal radiographs. Although calcification is common, it is much easier to detect on CT than on a

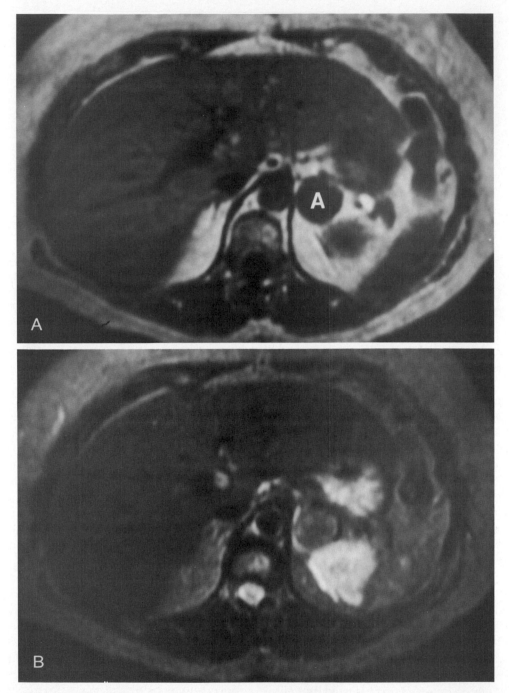

Figure 15.23. Benign adenoma. **A,** The left adrenal mass (*A*) is well defined on T1-weighted (TR = 500, TE = 25) images. **B,** The relatively low signal intensity on T2-weighted (TR = 2500, TE = 80) images distinguishes this benign tumor from an adrenal metastasis.

plain film. The urogram is usually abnormal. The ipsilateral kidney is displaced inferolaterally by the adrenal mass. Because the adrenal gland lies medial to the upper pole of the kidney, the renal axis is more vertical than normal. The kidney itself is normal, unless there is involvement of the left renal vein or direct extension into the kidney.

Ultrasound can demonstrate a suprarenal mass. Smaller lesions, up to 6 cm, often are homogeneous, whereas larger tumors have a heterogeneous texture with scattered echopenic areas representing tumor necrosis or hemorrhage. The tumors are characteristically well defined. Venous extension may occasionally be demonstrated.

The typical CT appearance of adrenal carcinoma is a

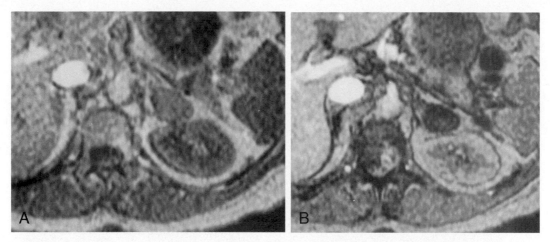

Figure 15.24.   Benign adenoma. **A,** An in-phase gradient-recalled echo (GRE) image shows a left adrenal mass that is isointense to paraspinal muscles. **B,** The mass becomes hypointense to the paraspinal muscles on opposed-phase GRE images. (From *Radiology* 197:411–418, 1995.)

large mass with central areas of low attenuation representing tumor necrosis (Fig. 15.25). Calcification is seen in approximately 30% of cases. Evidence of hepatic or regional lymph node metastases also may be seen on CT. Extension of tumor into the left renal vein or inferior vena cava may be detected by CT. If a bolus technique is used for contrast injection, the CT scan may define the extent of tumor thrombus. If this delineation is not clear, MRI may be needed.

The most difficult area for CT staging of adrenal carcinoma has been the detection of direct hepatic extension. If a fat plane exists between the tumor and the liver, there is no hepatic involvement. However, if there is no fat plane, it is impossible to predict the presence or absence of liver invasion.

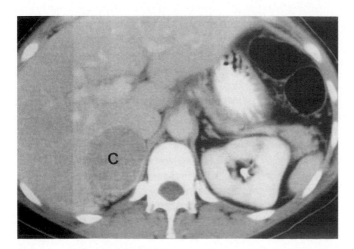

Figure 15.25.   Carcinoma. A heterogeneous 6-cm right adrenal mass (*C*) is seen on an enhanced computed tomography examination.

Arteriography is only infrequently needed for the evaluation of patients with suspected adrenal carcinoma. In patients with a huge mass in the region of the adrenal gland, it may be difficult to determine the tissue of origin. The adrenal gland may not be identified due to compression by the huge mass and fat planes no longer separate it from adjacent organs such as the kidney and liver. Selective arteriography can identify the primary vascular supply and determine the organ of origin of the mass. Selective renal, inferior phrenic, and celiac or hepatic artery injections should be performed. If possible, selective injection of the middle adrenal artery may also be helpful.

Adrenocortical carcinomas are typically hypovascular with large areas of central necrosis. The most vascular portion of the tumor is usually the periphery and the inferior phrenic artery provides the majority of the tumor vessels (Fig. 15.26).

The primary value of venography is delineation of intravenous tumor extension. However, dynamic bolus CT can usually detect and define caval extension. If this is inadequate such as patients in whom there is a contraindication to intravascular contrast media, MR can be performed.

MRI is often used to evaluate a suspected adrenal carcinoma. The high signal intensity on T2-weighted images further supports the malignant diagnosis (Fig. 15.27). The sagittal projection may be helpful in determining whether or not there is hepatic invasion. Venous extension can also be detected. Gradient echo techniques are most useful for this purpose.

Radionuclide examinations are seldom used for adrenal carcinoma. A cortical agent such as NP59 can detect the large tumor mass but does not add additional information.

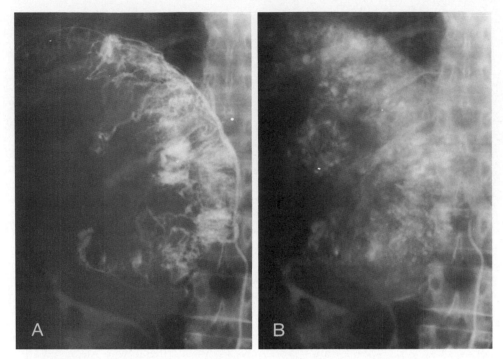

Figure 15.26. Adrenal carcinoma. **A** and **B,** A selective right inferior phrenic arteriogram demonstrates the peripheral vascularity of this adrenal carcinoma. Note the lateral displacement of the upper pole of the right kidney.

Myelolipoma

A *Myelolipoma* is a benign tumor comprised of mature adipose cells and hematopoetic tissue. The gross appearance resembles fatty tissue but may contain patchy red areas of blood-forming cells. It is an uncommon lesion with only approximately 250 cases reported in the literature.

The tumors are functionally inactive and are usually detected as an incidental finding. Occasionally large tumors may cause pain or present with displacement of adjacent organs. Retroperitoneal hemorrhage has been reported. The most common age at detection is the sixth decade. There is no sex predilection, and both glands are equally affected. Although some reports suggest an association with obesity, hypertension, or chronic illness, this probably reflects the patients being studied.

Radiology

The plain radiograph is not helpful except in large tumors where the low-density fatty mass may be detected. Calcification may be present but is nonspecific. Similarly, the excretory urogram will be normal unless the kidney is displaced by the adrenal mass.

Ultrasound reveals a highly echogenic mass (Fig. 15.28). If the tumor is 4 cm or larger, a propagation speed artifact may be present. This appearance is suggestive of a myelolipoma, however, it cannot be clearly distinguished from a retroperitoneal lipoma or liposarcoma. If the tumor is small or the patient has abundant retroperitoneal fat, the myelolipoma may be difficult to distinguish from perirenal fat.

The most definitive radiographic examination is CT (Fig. 15.29). A fatty adrenal mass is virtually diagnostic of a myelolipoma. However, two cases of adrenocortical carcinoma and one case of metastatic adenocarcinoma containing fat have been documented. Although not yet reported, an adrenal lipoma or liposarcoma could mimic this appearance. Unenhanced scans are usually adequate to make the diagnosis. Masking of the fat density of a myelolipoma by intravenous contrast injection may occur. MRI can also image myelolipomas but does not add information not gained with CT.

Treatment of myelolipomas is usually conservative. The clear diagnosis of this benign lesion does not usually require further confirmation although diagnosis by fine-needle aspiration has been reported. Symptomatic lesions should be excised. Large asymptomatic lesions are sometimes removed to avoid potential complications such as retroperitoneal hemorrhage.

Hemorrhage

Adrenal hemorrhage may be spontaneous, traumatic, or related to anticoagulation. Spontaneous adrenal hemorrhage often occurs in patients with septicemia, hy-

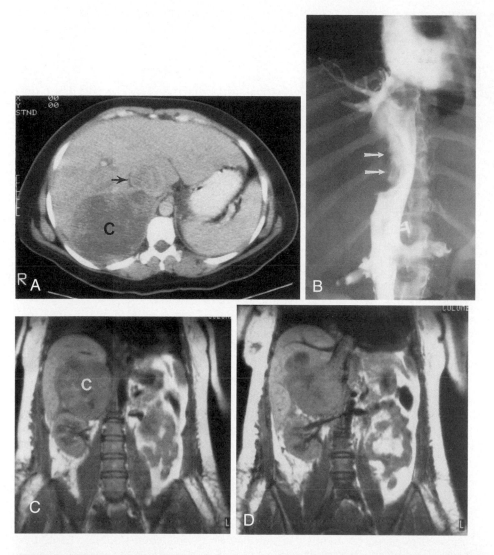

Figure 15.27. Adrenal carcinoma. **A,** A large right upper quadrant mass (*C*) is identified on this contrast-enhanced computed tomography examination. The enlarged, heterogeneous vena cava (*arrow*) is evidence of caval extension. **B,** Extension of the inferior vena cava is confirmed on cavography by a large tumor mass projecting into the vessel lumen (*arrows*). **C,** A magnetic resonance image in the coronal plane clearly shows a tissue plane between the mass (*C*) and the kidney. **D,** The same magnetic resonance exam demonstrates tumor extension into the inferior vena cava.

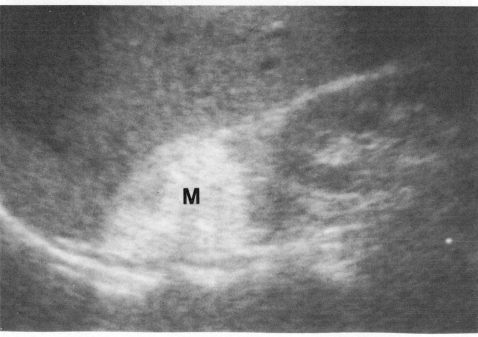

Figure 15.28. Myelolipoma. A highly echogenic adrenal mass (*M*) suggests a myelolipoma.

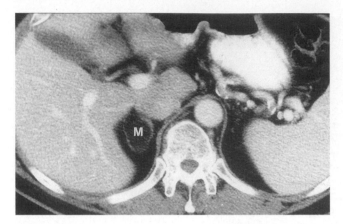

Figure 15.29. Myelolipoma. The right adrenal mass (*M*) is largely fat density.

pertension, renal vein thrombosis, or adrenal pathology, such as a tumor. It more commonly involves the right than the left adrenal gland.

Adrenal hemorrhage is more common in the newborn than in older children or adults. It may be due to the trauma of delivery, asphyxia, septicemia, or abnormal clotting factors. It is bilateral in only about 10% of cases. If the hemorrhage is large, a palpable mass, anemia, or prolonged jaundice may occur. Adrenal insufficiency is rare in the neonate. Hemorrhage can usually be distinguished from a tumor such as neuroblastoma and surgery avoided. Most adrenal hematomas will be resorbed, but some may liquify and persist as an adrenal pseudocyst.

When adrenal hemorrhage occurs in the older child or adult, it is often due to trauma or associated with systemic illness or anticoagulation. It has been seen with hypertension, septicemia, renal vein thrombosis, seizures, surgery, or treatment with ACTH, insulin, or corticosteroids. When related to anticoagulation therapy, it usually occurs during the first 3 weeks of therapy. However, it is not due to excessive anticoagulation, as associated hemorrhage does not occur in other areas.

Patients with the primary antiphospholipid syndrome (PAPS) have an increased frequency of thrombotic events, including deep venous thrombosis and strokes. Adrenal hemorrhage may occur in these patients, presumably due to adrenal vein thrombosis.

Adrenal hemorrhage may occur in up to 25% of severely traumatized patients and approximately 20% of cases are bilateral. The right adrenal gland is involved much more commonly than the left. This may be due to an acute rise in venous pressure, which is more directly transmitted to the right adrenal gland since the right adrenal vein enters the inferior vena cava directly. The hematoma is usually found in the adrenal medulla with stretching of the surrounding cortex.

Most adrenal hemorrhage is clinically silent. Only rarely is the endocrine function of the gland sufficiently impaired to cause adrenal insufficiency as both glands must be affected for this to occur.

Radiology

A large hematoma may be seen as a soft tissue mass on the plain radiograph, and the ipsilateral kidney may be displaced downward. The axis of the kidney becomes more vertical and the upper pole may even be lateral to the lower pole.

An adrenal mass can usually be seen with ultrasound (Fig. 15.30). The echogenicity varies with the state of the hematoma and may be hypoechoic, mixed, or moderately echogenic.

The most reliable method of identifying adrenal hemorrhage is CT (Fig. 15.31). Initially the hematoma has a high density, 50 to 90 HU. Follow-up studies usually show resorption of the hematoma and a gradual decrease in density to near water.

Magnetic resonance imaging of adrenal hemorrhage has also been reported. The MR appearance reflects the evolution from acute to chronic stages with hemoglobin breakdown. A heterogeneous signal intensity is seen on T1- and T2-weighted images of acute hemorrhage. There is no enhancement after administration of gadolinium-DTPA, but a peripheral rim may enhance if a vascular fibrous capsule has formed.

Cysts

Adrenal cysts are uncommon lesions that may occur at any age. They involve the right and left adrenal glands equally, but have a 3:1 female predilection.

Most adrenal cysts are asymptomatic and are found either at autopsy or as incidental findings. Large cysts may cause dull pain or symptoms because of compression on the stomach or duodenum.

There are several recognized etiologies of adrenal cysts. Endothelial cysts are the most common, accounting for approximately 45% of all adrenal cysts. They have an endothelial lining and may be lymphatic or angiomatous in origin. Lymphangiomatous cysts are more common and probably develop from blockage of a lymph duct.

Epithelial cysts are quite uncommon, because they comprise only 9% of adrenal cysts. They have a cylindrical epithelium and include cystic adenomas.

Parasitic cysts are the least common variety, comprising only 7% of the total. They are usually echinococcal in origin and are associated with widespread disease.

Pseudocysts are the second most common variety, as they comprise 39% of adrenal cysts. They are probably caused by adrenal hemorrhage into a normal or abnormal gland. The lining is not covered by epithelium.

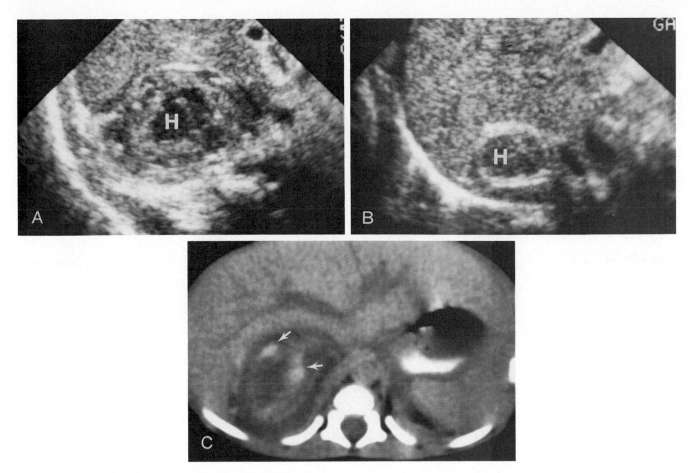

Figure 15.30.   Adrenal hemorrhage. **A,** A large mass (*H*) of mixed echogenicity is seen in the right adrenal gland. **B,** Six weeks later, the hematoma (*H*) is much smaller as it has started to resorb. **C,** Calcification (*arrows*) can be seen in the hematoma on computed tomography. (Courtesy of Kate Feinstein, M.D.)

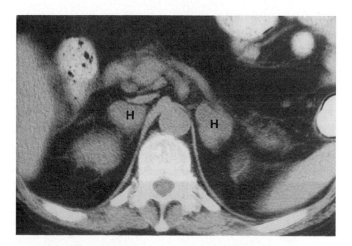

Figure 15.31.   Adrenal hemorrhage. Bilateral adrenal masses representing hemorrhage (*H*) are seen in this patient with meningococcemia and disseminated intravascular coagulopathy.

Pseudocysts are most commonly detected radiographically, because they tend to be larger than endothelial cysts.

Radiology

The abdominal radiograph will be revealing only if the cyst is calcified or very large. When present, calcification is curvilinear in the cyst wall. Urography is useful to exclude a renal origin.

Ultrasound demonstrates a cystic suprarenal mass (Fig. 15.32). Unlike renal cysts, adrenal cysts often exhibit a thick wall. Pseudocysts also may demonstrate internal septations. If a soft tissue mass–like component is present, surgery may be required to exclude a neoplasm.

Similar findings are detected with CT (Fig. 15.33). The density of the fluid can be measured, and calcification is easier to detect with CT than with ultrasound. However, it may still be difficult to exclude malignancy.

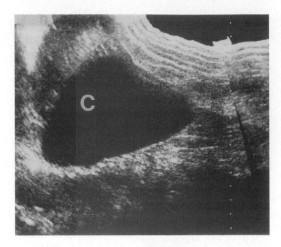

Figure 15.32. Adrenal cyst. Ultrasound demonstrates a huge cystic mass (*C*) in the left upper quadrant.

Cyst aspiration can be helpful if the fluid is clear and the cytology is benign.

Hemangioma

Adrenal hemangioma is a rare tumor of the adrenal cortex. Pathologically, adrenal hemangiomas are similar to hemangiomas of other organs. The vessels are lined with a vascular endothelium, and they may undergo degenerative changes including thrombosis, hemorrhage, and necrosis. They range in diameter from 2 to 22 cm. Patients have ranged from 25 to 79 years years of age. The tumors more often involve the right adrenal gland and show a female preponderance. None of the hemangiomas reported have shown evidence of hyperfunction, although adrenal insufficiency has been seen.

Most patients are asymptomatic, and the tumor is found at autopsy or during evaluation for another process. However, a dull pain and vague upper gastrointestinal tract symptoms may be present in very large lesions. An abdominal mass may be seen on a plain radiograph or may displace the ipsilateral kidney at urography. Calcification is common and may be phlebolith-like or may have an irregular stellate appearance.

Ultrasound demonstrates a complex mass and may reveal cystic areas. The CT appearance also depends on the tumor morphology. Typically, a large mass with a thick irregular wall and hypodense center is seen. There is patchy enhancement of the peripheral zone. Calcification is easily seen with CT.

The angiographic appearance of a hypovascular mass with contrast pooling and prolongation of the vascular stain is similar to hemangiomas in other organs. However, the radiographic findings often are not sufficiently characteristic, and surgical resection often is performed.

Metastases

The adrenal glands are a common site of metastatic disease. In a series of 1000 consecutive postmortem examinations of patients with an epithelial malignancy, Abrams and colleagues found 27% to have adrenal metastases. The incidence of adrenal metastases from the two most common primary tumors was even higher. Carcinoma of the breast metastasized to the adrenal glands in 54% of cases, whereas 36% of patients with lung carcinoma had adrenal metastases.

The radiographic appearance of adrenal metastases is not specific. They may be large or small, unilateral, or bilateral. A metastasis is a solid mass, and when less than 3 cm in diameter, is usually homogeneous (Fig. 15.34). Larger lesions may demonstrate central necrosis or areas of hemorrhage. Thus, an adrenal metastasis cannot be clearly distinguished from benign lesions such as adenomas, hematomas, pseudocysts, or inflammatory masses on the basis of morphology.

Nevertheless, several investigators have tried to identify criteria that would allow the diagnosis of a benign or malignant etiology based on CT criteria. Features that suggest a malignant lesion include a large size (>3 cm), poorly defined margins, invasion of adjacent structures, inhomogeneous attenuation, and thick irregular enhancing rim. Small ovoid lesions with a thin rim and homogeneous density are more likely to be benign.

Many patients have evidence of widespread metastatic disease involving the lungs, liver, and retroperitoneal lymph nodes, as well as the adrenal glands (Fig. 15.35). In these patients, whether or not the adrenal mass represents metastatic tumor is relatively unimportant. However, in some patients, an adrenal mass may be the only evidence of metastatic disease. This can be a critical distinction, because it may change the therapy from an attempt at cure to palliation.

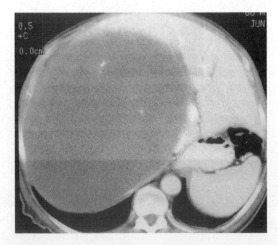

Figure 15.33. Adrenal pseudocyst. This huge right water-density adrenal mass contains calcification and several internal septations.

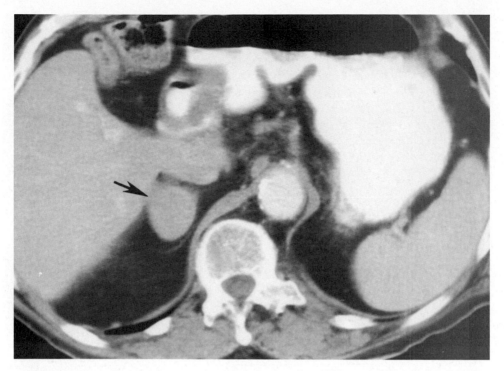

Figure 15.34.   Adrenal metastasis. This right adrenal metastasis (*arrow*) from an underlying hepatoma is small, well defined, and homogeneous.

Several radiographic procedures can be used in this setting.

The nature of an adrenal mass can be predicted with MRI. As discussed in the section on adenoma above, a calculated T2 relaxation time or signal intensity ratios of the adrenal mass to adjacent fat, muscle, or liver may be used to predict a benign or malignant nature of an adrenal mass (Fig. 15.36). However, this has met with only limited success. Similarly the use of gadolinium-DTPA to demonstrate the greater enhancement and

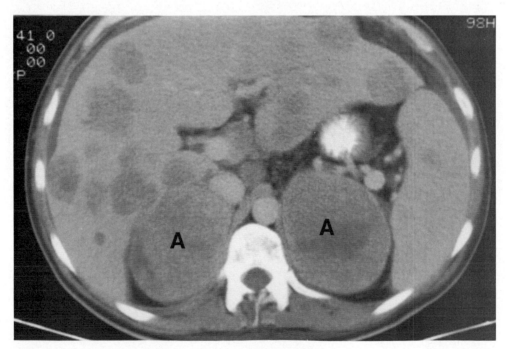

Figure 15.35.   Adrenal metastases. Widespread metastatic disease is evidenced by involvement of both adrenal glands (*A*) as well as liver, spleen, and lymph nodes.

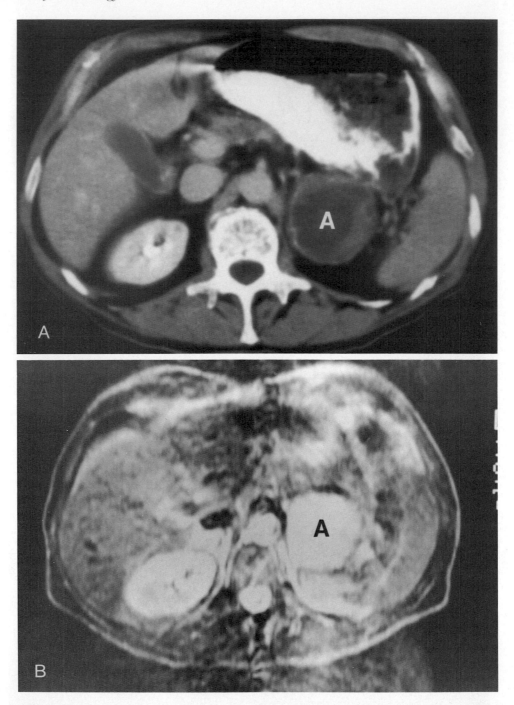

Figure 15.36. Adrenal metastasis. **A,** An enhanced computed tomography scan demonstrates an inhomogeneous right adrenal mass (*A*). **B,** The high signal intensity on a T2-weighted magnetic resonance image is consistent with metastasis.

more prolonged washout of metastases compared with adenomas has not proven to be sufficiently accurate to form the basis of clinical decisions.

The most useful MR technique is chemical shift imaging to detect lipids, which are found in adenomas but not in metastases. This same principle can be applied to CT, in which the density of adenomas is lower than that of metastases when viewed on unenhanced CT examinations. A common problem, however, is that oncologic patients are routinely scanned after intravenous contrast administration, and patients must return at a later time for an unenhanced scan.

Adrenal cortical scintigraphy also has been applied to this problem. Because benign adenomas absorb a cortical labeling agent such as NP59, they can be distinguished from nonadenomatous masses. Absence of uptake is not specific, however, as cysts, hematomas, and inflammatory masses will not take up the radionuclide. Thus, these benign masses cannot be distinguished from a metastasis with this examination.

Francis and coworkers applied NP59 scintigraphy to 28 oncologic patients who had a unilateral adrenal mass. Each of 14 patients with increased radionuclide uptake had an adenoma. None of the 11 patients with decreased uptake on the side of the mass had an adenoma; 9 had metastases and 2 had cysts. Uptake was indeterminate in three patients. Despite these encouraging results, adrenal scintigraphy is not used widely to distinguish benign from malignant adrenal masses.

Percutaneous aspiration biopsy is the most definitive method of confirming metastatic disease (Fig. 15.37). With experienced cytopathologists, the positive predictive value approaches 100%. A negative aspiration is not as diagnostic, because sampling error or an inadequate specimen may preclude a confident diagnosis. The overall accuracy reported for percutaneous adrenal biopsy ranges from 80 to 100%. The results vary with the patient population and the types of lesions aspirated. Positive results indicate malignancy. Negative aspirations can be repeated to increase the confidence that the lesion is benign.

Welch and colleagues recently reported their 10-year experience with 277 percutaneous adrenal biopsies. The overall accuracy improved from 85% in the first 5 years to 93% in the last 5 years. Their sensitivity was 81%, specificity 99%, positive predictive value 99%, and negative predictive value 80%. Thus, a positive biopsy is almost certainly metastatic tumor. A negative biopsy is much more reliable if normal adrenal cortical cells are present in the specimen.

Adrenal biopsy is an invasive procedure, and complications may occur. The most common complication is pneumothorax. These pneumothoraces are usually small and resolve spontaneously. Large or symptomatic pneumothoraces should be treated with a small chest tube that can be placed by the radiologist under fluoroscopic guidance. Tumor seeding of the needle tract and bacteremia are rare. When biopsy of the left adrenal gland is attempted from an anterior approach, pancreatitis may occur and can be a serious complication. Thus, the pancreas should be avoided if possible. Many patients will have a small amount of bleeding but this is seldom symptomatic. Welch and colleagues reported complications in 8 (2.8%) of their 277 adrenal biopsies.

The most worrisome complication of percutaneous needle biopsy of an adrenal mass is precipitation of a hypertensive crisis by a pheochromocytoma. This complication may be fatal despite regaining control of the blood pressure. Screening catecholamines may be useful in hypertensive patients, but may not be elevated in a nonfunctioning pheochromocytoma.

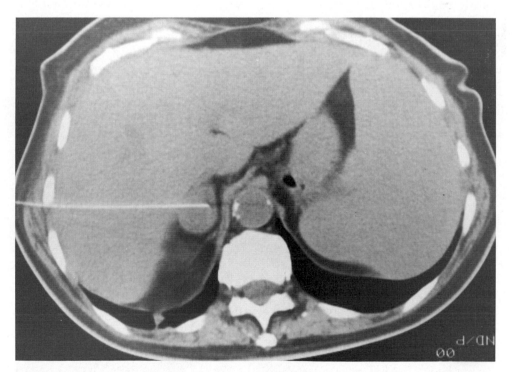

Figure 15.37.   Adrenal biopsy. Computed tomography is the most useful modality for directing percutaneous adrenal biopsies, particularly for small tumors. (From Dunnick NR: The adrenal gland. In Tavaras JM, Ferrucci JT (eds): *Radiology: Diagnosis, Imaging, Intervention.* Philadelphia: JB Lippincott, 1991.)

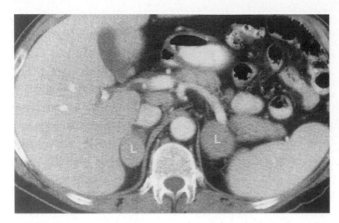

Figure 15.38. Lymphoma. The bilateral homogeneous adrenal masses (*L*) are consistent with lymphoma.

Lymphoma

Involvement of the adrenal gland by malignant lymphoma is more common in patients with non-Hodgkin's lymphoma than in those with Hodgkin's disease. Most patients have a diffuse rather than a nodular form of lymphoma. In a review of 173 patients with non-Hodgkin's lymphoma, Paling and Williamson, using CT, found evidence of adrenal involvement in seven (4%) patients during some portion of the course of their disease.

The adrenal glands are seldom an isolated site of disease, although other involvement may be distant. In most patients, however, retroperitoneal lymphoma also is present. Bilateral adrenal involvement is seen in approximately 50% of cases. Even with extensive disease, adrenal insufficiency is rare. The modalities in which adrenal lymphoma can be identified are ultrasound, CT, and MRI. On ultrasound, lymphoma appears as a well-defined, relatively echopenic homogeneous tissue mass. If extensive retroperitoneal disease is present, it may be difficult to identify the adrenal glands.

Computed tomography provides the best morphologic delineation (Fig. 15.38). The adrenal glands are enlarged with a rounded mass or more symmetric enlargement, preserving the basic glandular configuration. The tissue is usually homogeneous and demonstrates contrast enhancement. There is, however, no pathognomonic pattern to indicate lymphomatous involvement.

Pseudotumors

Retroperitoneal fat provides the contrast needed to demonstrate the adrenal glands. When there is a paucity of fat in the perirenal space, the adrenal glands are difficult to evaluate. Furthermore, large masses may compress the normal adrenal gland such that it is impossible to determine its organ of origin.

A number of abnormalities in the upper abdomen may simulate an adrenal mass. In addition to creating diagnostic confusion, percutaneous biopsy may be attempted. An appreciation of some of the etiologies of an adrenal pseudotumor may help avoid these pitfalls.

Lesions that may simulate an adrenal mass on either side include exophytic renal masses. A right-sided adrenal mass may be mimicked by a hepatic mass, interposition of the colon into the hepatorenal recess, or a dilated inferior vena cava.

Left-sided adrenal pseudotumors are more common. They include splenic lobulations, an accessory spleen, varices (Fig. 15.39), tortuous splenic vessels, and a

Figure 15.39. Adrenal pseudotumor. Gastric varices (*V*) may mimic an adrenal mass but can be differentiated by their serpiginous configuration and vascular enhancement.

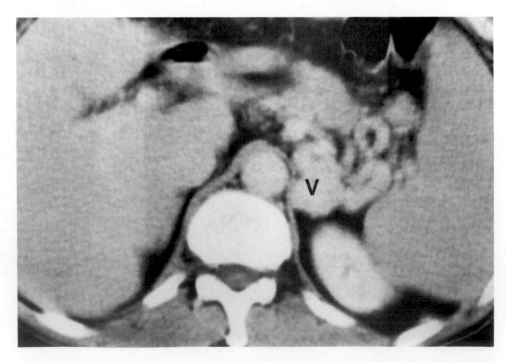

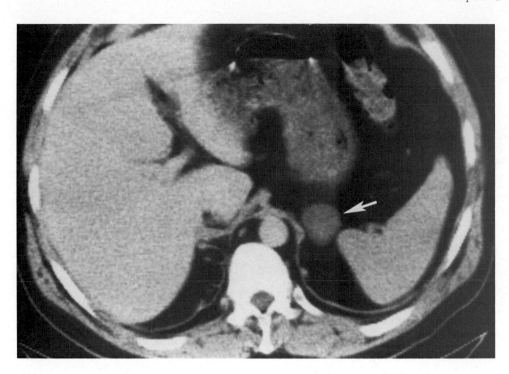

Figure 15.40. Pseudotumor. A mass (*arrow*) is seen in the region of the left adrenal gland. Subsequent barium study demonstrated this to be a gastric diverticulum.

splenic artery aneurysm. The tail of the pancreas may extend to the adrenal area and mimic a left adrenal lesion. While the stomach should be clearly distinguished by oral contrast medium, a gastric diverticulum may present a diagnostic problem (Fig. 15.40).

Careful attention to the adrenal glands and the use of oral contrast medium should distinguish most confusing structures. A bolus injection of intravenous contrast material should further delineate vascular structures. Repeat sections with narrow collimation also may help to elucidate the true nature of these lesions. If the diagnosis is still in doubt, however, an additional study such as ultrasound or MRI may be needed for a confident diagnosis.

SUGGESTED READING

Functional Diseases

Blevins LS, Wand GS: Primary aldosteronism: an endocrine perspective. *Radiology* 184:599, 1992.

Conn JW: Primary aldosteronism. *J Lab Clin Med* 45:661, 1955.

Doppman JL, Gill JR Jr: Hyperaldosteronism: sampling the adrenal veins. *Radiology* 198:309, 1996.

Doppman JL, Gill JR, Miller DL, et al.: Distinction between hyperaldosteronism due to bilateral hyperplasia and unilateral aldosteronoma: reliability of CT. *Radiology* 184:677, 1992.

Doppman JL, Miller DL, Dwyer AJ, et al.: Macronodular adrenal hyperplasia in Cushing disease. *Radiology* 166:347, 1988.

Doppman JL, Nieman L, Miller DL, et al.: Ectopic adrenocorticotropic hormone syndrome: localization studies in 28 patients. *Radiology* 172:115, 1989.

Dunnick NR: Adrenal imaging: current status. *AJR* 154:927, 1990.

Dunnick NR, Doppman JL, Mills SR, et al.: Preoperative diagnosis and localization of aldosteronomas by measurement of corticosteroids in adrenal venous blood. *Radiology* 133(2):331, 1979.

Dunnick NR, Leight GS, Roubidoux MA, et al.: CT in the diagnosis of primary aldosteronism: sensitivity in 29 patients. *AJR* 160:321, 1993.

Kenney PJ, Streeten DP, Anderson GH: Difficulties in the prospective diagnosis of functional adrenal diseases by CT. *Urol Radiol* 8:184, 1986.

Miyake H, Maeda H, Tashiro M, et al.: CT of adrenal tumors: frequency and clinical significance of low-attenuation lesions. *AJR* 152:1005, 1989.

Adrenal Insufficiency

Doppman JL, Gill JR, Nienhius AW, et al.: CT findings in Addison's disease. *J Comput Assist Tomogr* 6(4):757, 1982.

Eason RJ, Croxson MS, Perry MC, et al.: Addison's disease, adrenal autoantibodies and computerized adrenal tomography. *NZ Med J* 95(714):569, 1982.

Levine E: CT evaluation of active adrenal histoplasmosis. *Urol Radiol* 13:103, 1991.

Ling D, Korobkin M, Silverman PM, et al.: CT demonstration of bilateral adrenal hemorrhage. *AJR* 141:307, 1983.

Seidenwurm DJ, Elmer EB, Kaplan LM, et al.: Metastases to the adrenal glands and the development of Addison's disease. *Cancer* (Phila) 54:552, 1984.

Wilson DA, Muchmore HG, Tisdal RG, et al.: Histoplasmosis of the adrenal glands studied by CT. *Radiology* 150:779, 1984.

Pheochromocytoma

Carney JA, Sheps SG, Go VLW, et al.: The triad of gastric leiomyosarcoma, functioning extra-adrenal paraganglioma and pulmonary chondroma. *Medical Intelligence* 296:1517, 1977.

Cho KJ, Freier DT, McCormick TL, et al.: Adrenal medullary disease in multiple endocrine neoplasia type II. *AJR* 134:23, 1980.

Reinig JW, Doppman JL, Dwyer AJ, et al.: Adrenal masses differentiated by MR. *Radiology* 158:81, 1986.

Stefanaki A, Maris T, Gouliamos A, et al.: Characterization of pheochromocytomas using quantitative analysis of the parameter T2 of the mass (T2-QMRI). *Magma* 2:29, 1994.

Swensen SJ, Brown ML, Sheps SG, et al.: Use of ^{131}I-MIBG scintigraphy in the evaluation of suspected pheochromocytoma. *Mayo Clin Proc* 60:299, 1985.

van Gils APG, Falke THM, van Erkel AR, et al.: MR imaging and MIBG scintigraphy of pheochromocytomas and extraadrenal functioning paragangliomas. *RadioGraphics* 11:37, 1991.

Welch TJ, Sheedy PF, II, van Heerden JA, et al.: Pheochromocytoma: value of computed tomography. *Radiology* 148:501, 1983.

Whalen RK, Althausen AF, Daniels GH: Extra-adrenal pheochromocytoma. *J Urol* 147:1, 1992.

Neuroblastoma

Amundson GM, Trevenen CL, Mueller DL, et al.: Neuroblastoma: a specific sonographic tissue pattern. *AJR* 148:943, 1987.

Berdon WE, Ruzal-Shapiro C, Abramson SJ, et al.: The diagnosis of abdominal neuroblastoma: relative roles of ultrasonography, CT, and MRI. *Urol Radiol* 14:252, 1992.

Bissett GS III, Strife J, Kirks DR: Genitourinary tract. *In* Kirks DR (ed): *Practical Pediatric Imaging.* Boston, Little Brown & Co, 1991.

Bietrich RB, Kangarloo H, Lenarsky C, et al.: Neuroblastoma: the role of MR imaging. *AJR* 148:937, 1987.

Evans AE, D'Angio GJ, Randolph J: A proposed staging for children with neuroblastoma. *Cancer* 17:374, 1971.

Westra SJ, Zaninovic AC, Hall TR, et al.: Imaging of the adrenal gland in children. *RadioGraphics* 14:1323, 1994.

Adenoma

Berland LL, Koslin DB, Kenney PJ, et al.: Differentiation between small benign and malignant adrenal masses with dynamic incremented CT. *AJR* 151:95, 1988.

Bernardino ME: Management of the asymptomatic patient with a unilateral adrenal mass. *Radiology* 166:121, 1988.

Boland GW, Goldberg MA, Lee MJ, et al.: Indeterminate adrenal mass in patients with cancer: evaluation at PET with 2-[F-18]-fluoro-2-deoxy-D-glucose. *Radiology* 194:131, 1995.

Commons RR, Callaway CP: Adenomas of the adrenal cortex. *Arch Intern Med* 81:37, 1948.

Francis IR, Gross MD, Shapiro B, et al.: Integrated imaging of adrenal disease. *Radiology* 184:1, 1992.

Gross MD, Shapiro B, Francis IR, et al.: Scintigraphic evaluation of clinically silent adrenal masses. *J Nucl Med* 35:1145, 1994.

Hedeland H, Östberg G, Hökfelt B: On the prevalence of adrenocortical adenomas in an autopsy material in relation to hypertension and diabetes. *Acta Med Scand* 184:211, 1968.

Kloos RT, Gross MD, Shapiro B: Investigation of incidentally discovered, biochemically non-hypersecretory benign adrenal adenomas: a review of the current knowledge and areas for future investigation. *Internal Medicine* 2:9, 1994.

Korobkin M, Brodeur FJ, Yutzy GG, et al.: Differentiation of adrenal adenomas from nonadenomas using CT attenuation values. *AJR* 166:531, 1996.

Korobkin M, Lombardi TJ, Aisen AM, et al.: Characterization of adrenal masses with chemical shift and gadolinium-enhanced MR imaging. *Radiology* 197:411, 1995.

Krestin GP, Steinbrich W, Friedmann G: Adrenal masses: evaluation with fast gradient-echo MR imaging and Gd-DTPA-enhanced dynamic studies. *Radiology* 171:675, 1989.

McNicholas MMJ, Lee MJ, Mayo-Smith WW, et al.: An imaging algorithm for the differential diagnosis of adrenal adenomas and metastases. *AJR* 165:1453, 1995.

Mitchell DG, Crovello M, Matteucci T, et al.: Benign adrenocortical masses: diagnosis with chemical shift MR imaging. *Radiology* 185:345, 1992.

Outwater EK, Siegelman ES, Radecki PD, et al.: Distinction between benign and malignant adrenal masses: value of T1-weighted chemical-shift MR imaging. *AJR* 165:579, 1995.

van Erkel AR, van Gils APG, Lequin M: CT and MR distinction of adenomas and nonadenomas of the adrenal gland. *J Comput Assist Tomogr* 18:432, 1994.

Carcinoma

Bodie B, Novick AC, Pontes JE, et al.: The Cleveland Clinic experience with adrenal cortical carcinoma. *J Urol* 141:257, 1989.

Dunnick NR, Doppman JL, Geelhoed GW: Intravenous extension of endocrine tumors. *AJR* 135:471, 1980.

Dunnick NR, Heaston D, Halvorsen R, et al.: CT appearance of adrenal cortical carcinoma. *J Comput Assist Tomogr* 6(5):978, 1982.

Fishman EK, Deutch BM, Hartman DS, et al.: Primary adrenocortical carcinoma: CT evaluation with clinical correlation. *AJR* 148:531, 1987.

Hamper UM, Fishman EK, Hartman, DS, et al.: Primary adrenocortical carcinoma: sonographic evaluation with clinical and pathologic correlation in 26 patients. *AJR* 148:915, 1987.

Hutter AM, Kayhoe DE: Adrenal cortical carcinoma. *Am J Med* 41:572, 1966.

Smith SM, Patel SK, Turner DA, et al.: Magnetic resonance imaging of adrenal cortical carcinoma. *Urol Radiol* 11:1, 1989.

Myelolipoma

Cyran KM, Kenney PJ, Memel DS, Yacoub I: Adrenal myelolipoma. *AJR* 166:395, 1996.

Dieckmann KP, Hamm B, Pickartz H, et al.: Adrenal myelolipoma: clinical, radiologic and histologic features. *Urology* 29(1):1, 1987.

Gould JD, Mitty HA, Pertsemlidis D, et al.: Adrenal myelolipoma: diagnosis by fine-needle aspiration. *AJR* 148:921, 1987.

Greene KM, Brantly PN, Thompson WR: Adenocarcinoma metastatic to the adrenal gland stimulating myelolipoma: CT evaluation. *J Comput Assist Tomogr* 9(4):820, 1985.

Meaglia JP, Schmidt JD: Natural history of an adrenal myelolipoma. *J Urol* 147:1089, 1992.

Musante F, Derchi LE, Zappasodi F, et al.: Myelolipoma of the adrenal gland: sonographic and CT features. *AJR* 151:961, 1988.

Sato N, Watanabe Y, Saga T, et al.: Adrenocortical adenoma containing a fat component: CT and MR image evaluation. *Abdom Imaging* 20:489, 1995.

Hemorrhage

Bowen A, Kesler PJ, Newman, B, Hashide Y: Adrenal hemorrhage after liver transplantation. *Radiology* 176:85, 1990.

Hoeffel C, Legmann P, Luton JP, et al.: Spontaneous unilateral adrenal hemorrhage: computerized tomography and magnetic resonance imaging findings in 8 cases. *J Urol* 154:1647, 1995.

Khuri FJ, Alton DJ, Hardy BE, et al.: Adrenal hemorrhage in neonates: report of 5 cases and review of the literature. *J Urol* 124:684, 1980.

Ling D, Korobkin M, Silverman PM, et al.: CT demonstration of bilateral adrenal hemorrhage. *AJR* 141:307, 1983.

Murphy BJ, Casillas J, Yrizarry JM: Traumatic adrenal hemorrhage radiologic findings. *Radiology* 169:701, 1988.

Provenzale JM, Ortel TL, Nelson RC: Adrenal hemorrhage in patients with primary antiphospholipid syndrome: imaging findings. *AJR* 165:361, 1995.

Cysts

Cheema P, Cartagena R, Staubitz W: Adrenal cysts: diagnosis and treatment. *J Urol* 126:396, 1981.

Ghandur-Mnaymneh L, Slim M, Muakassa K: Adrenal cysts: pathogenesis and histological identification with a report of 6 cases. *J Urol* 122:87, 1979.

Johnson CD, Baker ME, Dunnick NR: CT demonstration of an adrenal pseudocyst. *J Comput Assist Tomogr* 9(4):817, 1985.

Sakamoto I, Nakahara N, Fukuda T, et al.: Atypical appearance of adrenal pseudocysts. *J Urol* 152:150, 1994.

Tung GA, Pfister RC, Papanicolaou N, Yoder IC: Adrenal cysts: imaging and percutaneous aspiration. *Radiology* 173:107, 1989.

Hemangioma

Derchi LE, Rapaccini GL, Banderali A, et al.: Ultrasound and CT findings in two cases of hemangioma of the adrenal gland. *J Comput Assist Tomogr* 13(4):659, 1989.

Salup R, Finegold R, Borochovitz D, et al.: Cavernous hemangioma of the adrenal gland. *J Urol* 147:110, 1992.

Metastases

Abrams HL, Spiro R, Goldstein N: Metastases in carcinoma: analysis of 1,000 autopsied cases. *Cancer* 3:74, 1950.

Baker ME, Blinder R, Spritzer C, et al.: MR evaluation of adrenal masses at 1.5 T. *AJR* 153:307, 1989.

Berland LL, Koslin DB, Kenney PJ, et al.: Differentiation between small benign and malignant adrenal masses with dynamic incremented CT. *AJR* 151:95, 1988.

Bernardino ME, Walther MM, Phillips VM, et al.: CT-guided adrenal biopsy: accuracy, safety and indications. *AJR* 144:67, 1985.

Bilbey JH, McLoughlin RF, Kurkjian PS, et al.: MR imaging of adrenal masses: value of chemical-shift imaging for distinguishing adenomas from other tumors. *AJR* 164:637, 1995.

Casola G, Nicolet V, vanSonnenberg E, et al.: Unsuspected pheochromocytoma: risk of blood-pressure alterations during percutaneous adrenal biopsy. *Radiology* 156:733, 1986.

Dunnick NR: CT and MRI of adrenal lesions. *Urol Radiol* 10:12, 1988.

Francis IR, Smid A, Gross MD, et al.: Adrenal masses in oncologic patients: functional and morphologic evaluation. *Radiology* 166:353, 1988.

Hussain S: Gantry angulation in CT-guided percutaneous adrenal biopsy. *AJR* 166:537, 1996.

Kane NM, Korobkin M, Francis IR, et al.: Percutaneous biopsy of left adrenal masses: prevalence of pancreatitis after anterior approach. *AJR* 157:777, 1991.

Koenker RM, Mueller PR, vanSonnenberg E: Interventional radiology of the adrenal glands. *Semin Roentgenol* 22(4):314, 1988.

Oliver TW Jr, Bernardino ME, Miller JI, et al.: Isolated adrenal masses in nonsmall-cell bronchogenic carcinoma. *Radiology* 153:217, 1984.

Pagani JJ: Non-small cell lung carcinoma adrenal metastases: computed tomography and percutaneous needle biopsy in their diagnosis. *Cancer* (Phila) 53:1058, 1984.

Reinig JW, Stutley JE, Leonhardt CM, et al.: Differentiation of adrenal masses with MR imaging: comparison of techniques. *Radiology* 192:41, 1994.

Schwartz LH, Panicek DM, Koutcher JA, et al.: Adrenal masses in patients with malignancy: prospective comparison of echoplanar, fast spin-echo, and chemical shift MR imaging. *Radiology* 197:421, 1995.

Silverman SG, Mueller PR, Pinkney LP, et al.: Predictive value of image-guided adrenal biopsy: analysis of results of 101 biopsies. *Radiology* 187:715, 1993.

Welch TJ, Sheedy PF, Stephens DH, et al.: Percutaneous adrenal biopsy: review of a 10-year experience. *Radiology* 193:341, 1994.

Whitney W, Dunnick NR: Biopsy techniques in uroradiology. *Radiology Rep* 2:302, 1990.

Lymphoma

Alvarez-Castells A, Pedraza S, Tallada N, et al.: CT of primary bilateral adrenal lymphoma. *J Comput Assist Tomogr* 17(3):408, 1993.

Paling MR, Williamson BRJ: Adrenal involvement in non-Hodgkin lymphoma. *AJR* 141:303, 1983.

Pseudotumors

Berliner L, Bosniak MA, Megibow A: Adrenal pseudotumors on computed tomography. *J Comput Assist Tomogr* 6(2):281, 1982.

16

The Ureter

The ureter is a thin-walled muscular tube that transports urine from the kidney to the bladder. The ureter keeps the pressure in the renal collecting system low, which is essential for normal function of the kidney. Radiologic studies are the primary methods for investigating morphologic and functional abnormalities of the ureter.

PHYSIOLOGY

The ureter transports urine from the renal pelvis to the bladder through a series of peristaltic contraction waves. Each contraction is preceded by a wave of depolarization of the smooth muscle membranes. These depolarization waves are generated from a site in the renal pelvis (the "pacemaker") and spread from this point throughout the collecting system and down the ureter to the bladder. The depolarization causes coordinated contraction of the smooth muscle. The frequency of the depolarization and contraction waves is proportional to the rate of urine output from the kidney, and is probably mediated by the degree of distention of the renal pelvic wall: the faster urine is made, the more rapidly the walls stretch, and the more frequently the pacemaker fires. In the normal ureter, each wave completely coapts the inner surfaces of the wall, so that the bolus of urine inferior to it is propelled ahead of the contraction wave.

The timing of the contraction waves in one ureter is independent of the other, and the ureter is usually empty between boluses, so that individual urographic images may reveal segments of ureter to be completely empty of urine. During maximal diuresis (a state that may be briefly achieved shortly after the administration of a large dose of contrast medium) the ureter may be filled with opacified urine so quickly that individual contraction waves do not form and the entire ureter fills with urine flowing from the pelvis to the bladder.

With normal rates of urine flow, the renal pelvic pressure stays low and coaptation of the ureteral walls prevents urine from flowing retrograde back into the renal pelvis. The ureterovesical junction (UVJ), which normally acts as a one-way valve and completely prevents retrograde flow, keeps urine from flowing from the bladder into the ureter, even when the ureteral musculature is relaxed. The ability of ureteral peristalsis and a competent ureterovesical valve to keep pressure in the renal pelvis low is crucial: elevated renal pelvic pressure reduces renal medullary blood flow, which normally takes place through the relatively low-pressure vasa recta, and thus compromises renal function.

URETERAL OBSTRUCTION

Acute Obstruction

Acute obstruction of the ureter leads almost immediately to an increase in urine pressure proximal to the obstruction. The level to which the pressure increases depends on the degree and duration of the obstruction, the health of the affected kidney, and whether forniceal rupture decompresses the system. A transient increase in renal blood flow may occur, but is quickly followed by reductions in renal blood flow, glomerular filtration, and renal concentrating ability.

High-grade acute obstruction may sufficiently increase calyceal pressure to rupture a calyceal fornix, with escape of urine into the renal sinus. This urine may dissect through the sinus, escape through the renal hilus, and diffuse along periureteral and other planes in the retroperitoneum. This escaped urine is usually absorbed into capillaries or lymphatics and returned to the general circulation. In most cases, the resorption is complete, but rarely the urine may form a discrete collection, become encapsulated, and persist as a urinoma. Rarely (usually in very young children) the urine may flow into the peritoneal cavity and form urinary ascites.

Peristalsis of the collecting system and ureter is diminished proximal to an acute obstruction. Distention of these structures is limited in acute obstruction, even if severe. Only long-standing elevation of intraluminal

Table 16.1.
Etiology of Chronic Ureteral Obstruction

Congenital lesions
  Ureteropelvic junction obstruction
  Ectopic ureterocele
Inflammatory conditions
  Tuberculosis
  Schistosomiasis
  Crohn's disease
  Pelvic inflammatory disease
  Pelvic abscess
Trauma
Tumors
  Primary ureteral tumors
  Retroperitoneal tumors
  Lymphadenopathy
  Metastases
Miscellaneous
  Ovarian vein syndrome
  Primary megaureter
  Pregnancy
  Retroperitoneal fibrosis
  Lymphocele
  Urinoma
  Calculus
  Iliac artery aneurysm
  Uterine prolapse
Lower urinary tract conditions
  Bladder tumor
  Neurogenic bladder
  Inflammatory lesions of the bladder
  Benign prostatic hypertrophy
  Prostate cancer
  Pelvic lipomatosis
  Urethral obstruction

pressure leads to marked dilation of the ureter and collecting system.

If acute obstruction is relieved within a few days, the anatomy and physiology usually return to normal. The ureter and collecting system reverse their distention and re-acquire a normal peristaltic pattern. There is little or no persistent renal anatomic abnormality, and blood flow and urine formation return to normal. However, urine concentrating ability may remain diminished for several days after relief of obstruction.

Chronic Obstruction

Long-standing, complete, ureteral obstruction progressively reduces renal blood flow and glomerular filtration. Urine production essentially ceases, and the kidney atrophies (Table 16.1).

Persistent partial obstruction causes changes that are quantitatively and qualitatively different. Some tubular atrophy appears, but glomerulae usually remain. Concentrating capacity is diminished, and although the urine flow may be variable, with persistent severe obstruction it tends to decrease. Initial loss of renal tissue is more severe in the medulla, so that even though the parenchyma thins, the outer dimensions of the kidney may not diminish and may even increase. The greatest degree of cortical thinning and renal expansion takes place with moderately severe obstruction that has been present since birth.

Chronic obstruction also produces increasing dilatation of the ureter and the collecting system proximal to the obstructing lesion. The amount of dilation varies greatly from case to case. In general, the dilation increases both with the duration of obstruction and as a direct function of the intraluminal pressure. The most severe dilation, therefore, does not happen with very mild obstruction or with complete obstruction (after which urine formation tends to cease), but rather at an intermediate state in which the degree of obstruction increases intraluminal pressure but does not cause immediate severe oliguria.

If a lesion causing chronic obstruction resolves or is cured, the dilatation tends to decrease. Morphologic changes in the renal parenchyma recover little, if at all, but the collecting system and ureter may diminish in diameter. They do not, however, return to normal if significant stretching of their walls has occurred.

Urinary obstruction at the level of the bladder outlet may cause abnormalities of the kidneys, collecting systems, and ureter similar to those produced by chronic partial ureteral obstruction. This process occurs when bladder pressure increases above the level at which ureteral peristalsis can completely expel each bolus into the bladder lumen; ureteral pressure begins to increase and the ureteral, pyelocalyceal, and renal changes described above begin to appear. Hydronephrosis is usually bilaterally symmetrical or nearly so when it is caused by bladder outlet obstruction.

Imaging of Acute Obstruction

Abdominal radiography rarely contains direct evidence of renal abnormalities, but may reveal ureteral stones that cause acute obstruction. The abnormalities seen at excretory urography are variable. If the obstruction is very mild, the nephrogram and calyceal opacification may be normal, with minimal ureterocaliectasis as the only sign of obstruction. With more severe ob-

struction, the nephrogram is delayed in onset, denser, and more persistent than the normal nephrogram (Fig. 16.1). This "obstructive nephrogram" may demonstrate faint radial striations due to contrast medium within the collecting ducts and tubules. The kidney often is slightly larger than normal.

When the obstruction is sufficiently severe to cause ipsilateral oliguria, the calyces opacify later than those of the normal kidney and the opacified urine proceeds through the collecting system and ureter at a slower rate than normal. This is due to the oliguria, the absence of

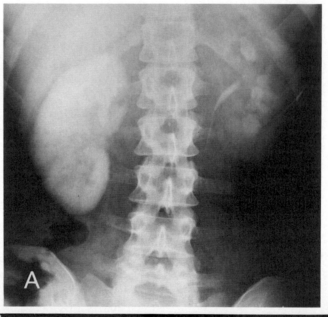

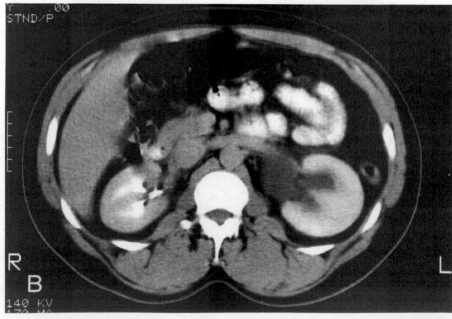

Figure 16.1. Obstructive nephrogram. **A,** A delayed film from an IVP demonstrates an obstructive nephrogram on the right. **B,** Computed tomography scan showing an obstructive nephrogram on the left with nonopacified urine filling the calyces and renal pelvis.

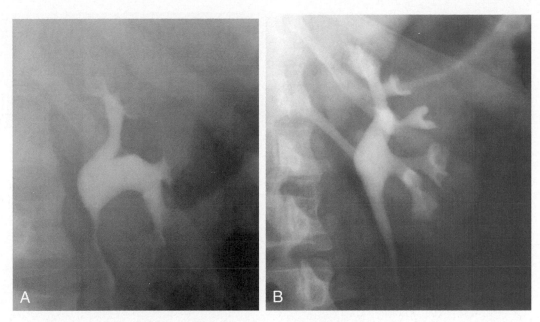

Figure 16.2. **A,** Normal excretory urogram. There is no obstruction and the fornices are very sharp. **B,** Minimal obstruction. Although there is no gross calyectasis, the fornices are blunted, which indicates mild obstruction.

peristalsis, and the increased intraluminal volume proximal to the obstruction. The contrast medium is less concentrated on the obstructed side, but may persist proximal to the obstruction for hours after the contralateral normal side has washed its contrast medium away.

A completely obstructed kidney that has become anuric may not opacify its collecting system at all, but if calyceal opacification occurs, serial films should be taken until the level of the obstructing lesion is demonstrated. This demonstration requires that two sequential films reveal no progression of opacification or that, on a single film, the level of opacification reaches a directly visualized obstructing lesion, such as a stone. Demonstration of opacification to the level of obstruction may require several hours. Delayed films may reveal opacification of the gallbladder as a sign of vicarious excretion of urographic contrast.

The collecting system and ureter are dilated as far inferiorly as the point of obstruction, but this dilatation is usually not severe in cases of acute obstruction, unless the obstruction is superimposed on a collecting system that has already been stretched by prior episodes of obstruction or vesicoureteral reflux. The calyceal fornices are always blunted to some degree. Indeed, visualization of sharply angular fornices virtually excludes even mild obstruction. (Fig. 16.2).

If forniceal rupture occurs, opacified urine dissects through the tissues of the renal sinus (pyelosinus extravasation) (Figs. 16.3 and 16.4). This opacified urine is usually feathery in appearance, and may dissect through the renal hilus into the perirenal (Fig. 16.5) and periureteral spaces in the retroperitoneum.

Retrograde ureterography may permit the diagnosis of acute complete obstruction if the ascending column of contrast medium encounters a lesion that completely occludes the ureter. When the obstructing ureteral lesion permits contrast medium to flow superiorly past it, the collecting system and ureter proximal to the obstructing lesion may be seen to be slightly dilated. Retrograde contrast injection may increase the pressure beyond that caused by the obstruction alone, with consequent exacerbation of the dilatation. Delayed films may reveal contrast medium injected superior to an obstructing lesion to wash out quite slowly, because of the increased volume

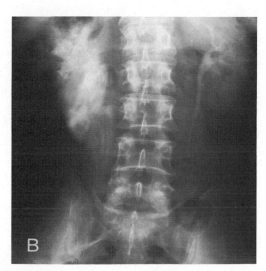

Figure 16.3. An excretory urogram demonstrates extensive pyelosinus extravasation in a patient with acute ureteral obstruction secondary to a ureteral calculus.

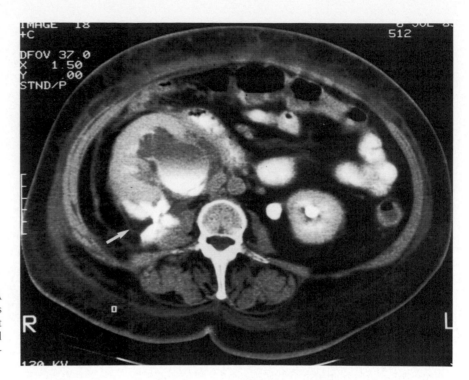

Figure 16.4. Pyelosinus extravasation. A computed tomography scan demonstrates a collection of extravasated contrast medium (*arrow*) adjacent to the renal pelvis in a patient with distal ureteral obstruction.

proximal to the obstruction and because of the associated oliguria.

During retrograde pyelography, the pressure of contrast medium in the collecting system may be transiently elevated by a vigorous injection so that the contrast flows retrograde into the tubules (pyelotubular backflow) (Fig. 16.6) or ruptures into the renal sinus. Under the latter circumstance, the contrast medium may be seen in the veins (pyelovenous backflow) (Fig. 16.7) or lymphatics (pyelolymphatic backflow) (Fig. 16.8).

Computed Tomography

Computed tomography (CT) reveals many of the same abnormalities that excretory urography demonstrates in patients with acute ureteral obstruction (*see* Figs. 16.1**B** and 16.4). The abnormal nephrogram, mild ureteral and pyelocalyceal dilation, and extracalyceal dissection of contrast from forniceal ruptures are well demonstrated. In unusual cases in which escaped urine forms a urinoma, CT may reveal a fluid-filled, thin-walled cystic structure near the kidney. Computed tomography has a lower spa-

Figure 16.5. Urinoma. A discrete extracalyceal collection of contrast material (*arrow*) is seen in this patient with ureteral obstruction due to a calculus.

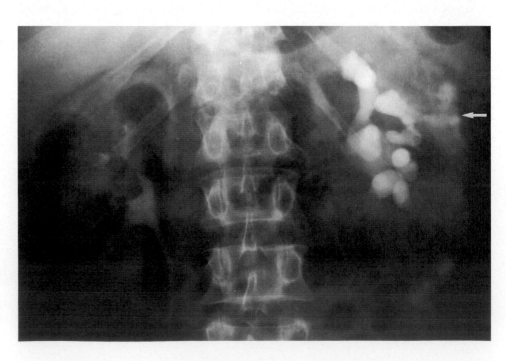

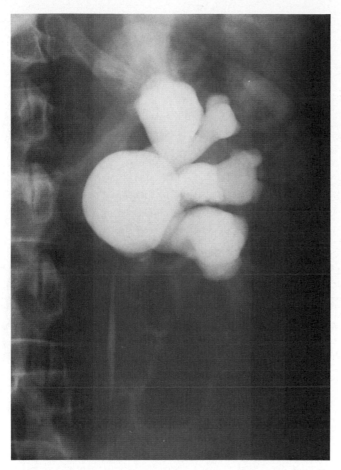

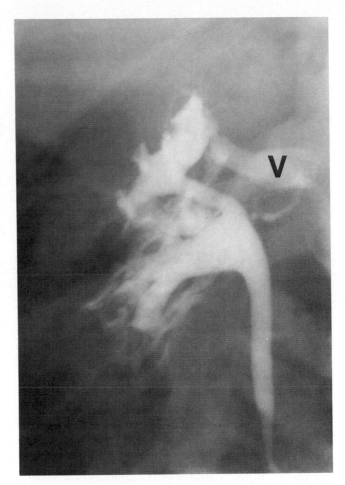

Figure 16.6. Pyelotubular backflow. A retrograde pyelogram demonstrates streaky collections of contrast medium in the distal collecting ducts extending from the minor calyces; this has occurred in the regions of the upper pole and superolateral segment.

Figure 16.7. Pyelovenous backflow. Contrast medium is seen in the renal vein (*V*) as well as the lymphatics and renal sinus during this retrograde pyelogram.

tial resolution than film–screen urography, so that the striations of the obstructive nephrogram and details of dilatation of the fornices are not seen. Because minimal forniceal dilation may be the only abnormality in patients with mild obstruction, CT is less accurate than urography in making this diagnosis.

Radionuclide Studies

The pharmacodynamics of diethylenetriaminepentaacetic acid (DTPA) are identical to those of urographic contrast agents, so that scintigraphy reveals abnormalities that reflect those seen on excretory urography. The activity in the renal parenchyma increases more slowly in an acutely obstructed kidney than in a normal one, and maintains its peak intensity longer. The peak intensity may or may not be greater than the peak of the normal side. The isotope appears in the collecting system more slowly than on the normal side, the peak calyceal activity is protracted, and its greatest intensity is variable. The advancing margin of isotope moves slowly along the ureter to the point of obstruction, and displays

a protracted washout. If forniceal rupture has occurred, the isotope may be seen in the perinephric space.

Ultrasound

With the introduction of duplex and color Doppler features, the ultrasound diagnosis of acute ureteral obstruction has become increasingly accurate. Pyelocalyectasis may be demonstrated in patients with acute ureteral obstruction (Fig. 16.9). Echo-free regions in the renal sinus corresponding to dilated calyces, infundibuli, and the pelvis may be observed. This is still the most useful finding, but it may produce both false-positive and false-negative results. The ranges of volumes of normal and acutely obstructed pyelocalyceal systems overlap. False-negative results may occur when a small, acutely obstructed collecting system has not sufficiently dilated to be recognized as abnormal. Furthermore, a normal system may be voluminous, or an abnormal system may be slightly dilated but not obstructed. Other fluid-filled structures may mimic dilated collecting systems, including renal hilar vessels (which may be identified by

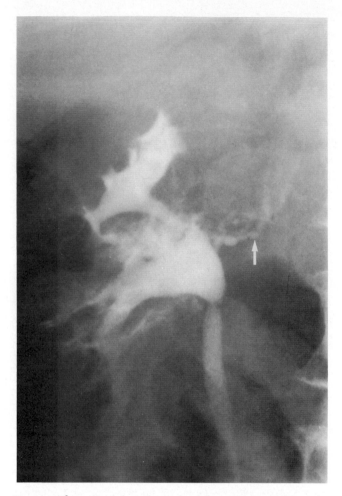

Figure 16.8. Pyelolymphatic backflow. Retrograde pyelogram demonstrating filling of lymphatic channels (*arrow*).

demonstrating flow using color Doppler), renal sinus cysts (which may be suspected from the inability to demonstrate dilated infundibuli connecting with a dilated pelvis), and a normal collecting system that has been slightly distended because of an extremely full bladder (which can be diagnosed by re-examination after voiding). These potential pitfalls notwithstanding, the demonstration of calyceal dilation by ultrasound remains the most useful sign of acute ureteral obstruction in patients whose clinical picture suggests it.

Dilation caused by obstruction usually involves the entire ureter proximal to the obstructing point. The most proximal ureter may be seen while the kidney is examined, but the midureter is usually obscured by overlying bowel. However, transvesical ultrasound of the distal ureters may demonstrate dilation when the obstruction is at or near the UVJ, and the lesion itself (e.g., a ureteral stone) may be demonstrated as well. Also, color Doppler ultrasound may be used to observe a jet of urine expelled into the bladder by a peristaltic wave. While such jets may be seen in cases of proximal partial ureteral obstruction, when prolonged observation fails to demon-

strate any jet, the ipsilateral kidney can be assumed to be anuric and (in the absence of other reasons for anuria) affected by high-grade or complete ureteral obstruction.

Pulsed Doppler ultrasound of intrarenal arteries may demonstrate abnormalities of arterial flow of kidneys affected by acute ureteral obstruction. In many acutely obstructed kidneys, diastolic flow velocity undergoes a relatively greater decrease than does systolic flow, with a consequent increase in the resistive index. Measurement of resistive indices alone cannot be used to diagnose obstruction; a chronically obstructed kidney may not have an elevated resistive index, and kidneys with a variety of intrinsic parenchymal or small-vessel diseases may have elevated resistive indices without obstruction. However, when resistive index measurements are combined with other ultrasound findings and when symmetry is analyzed, the measurement is of considerable aid in distinguishing obstructed from nonobstructed kidneys.

Magnetic Resonance Imaging

Relatively little work has been done with magnetic resonance imaging (MRI) in patients with acute ureteral obstruction. Pyeloureteral distention may be visualized and, because the pharmacokinetics of gadolinium-DTPA are the same as those of iodinated contrast media, renal parenchymal and calyceal signal changes might be expected with MRI using paramagnetic contrast agents. However, because of higher costs and more limited availability, MRI has not found a significant place in the clinical diagnosis or exclusion of ureteral obstruction.

Etiology of Acute Obstruction

The most common cause of acute ureteral obstruction is a calculus that becomes lodged in the ureter (Fig. 16.10). Calculi can obstruct the ureter at any point, but tend most frequently to obstruct at the ureteropelvic and

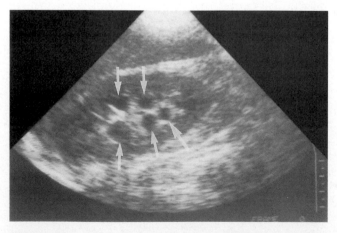

Figure 16.9. Mild ureteral obstruction. Sonography shows the dilated calyces as round, echo-poor regions (*arrows*) in the renal sinus. (From Amis ES Jr, Newhouse JH: *Essentials of Uroradiology.* Boston, Little, Brown and Co, 1991.)

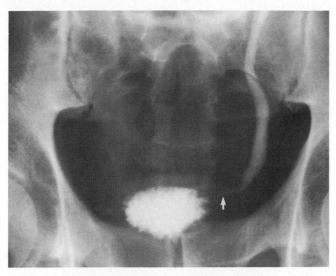

Figure 16.10. Distal ureteral calculus. The left ureter is slightly dilated owing to a stone (*arrow*) impacted at the ureterovesical junction.

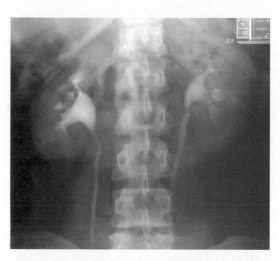

Figure 16.12. Postobstructive diminished concentration. A stone has recently passed down the left ureter. Although the configuration of the calyces reveals no persistent obstruction, the concentration of contrast on the left side in this urogram is diminished.

ureterovesical junctions. Excretory urograms must be carefully scrutinized at the region of the UVJ to find the small stones that frequently lodge there. Ureteral stones also must be distinguished from pelvic phleboliths, and stones that overlie the bony pelvis must not be missed. Ureterovesical junction stones may produce focal edema of the intramural ureter, which presents as a round filling defect in the bladder (Fig. 16.11) and is sometimes called a pseudoureterocele.

When an obstructing stone is passed, the clinical and urographic signs of obstruction frequently resolve immediately, although in some cases, the UVJ edema may briefly prolong the obstruction. Occasionally, a kidney whose ureter has been obstructed by a stone may not regain its full concentrating capacity for 1 day or so after the obstruction has been relieved, so that a urogram

reveals diminished concentration of contrast medium in that kidney's collecting system as the only sign of recently relieved obstruction (Fig. 16.12). Passage of a small calculus during urography is not uncommon, and may be aided by the diuretic effect of the contrast. When this happens, the patient's symptoms may resolve during the examination, the obstructive nephrogram may suddenly disappear, and the ureter may completely fill with contrast.

Blood clots that form in the kidney may cause acute ureteral obstruction similar to that produced by calculi. The findings are identical to those produced by a nonopaque calculus. Sloughed papillae and fungus balls may rarely cause acute ureteral obstruction.

Imaging of Chronic Obstruction

Radiography

If chronic obstruction has produced severe hydronephrosis, the kidney may be visible as a soft-tissue mass in the renal fossa. The plain-film radiograph also should reveal any opaque stones that might be responsible for the obstruction.

Excretory Urography

The obstructive nephrogram is not seen in cases of chronic obstruction (although it may appear if acute severe obstruction is superimposed on chronic milder obstruction). The nephrogram may show a diminished peak intensity. The nephrogram also reveals atrophy of the renal parenchyma, which appears first as loss of the medulla and then of the cortex; in the most severe cases, the parenchyma may be only a few millimeters thick. The opacification of extremely thinned parenchyma produces a "rim" sign.

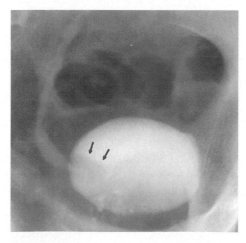

Figure 16.11. Edema of ureterovesical junction (*arrows*) due to an impacted stone. The ureter is slightly dilated.

Chronic obstruction produces various degrees of pye-localyceal dilation. During the nephrographic phase, before contrast medium enters the urine, the dilated lucent calyces are outlined by opacified remaining parenchyma and form a "negative pyelogram" (Fig. 16.13). The large volume of these calyces, combined with oliguria, may cause their opacification to be slow. Occasionally, contrast medium forms thin rings or crescents at the interfaces of the calyces and parenchyma (Fig. 16.14); these are called Dunbar's crescents, and they disappear when the calyces opacify. Kidneys whose collecting systems fill slowly because of chronic obstruction also display prolonged washout of contrast medium from the collecting system.

The ureter, as well as the collecting system, becomes dilated proximal to the obstructing lesion; it also tends to become more elongated and tortuous. Peristalsis may be seen, but the contraction waves frequently do not coapt the walls, so that the peristalsis is ineffective.

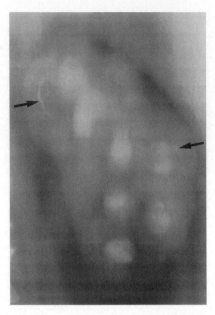

Figure 16.14. Chronic left ureteral obstruction. This nephro-tomogram shows calyceal crescents (*arrows*); these will disappear when the collecting system entirely fills with contrast medium. (From Amis ES Jr, Newhouse JH: *Essentials of Uroradiology.* Boston, Little, Brown and Co, 1991.)

Retrograde Ureteropyelography

Retrograde pyelography demonstrates the morphology of the dilated collecting system and ureter. As with acute obstruction, increased volume of these structures, along with oliguria, may produce delayed washout of the contrast medium introduced by retrograde injection.

Computed Tomography

Computed tomography reflects the same findings visualized on urography. The overall renal dimensions may be abnormal; varying degrees of renal parenchymal thinning, and calyceal and pelvic dilation may be seen (Fig. 16.15). As with urography, the obstructive nephrogram seen with acute ureteral occlusion is not demonstrated with chronic obstruction. Because CT is performed with the patient lying supine, the calyces may be shown to opacify from posterior to anterior, since contrast medium is heavier than urine and since there is no active peristaltic mixing.

Ultrasound

Sonography is highly reliable in the detection of chronic ureteral obstruction by demonstrating pyelo-caliectasis; sensitivities ranging from 93 to 100% have been reported. Pyelocaliectasis appears as echo-free regions in the center of the kidney conforming to the anatomy of the collecting system (Fig. 16.13**B**) and, as with acute obstruction, ureteral dilatation also may be

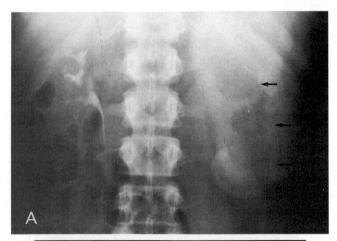

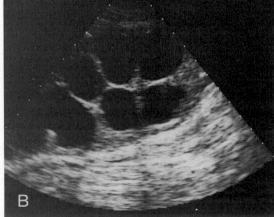

Figure 16.13. Negative pyelogram. **A,** An excretory urogram demonstrates lucent regions (*arrows*) in the nephrogram of a patient with chronic ureteral obstruction; these regions are dilated nonopacified calyces. **B,** Ultrasound image of the same patient confirms the hydronephrosis.

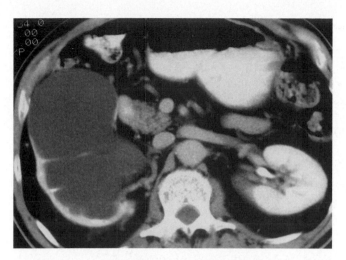

Figure 16.15. Severe obstructive hydronephrosis. The pyelocalyceal system of the right kidney is markedly dilated, and the renal parenchyma has been markedly thinned.

shown. Abnormal resistive indices may be seen, but are less reliable in chronic than acute obstruction, because chronically obstructed kidneys may lack the elevated intracalyceal pressure associated with abnormal Doppler measurements. False-positive ultrasound findings may occur: the collecting system may appear dilated in patients who are not obstructed but who have extrarenal pelves, vesicoureteral reflux, or persistent changes due to obstruction that has been relieved. Also, renal sinus cysts may masquerade as dilated calyces. Severe hydronephrosis and multicystic dysplastic kidneys may be difficult to distinguish from each other.

Radionuclide Studies

As in cases of acute obstruction, radionuclide examinations in chronic obstruction display findings similar to those seen on urography or CT as long as a compound is used that is excreted by the kidney in the same way as contrast medium (Fig. 16.16). The uptake of activity in the renal parenchyma may be slowed; its peak may be delayed when compared with that of the normal kidney, but the intensity of isotope in the parenchyma never exceeds that seen on the normal side. Activity appears within the collecting system more slowly than normal; by nature of the increased collecting-system volume, however, the total amount of activity seen within it may, at its peak, be considerably greater than that ever seen on the normal side. Washout from the collecting system is prolonged, and progression of the leading edge of isotope down the ureter may be slow.

Although in many patients with upper tract dilatation it is easy to determine whether the abnormalities are associated with ongoing obstruction, some cases with varying degrees of pyelocaliectasis or ureterectasis may not be accompanied by a partially obstructing lesion.

Most frequently, these patients had previously experienced ureteral obstruction that has subsequently been relieved but the dilatation has not completely resolved. Less frequently, patients may have upper tract dilatation caused by vesicoureteral reflux that has resolved or been repaired, or may even have innate ureteral abnormalities such as the prune-belly syndrome. In these patients, diagnosis or exclusion of concomitant obstructing lesions is important. If the ureters are obstructed, the offending lesion may need surgical correction to prevent deterioration of renal function. If the ureters are not obstructed, unnecessary surgery can be avoided. In these cases, a Whitaker test (ureteral perfusion) or a diuretic renogram may be used to distinguish obstructed from nonobstructed systems.

To perform the diuretic renogram, a diuretic is administered (usually furosemide, 40 mg intravenously) when a large amount of isotope has accumulated within the affected collecting system. If the isotope washes out very rapidly after the diuretic is administered, the system is not obstructed (Fig. 16.17). If the isotope in the collecting system remains at a high level or even increases in amount (Fig. 16.18), ureteral obstruction is presumed to be present. In some intermediate cases, very slow washout of isotope after diuretic administration produces an intermediate pattern of the time-activity curve, so that the presence or absence of obstruction cannot be determined. Some patients with indeterminate curves

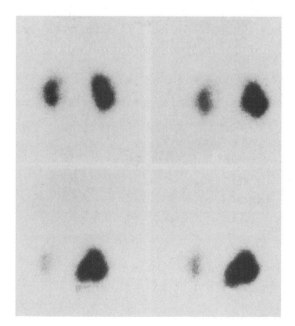

Figure 16.16. Right hydronephrosis: scintigram. The right kidney reveals hydronephrosis and activity which increases with time; the normal left side reaches its peak activity early and then diminishes in intensity. This pattern is consistent with chronic obstruction or hydronephrosis without obstruction. (From Amis ES Jr, Newhouse JH: *Essentials of Uroradiology.* Boston, Little, Brown and Co, 1991.)

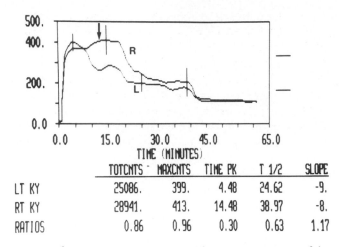

	TOTCNTS	MAXCNTS	TIME PK	T 1/2	SLOPE
LT KY	25086.	399.	4.48	24.62	-9.
RT KY	28941.	413.	14.48	38.97	-8.
RATIOS	0.86	0.96	0.30	0.63	1.17

Figure 16.17. Diuretic renogram. The renogram curve of the right kidney shows an ascending slope; however, after administration of the diuretic (*arrow*) a prompt decline in activity occurs. The left kidney shows a normal response to the diuretic.

may convert to diagnostic washout patterns if the test is repeated and the diuretic is administered 20 minutes before rather than several minutes after the isotope is given.

Diuretic-assisted scintigraphy rests on the proposition that nonobstructed kidneys respond to the drug with a diuresis, whereas partially obstructed kidneys cannot. This is not always the case. A severely damaged but nonobstructed kidney may not be able to increase its urine flow even when a diuretic is administered, and some mildly obstructed kidneys may respond with considerable diuresis. The test is, therefore, not perfectly accurate in distinguishing obstructed from nonobstructed dilated systems, but it is still commonly used, primarily because of its noninvasiveness.

Nuclear medicine studies also are useful in obstructive disease in conditions in which a severely hydronephrotic kidney may be resected or may have its

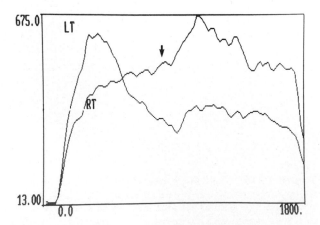

Figure 16.18. Diuretic renogram showing obstruction. Following administration of the diuretic (*arrow*), the activity in the right kidney shows an ascending slope.

obstructing lesion repaired. Measures of the accumulation of isotope within the two kidneys provides an estimate of the fraction of total renal function contributed by each kidney. When such surgical decisions need to be made, an alternate approach is to treat the obstruction temporarily with a percutaneous nephrostomy tube; after several weeks of relief, the obstructed kidney may have regained most of the function it might acquire after surgical repair, so that radioisotopic estimates of fractional renal function may be more accurate. Computed tomography, ultrasound, and nephrotomography may all contribute to this decision as well; each of these studies is able to provide an estimate of the volume of remaining parenchyma and provide at least a semi-quantitative estimate of the maximum amount of function an affected kidney might have.

Magnetic Resonance Imaging

Chronically obstructed kidneys may be demonstrated by MRI so that their morphologic characteristics become clear. The corticomedullary distinction usually seen on T1-weighted images may disappear, because the medulla often is destroyed. The dilated calyces are seen as low-signal-intensity regions on T1-weighted images and as bright regions on T2-weighted images.

Ureteral Perfusion

Ureteral perfusion was initially developed by Robert Whitaker, a British urologist, and often is called the Whitaker test. It is based on the proposition that the increased resistance to flow of fluid along the ureter caused by ureteral obstruction may be directly assessed by simultaneously measuring the pressures in the renal pelvis and bladder while fluid is flowing from the pelvis to the bladder at a known rate. Fluid is pumped through a nephrostomy tube into the renal pelvis at a given rate, and as it flows from the pelvis along the ureter to the bladder, the pressures in the pelvis and bladder soon reach constant levels at which they can be measured. The most commonly used perfusion rate is 10 ml per minute. This perfusion rate is sufficiently high that the addition of the kidney's urine to the fluid flowing along the ureter is relatively small, so that the total amount of fluid flowing along the ureter can be assumed to be almost identical to the 10 ml per minute pumped into the pelvis.

The test requires access to the renal pelvis and bladder. Access to the renal pelvis is usually gained by puncturing the collecting system with a 22-gauge needle or small catheter, whereas the bladder is reached by ureteral catheterization. The examination is preceded by a voiding cystourethrogram to exclude vesicoureteral reflux. The examination is usually performed with the patient prone on a fluoroscopy table. Fluid, usually normal saline to which enough contrast medium has been

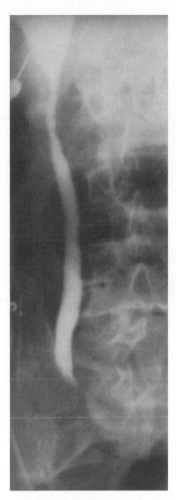

Figure 16.19. Right distal ureteral obstruction. Antegrade pyelography is performed through a needle in the collecting system. A Whitaker test also is being performed; as contrast medium is perfused through the ureter, the pressure in the right collecting system has increased, which confirms obstruction. (From Amis ES Jr, Newhouse JH: *Essentials of Uroradiology*. Boston, Little, Brown and Co, 1991.)

Differential pressures (renal pelvis pressure minus bladder pressure) of 10 cm of water or less are normal and those above 20 cm of water are abnormal. Whether pressures between 10 and 20 cm of water constitute an equivocal range or may contain a narrowly defined threshold denoting partial obstruction remains controversial, because relatively few studies have been conducted with normal ureters. Pfister and coworkers suggest that differential pressures of less than 12 cm of water are normal, those between 12 and 14 cm of water are equivocal, and those greater than 15 cm of water indicate at least some degree of obstruction.

Angiography

Angiography is not performed to assess ureteral obstruction, but occasionally an arteriogram performed for other reasons may demonstrate a hydronephrotic kidney. If the renal parenchyma has been severely reduced by obstructive atrophy, the main renal artery and its branches may be diminished in diameter to a degree reflecting the diminished renal blood flow. Arterial branches in the renal sinus may be splayed around the dilating collecting system. The nephrogram phase will reveal the parenchyma to be thinned, and the nephrogram intensity may be diminished.

IDIOPATHIC URETERAL DILATATION

Normal peristalsis produces changes in ureteral diameter; a bolus of urine in a noncontracted portion of ureter may expand the ureteral lumen to a diameter up to 8 mm. In some patients, a segment of the middle one third of the ureter superior to the crossing of the iliac vessels may be slightly dilated (Fig. 16.20); this appearance is called the *midureteral spindle*.

Primary megaureter, which refers to a dilated ureter not caused by obstruction or reflux is uncommon. It is probably caused by a functional abnormality of the juxtavesical ureter, which fails to transmit normal peristalsis and which is less distensible than normal. A characteristic beak-like configuration of the distal ureteral segment is seen during urography, and dilatation of the ureter proximal to this adynamic segment also is seen. This ureteral dilatation is characteristically more severe in the distal part of the ureter than in the proximal portions, but dilatation may extend as far proximally as the calyces. These cases have been classified as follows: (*a*) grade I, in which the dilatation is limited to the distal one third of the ureter (Fig. 16.21); (*b*) grade II, in which the dilatation extends into the proximal ureter (Fig. 16.22), with or without mild caliectasis; and (*c*) grade III, in which the entire ureter is dilated and there is moderate to severe caliectasis (Fig. 16.23). The most severe cases probably result from distal ureteral narrowing sufficiently severe to cause mild obstruction.

added that fluoroscopy and radiography during the exam can produce a high-quality pyeloureterogram (Fig. 16.19), is pumped into the renal pelvis at 10 ml per minute. Pressure in the renal pelvis and bladder should be measured frequently; either simple manometers or pressure transducers can be used. If a single needle has been used to puncture the collecting system, perfusion must be stopped for the few seconds necessary to measure pressure. Alternately, two needles or a dual-channel needle can be used, so that pressure can be monitored as perfusion continues. In either case, perfusion should be continued until the pressures in the renal pelvis and bladder reach a steady state, so that the difference between them is constant. In patients with massive hydronephrosis and hydroureter, as many as 15 to 20 minutes may be needed to reach steady state.

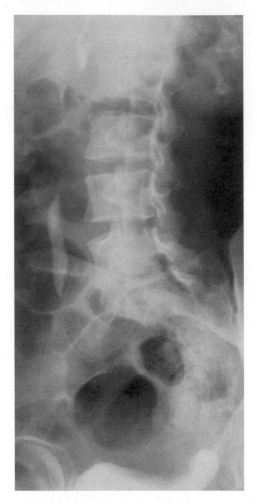

Figure 16.20.   Midureteral spindle.

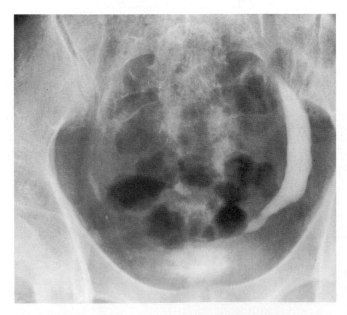

Figure 16.21.   Primary megaureter—grade 1.

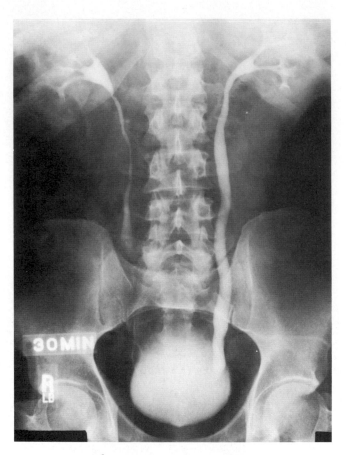

Figure 16.22.   Primary megaureter—grade 2.

A kind of primary megaureter may exist in certain congenital abnormalities, such as the Eagle-Barrett or prune-belly syndrome (Fig. 16.24), or because of chronically high urine flows, which may be encountered in patients with untreated diabetes insipidus.

URETERAL COURSE

The normal ureter begins at its junction with the renal pelvis, leaves the kidney through the hilus opposite the L1-L2 interspace, and descends to the true pelvis within the perirenal space. The proximal ureter often begins lateral to the psoas muscle, and, as it descends, moves anterior and then medial to it. It descends at first within Gerota's fascia, which it leaves at approximately L4-L5, where it crosses anterior to the common iliac artery. Urography in the anteroposterior projection usually reveals the midureter to be superimposed on the lateral portion of the transverse processes of the vertebrae; however, the position of the ureter is normally quite variable, and it may run as far medially as the vertebral pedicles or be lateral to the transverse processes. Within the true pelvis, the ureter takes a gentle posterolateral course approximately to the level of the iliac spine, and then runs anteromedially to enter the bladder.

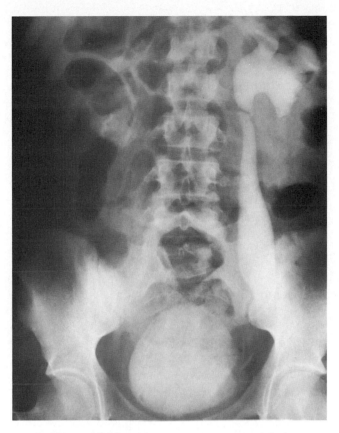

Figure 16.23.   Primary megaureter—grade 3.

In patients with ptotic kidneys the ureter may be tortuous in its proximal course. Tortuous ureters may undergo relatively sharp bends, and at points of maximum curvature, they may seem to have kinks or webs transversing them (Fig. 16.25); these kinks do not obstruct the ureter. Unusually large psoas muscles may deviate the course of the ureters. In this case, the proximal ureter lies at the lateral margin of the muscle, but then jogs medially to a position anterior to it; the proximal ureters thus seem to be laterally deviated, whereas the more distal portions are anteriorly and medially deviated (Fig. 16.26).

Ureteral deviations may be grouped according to whether the displacement affects the proximal, middle, or distal one third of the ureter.

Space-occupying lesions that arise from the medial aspect of the lower renal poles may deflect the ureters medially. Lateral displacement of the proximal one third of the ureter is most commonly caused by enlarged retroperitoneal lymph nodes (Fig. 16.27); malrotated kidneys also may laterally displace the proximal ureter.

The most common cause of lateral displacement of the middle one third of the ureter is retroperitoneal lymph node enlargement. An abdominal aortic aneurysm also may displace the midureter laterally, especially on the left; rarely, an abdominal aortic aneurysm may pull the ureter medially. As the ureter crosses the iliac artery, it may be displaced anteriorly, especially if the artery is tortuous or contains an aneurysm.

Medial deviation of the middle one third may be related to retroperitoneal tumors or fluid collections that are lateral to the ureter or to a congenital retrocaval ureter.

Deviations of the distal one third of the ureter are more common. Frequently, a bladder diverticulum may deviate the distal ureter anteromedially (Fig. 16.28). Enlarged iliac lymph nodes may medially displace the ureter, as may pelvic lipomatosis, retroperitoneal pelvic

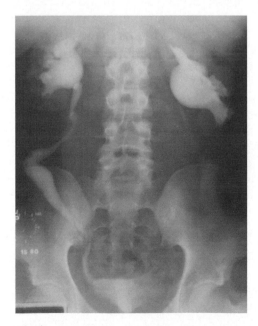

Figure 16.24.   Prune-belly syndrome. Excretory urography reveals tortuous dilated ureters.

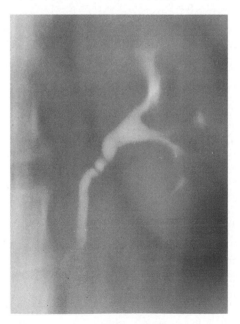

Figure 16.25.   Ureteral kinks. There is no obstruction.

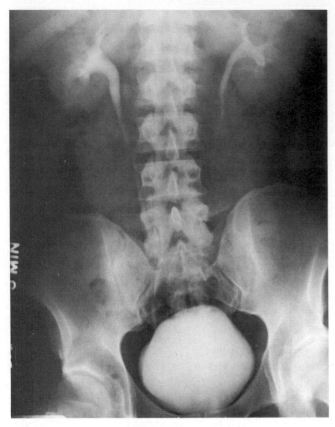

Figure 16.26. Medial deviation of the distal one third of the right ureter is caused by iliopsoas hypertrophy.

hematomas, and severe uterine and/or bladder prolapse. When there has been extensive retroperitoneal surgical dissection, as in radical abdominoperineal resection for rectal carcinoma, the ureters may follow an abnormally medial course, because the normal retroperitoneal support for them has been lost.

Lateral displacement of the pelvic ureter may accompany a variety of central pelvic masses, particularly those of gynecologic origin, such as uterine leiomyomata. Focal lateral deviations of the ureter may occur in patients with pelvic hernias that contain a segment of the ureter (Fig. 16.29).

VESICOURETERAL REFLUX

Normally, bladder urine is prevented from refluxing into the ureter by the UVJ, which acts as a one-way valve. The distal ureter traverses the muscular bladder wall at an angle, and then continues in the space just deep to the bladder epithelium and empties into the bladder at the ureteral orifice (Fig. 16.30). The pressure of bladder urine against the subepithelial tunnel effectively keeps the ureter closed, except when ureteral peristalsis actively pushes a bolus through it. This valve prevents reflux through a wide range of bladder pres-

sures: if the valve is anatomically normal, even the high pressure induced by voiding or retrograde instillation of fluid into the bladder does not cause reflux.

In infants, the bladder wall is thin and the intramural course of the ureter is short, so that only a small change from the normal anatomy may be sufficient to cause the valve mechanism to fail and reflux to occur. With normal growth and maturation, the UVJ approaches the normal adult configuration, so that vesicoureteral reflux diminishes in prevalence during early childhood. In some patients in whom reflux persists, vesicoureteral reflux may diminish in severity.

Primary vesicoureteral reflux is caused by an abnormality limited to the UVJ, and is congenital and familial. It is more commonly unilateral than bilateral, but appears bilaterally more frequently than would be accounted for by chance alone. The prevalence of this condition is not known, because it has not been sought in a large population of randomly selected children. Among infants and children with urinary tract infections, studies have found reflux in as many as one half of the tested patients.

Reflux also may be secondary; that is, associated with a disease that alters the anatomy of the UVJ. A diverticulum containing or immediately adjacent to the UVJ may produce reflux (Fig. 16.31). Male infants with posterior urethral valves have a high incidence of reflux. Bladder inflammatory processes, such as tuberculosis or schistosomiasis, may sufficiently alter the UVJ that reflux is acquired, as may diseases that produce neurogenic bladders. Ureteral duplication anomalies, imperforate anus, and other congenital urinary tract abnormalities are frequently accompanied by reflux. When a renal transplant is accompanied by a transplanted ureter, reflux often occurs. If the kidney that supplies a ureter becomes anuric or is resected, the nonfunctional ureter may acquire reflux.

Secondary changes in the urinary tract may be produced by the reflux. If the reflux is intermittent and mild, no changes may occur, but with more severe reflux, anatomic, physiologic, and pathologic changes may be severe. The bladder may be affected by high-volume reflux. During voiding, the detrusor contraction expels most of the urine into the refluxing ureter rather than through the urethra. This ureteral urine refills the bladder immediately after voiding, so that the additional urine produced before the next voiding distends the bladder to an abnormal degree.

The ureter itself may become abnormal. During voiding, a large-volume retrograde bolus travels up the ureteral lumen, stretching the ureter, which becomes dilated and tortuous. The muscular wall thins, peristalsis becomes less effective, and the ureter may become chronically distended. Children with severe bilateral ureterocalyectasis and a bladder distended by the mech-

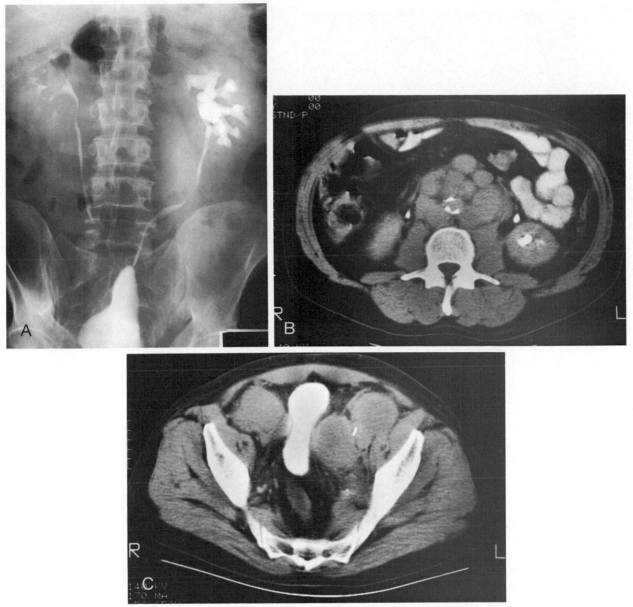

Figure 16.27. Ureteral deviation due to lymphadenopathy. **A,** An excretory urogram shows lateral deviation of the proximal left ureter and medial deviation of the distal left ureter. Computed tomography scans at the level of the kidneys (**B**) and bladder (**C**) demonstrate massive retroperitoneal lymphadenopathy.

anism described above have a condition known as the megaureter-megacystis syndrome. It has been ascribed to bladder outlet obstruction, and may be associated with posterior urethral valves, but severe vesicoureteral reflux may produce the syndrome without any obstruction.

A correlation exists between vesicoureteral reflux and urinary tract infection. This probably has to do with persistence and increased severity of infection, because it is unlikely that refluxing patients inoculate their urinary tracts any more frequently than normals. In patients with bacilluria, the concentration of bacteria

within the urine reflects a balance between the reproduction rate of the organisms and the rate at which they are washed out during voiding. If the ureters and bladder are normal, they are nearly empty at the end of micturition, so that sterile urine subsequently produced (assuming the kidneys are not infected) dilutes the small amount of remaining urine quickly and reduces the concentration of bacteria. This process becomes ineffective if a large volume of urine persists in the ureters and bladder after voiding. Also, in some patients, especially very young patients with high-pressure reflux, bacterial cystitis or pyelitis may become pyelonephritis if infected

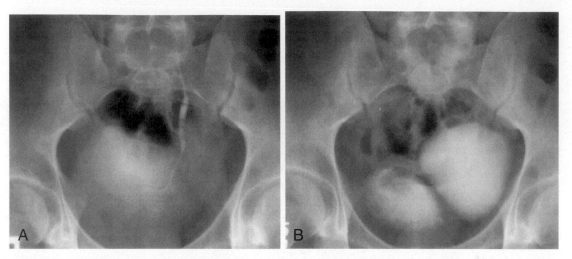

Figure 16.28. Bladder diverticulum. **A,** The left distal ureter courses medially. **B,** After the patient voids, the bladder diverticulum, which has displaced the ureter, is opacified.

urine is forced retrograde into renal tubules by reflux. For these reasons, urinary tract infections in young children often prompt investigation for vesicoureteral reflux.

Screening for Vesicoureteral Reflux

The most common reason for seeking reflux in a pediatric patient is urinary infection. Most authorities agree that even a single urinary infection should prompt screening in very young infants and in young male children, in whom posterior urethral valves are sufficiently frequent and dangerous that voiding cystourethrography should not be postponed. In young girls older than 2 years of age, urinary infections are so frequent that there is some difference of opinion regarding whether all patients should be screened. Some authorities believe that the first infection should prompt a search for

reflux, whereas others think that only a series of infections indicate workup. Studies have shown that as many as 50% of all children screened will display abnormalities, so we recommend earlier, rather than later, investigation. Screening young adult women with urinary infection, however, reveals reflux only in a small number. Reflux is demonstrated by cystourethrography, which may be radiographic, fluoroscopic, or radionuclide. Radionuclide cystourethrography has the highest sensitivity and lowest radiation dose, but fails to reveal intrinsic

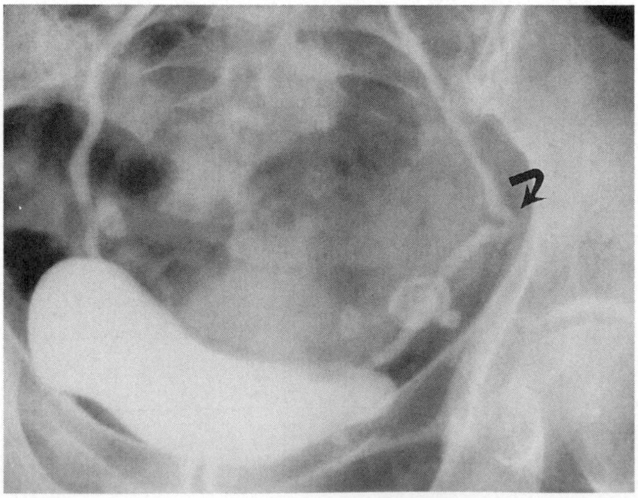

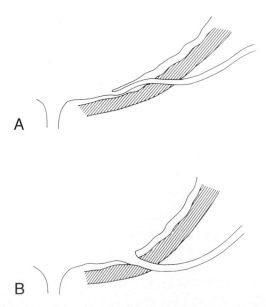

Figure 16.29. Sacrosciatic ureteral herniation. A "hair pin" deviation of the left distal ureter (*arrow*) is seen.

Figure 16.30. Diagram of ureterovesical junction. **A,** Normal—the ureter traverses the muscle wall (*shaded*) at an angle and courses submucosally before emerging at the orifice. This anatomy produces a competent valve. **B,** Refluxing—there is no submucosal ureteral course; vesicoureteral reflux occurs. (From Amis ES Jr, Newhouse JH: *Essentials of Uroradiology*. Boston, Little, Brown and Co, 1991.)

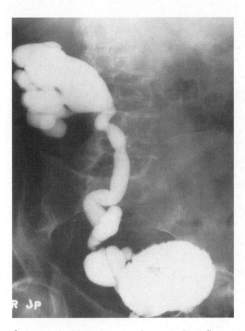

Figure 16.31. Bladder diverticulum with reflux. Cystography reveals a right-sided bladder diverticulum into which the right ureter empties. Contrast medium flows from the bladder through the diverticulum into the ureter and collecting system. This is not a periureteral diverticulum, which would be adjacent to, but would not include, the ureterovesical junction. (From Amis ES Jr, Newhouse JH: *Essentials of Uroradiology.* Boston, Little, Brown and Co, 1991.)

urethral or bladder-wall abnormalities, so it often is reserved for follow-up examinations.

Whichever method is used, several points are worth emphasizing. First, a voiding study is necessary; cystography alone is not sufficient to exclude reflux. The patient should be awake in order to void as normally as possible. A small urethral catheter will permit the patient to void around the catheter, so that the bladder can be filled and voiding can be observed more than once if necessary. Radiographic examinations should not be performed without fluoroscopy; transient reflux, functional details of micturition, and urethral abnormalities are easily missed in the absence of fluoroscopic control.

Whatever the examination type, vesicoureteral reflux is diagnosed by observing contrast medium or isotope in the ureter and/or collecting system after it has been instilled into the bladder. A patient may demonstrate low-pressure reflux (reflux that occurs during the early stage of bladder filling) or high-pressure reflux (reflux that occurs as the bladder detrusor muscle contracts). For radiographic and fluoroscopic examinations, a grading system to quantify the degree of reflux has been developed. Unfortunately, there is more than one such system. The international classification of vesicoureteral reflux is presented in Table 16.2 and Figure 16.32. Finally, voiding cystourethrography should not be per-

formed when contrast medium or isotope has been recently administered intravenously; residual material excreted into the calyceal system may be mistaken for reflux.

In patients with severe reflux, cystourethrography may occasionally demonstrate intrarenal reflux. Contrast medium that extends from the calyces into the renal collecting tubules may appear homogeneous or striated, and may extend as far as the renal capsule (Figs. 16.33 and 16.34). It is almost always focal, and has a predilection for the renal poles.

Radionuclide scintigraphy demonstrates reflux as streaks of activity extending from the bladder into the ureters and collecting systems. The international classification of reflux is not commonly applied to radionuclide studies, but the amount of activity that appears in the upper urinary tracts can be quantified and can produce a measurement useful in serial follow-up examinations.

URETERAL TUMORS

Tumors may develop in any of the tissues of the ureter or may develop outside the ureter and invade the ureter secondarily (Table 16.3). Primary ureteral tumors are relatively rare, accounting for approximately 1% of all urinary tract tumors. Most tumors develop in the ureteral epithelium, but they also may arise from the mesoderm. Ureteral neoplasms occur twice as frequently in men as in women and, for unknown reasons, seem to appear more frequently in the right ureter. Most primary neoplasms involve the distal one third of the ureter and are found in patients between 50 and 80 years of age.

Epithelial Tumors

Seventy five percent of all primary ureteral neoplasms are of epithelial origin. The most common of these neoplasms is transitional cell carcinoma, which may be of a papillary or nonpapillary type. Papillary tumors constitute 80 to 85% of transitional cell carcinomas and have a greater tendency to be multicentric than nonpapillary types.

Forty percent of papillary tumors, and most nonpapil-

Table 16.2.
International Classification of Vesicoureteral Reflux

Grade	Extent
I	Reflux only into ureter
II	Reflux into collecting system, without dilation
III	Reflux into collecting system, with mild dilation
IV	Reflux into collecting system, with moderate dilation
V	Reflux into collecting system, with severe dilation

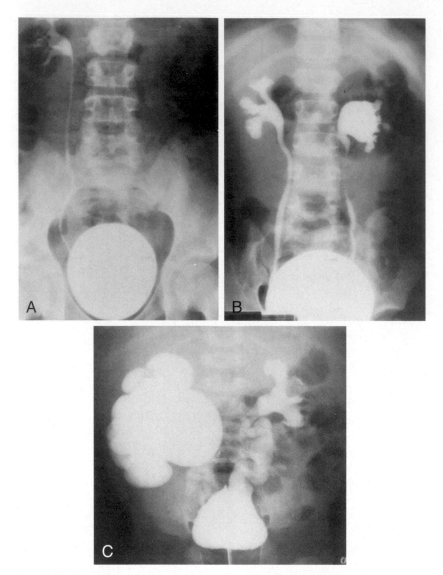

Figure 16.32. **A,** Grade II vesicoureteral reflux. In this cystogram, contrast flowed from the bladder into the entire ureter collecting system but has not caused dilation (courtesy of Robert Cleveland, M.D.). **B,** Grade III vesicoureteral reflux (bilateral). Cystography reveals bilateral opacification of the ureters and collecting systems with mild pyelocalyectasis (courtesy of Robert Cleveland, M.D.). **C,** Grade V vesicoureteral reflux on the right; grade III–IV on left. Cystography demonstrates reflux and severe upper tract dilation, especially on the right. (From Amis ES Jr, Newhouse JH: *Essentials of Uroradiology.* Boston, Little, Brown and Co, 1991.)

lary lesions, are invasive. Invasive tumors extend through subepithelial layers into the retroperitoneal tissues, and metastasize to regional lymph nodes, or more distantly to the liver, bones, lungs, mediastinum, and other sites. An associated transitional cell carcinoma of the bladder is found in approximately 25% of patients, and as many as 70% have an antecedent or subsequent urothelial lesions elsewhere. For this reason, complete nephroureterectomy is the standard therapy for lesions that are resectable at the time of diagnosis.

The stage of the tumor is very important in prognosis. In stage I, the tumor is limited to the urothelial layer; in stage II, invasion of the ureteral muscle occurs; in

stage III, invasion of the periureteral tissues occurs; and in stage IV, there are distant metastases. The prognosis also depends on the histologic characteristics of the tissue. Some authorities believe that extremely low-grade polypoid tumors represent benign papillomas, but most think they are malignant tumors with minimal potential for invasion and metastases.

Hematuria, pain due to ureteral obstruction, and malignant cells found on urine cytologic examination are common presenting features. As many as 40% of the patients may present with a nonfunctioning kidney because of ureteral obstruction.

When there is excretion of sufficient contrast medium

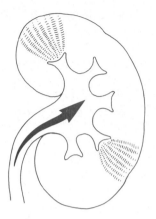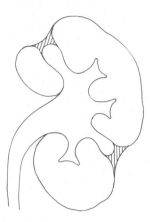

Figure 16.33. Intrarenal reflux. Diagram showing pattern of intrarenal reflux followed by scar formation, with focal parenchymal thinning and focal calyceal blunting. (From Amis ES Jr, Newhouse JH: *Essentials of Uroradiology*. Boston, Little, Brown and Co, 1991.)

Table 16.3.
Ureteral Tumors

Primary Tumors
  Epithelial tumors
    Transitional cell carcinoma
     Papillary
     Nonpapillary
    Squamous cell carcinoma
    Adenocarcinoma
  Nonepithelial tumors
    Fibroepithelial polyp
    Rare tumors
Secondary Tumors
  Direct invasion
    Cervical carcinoma
    Bladder carcinoma
    Prostate carcinoma
  Lymphadenopathy
    Lymphoma
  Hematogenous seeding
    Melanoma
    Lung carcinoma

at excretory urography to demonstrate the ureter, the lesion may present as a single filling defect or as multiple filling defects in the ureteral lumen. When the kidney is obstructed and fails to opacify the ureter, retrograde pyelography may be necessary. Solitary polypoid lesions frequently demonstrate slight dilatation of the ureter around and distal to the ureter, as well as above it (Fig. 16.35); this sign helps to differentiate the lesion from benign filling defects such as calculi or blood clots,

because these do not grow and progressively stretch the ureteral walls. The localized expansion of the ureter at the inferior margin of the lesion produces an appearance known as the "champagne glass" or "goblet" sign on retrograde ureterography. Coiling of a catheter in this dilated segment of ureter during retrograde ureterography is known as Bergman's sign. Intramural lesions may infiltrate the ureteral wall, so that the ureter becomes fixed; the lesion will demonstrate an irregular narrowing of the ureteral lumen with abrupt nontapering superior

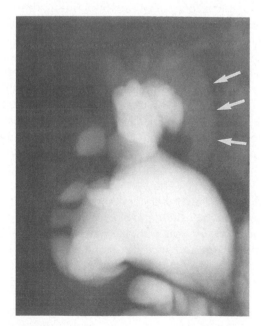

Figure 16.34. Voiding cystogram in a patient with reflux. The collecting system has been filled and dilated by contrast medium instilled into the bladder. Contrast medium has flowed from upper-pole calyces into the tubules of the upper-pole parenchyma, causing faint opacification (*arrows*). (Courtesy of Walter Berdon, M.D.) (From Amis ES Jr, Newhouse JH: *Essentials of Uroradiology*. Boston, Little, Brown and Co, 1991.)

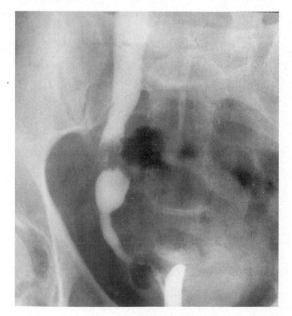

Figure 16.35. Transitional cell carcinoma of the ureter. Retrograde pyelogram reveals the tumor. The inferior portion of the surrounding ureter is dilated, creating a "champagne glass" or "goblet" sign.

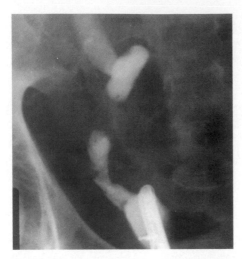

Figure 16.36. Transitional cell carcinoma of the ureter. Retrograde pyelogram reveals a circumferential lesion that nearly obliterates the ureteral lumen.

and inferior margins. The lesion may be eccentric, or it may encircle the ureter, producing an apple-core appearance (Fig. 16.36). In rare cases, the lesion may resemble a more benign ureteral stricture.

Computed tomography may be of value in the diagnosis of ureteral neoplasms (Fig. 16.37), particularly in those patients in whom urography or retrograde pyelography is unsuccessful. The technique also may be used to distinguish ureteral tumors from nonopaque ureteral calculi. Computed tomography may be of value in preoperative staging of transitional carcinomas of the ureter by revealing the presence or absence of periureteral invasion. However, CT is unable to distinguish stage A from stage B ureteral tumors.

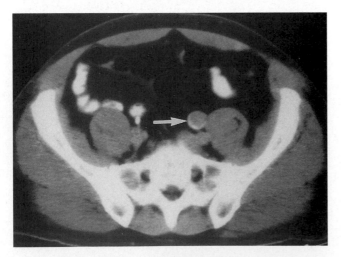

Figure 16.37. Polypoid left ureteral transitional cell carcinoma. Computed tomography reveals the tumor as a soft tissue-density lesion that has distended the left ureter; a rim of contrast medium (*arrow*) surrounds the lesion. (From Amis ES Jr, Newhouse JH: *Essentials of Uroradiology.* Boston, Little, Brown and Co, 1991.)

Squamous cell carcinoma is the most malignant of epithelial tumors of the ureter, but comprises less than 10% of primary ureteral epithelial neoplasms. It is frequently associated with chronic urinary tract infection and long-standing stone disease. Squamous cell carcinoma may present as a solitary filling defect or as a ureteral mural lesion; it is less likely to be clearly polypoid than transitional cell carcinoma.

Adenocarcinoma of the ureter is extremely rare. The lesion is thought to develop in the cell nests of von Brunn in the basal layer of the urothelium.

Ureteral tumors may require differential diagnosis. Intraluminal filling defects also may be produced by uric acid stones (which, unlike tumors, cast ultrasound shadows and are much denser than soft tissue on CT), ureteral clots (which are slightly denser than soft tissue and which resolve spontaneously), sloughed papillae (pieces of which may be recoverable in the urine and whose site of origin is usually visible by urography), and fibroepithelial polyps (which are usually longer and smoother than carcinomas).

Nonepithelial Tumors

The most common of the nonepithelial tumors of the ureter is the benign fibrous polyp, also known as the fibroepithelial polyp. The lesion consists of a core of fibrous and vascular tissue covered with normal transitional epithelium. The lesion is usually solitary, but multiple lesions have been reported. A nonepithelial tumor may occur in association with chronic urinary tract infection and may bleed slightly or cause obstruction and flank pain. It is not premalignant.

Urography may reveal the lesion to be mobile, owing to its long stalk. The polyps vary in size from a few millimeters to many centimeters in length. Most fibroepithelial polyps have a smooth cylindrical appearance (Fig. 16.38), but multilocular or frond-like appearances have been reported. Unlike primary malignant tumors, these polyps are most commonly found in the proximal one third of the ureter and typically occur in patients 20 to 40 years of age. They should be distinguished from vermiform clots in the ureteral lumen and the occasional pedunculated transitional cell carcinoma or papilloma.

Other primary nonepithelial tumors of the ureter are extremely rare, and include leiomyosarcomas, spindle cell sarcomas, hemangiosarcomas, lymphosarcomas, carcinosarcomas, and melanomas.

Secondary Tumors

These are much more common than primary ureteral neoplasms, because the latter are relatively uncommon and because the ureter is near many structures that frequently harbor malignancies. In many cases, obstruction of the ureter results from direct extension of the neoplasm from primary sites such as the cervix, prostate,

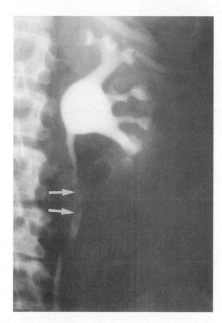

Figure 16.38. Fibroepithelial urothelial polyp. Urography shows a linear lucent filling defect (*arrows*) in the proximal ureter. (From Amis ES Jr, Newhouse JH: *Essentials of Uroradiology*. Boston, Little, Brown and Co, 1991.)

and bladder. Ureteral obstruction also may occur because of adjacent retroperitoneal lymph node enlargement due to lymphoma or other primary tumors (Fig. 16.39).

The ureter also may be indirectly obstructed from malignant disease, because some tumors invoke an intense periureteral desmoplastic reaction. In such cases, imaging studies may demonstrate extrinsic compression of the ureter by a soft tissue mass similar in appearance to retroperitoneal fibrosis. Occasionally, the obstructing lesion may be too small to be demonstrated by CT, in which case percutaneous biopsy or even surgery may be necessary to establish the diagnosis. Patients who experience ureteral obstruction after radiation therapy should not be assumed to have a benign radiation-induced stricture. The ureter is relatively resistant to radiation, so that postradiation ureteral obstruction usually means that the tumor had involved the ureteral wall before therapy or has recurred.

Much less commonly, hematogenous metastases to the ureter may present as solitary filling defects simulating primary ureteral tumors (Fig. 16.40); melanoma, carcinomas of the kidney, breast, lung and prostate, and multiple myeloma may be responsible.

INFLAMMATORY LESIONS

Leukoplakia

Leukoplakia is a rare inflammatory condition that involves the bladder more commonly than the ureter.

Ureteral involvement usually occurs in the proximal one third of the organ and is almost always associated with involvement of the renal pelvis. It results from squamous metaplasia of the urothelium and is frequently associated with chronic urinary tract infection or long-standing stone disease; it also may develop spontaneously. Leukoplakia is bilateral in approximately 10% of cases. Classically the condition has been thought to be a precursor of squamous cell carcinoma, but documentation of this association in the upper urinary tract is extremely rare.

The lesion consists of keratinization and desquamation of the involved epithelium, with proliferation of the deeper layers. When the keratinized epithelium forms a soft tissue mass, the condition is referred to as a cholesteatoma.

Leukoplakia occurs in middle-aged patients of both sexes. Hematuria is present in approximately one third

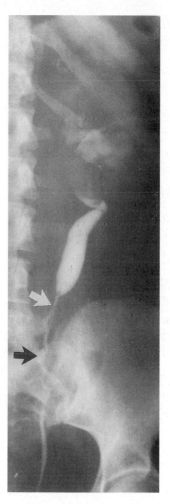

Figure 16.39. Metastatic retroperitoneal carcinoma involving the left ureter. The midureter is irregularly encased and narrowed (*arrows*); the proximal ureter is dilated. Insufficient contrast agent has been injected in this retrograde study to completely opacify the intrarenal collecting system. (From Amis ES Jr, Newhouse JH: *Essentials of Uroradiology*. Boston, Little, Brown and Co, 1991.)

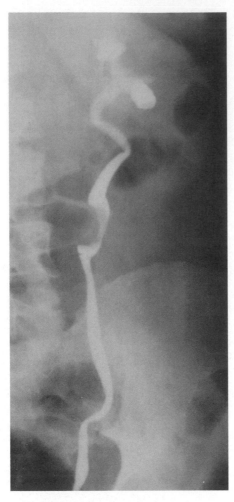

Figure 16.40. Malignant melanoma metastatic to the left ureteral wall.

of cases, and symptoms of chronic urinary tract infection with calculi have usually been present for years. The pathognomonic feature of leukoplakia is passage of pieces of white chalky, desquamated epithelium in the urine. These fragments may cause renal colic.

Radiographic features of ureteral leukoplakia include diffuse, irregular filling defects of the upper ureter and renal pelvis. There may be ridging of the mucosa of the ureter with evidence of ureteral obstruction. The radiologic appearance has only been described with urography; differentiation from malacoplakia and even from transitional cell carcinoma is difficult.

Malacoplakia

Malacoplakia is an uncommon inflammatory condition of the ureter that is usually associated with chronic urinary tract infection, often *Escherichia coli*. It is not a premalignant condition, but is more common among immunocompromised patients. The lesions consist of smooth, yellow, or brown subepithelial plaques com-

posed of inflammatory cells (histiocytes) that contain basophilic staining inclusions known as Michaelis-Gutmann bodies. These may represent collections of phagocytized bacteria or their fragments. Malacoplakia may result from a defect in intracellular digestion of bacteria.

The bladder is the most common site of urinary tract involvement, followed in frequency by the ureter, the renal pelvis, and the urethra. Most patients are middle-aged women with nonspecific complaints, including dysuria, flank pain and, occasionally, hematuria.

On urography, the lesions are demonstrated as a series of flat filling defects that characteristically involve the distal ureter, but may involve long segments of any part of the ureter (Fig. 16.41). Ureteral obstruction may or may not be present. The lesions are usually multiple and may coalesce, producing a cobblestone appearance. They may regress if treatment of the associated infection is successful, but there is a tendency for the disease to reappear after therapy, sometimes in another part of the urinary tract.

Differentiation of this condition from other lesions may be difficult. Ureteritis cystica may look similar, but the lesions of this condition are usually rounder and the ureter is rarely dilated. Tuberculosis may produce a thickening of the ureteral wall with focal strictures. Ma-

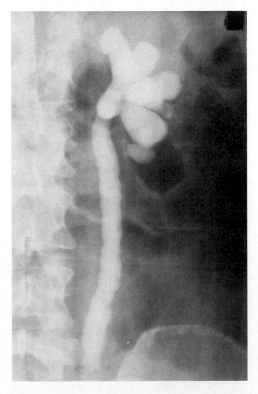

Figure 16.41. Ureteral malacoplakia. A retrograde pyelogram reveals a slightly dilated ureter with scalloped margins throughout its length. (Courtesy of Richard C. Pfister, M.D.) (From Amis ES Jr, Newhouse JH: *Essentials of Uroradiology.* Boston, Little, Brown and Co, 1991.)

lignant lesions of the ureter are rarely as widespread as malacoplakia.

Ureteritis Cystica

This condition consists of multiple, small, subepithelial fluid-filled cysts in the ureteral wall. They are thought to be caused by degeneration of the central cells of the basal layer of the urothelium, which results in proliferation of the surface epithelial cells; these become isolated from the epithelial surface and form fluid-filled cysts that project into the lumen of the ureter. This degeneration occurs with chronic urinary tract infection, which may or may not be present at the time of diagnosis. It may appear in the ureter, renal pelvis (pyelitis cystica), or bladder (cystitis cystica).

Ureteritis cystica is usually asymptomatic, but may be accompanied by hematuria and symptoms of urinary tract infection. The condition may or may not resolve when the infection is cured. Ureteritis cystica does not cause obstruction and is not premalignant. It may be unilateral or bilateral, and appears slightly more fre-

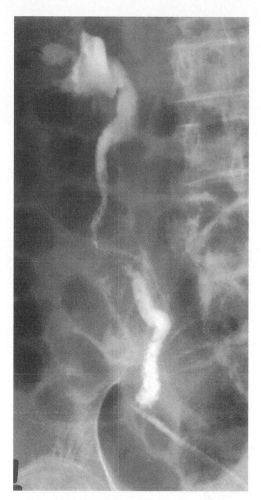

Figure 16.43. Ureteritis cystica. Retrograde pyelogram reveals multiple, small, well-defined ureteral lesions.

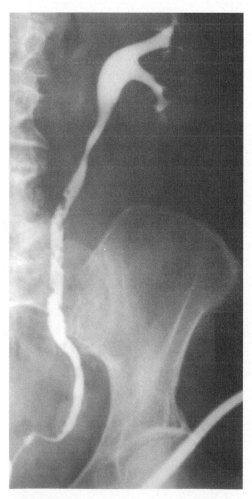

Figure 16.42. Ureteritis cystica. Multiple, small well-defined lesions are demonstrated on this retrograde pyelogram. Many lesions can be seen arising from the ureteral wall.

quently in women. Although this condition has been reported in all age groups, it is usually found in patients between 50 and 60 years of age.

The typical radiographic appearance is that of multiple small (2–3 mm) radiolucent filling defects that cause scalloping of the ureteral margins when seen in profile during excretory urography or retrograde pyelography (Figs. 16.42 and 16.43). These filling defects may appear anywhere in the ureter, but have a slight predilection for the proximal one third. When the cysts are numerous, they may produce a ragged appearance of the ureteral margin, but each cyst can be seen to have a smooth hemispherical surface. The differential diagnosis includes small air bubbles introduced at retrograde pyelography, hemorrhage into the ureteral wall (which usually produces filling defects that are not perfectly hemispherical and that resolve quickly), papillary neoplasms (which are rarely as numerous as the cysts of ureteritis cystica), and prolonged ureteral stenting (which may cause protrusion of the urothelium into the side holes of the stent and produces circular filling defects when the stent is removed)

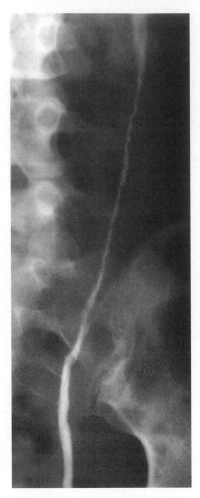

Figure 16.44. Ureteral mucosal irregularity due to recently-removed stent. The stent's multiple side holes have caused irregularity in the mucosa that conformed to the stent's surface.

(Fig. 16.44). However, the radiographic appearance of ureteritis cystica is usually sufficiently characteristic to allow a confident diagnosis.

Pseudodiverticulosis

Ureteral pseudodiverticulosis consists of one or more small (≤4 mm) outpouchings of the ureter. The lesions are hyperplastic buds of ureteral epithelium that project from the ureteral lumen into, but not entirely through, the muscular layers of the ureteral wall. Thus, they are not true diverticulae.

Ureteral pseudodiverticulosis may be associated with hematuria and urinary tract infection; it also has been found to co-exist with a wide range of urinary tract pathology, including calculi, benign prostatic hypertrophy, and transitional cell carcinoma. Cytologic examination of ureteral washings reveals cellular atypia in approximately 50% of cases.

Ureterography reveals small protrusions of the ureteral lumen (Fig. 16.45); the ureter may be otherwise normal, or there may be mild narrowing at the site of the diverticulae. The proximal and middle thirds of the ureter are more frequently affected than the distal third. The condition does not cause ureteral obstruction.

The association of ureteral pseudodiverticulosis and malignancy, usually transitional cell carcinoma, warrants careful evaluation of these patients. Wasserman and colleagues (1991) reported a uroepithelial malignancy in 17 (46%) of 37 patients with ureteral pseudodiverticula. The most common site of malignancy was the bladder. In two patients, the malignant tumors developed 2 and 3 years after demonstration of ureteral pseudodiverticulosis.

Eosinophilic Ureteritis

Inflammatory lesions characterized histologically by infiltration of eosinophils may occur in a variety of organ systems. The majority of cases in the urinary tract involve the bladder. Fewer than 60 cases involving the ureter have been reported under a variety of names, including nonspecific granuloma of the ureter, eosinophilic granuloma of the ureter, and eosinophilic ureteritis.

The lesion may be found at any level in the ureter and presents as a nodular defect within the ureteral lumen. There may be high-grade ureteral obstruction. Some cases have been associated with urinary tract calculi.

Schistosomiasis

Infection of the urinary tract by the fluke, *Schistosoma hematobium,* is endemic in areas where the specific type of snail necessary for asexual reproduction of the organ-

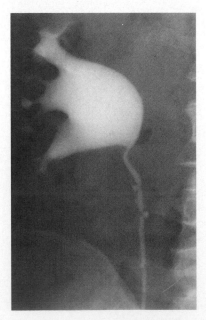

Figure 16.45. Ureteral pseudodiverticulosis. The small diverticulae are well demonstrated; notice the minimal ureteral narrowing at the site of the larger diverticulae.

ism is present. Endemic regions include parts of the Middle East, India, Puerto Rico, and a number of African countries, especially Egypt, Nigeria, South Africa, Tanzania, and Zimbabwe.

Infected humans excrete female eggs into stagnant fresh water, where they hatch into larvae or miracidia. The larvae enter the host snail and mature into mother sporocysts before dividing asexually into 20 to 40 daughter sporocysts. Each daughter sporocyst can produce 200 to 400 cerceriae, which are released into the stagnant water. When humans enter contaminated water, the cerceriae attach themselves and penetrate the skin. They enter the venous system and reach the heart, where they mature to adulthood. Male and female worms mate and migrate together against the flow of blood to the venous plexus of the bladder. The eggs are deposited in the subepithelial and muscular layers of the bladder and distal ureteral walls. Eggs that are excreted in the urine complete the cycle.

While the disorder most commonly affects the bladder, ureteral involvement is present in up to 30% of patients. The condition usually affects patients younger than 30 years of age and is more common in male than female patients. Symptoms of ureteral involvement may be absent or limited to flank pain. Ureteral disease is almost always bilateral, but is usually asymmetric. The disorder most commonly involves the distal ureters, but lesions at the level of the L3 vertebral body and, rarely, the ureteropelvic junction, also may be present. This infestation results in varying degrees of ureteral stenosis, thickening, and dilation. The ureter also may be obstructed by schistosomal involvement of the juxtaureteral bladder wall.

Radiologic findings of urinary bilharziasis are characteristic. Calcification, most commonly involving the pelvic portions of the ureters, is present in 75% of the cases. Calcification is usually linear (Fig. 16.46) or "tramtrack," but it also may be patchy, curvilinear, or diffuse. There is a characteristic deformity of the distal ureters consisting of medial and cephalic displacement of the ureters, which may then resemble cow's horns. There are various degrees of dilation and stenosis. In early stages of the disease, only mild distention of the distal ureters may be seen, but, in more advanced cases, a beaded appearance of the ureters secondary to multiple strictures may appear; this is similar to the abnormalities found in tuberculous ureteritis. Although the ureters are dilated, they are not tortuous; they tend to be straightened, especially in the midportions. Involvement of the UVJ commonly leads to vesicoureteral reflux. Solitary or multiple ureteral filling defects (bilharzial polyps) are reported in as many as 17% of patients and tend to appear in the early inflammatory stages of the disease rather than the later calcified stages. Although bilharzia of the bladder predisposes to bladder carcinoma, this compli-

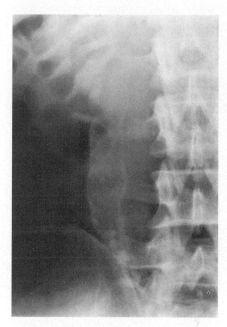

Figure 16.46. A diffusely calcified right ureter is seen in this patient with urinary schistosomiasis.

cation is very rare in the ureter. Ureteritis cystica may be present in patients with ureteral bilharziasis. Calcification of the cysts, presumably resulting from hemorrhage, may occur and may produce a stippled pattern termed ureteritis calcinosa.

Tuberculosis

Urinary tract infection with *Mycobacterium tuberculosis* is a result of hematogenous dissemination of the organisms to the kidney from other sites, usually the lungs. Although both kidneys are thought to receive the organisms, the disease usually progresses in only one. Ureteral involvement is the result of renal infection that spreads down from the collecting systems and pelvis. The bladder, seminal vesicles, and prostate also may become affected.

Tuberculosis may affect the urinary tract in patients of any age, but most are 40 years of age or older. Hematuria, sometimes gross, may be the first sign, but symptoms of lower urinary tract disease (frequency, dysuria, suprapubic pain) also may herald urinary tract involvement.

Radiographically demonstrable ureteral abnormalities are found in approximately 50% of patients with renal tuberculosis. The findings may be demonstrated on excretory urography if renal function is sufficient; otherwise, retrograde or antegrade pyelography may be necessary (Fig. 16.47). In patients with severe bladder disease, however, retrograde pyelography may be difficult or impossible to perform.

Ureteral infection produces ulcerations, fibrosis, stric-

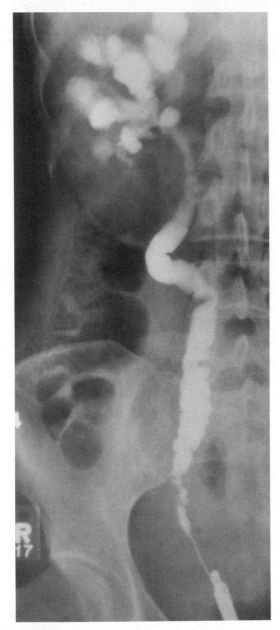

Figure 16.47. Ureteral tuberculosis. Retrograde pyelogram shows multiple strictures, as well as the characteristic calyceal changes.

straightened owing to periureteral fibrosis ("pipestem" ureter). Calcification of the ureters is considerably less common in tuberculous ureteritis than in bilharzial ureteritis and also is less common than calcification in the kidneys; when present, it may be linear or may appear as a faint putty-like calcification of inspissated material that fills the ureteral lumen (Fig. 16.48).

Amyloidosis

Amyloidosis is a disorder characterized by infiltration of the affected organ by a variety of insoluble proteins or protein-polysaccharide complexes. The disease is usually systemic and may accompany another systemic disorder, such as multiple myeloma. Rarely, amyloidosis may be localized to a specific organ. Ureteral amyloidosis is extremely rare; the few cases described show a slight predilection for elderly female patients. There are no specific clinical features; the disease may present with symptoms of chronic urinary tract obstruction. The radiographic features are nonspecific; a localized ureteral

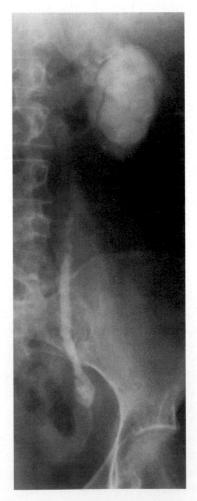

Figure 16.48. Urinary tract tuberculosis. A plain abdominal radiograph reveals putty-like calcification in the kidney and ureter.

ture, and calcification. The dilatation may involve the entire ureter and may be associated with hydronephrosis. Strictures may appear anywhere along the ureter, or ureteral dilatation may be caused by obstruction or reflux produced by abnormalities at the UVJ. The mucosal ulceration may produce a ragged appearance of the ureteral epithelium. If the ulcers are superficial, they may heal without sequela, but healing of deeper ulcerations often results in ureteral fibrosis. Multiple strictures may produce alternating segments of dilatation and narrowing; the resulting beaded appearance is characteristic of ureteral tuberculosis. The ureter is shortened and

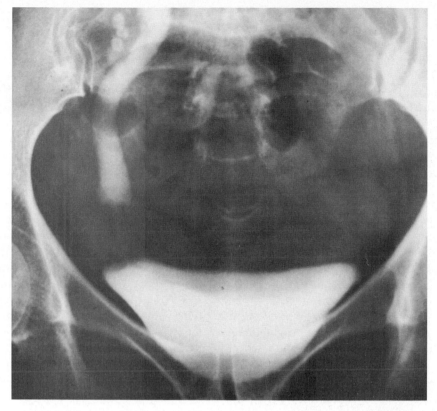

Figure 16.49.   Amyloidosis of the ureter. (Courtesy of John Hodson, M.D.)

stricture (Fig. 16.49), often in the distal ureter and often indistinguishable from neoplasm, is the usual finding.

Polyarteritis Nodosa

Polyarteritis nodosa is a systemic vasculitis that affects the kidneys in most patients and frequently results in renal infarction and renal failure. Ureteral involvement is quite rare; however, two distinct syndromes of ureteral involvement have been described. In the first, acute ureteral obstruction may be associated with acute systemic symptoms of fever, muscle pain, and the recent onset of hypertension. In the second, a stricture occurs, presumably caused by ischemia.

Suburothelial Hemorrhage

Suburothelial hemorrhage is exceedingly rare; only a few cases have been reported. It consists of hemorrhage within the wall of the ureter and is associated with coagulopathies. Patients usually present with hematuria. Urography reveals multiple filling defects projecting into the ureteral lumen that are less discrete than those seen in pyeloureteritis cystica and that resolve spontaneously when the coagulopathy is corrected. Computed tomography may reveal the focal urothelial thickening to be of relatively high attenuation, similar to that seen with hemorrhage elsewhere.

Endometriosis

Endometriosis is a condition of women of childbearing age in which endometrial tissue develops outside the endometrial cavity of the uterus. Ectopic endometrium undergoes the same cyclic changes as orthotopic tissue, and the periodic necrosis and hemorrhage that occurs produces hemorrhagic cystic lesions or masses. Although the active disease usually resolves with menopause, the lesions persist in postmenopausal women. The lesions most commonly appear within the myometrium, on the surface of the uterus, ovaries, or fallopian tubes, and on the peritoneal surfaces of other pelvic organs and the pelvic side walls; they may involve the bladder or ureters. The ectopic endometrial tissue may represent embryonic rests or an acquired condition in which retrograde menstruation through the fallopian tubes deposits endometrial tissues in the peritoneal surfaces.

Patients most commonly present with infertility and severe pelvic pain with menstruation. The endometriomas may be difficult to visualize by noninvasive techniques if they are small; if they are of moderate or large size, they display the characteristics of hemorrhagic cystic lesions or soft tissue masses, whether they are imaged by ultrasound, CT, or MRI. Only a small minority of patients have the urinary tract affected by endometriomas; the bladder is more frequently involved than the ureter. Ureteral involvement generally occurs in cases with widespread pelvic disease, although isolated cases in the ureter have been reported. When the ureter is involved, flank pain and hematuria (which may or may not be cyclic) are clues to the disease.

The ureter is usually involved in its distal portion. Endometriomas compress the ureter or involve the ureteral adventitia. Less frequently, intrinsic ureteral disease appears, in which there is direct invasion of the ureter by endometrial tissue that may lie within the lamina propria or muscular layers.

Ureteral involvement may result in hydronephrosis, narrowing of the pelvic ureter and, occasionally, intraureteral masses. Ureterography usually reveals a short or medium-length ureteral stricture in the distal segment (Fig. 16.50); the involved segment is usually within a few centimeters of the inferior aspect of the sacroiliac joint. The stricture is usually smooth but abruptly tapered, and there may be sharp medial angulation of the ureter in the region of the narrowed segment. The ureter distal to the site of involvement is normal. The intrinsic

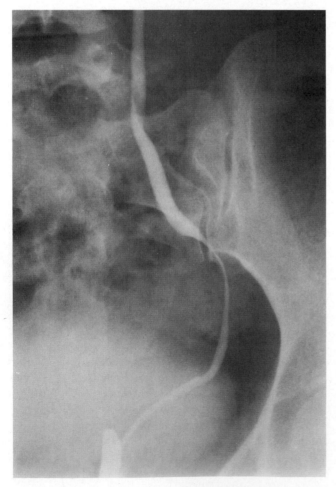

Figure 16.50. Ureteral endometriosis. Retrograde pyelogram shows a medium-length stricture at the pelvic brim.

and extrinsic forms of ureteral involvement by endometriosis cannot be distinguished by radiographic appearance alone. Computed tomography may demonstrate envelopment of the ureter by a soft tissue mass.

Inflammatory Bowel Disease

Genitourinary complications may occur in up to 25% of all patients with inflammatory bowel disease. Nephrolithiasis is the most common complication; obstruction due to direct ureteral involvement with inflammatory bowel processes is the second most common complication. In most patients, urinary tract involvement appears after the gastrointestinal disease has been present for years; rarely urinary pathology may be the initial manifestation of the disorder.

Ureteral involvement by Crohn's disease usually occurs on the right and is almost always at the level of the pelvic brim. The process may involve the ureter by direct extension of bowel inflammation to the pericolic or retroperitoneal regions, or by fistulae that extend from an involved bowel segment to the retroperitoneum, with periureteral inflammation that may or may not involve a flank abscess. Rarely, the left ureter may be involved in patients with granulomatous colitis or with Crohn's disease that involves the jejunum. Ureteral involvement often is asymptomatic; clinical evidence of psoas irritation may be present if there is a retroperitoneal abscess.

On urography, the involved ureter usually displays a sharply tapered smooth area of narrowing over several centimeters; and may cause varying degrees of obstruction (Fig. 16.51). A soft tissue inflammatory mass can usually be demonstrated by CT, which may simultaneously display the narrowing and wall thickening characteristic of Crohn's disease. When ureteral narrowing and obstruction have been caused by an acute exacerbation of inflammatory bowel disease, the obstruction usually diminishes with resolution of active bowel inflammation or surgical bypass of the abnormal segment. When the process has become chronic, however, dense periureteral fibrosis requiring ureterolysis may be present.

A small fraction of patients with diverticulitis have involvement of the ureter, usually on the left. As in patients with Crohn's disease, a focus of inflammation or frank abscess appears adjacent to the involved bowel and includes the ureter; the ureter itself may be displaced, compressed, or surrounded by the mass, and the specific diagnosis depends on the clinical or imaging diagnosis of diverticulitis.

Rarely, appendicitis and periappendiceal abscesses may involve and narrow the ureter. The specific appearance of the ureter on urography often does not offer a specific diagnosis of appendicitis, but if the clinical and imaging studies provide other indications of appendiceal inflammation or abscess formation, the diagnosis becomes apparent.

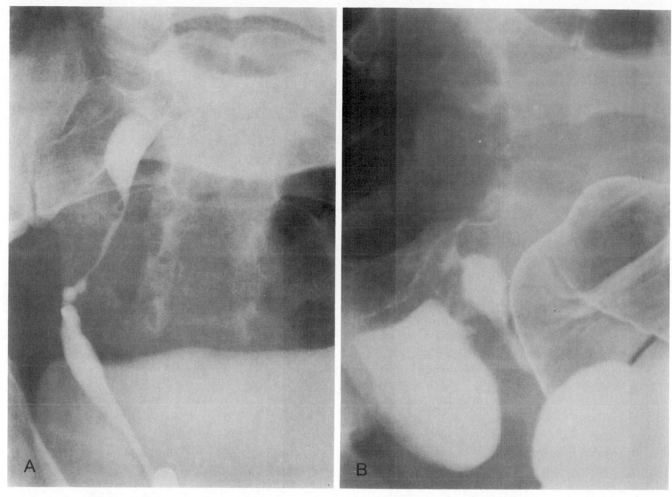

Figure 16.51. Crohn's disease. **A,** Retrograde pyelogram shows a long ureteral stricture involving the right ureter at the level of the pelvic brim. **B,** Barium enema shows characteristic changes of Crohn's disease involving the terminal ileum.

MISCELLANEOUS CONDITIONS

Pelvic Inflammatory Disease

Pelvic inflammatory disease and tuboovarian abscesses may produce extrinsic ureteral obstruction by surrounding the ureter with inflammation or by producing an abscess that compresses the ureter. This complication is more likely to occur in cases of chronic or recurrent pelvic inflammation, than in the acute stages of the disease. The obstruction usually occurs at the pelvic brim, and its radiologic appearance is similar to that produced by inflammatory bowel disease. In some cases, the ureteral obstruction resolves after conservative therapy, but when scarring and fibrosis are present, ureterolysis may be necessary.

Retroperitoneal Fibrosis

Retroperitoneal fibrosis is a disease in which a fibrous soft tissue mass develops in the retroperitoneum. It most frequently appears between the kidneys and pelvic brim and, by involving the ureters, becomes a disease primarily of urologic importance. However, retroperitoneal fibrosis may extend anywhere from the pelvic floor through the entire retroperitoneum into the mediastinum and even into the neck. In at least 70% of the cases, the etiology of the condition is unclear; idiopathic retroperitoneal fibrosis also is known as Ormond's disease.

The ingestion of methysergide (Sansert, Sandoz Pharmaceuticals, East Hanover, NJ) for relief of migraine headache is common among the specific conditions that predispose to retroperitoneal fibrosis. The disease may occur after several months of treatment and may regress when the drug is discontinued. It also is seen after administration of ergotamine and methyldopa. Other benign retroperitoneal processes may produce retroperitoneal fibrosis, including adjacent inflammatory disease of the kidneys, pancreas, and gastrointestinal tract. Retroperitoneal fibrosis has been reported after retroperitoneal involvement with collections of blood, urine, and contrast medium. The disease has been reported in association with abdominal aortic aneurysms; there has been controversy regarding whether or not retroperitoneal bleeding from the aneurysms is necessary to produce fibrosis. Retroperitoneal surgery and radiation therapy have produced the condition. Desmoplastic reactions may occur in response to a number of tumors, including Hodgkin's disease and other lymphomas, certain sarcomas and various anaplastic carcinomas (breast, stomach, colon, prostate, lung, and kidney). The radiographic findings in malignant retroperitoneal fibrosis may be sufficiently difficult to distinguish from the benign variety that biopsy may be required. Because many authorities believe that retroperitoneal fibrosis is an immunologic process, therapy with corticosteroids has been advocated as a major form of treatment; however, a combination of ureterolysis and steroid therapy is generally used in patients who need to be treated to salvage renal function.

The disease tends to appear clinically in patients between 50 and 70 years of age; there is a 3:1 male predilection. Flank or back pain, weight loss, nausea, vomiting, oliguria, and malaise are the most frequent presenting symptoms. In some cases, symptoms of lower-extremity venous obstruction or claudication are present. Hyper-

tension, anemia, and an elevated erythrocyte sedimentation rate are commonly found.

Pathologically, the lesion consists of a plaque-like soft tissue mass several centimeters thick that is seldom encapsulated but is well delineated; it has a woody consistency and a gray-white color. The lesion is composed primarily of fibrous tissue infiltrated to varying degrees by mononuclear cells and other blood elements. The mass surrounds, but usually does not invade, adjacent hollow viscera, muscles, blood vessels, lymphatics, and retroperitoneal nerves. It restricts the lumen of involved structures as a result of contraction of collagen fibers. Because the ureters are relatively sensitive to such compression, urinary obstruction often brings the condition to light.

Retroperitoneal fibrosis may be diagnosed radiologically by demonstrating the fibrotic mass and its effects on the ureter, blood vessels, and lymphatics. Plain-film findings are not specific. On urography, varying degrees of extrinsic ureteral narrowing may be observed (Fig. 16.52). The abnormalities may be unilateral or bilateral, and the length of the narrowed areas and degree of obstruction and proximal calyectasis is variable. Any portion of the ureter may be involved, but the middle one

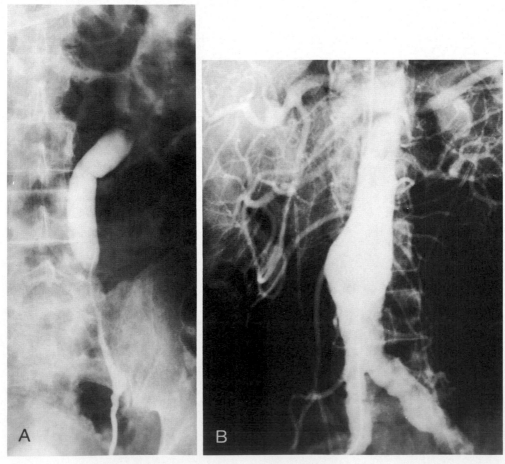

Figure 16.52. Retroperitoneal fibrosis. **A,** Retrograde pyelogram shows obstruction of the left ureter just above the pelvic brim. **B,** Abdominal aortogram shows an abdominal aortic aneurysm.

third is the most classic location. Peristalsis through the affected areas may be diminished or absent, and this peristaltic abnormality, as well as the obstruction, contributes to the renal impairment. Although the classic description includes medial displacement of the affected portions of the ureter, in most cases the ureteral course is not deviated beyond the range of normal. When azotemia precludes satisfactory excretory urography, retrograde or antegrade pyelography is necessary to demonstrate the characteristic ureteral changes. As in cases of primary megaureter, there is little resistance to passage of a retrograde catheter through the narrow regions of the ureter.

On ultrasound, retroperitoneal fibrosis is usually demonstrated as clearly marginated and extremely echopenic fibrotic masses. Nearly all patients have ultrasonographic evidence of calyectasis; when the retroperitoneum is obscured by obesity or intestinal gas, unilateral or bilateral hydronephrosis may be the only sign of the disease.

Computed tomography demonstrates the mass to be homogeneous; it usually demonstrates a relatively sharp anterior margin (Fig. 16.53). The mass may envelop the aorta, vena cava, and ureters, but, in contrast to retroperitoneal tumors such as lymphoma, does not displace these structures. The typical fibrous lesion may be seen on CT to be slightly denser than adjacent soft tissue structures, and may enhance with intravascular contrast administration.

On MRI, the fibrous tissue is usually of slightly greater signal intensity than retroperitoneal muscle on T1-weighted spin-echo images, but is distinctly less intense than fat. On T2-weighted images, the fibrous tissue may be quite low in intensity, especially if the fibrosis is benign and the process is long standing. This finding may be of use in distinguishing benign retroperitoneal fibrosis from retroperitoneal neoplasm or desmoplastic responses to tumor, which tend to be moderately heterogeneous. However, even benign retroperitoneal fibrosis, if rapidly growing, may display bright regions on T2-weighted images, so that MRI may not always obviate the need for biopsy. If the vena cava is compressed, flow phenomena may display lumenal abnormalities on MRI as contrast enhancement does on CT.

Ovarian Vein Syndrome

The right ovarian vein crosses the ureter at the level of the L3, but usually does not cause a distinct vascular impression. Cases of ureteral dilatation and hydronephrosis, sometimes in association with urinary tract infection, have been attributed to thrombosis of the vein. The syndrome typically occurs in young women who have had one or more pregnancies. The hydronephrosis of pregnancy, however, is probably not caused by the ovarian vein. Rarely, varicosities of the ovarian vein may produce multiple notched defects in the ureter.

Other vascular structures may produce impressions on the ureters. Tortuosity or aneurysms of the iliac vessels or aorta may deflect the ureters. Rarely, hemorrhage occurs from an abdominal aortic aneurysm and, if a

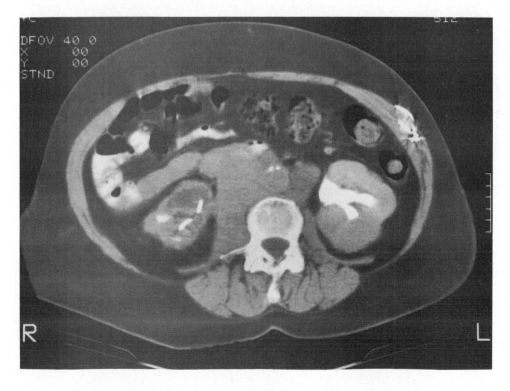

Figure 16.53. Retroperitoneal fibrosis. Computed tomography shows a large retroperitoneal mass that envelops the aorta and inferior vena cava. Bilateral hydronephrosis, worse on the right, is present; portions of a stent are seen in the right collecting system.

pseudoaneurysm forms, the ureter may be involved in its wall and become partially obstructed. Patients with severe renal artery stenosis may form collaterals that produce vascular notching on the ureter. Retroperitoneal branches from the aorta supply the ureteral artery, which enlarges and supplies flow that enters the renal artery distal to the stenosis. Although ureteral notching may be a sign of renal artery stenosis, it is not specific or sensitive. Venous collaterals associated with inferior vena cava or renal vein obstruction, vascular malformations, or congenital abnormalities also may be found. However, in most cases in which ureterography displays a vascular impression on the ureteral lumen, the finding is not associated with significant pathology.

An association exists between congenital ureteropelvic junction obstruction and impingement or entrapment of the ureteropelvic junction by a crossing vessel. Rarely, impressions on the ureters related to dilated lymphatics also may be found. Such cases occur in association with lymphatic obstruction or lymphangiectasia.

Dilatation of Pregnancy

Physiologic dilatation of the upper urinary tract occurs during pregnancy. The etiology of this dilatation has long been a matter of dispute; some believe that this phenomenon is a hormonal effect on the ureters, and others believe that it is primarily obstructive. The weight of opinion has supported the latter hypothesis. The changes of pregnancy are characterized by dilation of the proximal two thirds of the ureters, with more pronounced changes seen on the right (Fig. 16.54). The distal ureters are normal in caliber. Dilatation extends inferiorly to the point at which the ureter crosses the iliac artery at the pelvic brim. Slight differences in the angles at which the arteries and ureters cross may be responsible for the asymmetrical degrees of dilatation. The changes are presumed to be related to compression by the gravid uterus of the ureters against the iliac arteries. The changes usually resolve after delivery, but may persist to a slight degree. Pelvic masses in both sexes can produce changes in the ureters identical to those produced by pregnancy.

Pseudoureterocele

A ureterocele is a congenital cystic dilatation of the intramural segment of the intravesical ureter. On urography, these lesions produce bladder filling defects at the UVJ, which may be lucent throughout if the ureterocele is obstructed, or may have a lumen filled with contrast medium if there is no obstruction. Lesions that cause similar lucent filling defects at the UVJ are called pseudoureteroceles and are virtually always acquired lesions. They may represent edema caused by impaction at (or recent passage through) the UVJ of a small stone (Fig. 16.55), transitional cell carcinoma of the bladder, focal radiation cystitis, or even local invasion of part of

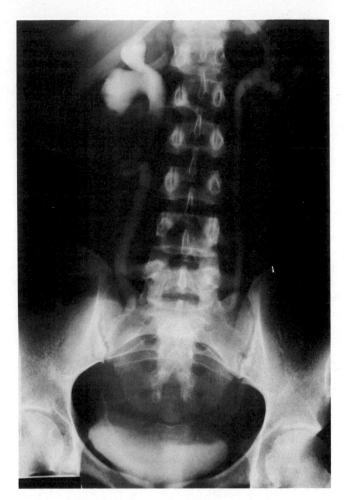

Figure 16.54. Dilatation of pregnancy. An excretory urogram shows bilateral ureterectasis, worse on the right, in this recently pregnant patient. The soft tissue mass in the pelvis is the still-enlarged uterus.

the bladder trigone by a secondary malignancy. Depending on the duration of the obstruction and the size of the abnormality within the bladder, these lesions may appear as primarily lucent UVJ masses with varying degrees of ureterectasis or as a "halo sign," which is a lucent rim surrounding a dilated intramural ureteral lumen. Distinction among the various etiologies of pseudoureterocele can be made using a combination of radiographic findings (smooth versus ragged margin of the filling defect, presence or absence of a calcified stone), clinical information (recent or ongoing colic), or cystoscopy.

Procidentia

Procidentia of the uterus is an uncommon cause of bilateral ureteral obstruction; in severe cases, it has led to hydronephrosis and progressive renal failure. The patients are usually elderly females with severe uterine prolapse. Urography may demonstrate the abnormality, especially if an upright film is included. The ureters are

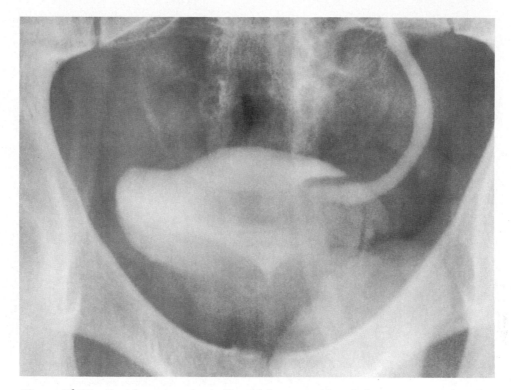

Figure 16.55.   Pseudoureterocele. A dilated left ureter with a "halo sign" surrounding the ureteral orifice is seen in this patient with a calculus impacted at the ureterovesicle junction.

seen to descend through the pelvic floor (Fig. 16.56), and may or may not be accompanied by urographic signs of bladder prolapse. The mechanism of ureteral obstruction is poorly understood; ureteral kinking, obstruction produced by the uterine artery, pressure from the levator ani muscles, and mechanical deformity of the ureteral meati in the bladder have all been proposed.

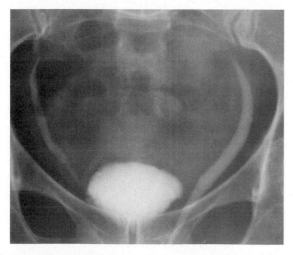

Figure 16.56.   Prolapsed bladder and distal ureter. This urogram reveals the nonprolapsed portion of the bladder; the prolapsed portion was not included on the film. The left ureter descends through the pelvic floor toward the prolapsed segment of the bladder.

Ureteral Herniation

Hernia of the ureter is rare, but is usually recognized on urograms. Occasionally, a herniated ureter may be obstructed. Inguinal, femoral, or sciatic hernias may include the ureter. The ureter accompanies hernias into the groin or scrotum only rarely and, of these cases, only a few are obstructed. Sciatic herniation is recognized by the characteristic ureteral course: the pelvic ureter extends laterally through the sacrosciatic notch, producing a hairpin-shaped redundancy (Fig. 16.29), which is only rarely obstructed.

Ureteral Stricture

Strictures of the ureter, not associated with a known pathogen or neoplasm, commonly result from some form of ureteral injury, either iatrogenic, after radiation therapy, or from external violence. The stricture is caused by damage to the blood supply of the ureter with resultant fibrosis. Approximately 10% of patients who undergo ureteroileal conduit diversion after cystectomy will develop a benign stricture at the ureteroileal anastomosis.

Antegrade transluminal dilatation now offers an attractive alternative to surgical therapy for the treatment of such strictures (Fig. 16.57). The long-term results of balloon catheter dilatation of ureteral strictures have been reported in several series. Johnson and associates report that for strictures less than 7 months old, an approximate

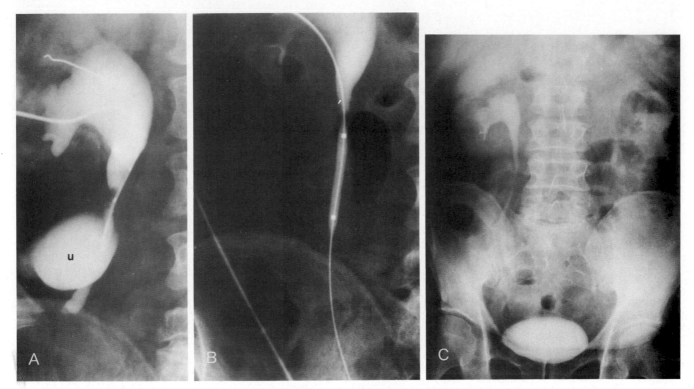

Figure 16.57. Balloon dilatation of a ureteral stricture. **A,** Antegrade pyelogram demonstrates complete occlusion of the midportion of the right ureter associated with a large urinoma (*U*) in a patient who underwent a traumatic midureteral stone basketing. After a period of nephrostomy drainage, the uri-noma resolved. **B,** A guidewire has been advanced through the stricture and a 6-mm balloon catheter inflated to dilate the stricture. A stent was then placed for 6 weeks. **C,** Follow-up urogram shows patency of the ureter with minimal residual dilatation of the right collecting system

65% success rate was achieved; in strictures present for longer than 7 months, however, balloon ureteroplasty was not successful. Lang and Glorioso reported an overall success rate of 50% for long-term patency. In this series also, procedures for strictures of short duration and those not associated with a compromised vascular supply of the ureter (i.e., after radiation therapy) had a higher success rate. Shapiro and coworkers have reported, however, that long-term success with the subgroup of patients having ureteroileal stricture dilatation is only 16% in patients followed for at least 1 year.

Ureteral fistulae may develop as a result of penetrating trauma or as a complication of ureteral surgery involving or adjacent to the urinary tract. They may also develop as a result of adjacent malignant or inflammatory disease.

Most ureteral fistulae present with associated urinary tract infection or with clinical evidence of urine flow through the fistula. Rarely, fistulae between the ureter and a blood vessel may result in massive gross hematuria.

The diagnosis of ureteral fistula is usually established by ureterography. Direct (antegrade or retrograde) injection of contrast medium into the ureter is more likely to demonstrate the fistula than excretory urography, because of the higher contrast concentration and greater in-

traureteral pressures that can be achieved. Rarely, contrast studies of the gastrointestinal tract in patients with ureteroenteric fistulae demonstrate a communication with the ureter. Computed tomography may demonstrate the primary lesion and movement of contrast medium through the fistula to or from the ureteral lumen.

Interventional uroradiologic procedures using a variety of catheters and guidewires to cross the segment of the ureter containing the fistula with subsequent antegrade ureteral stenting now play a major role in the management of such fistulas. Mitty and coworkers reported successful healing of ureteral fistulas in each of six patients in whom the procedure was technically successful. Lang reported a larger series of patients with ureteral leaks and fistulae; although the injured area of the ureter was successfully crossed in 41 of 50 patients, renal function was preserved for at least 6 months in only 30 patients.

SUGGESTED READING

General References

Bergman H (ed): *The Ureter,* ed 2. New York, Springer-Verlag, 1981.

Pfister RC, Newhouse JH: Radiology of ureter. *Urology* 12(1):15, 1978.

Weiss RM: Physiology of the upper urinary tract. *Semin Urol* 5(3):148, 1987.

Ureteral Obstruction

Amis ES, Cronan JJ, Pfister RC, et al.: Ultrasonic inaccuracies in diagnosing renal obstruction. *Urology* 19:101, 1982.

Bosniak MA, Megibow AJ, Ambos MA, et al.: Computed tomography of ureteral obstruction. *AJR* 138:1107, 1982.

Cremin BJ: Urinary ascites and obstructive uropathy. *Br J Radiol* 48:113, 1975.

Cronan JJ: Contemporary concepts for imaging urinary tract obstruction. *Urol Radiol* 14:8, 1992.

Dyer RB, Gilpin JW, Zagoria RJ, et al.: Vicarious contrast material excretion in patients with acute unilateral ureteral obstruction. *Radiology* 177:739, 1990.

Elkin M, Boyarsky S, Martinez J, et al.: Physiology of ureteral obstruction as determined by roentgenologic studies. *Radiology* 92(2):291, 1964.

Hay AM, Normal WJ, Rice ML, et al.: A comparison between diuresis renography and the Whitaker test in 64 kidneys. *Br J Urol* 56:561, 1984.

Hill MC, Rich JI, Mardiat JG, et al.: Sonography vs. excretory urography in acute flank pain. *AJR* 144:1235, 1985.

Hodson CJ, Craven JD: The radiology of obstructive atrophy of the kidney. *Clin Radiol* 17:305, 1966.

Howman-Giles R, Uren R, Roy LP, et al.: A comparison between diuresis renography and the Whitaker test in 64 kidneys. *Br J Urol* 56:561, 1984.

Kamholtz RG, Cronan JJ, Dorfman GS: Obstruction and the minimally dilated renal collecting system: US evaluation. *Radiology* 170:51, 1989.

Koff SA, Thrall JA, Keyes JW: Diuretic radionuclide urography: a noninvasive method for evaluating nephroureteral dilatation. *J Urol* 122:451, 1979.

Krueger RP, Ash JA, Silver MM, et al.: Primary hydronephrosis: Assessment of diuretic renography, pelvis perfusion pressure, operative findings and renal and ureteral histology. *Urol Clin North Am* 7:231, 1980.

Laing FC, Jeffrey RB Jr, Wing VW: Ultrasound versus excretory urography in evaluating acute flank pain. *Radiology* 154:613, 1985.

Levine M, Allen A, Stein JL, et al.: The crescent sign. *Radiology* 81:971, 1963.

McInerny D, Jones A, Roylance J: Urinoma. *Clin Radiol* 28:345, 1977.

Newhouse JH, Pfister RC: The nephrogram. *Radiol Clin North Am* 17:213, 1979.

Newhouse JH, Pfister RC, Hendren WH, et al.: Whitaker test after pyeloplasty: establishment of normal ureteral perfusion pressures. *AJR* 137:223, 1981.

O'Reilly PH, Testa HJ, Lawson RS, et al.: Diuresis renography in equivocal urinary tract obstruction. *Br J Urol* 50:76, 1978.

Pfister RC, Newhouse JH: Interventional percutaneous pyeloureteral techniques: I. Antegrade pyelography and ureteral perfusion. *Radiol Clin North Am* 17:341, 1979.

Platt JF, Puchin JM, Ellis JH: Acute renal obstruction: evaluation of intrarenal duplex Doppler and conventional ultrasound. *Radiology* 186:685, 1993.

Senac MO Jr, Miller JH, Stanley P: Evaluation of obstructive uropathy in children: radionuclide renography vs. the Whitaker test. *AJR* 143:11, 1984.

Talner LB, Scheible W, Ellenbogen PH, et al.: How accurate is ultrasonography in detecting hydronephrosis in azotemic patients? *Urol Radiol* 3:1, 1981.

Thrall JH, Koff SA, Keyes JW: Diuretic radionuclide renography and scintigraphy in the differential diagnosis of hydroureteronephrosis. *Semin Nucl Med* 11(2):89, 1981.

Vaughan ED Jr, Gillenwater JY: Recovery following complete chronic unilateral ureteral occlusion: functional radiographic and pathological alterations. *J Urol* 106:27, 1971.

Wacksman J, Brewer E, Gelfand MJ, et al.: Low grade pelviureteric junction obstruction with normal diuretic renography. *Br J Urol* 58:364, 1986.

Whitaker RH: Investigating wide ureter and ureteral pressure flow studies. *J Urol* 116:81, 1976.

Whitaker RH, Buxton-Thomas MS: A comparison of pressure flow studies and renography in equivocal upper urinary tract obstruction. *J Urol* 131:446, 1984.

Ureteral Dilatation

Hamilton S, Fitzpatrick JM: Primary non-obstructive megaureter in adults. *Clin Radiol* 38:181, 1987.

King LR: Megaloureter: definition, diagnosis and management. *J Urol* 123:222, 1980.

Pfister RC, Hendren WH: Primary megaureter in children and adults. *Urology* 12(2):160, 1978.

Sherwood T: The dilated upper urinary tract. *Radiol Clin North Am* 17:333, 1979.

Ureteral Course

Bree RL, Green B, Keiller DL, Genet EF: Medial deviations of the ureters secondary to psoas muscle hypertrophy. *Radiology* 118:691, 1976.

Cunat JS, Goldman SM: Extrinsic displacement of the ureter. *Semin Roentgenol* 21(3):188, 1986.

Ney C, Friedenberg RM: *Radiographic Atlas of the Genitourinary System*. Philadelphia, JB Lippincott, p 1295, 1981.

Pollack HM, Popky GL, Blumberg ML: Hernias of the ureter-an anatomic-roentgenographic study. *Radiology* 117:275, 1975.

Saldino RM, Palubinskas AJ: Medial displacement of the ureter: a normal variant which may simulate retroperitoneal fibrosis. *J Urol* 107:582, 1972.

Vesicoureteral Reflux

Blickman JG, Taylor GA, Lebowitz RL: Voiding cystourethrography: the initial study in children with urinary tract infection. *Radiology* 156:659, 1985.

Bourchier D, Abbott GD, Maling TMJ: Radiological abnormalities in children with urinary tract infection. *Radiology* 156:659, 1985.

Conway JJ, King LR, Belman AB, Thorson T: Detection of vesicoureteral reflux with radionuclide cystography. *AJR* 115:720, 1972.

Elo J, Tallgren LG, Sarna S, Alfthan O, Stenstrom R: The role of vesicoureteral reflux in pediatric urinary-tract infection. *Scand J Urol Nephrol* 15(3):243, 1981.

Gillenwater JY, Harrison RB, Kunin CM: Natural history of bacteriuria in schoolgirls: a long-term case-control study. *N Engl J Med* 301:346, 1979.

Hawtrey CE, et al.: Ureterovesical reflux in an adolescent and adult population. *J Urol* 170:1067, 1983.

Kincaid-Smith PS: Natural history and treatment of reflux nephropathy. In *Proceedings of the Ninth International Congress of Nephrology* (Los Angeles, June 1984). Berlin: Springer-Verlag, pp. 959–979, 1984.

Manley CB, Newman N, McAlister WH: Prognosis for resolution of moderate, primary reflux in girls. *J Urol* 115:307, 1976.

Newhouse JH, Amis ES Jr: The relationship between renal scarring and stone disease. *AJR* 151:1153, 1988.

Sirota L, Hertz M, Laufer E, et al.: Familial vesicoureteral reflux. A study of 16 families. *Urol Radiol* 8:22, 1986.

Strife JL, Bissett GS III, Kirks DR, et al.: Nuclear cystography and renal sonography: Findings in girls with urinary tract infection. *AJR* 153:115, 1989.

Thomsen HS: Vesicoureteral reflux and reflux nephropathy. *Acta Radiol Diagn* 26:3, 1985.

Wikstad I, Aperia A, Broberger D, Löhr G: Long-term effect of large vesicoureteral reflux. *Acta Radiol Diagn* 20:292, 1979.

Ureteral Tumors

Ambos MA, Bosniak MA, Megibow AJ, et al.: Ureteral involvement by metastatic disease. *Urol Radiol* 1:105, 1979.

Anderstrom C, Johnson SL, Petterson S, et al.: Carcinoma of the ureter: a clinicopathologic study of 49 cases. *J Urol* 142:280, 1989.

Babaian RJ, Johnson DE: Primary carcinoma of the ureter. *J Urol* 123:357, 1980.

Banner MP, Pollack HM: Fibrous ureteral polyps. *Radiology* 130: 73, 1979.

Baron RL, McClennan BL, Lee JKT, et al.: Computed tomography of transitional cell carcinoma of the renal pelvis and ureter. *Radiology* 144:125, 1982.

Debruyne FMJ, Moonen WA, Daenkindt AA, DeLaere KPJ: Fibroepithelial polyp of ureter. *Urology* 16:355, 1980.

Ghazi MR, Morales PA, Al-Askari S: Primary carcinoma of ureter. *Urology* 14:18, 1979.

Hughes FA, Davis CS: Multiple benign ureteral fibrous polyps. *Radiology* 126(4):723, 1976.

Kenney PJ, Stanley RJ: Computed tomography of ureteral tumors. *J Comput Assist Tomogr* 11(1):102, 1987.

Richie JP, Withers G, Ehrlich RM: Ureteral obstruction secondary to metastatic tumors. *Surg Gynecol Obstet* 148:355, 1979.

Winalski CS, Lipman JC, Tumeb SS: Ureteral neoplasms. *RadioGraphics* 10:271, 1990.

Witters S, Vereecken RL, Baert AL, et al.: Primary neoplasm of the ureter: a review of twenty eight cases. *Eur Urol* 13:256, 1987.

Yousem DM, Gatewood OMB, Goldman SM, et al.: Synchronous and metachronous transitional cell carcinoma of the urinary tract: prevalence, incidence, and radiographic detection. *Radiology* 167:613, 1988.

Leukoplakia

Benson RC Jr, Swanson SK, Farrow GM: Relationship of leukoplakia to urothelial malignancy. *J Urol* 131:507, 1984.

Hertle L, Androulakakis R: Keratinizing desquamative squamous metaplasia of the upper urinary tract: leukoplakia-cholesteatoma. *J Urol* 127:631, 1982.

Willis JS, Pollack HM, Curtis JA: Cholesteatoma of the upper urinary tract. *AJR* 136:941, 1981.

Malacoplakia

Arap S, Denes FT, Silva J, et al.: Malakoplakia of the urinary tract. *Eur Urol* 12:113, 1986.

Stanton MJ, Maxted W: Malacoplakia: a study of the literature and current concepts of pathogenesis, diagnosis and treatment. *J Urol* 125:139, 1981.

Ureteritis Cystica

Loitman BS, Chiat H: Ureteritis cystica and pyelitis cystica: a review of cases and roentgenologic criteria. *Radiology* 68:345, 1957.

Parker MD, Clark RL: Urothelial striations revisited. *Radiology* 198: 89, 1996.

Thompson JS, McAlister WH: Subepithelial hemorrhage in the renal pelvis and ureter simulating pyeloureteritis cystica. *Pediat Radiol* 3:156, 1975.

Pseudodiverticulosis

Cochran ST, Waisman J, Barbaric ZL: Radiographic and microscopic findings in multiple ureteral diverticula. *Radiology* 137: 631, 1980.

Wasserman NF: Pseudodiverticulosis: unusual appearance for metastases to the ureter. *Abdom Imaging* 19(4):376, 1994.

Wasserman NF, La Pointe SL, Posalaky IP: Ureteral pseudodiverticulosis. *Radiology* 155:561, 1985.

Wasserman NF, Posalaky IP, Dykoski R: The pathology of ureteral pseudodiverticulosis. *Invest Radiol* 23(8):592, 1988.

Wasserman NF, Zhang G, Posalaky IP, Reddy PK: Ureteral pseudodiverticula: frequent association with uroepithelial malignancy. *AJR* 157:69, 1991.

Eosinophilic Ureteritis

Uyama T, Moriwaki S, Aga Y, et al.: Eosinophilic ureteritis. *Urology* 18(6):615, 1981.

Schistosomiasis

Abdel-Wahab MF, Ramzy I, Esmat G, El Kafass H, Strickland GT: Ultrasound for detecting Schistosoma hematobium urinary tract complications: comparison with radiographic procedures. *J Urol* 148:346, 1992.

Al-Ghorab MM: Radiological manifestations of genito-urinary bilharziasis. *Clin Radiol* 19:100, 1968.

Jorulf H, Lindstedt E: Urogenital schistosomiasis: CT evaluation. *Radiology* 157:745, 1985.

Young SW, Khalid KH, Farid Z, et al.: Urinary tract lesions of schistosoma haematobium. *Radiology* 111:81, 1974.

Tuberculosis

Friedenberg RM, Ney C, Stachenfeld RA: Roentgenographic manifestations of tuberculosis of the ureter. *J Urol* 99:25, 1968.

Kollins SA, Hartman GW, Carr DT, et al.: Roentgenographic findings in urinary tract tuberculosis. *AJR* 121(3):487, 1974.

Roylance N, Penry JB, Davies ER, et al.: The radiology of tuberculosis of the urinary tract. *Clin Radiol* 21:163, 1970.

Amyloidosis

Davis PS, Bararia A, March DE, et al.: Primary amyloidosis of the ureter and renal pelvis. *Urol Radiol* 9:158, 1987.

Robinson CR, Fowler JE Jr: Localized amyloidosis of the ureter. *J Urol* 131:112, 1984.

Endometriosis

Kane C, Dronin P: Obstructive uropathy associated with endometriosis. *Am J Obstet Gynecol* 151:207, 1985.

Laube DW, Calderwood GW, Benda JA: Endometriosis causing ureteral obstruction. *Obstet Gynecol* 65:695, 1985.

Pollack HM, Wills JS: Radiographic features of ureteral endometriosis. *AJR* 131:627, 1978.

Inflammatory Bowel Disease

Banner MP: Genitourinary complications of inflammatory bowel disease. *Radiol Clin North Am* 25(1):199, 1987.

Demos TC, Moncada R: Inflammatory gastrointestinal disease presenting as genitourinary disease. *Urology* 13:115, 1979.

Shield DE, Litton B, Weiss RM, Schiff M, Jr: Urologic complications of inflammatory bowel disease. *J Urol* 115:701, 1976.

Retroperitoneal Fibrosis

Baker LRI, Mallinson WJW, Gregory MC, et al.: Idiopathic retroperitoneal fibrosis: a retrospective analysis of 60 cases. *Br J Urol* 60:497, 1988.

Degesys GE, Dunnick NR, Silverman PM, et al.: Retroperitoneal fibrosis: use of CT in distinguishing among possible causes. *AJR* 146:57, 1986.

Fagan CJ, Amparo EG, Davis M: Retroperitoneal fibrosis. *Semin Ultrasound* 3(2):123, 1982.

Graham JR, Suby HI, LeCompte PR, et al.: Fibrotic disorders associated with methysergide therapy for headache. *N Engl J Med* 274(7):359, 1966.

Hricak H, Higgins CB, William RD: Nuclear magnetic resonance imaging in retroperitoneal fibrosis. *AJR* 141:35, 1983.

Labardini MM, Ratliff RK: The abdominal aortic aneurysm and the ureter. *J Urol* 98:590, 1967.

Lepor H, Walsh PC: Idiopathic retroperitoneal fibrosis. *J Urol* 122:1, 1979.

Rubenstein WA, Gray G, Auh YH, et al.: CT of fibrous tissues and tumors with sonographic correlation. *AJR* 147:1067, 1986.

Ovarian Vein Syndrome

Angel JL, Kruppel RA: Computed tomography in diagnosis of puerperal ovarian vein thrombosis. *Obstet Gynecol* 63:61, 1984.

Dure-Smith P: Ovarian syndrome: Is it a myth? *Urology* 13:335, 1979.

Dykhvizen RF, Roberts JA: The ovarian vein syndrome. *Surg Gynecol Obstet* 130:443, 1970.

Dilatation of Pregnancy

Dure-Smith P: Pregnancy dilatation of the urinary tract. *Radiology* 96:545, 1970.

Peake SL, Roxburgh HB, Langlois S, Le P: Ultrasonic assessment of hydronephrosis of pregnancy. *Radiology* 146:167, 1983.

Watzer WC: The urinary tract in pregnancy. *J Urol* 125:271, 1981.

Pseudoureterocele

Thornbury JR, Silver TM, Vinson RK: Ureteroceles vs. pseudoureteroceles in adults. *Radiology* 122:81, 1977.

Procidentia

Chapman RH: Ureteric obstruction due to uterine prolapse. *Br J Urol* 47:531, 1975.

Stabler J: Uterine prolapse and urinary tract obstruction. *Br J Radiol* 50:493, 1977.

Ureteral Strictures

Banner MP, Pollack HM, Ring EJ and Wein AJ: Catheter dilatation of benign ureteral strictures. *Radiology* 147:427, 1983.

Beckman CF, Roth RA, Bihrle W III: Dilation of benign ureteral strictures. *Radiology* 172:432, 1989.

Johnson CD, Oke EJ, Dunnick NR, et al.: Percutaneous balloon dilatation of ureteral strictures. *AJR* 148:181, 1987.

Lang EK: Antegrade ureteral stenting for dehiscence, strictures and fistulae. *AJR* 143:795, 1984.

Lang EK, Glorioso LW III: Antegrade transluminal dilatation of benign ureteral strictures: long term results. *AJR* 150:131, 1988.

Mitty HA, Train JS, Dan SJ: Antegrade ureteral stenting in the management of fistulas, strictures and calculi. *Radiology* 149:433, 1983.

Shapiro MJ, Banner MP, Amendola MA, et al.: Balloon catheter dilatation of ureteroenteric strictures: long term results. *Radiology* 168:385, 1988.

17

The Urinary Bladder

BENIGN BLADDER CONDITIONS

Filling Defects

Filling defects in the bladder must be differentiated from contour defects. The term *filling defect* denotes something lying free within the bladder lumen and resulting in a lucent defect in the contrast-filled bladder on urography or cystography. Filling defects in the bladder also can be seen on plain films if they are intrinsically radiopaque or if they become encrusted with calcium. Examples include calculi, blood clots, and foreign bodies. Contour defects, however, are mural or mucosal lesions that alter the contour of the contrast-filled bladder; examples include urothelial tumors, metaplastic and inflammatory masses, and wall thickening from any cause.

Blood clots within the bladder may arise from a bleeding renal, ureteral, bladder, or prostate lesion. On excretory urography, a blood clot usually appears as an irregular mobile filling defect, but occasionally may ap-

pear fixed in position and therefore may not be distinguishable from a tumor. Clots in the bladder may have a vermiform or worm-like appearance if bleeding has occurred in the upper urinary tract and clot has formed in the ureter. Ultrasound shows that the blood clot is quite echogenic, unlike a bladder tumor, which has an echogenicity similar to the bladder wall or other soft tissue. Computed tomography (CT) may help to distinguish blood clot from tumor by demonstrating the typical high attenuation of blood (60–80 Hounsfield units [HU]), and also is useful to exclude a radiolucent stone.

Foreign bodies within the bladder are most commonly inserted by the patient. Among other items, pens, pencils, matches, wire, tubing, and string are seen within the bladder lumen. Foreign bodies also may be iatrogenic in origin or may result from penetrating trauma (e.g., bullets). Broken or shorn catheter fragments have been seen within the bladder. Another complication of bladder catheterization is the introduction of pubic hairs into the bladder. These may become encrusted with calcium (Fig. 17.1).

Most foreign bodies within the bladder are radiopaque. Long-standing intravesical radiolucent foreign bodies commonly have a deposit of encrusted calcium and may become apparent on plain films. Foreign bodies also are usually well seen on excretory urography and ultrasonography.

Edema

Mucosal edema around one ureteral orifice is most often caused by a stone impacted at the ureterovesical junction, but may also be due to the recent passage of such a stone (Fig. 17.2). Focal mucosal edema also may result from bladder irritation by extravesical conditions such as acute appendicitis, Crohn's disease, or sigmoid diverticulitis. Another cause of focal edema is an indwelling catheter, whose tip may irritate the bladder wall, typically near the dome. Generalized bullous edema may accompany acute cystitis secondary to infectious or inflammatory (irritative) etiologies.

Excretory urography and cystography show the irregularity of the bladder wall (Fig. 17.3**A**) when the bladder is filled with contrast medium; this is known as a contour defect, as opposed to a filling defect, which is an object in the bladder lumen and free of the wall.

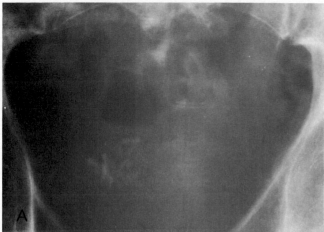

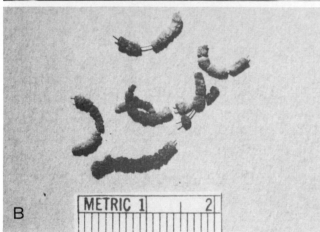

Figure 17.1.   A, A plain-film radiograph of the pelvis showing multiple irregular elongated calcifications within the bladder outline. **B,** Gross specimen on calcific encrusted hairs after removal at cystoscopy. (From Amendola MA, Sonda LP, Diokno AC, et al.: Bladder calculi complicating intermittent clean catheterization. *AJR* 141:751, 1983.)

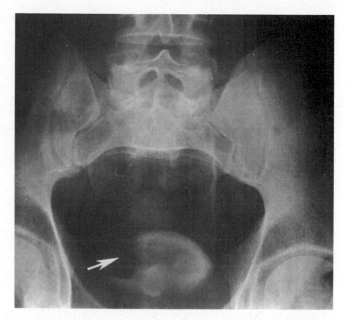

Figure 17.2.   Excretory urogram in a patient with severe right renal colic. A faintly opacified stone (*arrow*) is seen at the right ureterovesical junction. The filling defect in the bladder outline represents edema. (From McCallum RW, Colapinto V: *Urological Radiology of the Adult Male Lower Urinary Tract.* Springfield, IL, Charles C Thomas, p 271, 1976.)

The etiology of bladder edema cannot always be ascertained by imaging, and a malignant bladder infiltration should be excluded in such cases. Ultrasound may show an extravesical cause for localized bladder edema, such as an appendiceal abscess, a diverticular abscess, or a mass due to Crohn's disease. If no localized extravesical mass is seen, care should be taken to visualize the bladder wall for localized thickening, which may indicate a bladder tumor causing localized edema. Computed tomography may likewise show an associated extravesical mass. The density of the edematous mucosa is only slightly less than that of soft tissue and presents as a contour defect of the bladder wall. Computed tomography is unlikely to distinguish edema from other causes of bladder wall thickening, including the presence of infiltrating bladder tumor (Figs. 17.3**B** and 17.3**C**).

Infections

Virtually all acute infections of the bladder can, if severe, result in diffuse bullous edema of the urothelium, resulting in a nodular irregular contour of the bladder on imaging studies. In many instances, with proper therapy, this acute pattern will resolve in a matter of days and the bladder will return to its normal smooth appearance. However, severe infections can progress to a chronic phase, in which the bladder capacity is significantly reduced by fibrosis and contraction of the bladder wall. An identical chronic cystitis occurs with many of the inflammatory (irritative) processes discussed later in this chapter.

Acute Bacterial Cystitis

Acute cystitis is present when more than 100,000 bacteria are present in 1 ml of fresh urine. Most bacteria causing cystitis enter the bladder through the urethra. *Escherichia coli* is the most commonly encountered organism, but other common agents include species of *Staphylococcus, Streptococcus, Proteus, Pseudomonas, Aerobacter,* and *Candida.* Tuberculosis typically infects the bladder by descent down the ureter from a granulomatous focus in one or both kidneys.

Several factors contribute to the resistance of the bladder to becoming infected. These include a natural resistance of the bladder mucosa to invasion by infec-

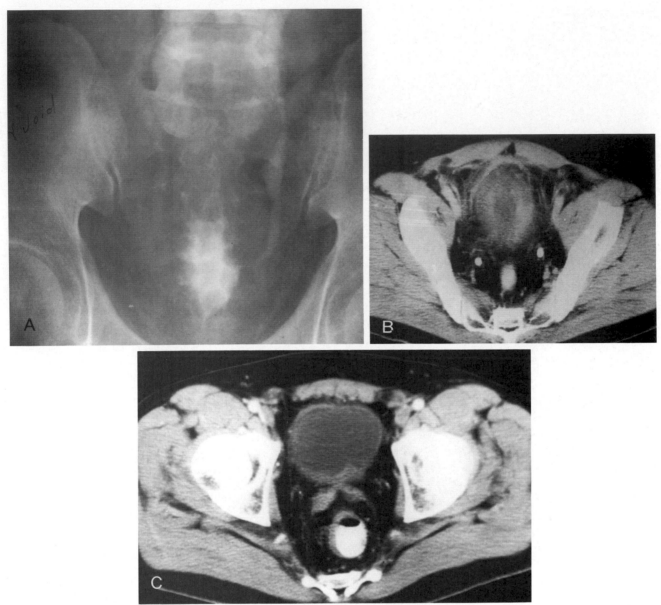

Figure 17.3. **A,** Excretory urogram in a patient with acute fulminating cystitis and severe bladder edema. Note the markedly reduced bladder capacity due to edema. **B,** Computed tomography of the same patient showing marked blad-der wall thickening. **C,** Computed tomography 1 month later. The edema has subsided, but the bladder wall remains irregularly thickened. Multiple bladder biopsies showed infiltrating transitional cell carcinoma. (Courtesy of P. Poon, M.D.)

tion, the washing of organisms out of the bladder by normal voiding, and trapping of organisms entering the bladder through the urethra by mucous secretion of the periurethral glands or the bactericidal effect of prostatic secretions. Bladder infection is almost invariably the result of interference with one or more of these factors. For example, the bladder mucosa may be damaged by trauma, stone, or tumor; outlet obstruction results in residual urine, so that bacteria are not completely washed out; and bladder catheterization or instrumentation may introduce infection by bypassing the protective mechanisms of the urethra and prostate. Acute cys-

titis can present with varying degrees of severity. In women, associated hemorrhage is common.

The excretory urogram is typically normal. However, in more severe cases, generalized bullous edema may result in a cobblestone appearance of the bladder wall. This finding is usually more apparent on films with the bladder partially filled or on the postvoid film if some residual contrast medium is present (Fig. 17.3A). Acute cystitis usually responds well to antibiotic therapy, and in uncomplicated cases with common organisms, does not progress to chronic disease. While cystitis may recur two or three times a year in sexually active women, more

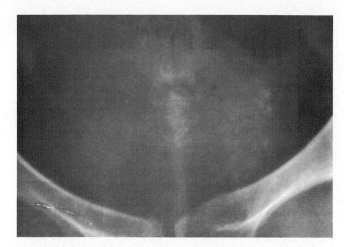

Figure 17.4. Early film from an excretory urogram in a patient with renal tuberculosis. Very little contrast medium has entered the bladder at this time. Multiple densities in the left bladder outline represent bladder tuberculous calcifications. (Courtesy of G. Hartman, M.D.)

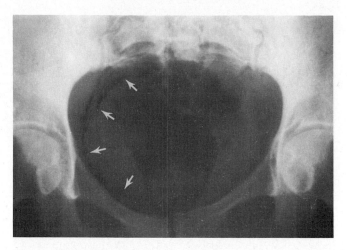

Figure 17.5. Emphysematous cystitis. Linear collections of gas within the bladder wall (*arrows*) indicate infection in this patient with diabetes mellitus.

frequent recurrence of acute cystitis and cases that are resistant to antibiotic therapy should raise the possibility of an underlying causative lesion within the urinary tract or from a source outside but adjacent to the bladder. In such cases, imaging of the entire urinary tract and cystoscopic evaluation of the bladder are usually indicated to exclude causes such as urinary stone disease, bladder diverticulum, colovesical fistula, and perivesical abscess.

Cystitis due to tuberculosis is an interstitial process initially associated with mucosal edema and later progressing to bladder wall thickening and fibrotic contraction with reduced bladder capacity and a predisposition to vesicoureteral reflux. Rarely there is calcification of the bladder wall (Fig. 17.4) as well as of the vasa deferentia, the seminal vesicles, the prostate, and the epididymides. However, calcification of the vas deferens (and sometimes of the seminal vesicles) is more commonly found as a result of diabetes mellitus, and is almost pathognomonic of that disease.

Emphysematous Cystitis

Emphysematous cystitis is a rare condition almost always found in diabetic or immunocompromised patients. This is a true infectious cystitis most often due to *E. coli,* which ferments glucose to produce carbon dioxide and hydrogen. This gas is initially formed in the bladder wall and subsequently transgresses the mucosa into the lumen of the bladder. Emphysematous cystitis is associated with the same type of irritative symptoms as any other acute bladder infection. Cystoscopic examination reveals a red and edematous mucosa with multiple blebs that rupture easily, releasing gas.

Gas within the bladder but not in the bladder wall is usually not caused by cystitis, but rather results from a

fistula between the bladder and the small bowel, colon, or vagina, or from catheterization or instrumentation of the bladder, during which air is introduced into the bladder.

In patients with emphysematous cystitis, the plain film typically shows gas within the bladder and irregular streaky radiolucencies within the bladder wall (Fig. 17.5). Gas may occasionally be seen in the ureters, which should raise the possibility of vesicoureteral reflux; however, it is possible for gas to pass through a competent vesicoureteral junction. Air within the bladder should not be mistaken for rectal air. Air within the bladder conforms to the bladder shape (i.e., ovoid with

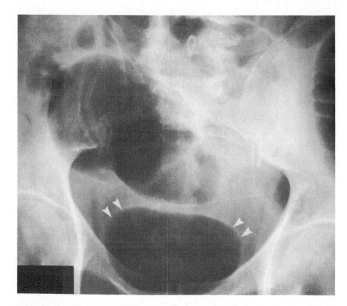

Figure 17.6. Gas within the bladder outline (*arrows*) resulting from colovesical fistula. (Modified from McCallum RW, Colapinto V: *Urological Radiology of the Adult Male Lower Urinary Tract.* Springfield, IL, Charles C Thomas, p 302, 1976.)

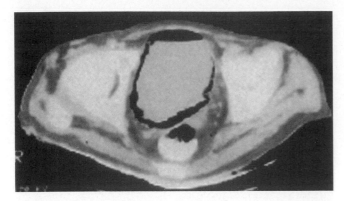

Figure 17.7. Computed tomography section through the bladder in a patient with emphysematous cystitis clearly shows gas within the bladder wall. The gas has ruptured into the bladder lumen, resulting in a gas/fluid level anteriorly. (From Amis ES Jr, Newhouse JH: *Essentials of Uroradiology.* Boston, Little, Brown and Co, 1991.)

the long axis horizontal [like an egg on its side] and in central position low in the pelvis) (Fig. 17.6). Gas within the rectum has a vertical orientation, and the rectal folds often may be recognized. A lateral radiograph often is definitive by distinguishing the anterior position of the bladder from the posterior location of the rectum. Computed tomography clearly shows the mural and luminal location of the gas (Fig. 17.7).

Emphysematous cystitis almost always responds rapidly to appropriate antibiotic therapy and control of underlying diseases such as diabetes; it does not progress to a chronic condition.

Schistosomiasis

Schistosomiasis (Bilharzia) is one of the most common parasitic infections in the world. It can be contracted in many parts of Africa and is especially prevalent in the Nile Valley. Only *S. haematobium* affects the urinary tract. The definitive host is a human and the intermediate host is a fresh water snail. Because the disease typically involves the intestines and bladder, eggs escape the human host in the feces and urine. These eggs, when deposited in fresh water, hatch into miricidia which infest snails, develop, and emerge as infective cercariae. These cercariae infect humans during swimming, wading, or bathing in infested waters. After the skin is penetrated, they enter peripheral capillaries, drain to the lung, squeeze through the alveolar capillaries, and enter the systemic circulation. The only cercariae that survive enter the mesenteric arteries, and hence pass through the portal venous system. They develop into adolescent flukes in the portal blood and then migrate against the flow in the portal system using two suckers, which they alternately attach to the wall of a vein. They eventually reach the smallest venules in the

walls of the bladder and ureters, probably through the hemorrhoidal plexus. From there, millions of eggs enter the urine, or are trapped in the ureteral and bladder walls where they die, producing a severe granulomatous reaction. The granulomas calcify, causing linear streaks of calcium in the ureteral and bladder walls. Large conglomerations of eggs in the bladder wall produce masses known as bilharzioma, which may eventually calcify.

The clinical presentation of urinary schistosomiasis is typically hematuria. In initial stages, the bladder mucosa is edematous and hemorrhagic. Later, the bladder becomes fibrotic with a reduced volume and calcified wall. Cystoscopic examination is mandatory to exclude bladder cancer, which has a markedly increased incidence in patients with schistosomiasis. These tumors are typically squamous cell carcinomas. Biopsy may be necessary to distinguish bilharzioma from carcinoma, although carcinoma usually presents as a later complication. Schistosomiasis rarely affects the kidneys or collecting systems, except by obstruction due to ureteral and bladder disease.

Urographic findings in patients with early schistosomiasis may show an irregular bladder outline caused by edema and granulomatous reaction. No bladder or ureteral calcification is evident. As the disease progresses, faint hazy calcification of the bladder wall can be seen. Later in the disease, plain-film radiography may show dense calcification of the bladder wall, bladder stones, and ureteral calcification (Figs. 17.8 and 17.9). A bladder tumor should be suspected when follow-up studies show absence of wall calcification in areas that were previously calcified (Fig. 17.10). While there are other causes of bladder calcification (Table 17.1), none

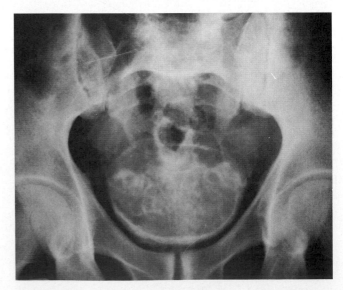

Figure 17.8. Plain-film radiograph of the pelvis showing marked bladder wall calcification. Seminal vesicle calcification also is seen through the bladder outline. (Courtesy of S. Sejeni, M.D.)

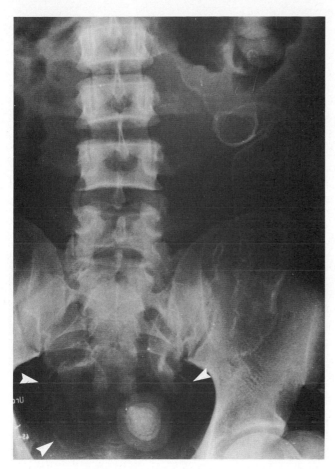

Figure 17.9. Plain-film radiograph in a patient with schistosomiasis. Crescentic calcifications are seen in the bladder wall (*arrows*). A large laminated stone is seen within the bladder. The ureter is dilated and calcified. (Modified from McCallum RW, Colapinto V: *Urological Radiology of the Adult Male Lower Urinary Tract.* Springfield, IL, Charles C Thomas, p 272, 1976.)

is as common or as dramatic as schistosomiasis. The ureterovesical junction may be partially obstructed by the changes in the bladder wall, resulting in ureteral dilation. Excretory urography may show obstructive dilatation of the upper urinary tracts in such cases. Schistosomiasis also may affect the prostate and urethra. The disease is destructive and results in urethral fistula formation, producing a pattern similar to that seen with advanced tuberculosis. Fistulae may drain into the perineum, scrotum, suprapubic skin, or buttocks.

Computed tomography is more sensitive than excretory urography in visualizing faint calcifications in the walls of the ureters and bladder in patients with suspected schistosomiasis.

Candidiasis

Candidiasis of the bladder, typically seen in poorly controlled diabetics causes fermentation of sugars in the urine, forming gas in the bladder lumen. It also may pre-

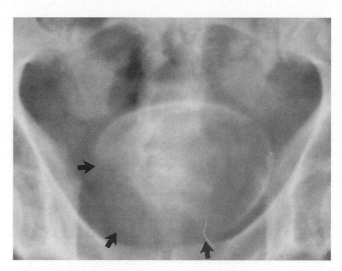

Figure 17.10. Plain-film radiograph of the pelvis reveals a faintly calcified wall in a somewhat contracted bladder in a patient with schistosomiasis. Note that the right inferolateral wall of the bladder is not calcified (*arrows*). This loss of calcification in a previously calcified bladder is indicative of the development of a tumor in this region.

sent as a fungus ball in the lumen. These fungus balls may be single or multiple, and are seen as laminated, gas-containing filling defects within the bladder.

Inflammatory Conditions

Radiation Cystitis

Usually seen after external beam irradiation doses of 3000 rads or more, the acute form of radiation cystitis is associated with edema and hemorrhage. This acute phase is usually self-limiting and resolves completely. However, it may progress to mucosal ulceration, fibrosis, and a small capacity bladder. Rarely, calcification of the bladder wall may occur. Hemorrhage in the acute phase may be severe, and angiographic embolization may be necessary to control bleeding. Cystography and excretory urography show contour irregularity of the bladder wall due to edema that is indistinguishable from other causes of bladder mucosal edema (Fig. 17.11). Fortunately, severe cystitis as a complication of radiation therapy is uncommon.

Table 17.1.
Causes of Bladder Calcification

Schistosomiasis
Tuberculosis
Radiation cystitis
Cytoxan cystitis
Alkaline encrustation cystitis
Amyloidosis
Tumor

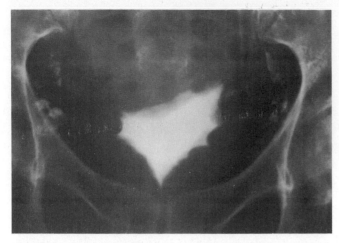

Figure 17.11. Radiation cystitis. Bladder irradiation has resulted in marked thickening of the bladder wall with edema.

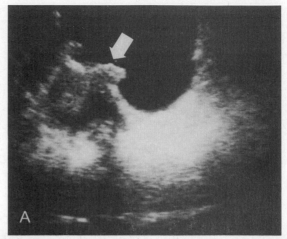

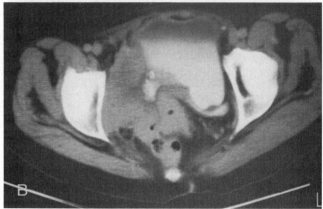

Figure 17.12. **A,** This 38-year-old woman had a renal transplant and was treated with cyclophosphamide. The ultrasound study shows a bladder mass (*arrow*) at the ureterovesical junction that proved to be transitional cell carcinoma. **B,** Computed tomography on the same patient. The transitional cell carcinoma extends through the bladder wall producing a large extravesical mass.

Cyclophosphamide Cystitis

Up to 40% of patients treated with cyclophosphamide (Cytoxan, Bristol-Myers Squibb, Princeton, NJ) may develop an acute cystitis. The inflammatory change is caused by exposure of the bladder mucosa to the metabolic end products of this chemotherapeutic agent. Marked bladder edema and hemorrhage can occur; hemorrhage may be so severe that angiographic embolization may be required. Massive bleeding may require heroic measures for control, including instillation of formalin into the bladder or even cystectomy. The acute form, usually following high-dose intravenous injections of cyclophosphamide, tends to resolve with symptomatic therapy. A chronic form can occur after many months of oral cyclophosphamide therapy, progressing to a contracted bladder. Bladder wall calcification is a rare finding in these patients. There is an increased incidence of bladder carcinoma in patients being treated with cyclophosphamide (Fig. 17.12).

Eosinophilic Cystitis

Eosinophilic cystitis occurs in patients with severe allergic conditions and is more common in women. Rarely it is seen in elderly men in association with chronic outlet obstruction. Eosinophilic infiltration of the bladder mucosa and submucosa results in edema, hemorrhage, and ulceration. Imaging of the bladder shows mucosal irregularity associated with focal or diffuse wall thickening. The condition usually responds well to steroids.

Alkaline Encrustation Cystitis

Alkaline encrustation cystitis may occur in association with bladder infection, typically *P. mirabilis*. Urea-splitting bacteria may cause a virulent cystitis, resulting

in areas of necrosis and sloughing in the mucosa and a severe inflammatory reaction in the muscularis and adventitia. An alkaline urine is produced by the release of ammonia from urea, which leads to calcium salt deposition in the necrotic areas of the mucosa; calcification may then be seen in the bladder wall (Fig. 17.13).

Interstitial Cystitis

Interstitial cystitis is seen only in women, usually after menopause. The mucosa is hemorrhagic, and a typical finding at cystoscopy is ulceration near the bladder dome that cracks and bleeds with bladder distention. This lesion is known as a Hunner's ulcer. Infiltration of the bladder wall with chronic inflammatory cells results in fibrosis and a very small bladder, often with a capacity of no more than 30 to 50 ml. Interstitial cystitis has no known etiology, and no associated conditions have been identified. The condition is extremely debilitating

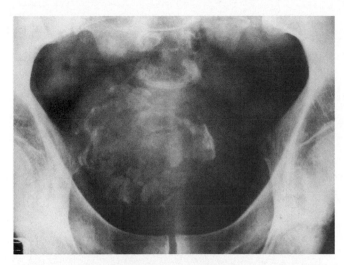

Figure 17.13. Alkaline encrustation cystitis. Plain-film radiograph of the pelvis reveals irregular sheet-like calcification in the region of the bladder. This elderly man proved to have a grossly enlarged prostate with severe outlet obstruction.

because of the small bladder capacity and the pain associated with overfilling.

Malacoplakia

Malacoplakia of the bladder is of unknown etiology, but is associated with conditions such as pulmonary tuberculosis, chronic osteomyelitis, and long-standing malignant disease elsewhere in the body. Malacoplakia may be associated with coliform bladder infection. The bladder mucosa is involved with multiple yellow-gray plaques that tend to occur in the bladder base. The histology of these plaques shows histiocytes, lymphocytes, and plasma cells. Michaelis-Gutmann bodies in the biopsy specimen are diagnostic; these calcospherules

are thought to result from phagocytized bacteria. Radiographically, rounded contour defects predominantly in the region of the trigone may be difficult to differentiate from cystitis cystica. Occasionally this benign process may resemble a tumor, requiring biopsy for diagnosis.

Infiltrating Lesions

Amyloidosis

Amyloidosis of the bladder is extremely rare. It may be primary or secondary and may be associated with amyloidosis elsewhere. The patient presents with hematuria and urinary frequency. Cystoscopy shows irregular infiltrating lesions in the mucosa and submucosa that bleed readily. Biopsy is necessary for diagnosis. Excretory urography, ultrasound, and CT may show multiple contour defects projecting into the bladder from the bladder wall, but the appearance is nonspecific and cannot be distinguished from other mucosal lesions. The bladder base often is spared. Rarely bladder wall calcification develops within the submucosal infiltrations.

Endometriosis

Endometriosis affecting the bladder is rare. Endometrial tissue may infiltrate through the bladder muscle and produce mural masses projecting into the bladder lumen. This condition results in cyclic hematuria that is more prominent at menstruation. The diagnosis is based on historical and cystoscopic findings. Ultrasound, CT, and magnetic resonance imaging (MRI) may be helpful in showing a mural mass protruding into the bladder, typically near the dome, as a direct extension of an extrauterine endometrial mass (Fig. 17.14). Other masses may be seen elsewhere in the pelvis and in the peritoneal space.

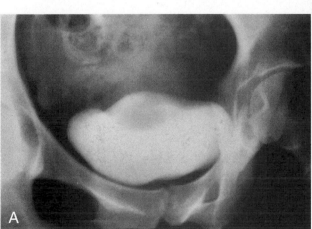
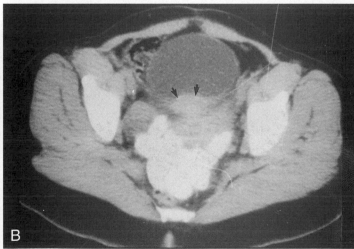

Figure 17.14. Endometriosis of the bladder. **A,** bladder phase of an excretory urogram reveals a smooth ovoid contour defect in the dome of the bladder. **B,** Computed tomography shows that this soft tissue mass involving the bladder wall (*arrows*) extends directly from an irregular pelvic mass. This proved to be endometriosis. (From Amis ES Jr, Newhouse JH: *Essentials of Uroradiology.* Boston, Little, Brown and Company, 1991.)

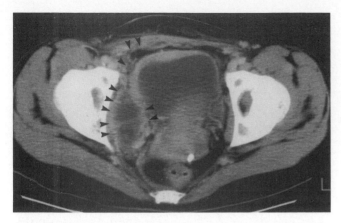

Figure 17.15. Computed tomography of the pelvis in a patient with an extensive thick-walled appendiceal abscess (*arrows*). Note the marked adjacent bladder wall thickening.

Perivesical Inflammatory Lesions

Inflammatory lesions in the pelvis can abut the bladder and produce reactive thickening of the bladder wall (Fig. 17.15) and mucosal irregularities. Mucosal changes may at times be so severe as to appear tumefactive (Fig. 17.16). If untreated, fistulization can occur. Typical conditions that can involve the bladder include appendiceal, diverticular, and tuboovarian abscesses. The bladder changes caused by such conditions may at times be difficult to differentiate from metaplastic processes or urothelial neoplasms originating in the bladder. Direct extension of tumor into the bladder from adjacent organs also can have a similar imaging appearance. However, the clinical presentation of a perivesical abscess should

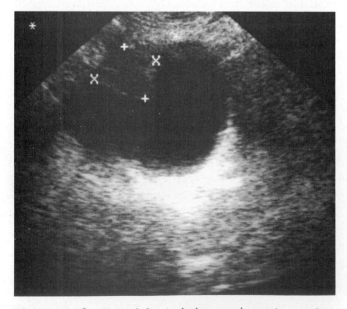

Figure 17.16. Transabdominal ultrasound scan in a patient with Crohn's disease. The inflammatory bowel process abuts the bladder, causing localized bladder wall edema (*markers*). Proven at cystoscopy.

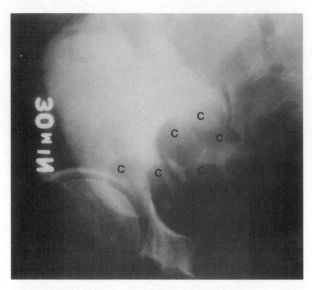

Figure 17.17. Cystitis cystica. Bladder phase of urogram (oblique view) shows smooth rounded contour defects in region of bladder base. c = cysts.

suggest an infectious process, and ultrasound or CT can be helpful in establishing the definitive diagnosis.

Proliferative/Metaplastic Conditions

Cystitis Cystica

Cystitis cystica is a benign condition, most commonly found in women with recurrent or chronic cystitis secondary to *E. coli* infection. Domelike cystic lesions 1 to 2 cm in diameter tend to occur in the bladder base and on the trigone; these lesions result from degeneration of subepithelial clusters of transitional cells known as Brunn's nests. Radiographically, the bladder base shows multiple rounded contour defects (Fig. 17.17), a finding suggestive of, but not specific for, cystitis cystica.

Cystitis Glandularis

Cystitis glandularis, also associated with chronic or recurrent infections, occurs with further metaplasia of the Brunn's nests into glandular structures resembling intestinal epithelium. These lesions are considered premalignant because they occasionally transform into adenocarcinomas. On cystoscopy, typically one or more irregular mucosal lesions grossly resemble bladder cancer. Radiographically, these lesions can not be clearly differentiated from cancer (Fig. 17.18) and often require biopsy to establish the diagnosis.

Nephrogenic Adenoma

Nephrogenic adenoma is a very rare proliferative response of the bladder epithelium to chronic infection or irritation. The name derives from the histologic appearance of the lesions, which is similar to that of the prox-

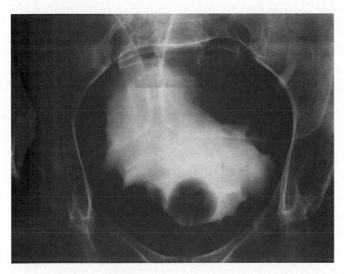

Figure 17.18. Multiple rounded masses are appreciated in the bladder wall in this patient with cystitis glandularis.

imal tubules of the nephron. This lesion is more common in the bladder than in other locations in the urinary tract, and can have diverse gross and radiographic appearances. Typically, the lesions may range from mucosal irregularities to large malignant-appearing masses arising from the bladder wall. No specific findings allow differentiation of nephrogenic adenoma from bladder cancer, and biopsy is necessary to establish the diagnosis. While this condition is not considered premalignant, it can involve the bladder extensively and is difficult to eradicate.

Diverticula

Bladder diverticula usually occur as a result of bladder outlet obstruction. Rarely a congenital deficiency in bladder musculature adjacent to the ureterovesical junction results in a diverticulum adjacent to the ureteral orifice. This is termed a "Hutch" diverticulum and is commonly associated with ipsilateral vesicoureteral reflux.

Bladder diverticula due to outlet obstruction are rare in children, but may occur in the clinical setting of urethral valves. Neurogenic dysfunction of the bladder is another cause of multiple diverticula in children. In men, diverticula can be found associated with any cause of bladder outlet obstruction, including urethral stricture (Fig. 17.19), prostatic hypertrophy, or prostatic carcinoma, although hypertrophy is the most common cause. Acquired bladder diverticula are rare in women.

Multiple bladder diverticula are common, usually arising from the lateral walls and rarely arising near the bladder dome. A wide-necked diverticulum empties readily when the bladder empties. A narrow-necked diverticulum empties slowly as the bladder empties and is therefore more likely to have residual urine and urinary

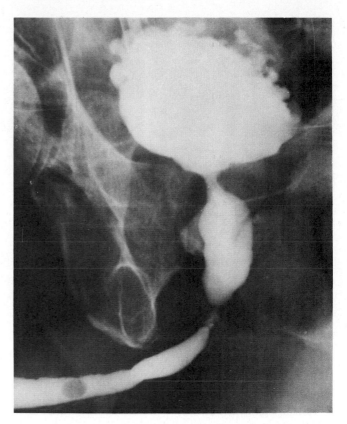

Figure 17.19. Severe bulbous urethral stricture causing outlet obstruction. Multiple bladder diverticulae and saccules are seen.

stasis. A large bladder diverticulum may displace the bladder to the opposite side and may be larger than the bladder. In such cases, the bladder is identified on urography by its irregular trabeculated contour and on CT by its thickened wall, while the diverticulum has a smooth thin wall. A large lateral wall diverticulum tends to deviate the ipsilateral distal ureter medially.

There may be a higher incidence of tumor in bladder diverticula than in the bladder lumen itself, explained by stasis of carcinogen-laden urine in the diverticulum. There is a tendency for such tumors to spread outside the bladder more rapidly than bladder lumen tumors because the wall of the diverticulum is not surrounded by detrusor muscle, rather consisting only of urothelium protruding between muscle bundles.

The plain film is seldom helpful in evaluating for bladder diverticulum, unless it contains a radioopaque calculus. Excretory urography commonly shows a diverticulum well (Fig. 17.20), but occasionally a narrow-necked diverticulum does not fill with contrast medium and can be overlooked. Anteroposterior and oblique views should be obtained during urography or cystography to evaluate the back of the bladder. A film should be obtained after voiding. If a bladder diverticulum is

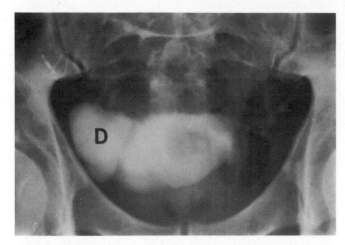

Figure 17.20. Bladder diverticulum. The irregular contour of the bladder is easily distinguished from the smooth contours of the diverticulum (*D*) on this excretory urogram.

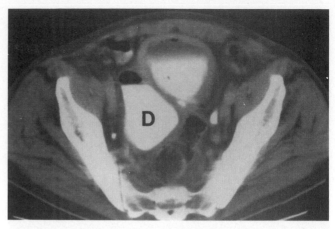

Figure 17.22. Computed tomography section clearly shows the bladder diverticulum (*D*). Air within the diverticulum and bladder are caused by recent instrumentation.

suspected but is not visualized, cystography is indicated. Cystography may be performed with a catheter in the bladder, but retrograde urethrography can provide information regarding the cause of outlet obstruction. A filling defect in a diverticulum is usually caused by stone, debris, or tumor.

Ultrasound also is effective in the assessment of bladder diverticula. Echo-free outpouchings from the bladder are readily seen (Fig. 17.21), and filling defects within a diverticulum such as stones or tumor also are visible. Tumor within a diverticulum may present as a soft-tissue mass in the diverticulum or only as a thick-

ening of the diverticulum wall, while stones produce typical shadowing.

Computed tomography also is an excellent method of assessing bladder diverticula (Fig. 17.22), but is usually

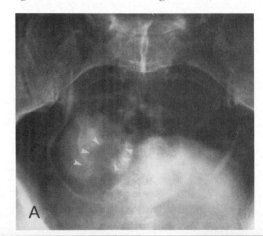

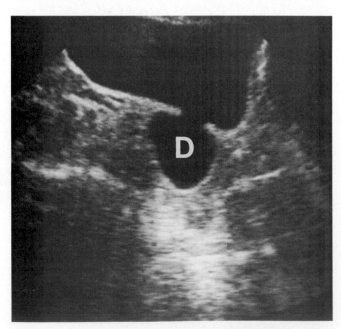

Figure 17.21. Transabdominal ultrasound showing the urine-filled bladder with a urine-filled wide-necked diverticulum (*D*).

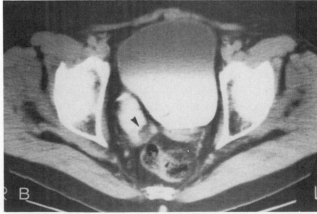

Figure 17.23. **A,** Excretory urogram showing a bladder diverticulum containing a lobulated filling defect (*arrows*). **B,** Computed tomography clearly showing the filling defect within the contrast medium–filled diverticulum (*arrow*). Proven transitional cell carcinoma.

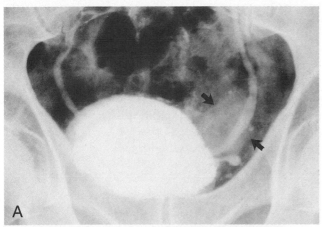

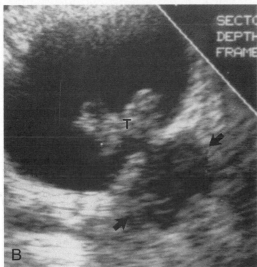

Figure 17.24. Bladder diverticulum filled with tumor. **A,** Bladder phase of excretory urogram reveals soft tissue mass (*arrows*) deviating bladder slightly to right. **B,** Sonogram shows tumor filling the diverticulum (*arrows*) with exophytic tumor (*T*) extending into bladder lumen. This part of the tumor was not appreciated on the urogram because of the opacity of the contrast in the bladder.

unnecessary. Stones are easily seen on unenhanced CT images as high-attenuation filling defects, whereas a tumor presents as a soft tissue mass arising from the diverticular wall and protruding into the contrast medium–filled diverticulum (Fig. 17.23). Occasionally a diverticulum may not fill with contrast medium because a tumor completely occupies its lumen or obstructs its neck (Fig. 17.24). Magnetic resonance imaging has been recently described as useful in evaluating tumors arising in bladder diverticula.

Herniation

Patients with herniation of the bladder into or through the inguinal canal present with swelling in the groin or scrotum that increases as the urinary bladder fills and subsides as the patient voids. This may cause painful, partly obstructed micturition because the trigone tends to remain in normal position, resulting in a sharp angle at the inguinal canal. Bladder herniation most commonly is paraperitoneal in location, with the bladder remaining extraperitoneal and medial to a true inguinal hernia sac. Herniation of the bladder also can be within a true hernia sac, or can occur totally extraperitoneally with the peritoneum remaining in the abdomen. The bladder also may herniate through the femoral canal into the thigh or through various incisional hernias.

Bladder herniation can occur in varying degrees and can usually be seen when the bladder is filled with contrast medium during excretory urography or cystography (Fig. 17.25), although an upright film is occasionally necessary to make the diagnosis. A prevoid and postvoid ultrasound examination also is useful for examination of suspected bladder herniation. Bladder herniation may occasionally be seen as an incidental finding on CT (Fig. 17.26).

Cystocele and Stress Incontinence

Cystocele occurs almost exclusively in multiparous women. Prolapse of the anterior vaginal wall and slackness of the pelvic floor muscles due to stretching during childbirth contribute to lack of support for the posteroinferior bladder wall, resulting in prolapse of that part of the bladder along with the anterior vaginal wall. Prolapse may be mild or severe enough that a large portion of the bladder protrudes through the introitus.

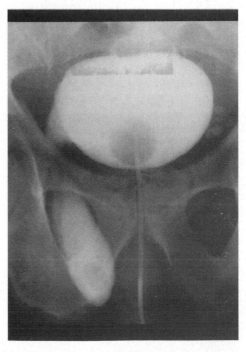

Figure 17.25. Bladder herniation. Cystogram shows part of bladder herniated into scrotum.

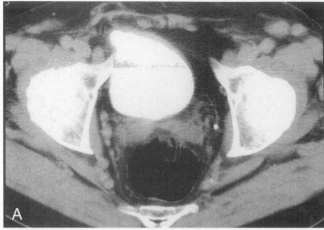

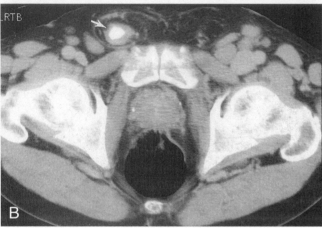

Figure 17.26. **A** and **B,** Bladder herniating into the inguinal canal (*arrow*) was found as an incidental finding on this contrast-enhanced computed tomography examination.

While cystocele has been related to stress incontinence of urine in some reports, this type of incontinence is probably caused by the angle at which the urethra joins the bladder. The posterior urethrovesical (PUV) angle should not be more than 100° in normal patients; the anterior angle of inclination (i.e., the angle formed by the urethra and a vertical line) should not exceed 40° (Fig. 17.27). Mild stress incontinence results from gradual increase of the PUV angle due to backward and downward rotation of the posterior bladder wall (Green type I); eventually this rotation becomes so severe that the PUV angle is virtually reversed, resulting in severe stress incontinence (Green type II).

In the past, chain cystourethrography was recommended to determine the PUV angle. This required the placement of a flexible chain throughout the urethra into the bladder lumen, filling the bladder with diluted contrast medium, and exposing films with the patient in standing, straining, and lateral positions. The radioopaque chain clearly showed the angle between the urethra and bladder. Currently, clinical evaluation is usually considered

satisfactory for determining the severity of stress incontinence and predicting the results of surgical correction.

Bladder Fistulae

Fistulae may develop between the bladder and the large or small bowel, or between the bladder and the vagina. Fistulae to the bowel are by far more difficult to detect unless the communication is large, resulting in the need for a high index of suspicion in patients with diseases predisposing to the formation of fistulae.

Enterovesical and Colovesical Fistulae

Fistulae to the bowel are classically described as presenting with fecaluria and pneumaturia. In fact, another common presentation is persistent urinary tract infection, resulting from a microscopic communication between the bladder and bowel that allows passage of bacteria, but not gas or stool.

When small bowel is involved, the term enterovesical fistula is preferred. Such fistulae are usually caused by Crohn's disease. The rectosigmoid colon is the most frequently involved segment of the large bowel in fistula development. These are called colovesical fistulae, and the most common cause in the United States is diverticulitis. Colon cancer is the second most common cause. Other causes of fistulae between the bladder and the bowel include penetrating trauma, surgical misadventures, other inflammatory processes such as appendiceal abscess or pelvic inflammatory disease, and bladder infections with granulomatous conditions such as schistosomiasis and tuberculosis.

The presence of gas in the bladder on plain films may indicate a fistula. However, recent instrumentation by catheterization or cystoscopy, or acute cystitis with *E. coli* also may produce such a finding. Gas in the bladder wall is only found in emphysematous cystitis.

Of the contrast studies, excretory urography is disappointing because it often fails to demonstrate any but the most gross fistulae, probably because the bladder is not distended during the procedure. Findings suggestive of a fistula on urography are focal irregularity and thickening of the bladder wall. Even using multiple studies, the likelihood of demonstrating the flow of contrast medium from bladder to bowel or bowel to bladder is not high. Cystography is positive in approximately 50% of cases, and barium enema or small bowel studies are positive in even fewer cases. However, when the fistulous tract is widely patent, imaging of the contrast-filled bladder or bowel dramatically demonstrates the communication (Fig. 17.28). Cystoscopy may show the actual fistula in gross cases; the more typical finding is an isolated area of inflammation of the bladder wall.

When fistula is suspected but cannot be demonstrated by standard examinations, CT has proved to be a sensitive modality for detecting the condition. A small

CHAIN CYSTOURETHROGRAPHY

GREEN'S CLASSIFICATION OF STRESS INCONTINENCE

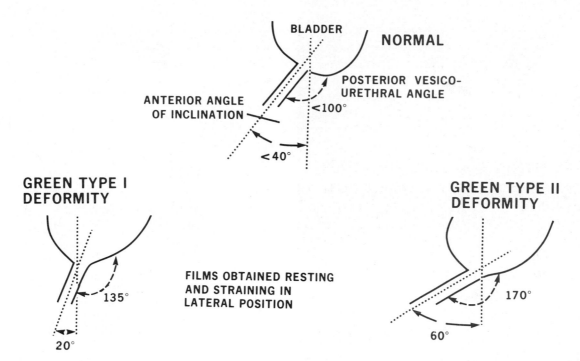

Figure 17.27.   Diagrammatic representation of normal and abnormal angles in the assessment of stress incontinence.

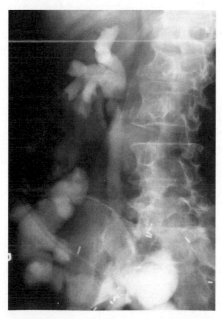

Figure 17.28.   Fistula from ileal conduit to colon. Opacification of colon is seen during this loopogram. Note expected reflux into the right renal collecting system.

amount of air in the bladder lumen can be seen in 90% of patients (Fig. 17.29) and an equal number exhibit focal bladder wall thickening, associated with focal thickening of a loop of small or large bowel adjacent to the bladder (Fig. 17.30). In approximately 75% of patients, a soft tissue mass is seen adjacent to the bladder. The diagnosis can usually be inferred from these findings in patients with predisposing conditions. As in cystography and barium enema, CT shows flow of contrast medium through the fistula in only about 50% of cases.

Vesicovaginal Fistula

Vesicovaginal fistulae result in painless constant dribbling of urine from the vagina. They may result from surgical misadventures and are a known complication in patients undergoing radical surgery for pelvic malignancies, especially after preoperative radiation. A rare cause of fistulization between the bladder and female genital tract is gynecologic malignancy that invades the bladder. Such patients may be treated with percutaneous occlusion of the ureteral lumen and permanent nephrostomy drainage as an alternate to surgery.

Vesicovaginal fistulae are usually relatively easy to demonstrate during urography or cystography. To visualize the contrast-filled vagina better, oblique, lat-

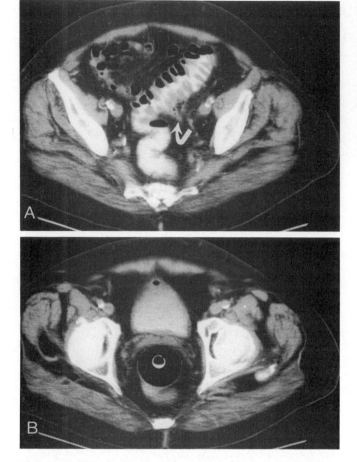

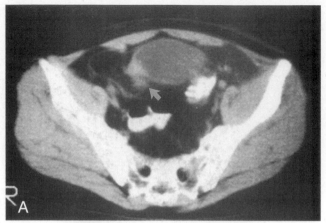

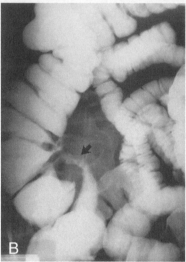

Figure 17.29.   **A,** Computed tomography examination in a patient with diverticulitis and paracolic abscess. The examination clearly shows evidence of diverticulitis and an irregular leak of barium (*arrow*) from the sigmoid colon. **B,** Same patient showing small pocket of air within the bladder.

Figure 17.30.   Enterovesical fistula secondary to Crohn's disease. **A,** Computed tomography section through the bladder shows right focal bladder wall thickening with an adjacent loop of small bowel (*arrow*). (From Amis ES Jr, Newhouse JH: *Essentials of Uroradiology.* Boston, Little, Brown and Company, 1991.) **B,** Barium study of the terminal ileum shows changes consistent with Crohn's disease (*arrow*).

eral (Fig. 17.31), or postvoiding (Fig. 17.32) films may be necessary.

Deviations and Impressions

Various conditions in the pelvis extrinsic to the bladder can cause impression (mass effect) of the bladder wall, can circumferentially compress the bladder, or can deviate the bladder to one side or the other.

Displacement or compression of the bladder implies a pelvic mass. There may be only a subtle mass effect on one wall, or the entire bladder may be dramatically deviated in virtually any direction depending on the location of the mass. Common lesions that may indent the bladder include enlarged pelvic lymph nodes, tumors arising from the colon, reproductive organs, or mesenchymal tissues, presacral teratomas, iliac artery aneurysms, hematomas, and abscesses. As previously discussed, a bladder diverticulum may become large enough to actually displace the bladder to one side; such a lesion is usually opacified during urography.

While a posterior bladder diverticulum can deviate the bladder anteriorly, another cystic mass that can occur behind the bladder is an anterior meningomyelocele. These masses are usually accompanied by pathognomonic change in the sacrum: a well-corticated concavity on one side of the sacrum, and deviation of the sacrum to the contralateral side. This is known as the "scimitar sacrum." Yet other cystic lesions that can indent the bladder from behind are seminal vesicle and müllerian duct cysts.

The female bladder may be impressed on its base, resulting in a radiographic pattern similar to that of an enlarged prostate in an older man as seen on excretory urography (Fig. 17.33). This has been termed the "female prostate." A variety of processes can produce this finding, the most common being a urethral diverticulum

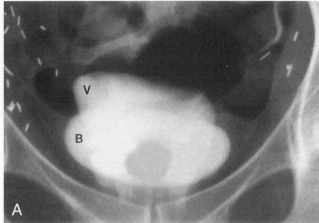

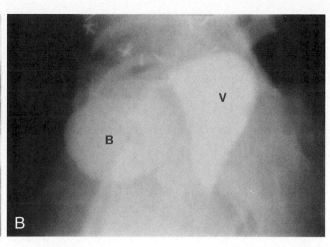

Figure 17.31. **A,** Contrast enhancement is seen in both the bladder (*B*) and vagina (*V*). **B,** The lateral view demonstrates the fistulous tract between the bladder (*B*) and vagina (*V*).

of the proximal urethra. These can extend cephalad in the urethrovaginal septum and indent the bladder base. Other causes of the "female prostate" include periurethral inflammation, urethral tumor, benign and malignant tumors of the anterior vaginal wall, degenerative or malignant changes of the pubic symphysis, and postoperative change after repair of urinary stress incontinence.

Circumferential compression of the bladder results in a configuration commonly known as a "teardrop," "vertical," or "pear-shaped" bladder. Several processes can involve the entire pelvis and can surround the bladder (Table 17.2), including the normal variant of a narrow pelvis with prominent iliopsoas muscles such as can be found in young male patients. Diffuse pelvic hematoma, another cause of teardrop bladder, is almost always seen in the setting of recent surgery or trauma (Fig. 17.34), although spontaneous bleeding can occur in patients with bleeding diatheses or on anticoagulation

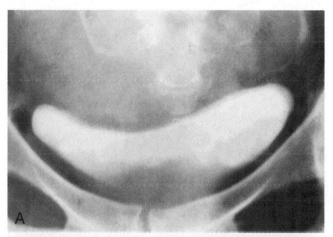

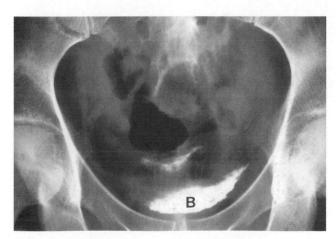

Figure 17.32. A postvoid film separates the contrast medium remaining in the bladder (*B*) from that in the vagina.

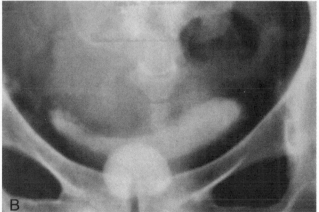

Figure 17.33. "Female prostate." **A,** Bladder phase of an excretory urogram in a middle-aged woman reveals an indentation on the base similar to that seen with an enlarged prostate in a man. **B,** Postvoid film shows filling of a urethral diverticulum, the etiology of the bladder base indentation. (From Amis ES Jr, Newhouse JH: *Essentials of Uroradiology.* Boston, Little, Brown and Co, 1991.)

Table 17.2.
Causes of Teardrop (Vertical) Bladder

Perivesical fluid (hematoma)
Pelvic lymphadenopathy (lymphoma)
Pelvic lipomatosis
Pelvic venous collaterals due to inferior vena cava
   obstruction
Retroperitoneal fibrosis
Pancreatic pseudocyst
Prominent ileopsoas muscles (normal variant)

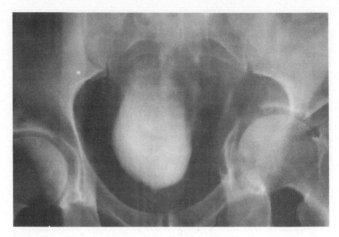

Figure 17.34.   Pelvic fracture. Hematomas from pelvic fracture create bilateral pelvic masses and a teardrop configuration of the bladder.

therapy. Other pelvic fluid collections, such as urinoma or rarely, abscesses, can surround and compress the bladder.

A common condition resulting in bladder compression is pelvic lipomatosis. This results from a proliferation of mature, unencapsulated fat within the pelvis, typically in middle-aged black men, although it also has been found in women and children. No etiology for this condition has been identified. Radiographically, plain films may show a lucency in the pelvis corresponding to the increased fat. Excretory urography shows the teardrop shape of the bladder, which may be extreme and elevated well above the pubic symphysis (Fig.

17.35**A**). The distal ureters are medially deviated, but the midureters may be laterally displaced due to the elevation of the lower urinary tract. Additionally, the ureters may be obstructed in severe cases. On barium enema, the rectosigmoid colon is straightened and narrowed (Fig. 17.36).

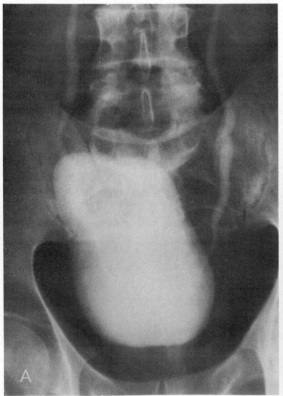

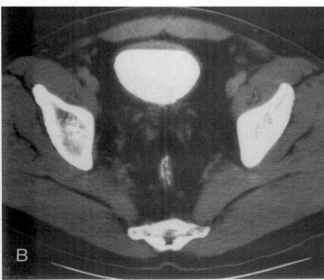

Figure 17.35.   Pelvic lipomatosis. **A,** On an excretory urogram, the bladder is vertically oriented and the base is elevated. Both ureters are deviated medially. **B,** Computed tomography demonstrates excess pelvic fat and the absence of soft tissue masses to explain the bladder deformity.

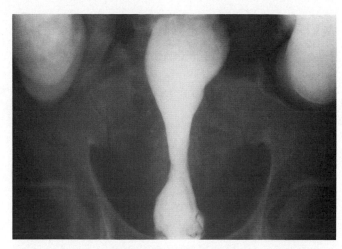

Figure 17.36. Pelvic lipomatosis. A barium enema demonstrates elevation of the rectosigmoid colon from the pelvis.

On ultrasound, pelvic lipomatosis is seen as compressed echo-free bladder floating in a sea of echogenic fat. The diagnosis can be easily confirmed with CT or MRI. On CT, the fat shows low attenuation values (Fig. 17.35**B**), and on MRI the fat has high signal intensity on T1-weighted images and intermediate high signal on T2-weighted images. A rare condition, lipoplastic lymphadenopathy, in which the pelvic nodes are filled with massive amounts of fat, may be difficult to differentiate from pelvic lipomatosis.

Bilateral pelvic lymphadenopathy due to metastatic disease also may result in a teardrop configuration of the bladder (Fig. 17.37). This is usually found in patients with lymphoma. Other tumors that drain to the pelvic lymph nodes, such as prostate cancers, do not typically produce bulky metastases. Other causes of teardrop bladder include development of massive venous collat

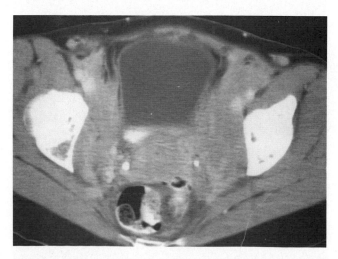

Figure 17.37. Lymphoma. Bilateral external iliac lymph node enlargement compresses the bladder resulting in a vertical orientation. This is easily distinguished from pelvic lipomatosis by computed tomography.

erals in the pelvis in patients with inferior vena caval obstruction, retroperitoneal fibrosis occurring deep in the pelvis, and lymphoceles that form after extensive pelvic lymph node dissection. Rarely, an extensive pancreatic pseudocyst may extend into the pelvis and compress the bladder. Diagnosis of these conditions also usually can be made using CT or MRI.

BLADDER TUMORS

Benign Tumors

Benign bladder tumors are rare, and the definitive diagnosis is cystoscopic and pathologic rather than radiologic. Most benign bladder tumors are mesenchymal in origin, and leiomyomas are the most common.

Leiomyoma

Leiomyoma of the bladder is most commonly found in women from 30 to 50 years of age. This lesion usually arises at the trigone, but may be found on the lateral or posterior walls. The dome and anterior bladder wall are infrequent sites. More than 60% of tumors project intravesically, 30% project extravesically, and the remainder have both intra- and extravesical components. Patients with intravesical leiomyoma commonly present with hematuria and irritative symptoms. Outlet obstruction due to trigonal leiomyoma at the bladder neck has been reported. Extravesical leiomyomas are usually asymptomatic until they reach a large size, and patients present with a palpable mass.

Radiographically, an intravesical leiomyoma is seen as a smooth mural mass protruding into the bladder lumen (Fig. 17.38). If there is a large extravesical component, the bladder will be compressed or displaced. Extravesical leiomyoma is seen as an extrinsic mass, and it may be difficult to discern that it originates in the bladder wall or to distinguish it from a uterine leiomyoma (Fig. 17.39).

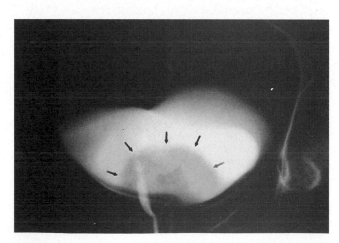

Figure 17.38. Leiomyoma. A smooth mural mass (*arrows*) is seen projecting into the bladder lumen.

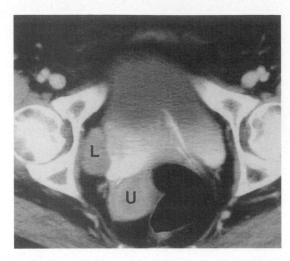

Figure 17.39. Leiomyoma. A soft tissue mass (*L*) arises from the lateral wall and projects outside the bladder lumen. The uterus (*U*) is seen posteriorly.

Ultrasound, CT, and MRI have all proven useful in evaluating such tumors.

Hamartoma

The few reported cases of bladder hamartoma are associated with hamartomas elsewhere, especially in the intestinal tract as found in patients with Peutz-Jeghers syndrome. Malignant change is well recognized in the intestinal hamartomas of Peutz-Jeghers syndrome, but no malignant potential has been recorded in bladder hamartomas. Local excision appears to be adequate therapy. The few reported cases have occurred in children or young adults. The lesion arises submucosally, and the overlying urothelium is commonly ulcerated.

Nephrogenic Adenoma

Nephrogenic adenoma is associated with metaplastic processes resulting from chronic urinary tract infection, bladder stones, an indwelling catheter, previous bladder trauma, and interstitial cystitis. Nephrogenic adenoma occurs as a localized polypoid lesion after a latent period of some years after the initial bladder insult. Unsuspected neoplastic processes, such as adenocarcinoma and transitional cell carcinoma, may be concomitantly present, and patients with nephrogenic adenoma require close follow-up. Radiologic examination is nonspecific and indistinguishable from other polypoid lesions.

Fibrous Polyp (Fibroepithelial Polyp)

A fibrous polyp is a small solitary polypoid lesion on a stalk consisting of a fibrovascular core covered by normal or slightly hyperplastic urothelium. The lesion is rare, but is found in children and young adults. The length of the stalk may allow the polyp to prolapse into the vesicourethral orifice, causing intermittent outlet obstruction or difficulty in micturition. The lesion is benign without malignant potential.

Bladder Papilloma

Bladder papilloma is epithelial in origin and is thought by many to be stage 0 bladder cancer. However, a few patients have had papillary lesions lined by transitional cells that are normal on cytology examination without the presence of mitoses. The lesions are benign at the time of local resection, but have a recurrence rate approximating 50%, and 10% of patients develop transitional cell carcinoma. Fifty percent of women and 30% of men with bladder papilloma will develop malignancy in a nonurologic site.

Pheochromocytoma

The bladder is a rare location for an ectopic pheochromocytoma. These tumors arise from chromaffin cells of the sympathetic plexus in or near the bladder wall. Most are found near the trigone. During cystoscopy, pheochromocytomas are seen as a small bulge in the bladder wall covered by transitional epithelium. A slight female predilection is reported.

Most patients with ectopic pheochromocytoma of the bladder are hypertensive and many have characteristic attacks of palpitations, sweating, headache, and blurred vision on micturition. The diagnosis should be suspected by this classic history and can be confirmed by measuring serum catecholamine levels.

An intramural mass may be detected on excretory urography. On CT examination, a soft tissue mass is seen in the wall of the bladder (Fig. 17.40). Because these tumors have a high signal intensity on T2-weighted images, they are readily identified on MRI as well.

Malignant Tumors

Malignant neoplasms involving the bladder are classified as primary or secondary. Primary tumors develop

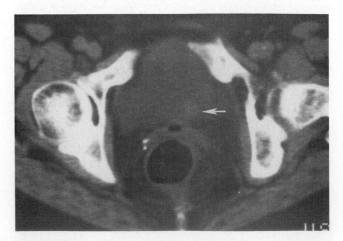

Figure 17.40. Pheochromocytoma. A small tumor mass (*arrow*) is seen in the bladder wall.

in the muscle wall or urothelium. Tumors of the urothelium are by far the more common bladder malignancies, comprising approximately 95% of all such lesions. Of the urothelial tumors, 90 to 95% are transitional cell carcinomas, 4 to 8% are squamous cell carcinomas, and 1 to 2% are adenocarcinomas. Bladder cancer is responsible for 4.5% of all new malignant tumors and 1.9% of cancer deaths in the United States.

Transitional Cell Carcinoma

There is a well known association of transitional cell carcinoma (TCC) with chemical carcinogens. These carcinogens include the aromatic amines, nitrosamines, and particular aldehydes such as acrolein that are common use in the textile, rubber, dye, and chemical industries. The latent period between occupational exposure and the development of clinical cancer is quite long, varying from 15 to 40 years.

Other causes of TCC include smoking and treatment with cyclophosphamide, a chemotherapeutic agent that results in the excretion of acrolein in the urine. A significant proportion of bladder tumors are found in cigarette smokers, probably because of aromatic amines, nitrosamines, and acrolein present in cigarette smoke.

Recent studies indicate that genetic factors in the host are responsible for regulating the response of the urothelium to carcinogens, probably by enzymatic degradation of the carcinogens as well as less understood changes in the urothelium itself.

Patients with TCC usually present with hematuria, although irritative symptoms from a secondary infection may be the initial complaint. When the tumor has obstructed one or both ureteral orifices, there may be aching loin pain, although the upper urinary tract obstruction is usually clinically silent because of its insidious onset.

While TCC can occur anywhere in the urinary tract where urothelium is present, it occurs most commonly in the bladder. This is because of the large surface area of the bladder and the fact that the bladder acts as a reservoir of urine. Therefore, any urine carcinogens are in contact with bladder urothelium longer than elsewhere in the urinary tract. In the bladder, TCC is most commonly found on the lateral walls (up to 50% of patients), followed in decreasing frequency by the trigone and bladder dome.

Transitional cell carcinoma spreads by invading through the bladder wall into the perivesical lymphatics and capillaries. Involvement of pelvic lymph nodes is common, and hematogenous spread is most frequent to liver and lungs, although lytic bone metastases also can be found in a small percentage of cases. Direct extension into the prostatic urethra and seminal vesicles in men and into the vagina in women can occur.

Staging of bladder carcinoma is an attempted assessment of the extent of tumor spread, in particular the degree of bladder wall penetration. Approximately 70% of all newly diagnosed TCC is superficial, 25% is already muscle invasive, and the remaining 5% has metastasized. Both the Jewett-Strong-Marshall (ABCD) and the tumor, nodes, metastases (TNM) staging classifications are based on the involvement by tumor of the various layers of the bladder wall, the perivesical fat, and more distant organs. Staging is diagrammatically illustrated in Figure 17.41.

The major difficulties in staging TCC are assessment of the degree of invasion of the muscle layers of the bladder wall, and whether or not microscopic spread of tumor into the perivesical fat has occurred. The TNM classification has been applied to bladder cancer, but many investigators believe that it is overcomplicated and does not clarify the difficulty in the staging of bladder cancer invading muscle.

Cellular grading of bladder cancer is a histologic assessment of malignant change. A recent emphasis on simplification of tumor grading seeks to classify tumors into three grades: well-differentiated (grade 1), moderately differentiated (grade 2), and poorly differentiated (grade 3). Grading of bladder carcinoma usually correlates well with staging: 80% of grade 3 lesions are invasive into muscle compared with only 50% of grade 2 lesions, and only 10% of grade 1.

Both staging and grading should be considered in the management of bladder carcinoma. Grades 1 and 2, stage 0, A, or B_1 are usually managed by local resection. Higher grades and stages may require partial or total cystectomy. Carcinoma in situ, although fitting into the staging classification as stage 0, commonly has histo-

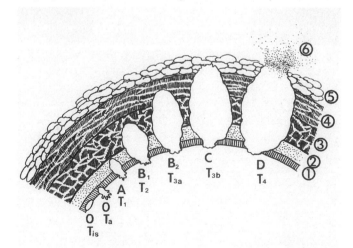

Figure 17.41. Staging of transitional cell carcinoma of the bladder. Both ABCD and TNM systems are shown. Layers of the bladder wall are as follows: *1,* mucosa; *2,* submucosa; *3,* superficial muscle; *4,* deep muscle; *5,* perivesical fat; and *6,* denoting adjacent organs or distant metastases. (From Amis ES Jr, Newhouse JH: *Essentials of Uroradiology.* Boston, Little, Brown and Company, 1991).

logic evidence of a higher grade. Approximately 12% of patients with carcinoma in situ develop invasive carcinoma.

In imaging TCC, the plain film is usually normal, and stippled or floccular dystrophic calcifications (Fig. 17.42) occur in less than 1% of cases. In some instances, tumoral calcification may be better appreciated on CT (Fig. 17.43).

Excretory urography should be performed in all cases of suspected or proven bladder cancer to exclude urothelial lesions in the collecting system and ureters, because multicentricity, although uncommon, is well documented in TCC. In slightly more than 2% of patients with bladder TCC, metachronous lesions of the upper urinary tract can be detected, usually after an average delay of 70 months; conversely, approximately 20% of patients with TCC of the upper urinary tract have a history of antecedent bladder tumor.

The bladder tumor may obstruct the ureteral orifice (Fig. 17.44); this is a poor prognostic sign, because such

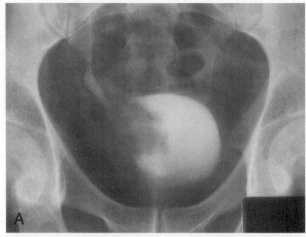

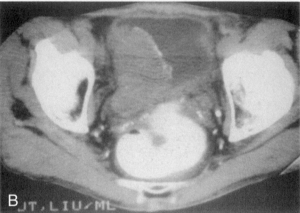

Figure 17.43. Calcified bladder tumor. **A,** Bladder phase of excretory urogram reveals a large irregular mass arising from right bladder wall. **B,** Computed tomography confirms the mass and also shows faint calcification on its surface. Note that the tumor has extended into the region of the right seminal vesicle and that another small focus on the left bladder wall is seen.

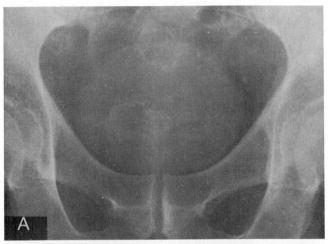

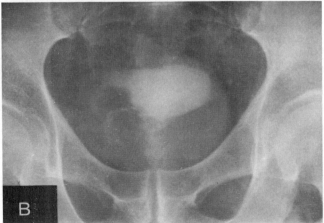

Figure 17.42. **A,** Plain-film radiograph demonstrating irregular crescentic calcification. **B,** Excretory urogram showing some contrast medium within the bladder. The calcification on the plain film is seen to be part of a lobulated filling defect, which proved to be transitional cell carcinoma.

tumors are usually invasive into the muscle around the involved ureteral orifice. Bladder cancers more than 1.5 cm in size can typically be seen on the bladder phase of an excretory urogram. Occasionally cancer is found within a bladder diverticulum; oblique views may be necessary for better visualization.

Overlying bowel gas may be difficult to distinguish from an intraluminal bladder filling defect, although oblique views also may be helpful. Because of this and other reasons, excretory urography is an insensitive modality for diagnosis of TCC, and cystoscopy remains the gold standard for evaluating the bladder of patients with hematuria. Cystography does not add significantly to the information obtained from urography, and it is rarely requested.

Suprapubic ultrasound has been reported of some use in visualizing bladder cancer. The filled bladder and bladder wall are well visualized in the normal patient.

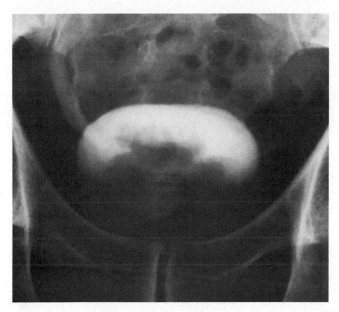

Figure 17.44. Excretory urogram showing dilated right ureter due to irregular transitional cell carcinoma. The bladder base is elevated by enlarged prostate.

Exophytic TCC is seen as a soft tissue mass projecting into the lumen from the bladder wall (Fig. 17.45). Stage 0 or stage A bladder cancers do not alter the normal echogenicity of the bladder muscle, whereas tumor invasion of bladder muscle may disrupt the normal echo pattern of the bladder wall.

The main advantage of CT over ultrasound is better definition of pelvic structures for staging. In addition, CT of the abdomen can delineate paraaortic lymph node enlargement (Fig. 17.46**A**) and can be used for guided biopsy of these nodes. Paraaortic node enlargement due to cancer of the bladder places the cancer in an ad-

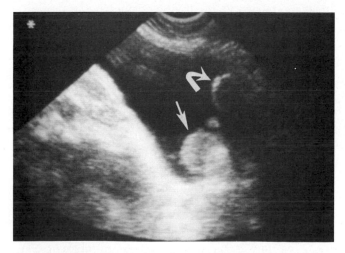

Figure 17.45. Suprapubic ultrasound showing a filling defect of irregular echogenicity (*straight arrow*) in the bladder producing thickening of the adjacent bladder wall. Proven transitional cell carcinoma. The curvilinear echogenic area (*curved arrow*) is a bladder catheter.

vanced stage D, which alters management. As with transabdominal ultrasound an exophytic TCC or wall thickening is usually readily visualized (Fig. 17.46**B**).

Tumor invading through the wall into perivesical fat and surrounding structures (Fig. 17.47) is better assessed by CT than by ultrasound. Anatomic detail of tumor involving pelvic muscles, vessels, and adjacent viscera is better seen with CT. When enlarged lymph nodes are identified, confirmation of the metastatic disease can be obtained with CT-guided thin needle biopsy. Dynamic scanning can identify tumor capillary enhancement, which may help detect tumors invading the bladder musculature or extending into perivesical fat.

Computed tomography also has proven helpful in following patients after treatment of TCC with radical cystectomy. Approximately one third of recurrences are at the cystectomy site, and two thirds are in the pelvic lymph nodes. Computed tomography in such patients

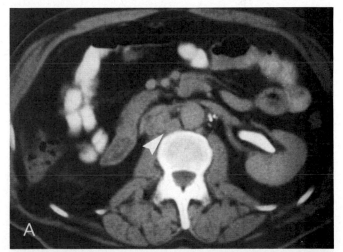

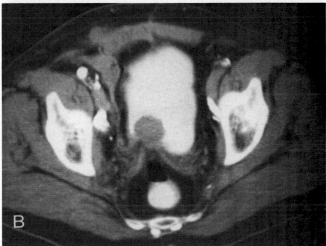

Figure 17.46. A, The right kidney has been removed for transitional cell carcinoma 1 year previously. Enlarged right paraaortic nodes are present (*arrowhead*). **B,** Same patient. The filling defect in the bladder is a second transitional cell carcinoma that has invaded through the bladder wall.

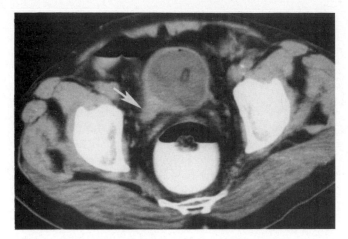

Figure 17.47. Computed tomography scan of pelvis in a patient with hematuria. The bladder wall is irregularly thickened and a mass is present at the ureterovesical junction (*arrow*) with invasion into the ureter. There also is early invasion of perivesical fat.

should not only include the upper abdomen to evaluate the liver for metastases, but also should extend to the deep perineum, because this is a common area for recurrence.

Magnetic resonance imaging is a promising modality for staging bladder cancer. T1-weighted images provide excellent anatomic detail. The fact that malignant tumors contain more water than normal tissue allows excellent tumor visualization on T2-weighted images (Fig. 17.48). Views can be obtained in the transverse, sagittal, and coronal planes, which may aid in the staging of bladder cancer. Muscle wall invasion may be clearly seen with MRI, possibly solving the problem of accurate differentiation of stage B_1 and stage B_2 tumors. The bladder should be filled with urine for this examination. On T2-

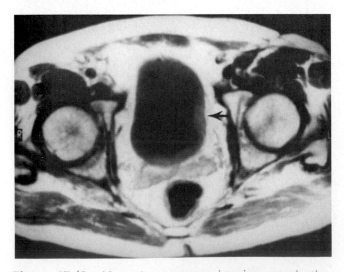

Figure 17.48. Magnetic resonance imaging examination showing a left bladder wall mass (*arrow*) extending to the posterior bladder wall on a T2-weighted image.

weighted images, normal low signal intensity of the bladder wall is increased in an area of tumor invasion, whereas transmural invasion presents as an area of lower intensity in the perivesical fat. Recent studies have shown that gadolinium-enhanced dynamic MR studies improve the assessment of extent of bladder wall invasion by TCC. In fact, one study comparing this technique with CT found an overall staging accuracy of 85% for enhanced MRI as opposed to 55% for CT. However, because MRI is expensive and still not universally available, and because many urologists rely on biopsy specimens to assess microscopic muscle invasion, CT remains the most widely used method for staging bladder tumors.

Squamous Cell Carcinoma

Most patients with squamous cell carcinoma have a history of chronic or recurrent bladder infections, bladder calculi, or both. The incidence of squamous cell tumors is higher in bladder diverticula than in the bladder lumen, probably because of stasis and infection. Patients with schistosomiasis are at increased risk for squamous cell tumors.

Squamous cell carcinomas are multifocal in 25% of patients and tend to be poorly differentiated and invasive. The 5-year survival rate for these patients is a dismal 10%.

Radiographically, squamous cell carcinoma cannot be differentiated from other urothelial tumors. As with TCC, staging is currently best accomplished with CT.

Adenocarcinoma

While bladder adenocarcinoma can be an isolated finding, this tumor is typically associated with metaplastic change in extrophic bladders, as a malignant transformation in patients with cystitis glandularis, and with urachal remnants in the region of the bladder dome.

Urachal Carcinoma

In adults, the urachus is a musculofibrous band 5 to 6 cm long extending from the umbilicus to the anterosuperior surface of the bladder. It lies in the extraperitoneal space of Retzius, between the transversalis fascia anteriorly and the peritoneum posteriorly. The urachus represents a vestigial remnant of the obliterated umbilical arteries and the allantois. It retains a minute lumen lined by transitional epithelium in 70% of adults. The bladder attachment of the urachus consists of supravesical, intramuscular, and intramucosal segments.

Numerous anomalies of urachal closure may occur. Patent urachus is failure of closure along the entire length of the urachus, resulting in urine draining from the umbilicus. Urachal cysts occur anywhere along the urachus and are caused by cystic dilation of an isolated section of urachal lumen. Urachal sinus is a blind-ending dilatation of a remaining segment of urachal lumen at the umbilical end. Urachal diverticulum is dilation of an isolated urachal lumen adjacent to the bladder, resulting in a diverticulum of the anterior superior aspect of the bladder. Patent urachus is rare and presents in infancy. Urachal cysts and sinuses usually present in adults and are not clinically recognized unless infection occurs in the cyst or sinus. Urachal diverticulum more commonly presents in adults and the diagnosis should be made when a single diverticulum is seen in the midline bladder dome.

The transitional epithelium lining the urachus may undergo metaplasia to glandular epithelium that can produce mucin. Consequently, malignant change in urachal epithelium includes mucin-producing adenocarcinoma (approximately 70%), nonmucin-producing adenocarcinomas (15%), transitional cell carcinomas, squamous cell carcinomas, or sarcomas. Squamous cell carcinomas are occasionally associated with urachal cysts and calculi in urachal diverticula. Approximately 70% of urachal sarcomas occur in patients younger than 20 years of age. Urachal carcinomas may occur at any age, but most occur in patients between 40 and 70 years of age. Sixty-five percent of urachal carcinomas occur in male patients, and 90% are juxtavesical.

Patients with urachal carcinoma usually present with hematuria. Mucus is found in the urine in 25% of patients and is an almost pathognomonic finding. Abdominal pain, a lower abdominal palpable mass, and dysuria also are presenting symptoms. Umbilical discharge is rare. Urachal carcinoma may invade the bladder and is visible cystoscopically in the bladder dome in the large majority of cases.

Calcification is common, but may be difficult to detect on the plain-film radiograph. The calcification may be stippled, granular, or curvilinear. Stippled calcification associated with deformity of the bladder dome is virtually pathognomonic of urachal carcinoma.

Ultrasound may show a supravesical complex mass. Computed tomography offers the most hope for a definite preoperative diagnosis, since this modality is capable of demonstrating the extravesical location and extent of the tumor. Calcification detected by CT has been reported in 70% of patients. Computed tomography demonstration of a calcified mass above or anterior to the bladder is highly suggestive of urachal carcinoma (Fig. 17.49). The mass may invade the bladder, extend anterosuperiorly to the umbilicus, or both.

The prognosis of patients with urachal carcinoma is poor, as 5-year survival rate is less than 15%. The poor prognosis is likely the result of late presentation of symptoms after the tumor is well-established, an early tendency for local infiltration, and the early development of lung and bone metastases.

The differential diagnosis includes a urothelial malignancy of the bladder (14% occur in the bladder dome)

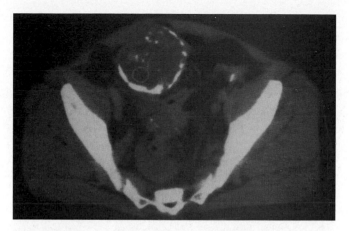

Figure 17.49.   Computed tomography demonstrating an anterior abdominal mass with a thick rim of irregular calcification and invasion of the right anterior abdominal wall musculature. Proven urachal carcinoma. (Courtesy of E. Fitzgerald, M.D.)

and a metastasis to the bladder from adenocarcinoma of the rectum, stomach, ovary, uterus, cervix, and prostate.

Malignant Mesenchymal Tumors of Bladder Muscle

These are rare tumors, the most common being leiomyosarcoma and rhabdomyosarcoma. Leiomyosarcomas have a tendency to grow quite large and ulcerate. If they are undifferentiated, they become less smooth, and may be difficult to distinguish from rhabdomyosarcomas.

Rhabdomyosarcomas have a biphasic age distribution. In adults, they and leiomyosarcomas tend to occur in the older age groups. The embryonal variety occurs during the first few years of life, and is quite similar to the rhabdomyosarcoma that arises from the prostate in boys and the vagina in girls. In fact, it often is very difficult to detect the organ of origin in rhabdomyosarcomas. The tumors frequently have a lobulated appearance resembling a cluster of grapes, resulting in the term "sarcoma botryoides". Patients with these highly malignant tumors have poor survival rates, even after radical extirpative surgery.

Radiographically, mesenchymal malignancies of the bladder typically present as irregular, ulcerating mural masses, unlike the smooth masses that typify benign lesions. Extension through the bladder wall into adjacent pelvic organs may make it difficult to determine the organ of origin. At any rate, biopsy is virtually always indicated to establish the diagnosis and to determine appropriate therapy. As noted above, a botryoid appearance of a bladder tumor is characteristic of rhabdomyosarcoma; these tumors may grow so large that they almost fill the bladder.

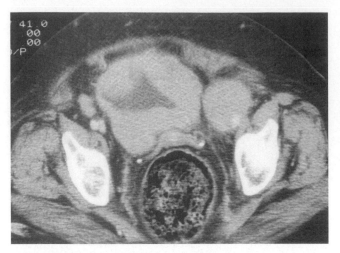

Figure 17.50. Lymphoma. Multiple soft tissue masses are seen in the bladder wall. Note the left iliac adenopathy.

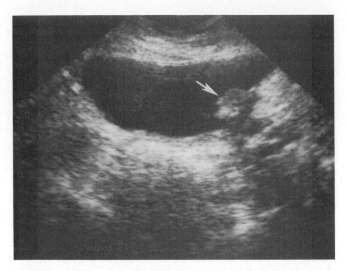

Figure 17.52. Transabdominal ultrasound showing a soft tissue mass projecting into the left side of the bladder (*arrow*). Proven carcinoma of sigmoid colon.

Lymphoma

Lymphoma involving the bladder is rare. However, this tumor can primarily occur in the bladder as a mural-based nodular mass, usually in the region of the bladder base (Fig. 17.50). It cannot be grossly or radiographically distinguished from other metaplastic or malignant lesions of the bladder.

Secondary Bladder Tumors

Metastases to the bladder constitute approximately 1% of all malignant vesical lesions. Furthermore, the bladder is only involved in 3 to 4% of patients with terminal carcinomatosis. The most common secondary tumor found in the bladder is malignant melanoma, usually presenting as multiple foci. Other tumors that commonly metastasize to the bladder through a hematogenous route include carcinomas of the stomach, colon, pancreas, ovary, breast, kidney, and lung. It is more common, however, for the bladder to be directly invaded by tumors in adja-

cent pelvic organs, such as prostate, sigmoid, and cervical cancers.

Radiographically, these tumors are seen as one or more mural masses projecting into the bladder lumen (Figs. 17.51–17.53). With the history of a primary tumor elsewhere, the diagnosis of secondary spread should be suspected when such a pattern is seen, but the possibility of a metaplastic process or primary urothelial tumor should not be discarded without biopsy if the patient's condition warrants.

BLADDER CALCULI

There are multiple causes of bladder calculi, the most common being bladder outlet obstruction. Other etiologies include infections with urea-splitting organisms

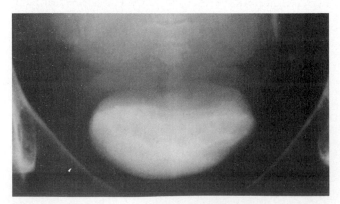

Figure 17.51. Cervical carcinoma invading bladder. Bladder phase of urogram shows gross mucosal nodularity. Note soft tissue tumor mass above bladder.

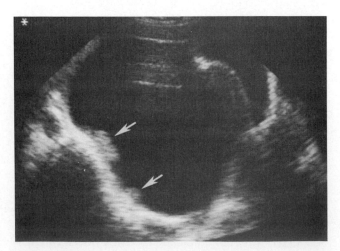

Figure 17.53. Transabdominal ultrasound scan showing nodular lesions (*arrows*) in a thickened bladder wall, due to invasion of the bladder wall by ovarian cystadenocarcinoma.

(triple phosphate stones), cystinuria (cystine stones), and hyperuricosuria (uric acid stones). In some cases, there may be more than one cause, such as bladder infection associated with outlet obstruction. Bladder stones are more common in men than in women.

In adult patients, outlet obstruction accounts for 70% of bladder stones. Outlet obstruction is most commonly the result of prostatic hypertrophy, but also may be seen with urethral stricture, bladder neck contracture, or neurogenic bladder dysfunction. The large majority of bladder stones due to obstruction are calcium oxalate, calcium phosphate, or a mixture of both. The remainder include triple phosphate "infection stones," uric acid stones, and cystine stones, which also may occur in the absence of bladder outlet obstruction.

An indwelling bladder catheter, although fulfilling its function of bladder drainage, will lead to bladder infection and may result in stone formation if left in position long enough. Catheter-associated stones are most frequently found in neurogenic bladders. Fortunately, modern treatment of such patients includes intermittent catheterization, bladder training, or continent urinary diversions, all of which preclude the need for long-term indwelling catheters. However, intermittent clean catheterization may introduce pubic hairs into the bladder that act as nidi for calcareous deposits resulting in stone formation.

Other unusual causes of bladder calculi are sutures in the bladder wall, which can act as a foreign body on which a stone may form, and foreign bodies (usually self-introduced via urethra as a form of sexual stimulation), which form a nidus for stone formation.

Most renal stones that migrate down the ureter into the bladder are quickly passed per urethra. Consequently, calculi only remain in the bladder when there is some degree of outlet obstruction; over a period of years, such stones may grow quite large.

Endemic calculi occur in infants and young children. Documentation of idiopathic stone disease first occurred in England in the nineteenth century. Such stone formation is usually caused by dietary factors, possibly replacement by carbohydrate food in the first few weeks of life. Although idiopathic stone disease has been eradicated in the Western world, it still occurs in underdeveloped countries.

A significant number of bladder stones are asymptomatic and are only discovered incidentally. Symptomatic patients present with bladder pain, which may be a dull ache suprapubically. Referred pain to the penis, buttock, perineum, or scrotum also may occur. Microhematuria in bladder stone disease may occur as a result of chronic irritation of bladder mucosa, but gross hematuria is rare.

Bladder stones may be visualized with plain radiography, excretory urography, ultrasound, and CT. Blad-

der stones vary from very dense to radiolucent (Fig. 17.54). An exacting radiographic technique is essential for stone visualization. A low kilovoltage of 60 to 70 kV to increase image contrast is generally best for plain-film studies. Bladder stones vary in size from a few millimeters in diameter to large stones that fill the bladder (Fig. 17.55). Well-calcified stones over a few millimeters in diameter are usually apparent on the plain film. They may be obscured by overlying fecal material in the rectosigmoid colon, or they may overlie the sacrum and coccyx, where they are difficult to identify. Consequently, any suspected calcification seen on the plain

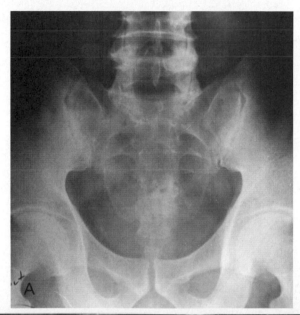

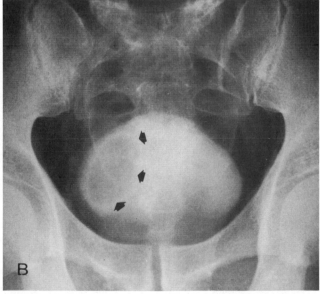

Figure 17.54.   A, Plain-film radiograph of the pelvis. No radiopaque calculus is visualized. **B,** Excretory urogram on the same patient showing the contrast-filled bladder with an oval filling defect (*arrowheads*) in the right side of the bladder that proved to be a uric acid stone.

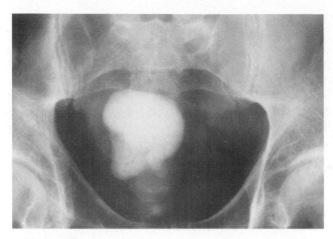

Figure 17.55. A huge bladder stone is evident on this plain-film radiograph.

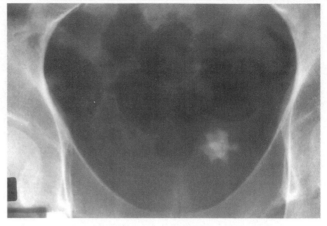

Figure 17.57. Bladder jackstone. This terminology is due to the multiple spiculations. (From Amis ES Jr, Newhouse JH: *Essentials of Uroradiology*. Boston, Little, Brown and Co, 1991.)

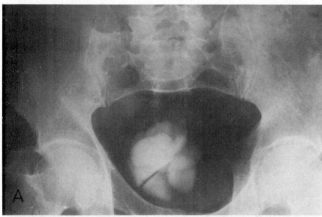

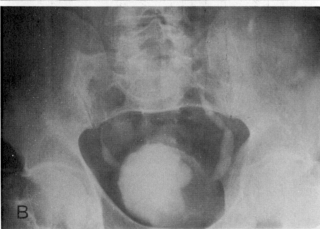

Figure 17.56. **A,** Plain-film radiograph of the pelvis showing multiple multifaceted stones lying to the right of midline. **B,** Same patient. Excretory urogram showing large filling defect in the left side of the bladder due to transitional cell carcinoma causing mild left ureteric dilatation. (From McCallum RW, Colapinto V: *Urological Radiology of the Adult Male Lower Urinary Tract*. Springfield, IL, Charles C Thomas, 1976.)

film should be pursued before the injection of contrast medium. Oblique views of the pelvis often are helpful in separating a calcified stone from the sacrum and coccyx, and colonic or rectal fecal material. Bladder stones should lie in the midline with the patient supine. Bladder stones identified on the plain film not lying in the midline may lie within a bladder diverticulum or may be displaced to one side by a large prostatic adenoma. Rarely, a large carcinoma resulting from long-standing chronic irritation may displace a stone (Fig. 17.56).

Bladder calculi may assume a variety of configurations. A laminated appearance is not unusual in bladder stones; these can grow to quite large sizes and can be single or multiple. Stones with multiple spicules are termed "jackstones" (Fig. 17.57), and those with a bumpy margin are known as "mulberry stones" (Fig. 17.58). Stones associated with bladder outlet obstruction

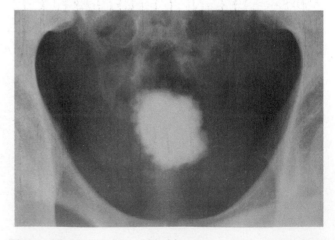

Figure 17.58. Mulberry bladder stone. (From Amis ES Jr, Newhouse JH: *Essentials of Uroradiology*. Boston, Little, Brown and Co, 1991.)

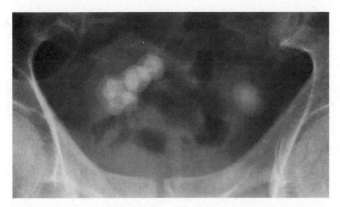

Figure 17.59. Multiple faceted stones in man with enlarged prostate. Note that the stones are displaced by the enlarged prostate elevating the bladder base.

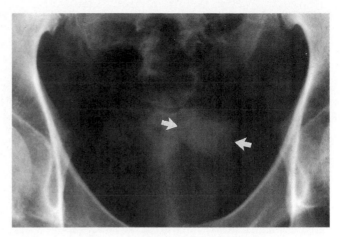

Figure 17.60. Cystine bladder stone. The oval stone (*arrows*) is only faintly seen on this plain film of the pelvis.

may be numerous, usually small and round (Fig. 17.59). Multiple stones also may have a faceted configuration.

Pure uric acid stones are radiolucent and are not seen on plain-film studies. Occasionally bladder calculi composed of struvite are faintly calcified, producing a shadow of low density. Even after careful scrutiny and oblique views, it may be impossible to be certain that a bladder stone is present. Cystine stones contain sulfur rather than calcium and are generally smoothly round or oval. If greater than 1 cm in diameter, they should be visible on the plain film (Fig. 17.60).

Calcified bladder calculi easily seen on the plain film may be completely obscured by contrast medium in the bladder during urography. Consequently, calcifications

in the pelvis raising the suspicion of bladder stones on the plain film may require oblique views of the contrast-filled bladder to prove they are intravesical and do not lie outside the filled bladder. Many calcified bladder stones are less dense than contrast medium, and therefore, cast a negative shadow within the bladder on the contrast-filled films (Fig. 17.61). However, oblique films may be necessary to distinguish bowel gas overlying the bladder from an intraluminal filling defect. Radiolucent stones cast negative shadows within the contrast-filled bladder. The bladder phase of all urograms should be carefully scrutinized for stones, because small calculi may be easily missed.

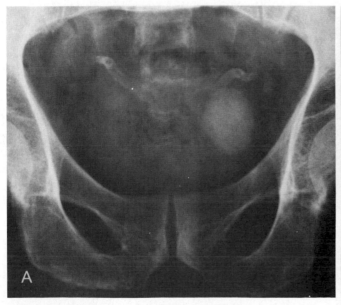

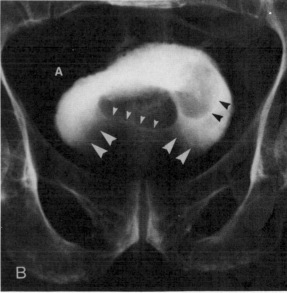

Figure 17.61. **A,** Plain-film radiograph of the pelvis in a diabetic male patient showing calcification in the vas deferens due to diabetes mellitus and an oval, faintly calcified stone on the left side of the bladder. **B,** Excretory urogram showing the stone as a filling defect (*black arrowheads*) surrounded by denser contrast medium. The stone is pushed to the left of the bladder by an enlarged prostate (*large white arrowheads*). The radiolucent area in the center of the bladder outline is gas in the bowel emphasized by Simpson's white line (*small white arrowheads*). The ampulla (*A*) of the vas deferens is again seen.

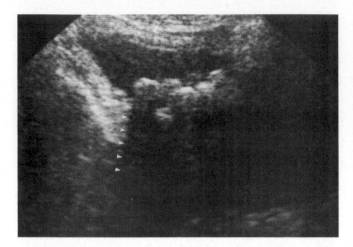

Figure 17.62. Transabdominal ultrasound in a patient with multiple bladder stones seen as bright echoes with acoustic shadowing (*arrows*).

Ultrasound demonstrates bladder stones as echogenic foci with acoustic shadowing (Figs. 17.62 and 17.63). Radiolucent or poorly calcified stones on radiography are well-seen on ultrasound and are not significantly different from well-calcified stones. Mobility of a shadow-producing lesion within the bladder distinguishes stone from calcified bladder tumor.

Computed tomography shows all bladder calculi, whatever their composition, as highly attenuated. Tumors with calcification are easily distinguished from stones (Fig. 17.64).

Small bladder stones seen at cystoscopy can be easily grasped by forceps and removed through the cystoscope. Larger stones must be crushed (litholapaxy) using a lithotrite or must be disintegrated to small fragments

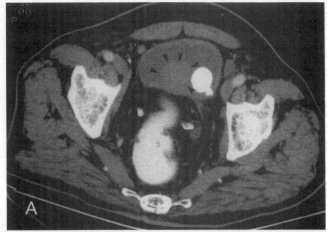

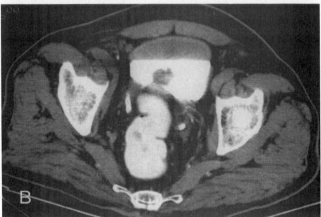

Figure 17.64. **A,** Computed tomography of the pelvis before contrast medium enters the bladder. Two dense stones are well seen. In addition, there is a faintly seen mass centrally (*arrows*). **B,** The bladder contains contrast medium, which obliterates the stones. The faintly seen mass is now obvious as a soft tissue mass arising from the posterior bladder wall. Proven transitional cell carcinoma.

using electrohydraulic lithotripsy. Fragments are washed out per urethra by continuous irrigation throughout the procedure. Very large stones are usually removed surgically. Pure uric acid stones too large for simple cystoscopic removal may be dissolved by systemic urinary alkalinization.

POSTOPERATIVE BLADDER CHANGES

Bladder Surgery to Compensate for Distal Ureteral Loss

An unfortunate circumstance of pelvic surgery can be the loss of viability of the distal portion of one ureter. This rare complication is typically seen after gynecologic surgery or after urologic procedures that involve manipulation or surgery on the distal ureter. Stricturing or sloughing of the distal ureter can occur, necessitating

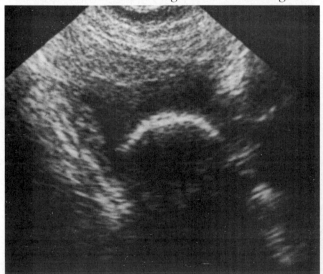

Figure 17.63. Transabdominal ultrasound. A single large bladder stone is present producing acoustic shadowing.

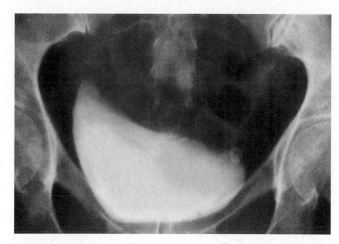

Figure 17.65. Psoas hitch. The bladder has been elevated and sutured to the iliopsoas fascia.

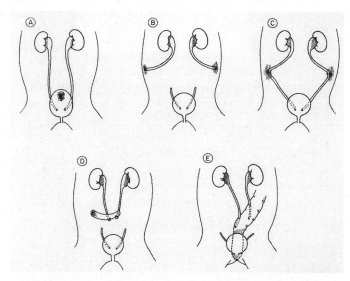

Figure 17.66. Types of urinary diversion. **A,** Vesicostomy. An opening is created between the bladder and the lower abdominal wall in the midline. **B,** End cutaneous ureterostomies. These are uncommonly used and are difficult to keep open unless the ureters are grossly dilated. **C,** Loop cutaneous ureterostomies. This temporary diversion involves creating an opening in the midportion of one or both ureters and bringing that portion of the ureter to the skin in the flank. **D,** Ileal conduit. This is a permanent diversion that has been popular since 1950. **E,** Ureterosigmoidostomy. This type of diversion is no longer commonly performed because of the increased incidence of bowel tumors. (From Amis ES Jr, Pfister RC, Hendren WH: Radiology of urinary undiversion. *Urol Radiol* 3:161, 1981.)

a procedure to bridge this ureteral deficiency. The bladder itself can be involved in this process, and at least two procedures result in distinctive appearances of the bladder postoperatively.

Psoas Hitch

The psoas hitch involves mobilization of the bladder so that the posterior wall and dome can be stretched toward the side of ureteral loss. The posterior bladder wall is sutured to the iliopsoas fascia above the level of the iliac vessels, resulting in a much more cephalad placement of the bladder base into which the remaining ureter can be reimplanted. This results in a characteristic bladder appearance on urography, often resembling a banana after significant mobilization and high fixation (Fig. 17.65). Distal ureteral gaps of 5 cm or more can be overcome using this procedure.

Boari Flap

The Boari flap is another method for bridging distal ureteral defects. In this technique, an anterior bladder flap is created, with the base of the flap on the side of ureteral deficiency. The flap is then rotated superiorly and rolled into a tube that will replace the distal ureter. Radiographically, a Boari flap is seen as a finger-like protrusion extending superolaterally from one side of the bladder. This protrusion fills with contrast on cystography, but because the ureter can be implanted into the tube in a nonrefluxing fashion, reflux into the upper urinary tract should not be seen.

Urinary Diversion

There are several methods for diverting urine from the kidneys to the skin above the level of a defunctionalized or surgically absent bladder (Fig. 17.66).

Temporary Diversions

A simple diversion is the end-cutaneous ureterostomy, in which the ureter or ureters are transected and the proximal ends brought to the skin. This procedure is rarely used, because ureters that are not significantly dilated tend to stenose at their anastomosis with the skin. A variation is the loop-cutaneous ureterostomy in which the exteriorized ureter drains into a collecting device. Yet another relatively simple way of diverting urine is to create a vesicostomy, in which an opening is created between the anterior bladder and the skin. These methods are temporizing measures for patients whose bladder function can be expected to improve.

Ileal Conduit

An acceptable permanent form of supravesical urinary diversion was described by Bricker in 1950. The ileal conduit, initially used for women undergoing pelvic exenteration, involves isolating a 15-cm length of terminal ileum to act as a urinary conduit. The mesentery of this bowel loop is left intact to ensure its viability, the proximal end is closed, and the ureters are anastomosed end-to-side to the loop. The distal open end of

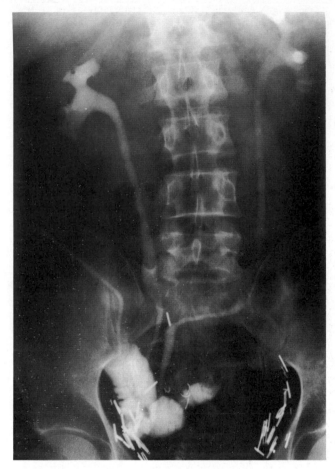

Figure 17.67. Ileal loop. A loopogram opacifies the ileal loop, and contrast medium refluxes into both upper urinary tracts.

the loop is tunneled through the abdominal wall in the right lower quadrant, and a nippled ostomy is formed, over which a collecting device can be placed. The ileal conduit is not a reservoir system and drains continuously into the collecting device, which must be worn at all times; this is a freely refluxing system. Ileal conduits are typically studied by loopography (*see* Chapter 3), in which a medium Foley catheter is inserted through the ostium and the balloon is inflated in the conduit just below the internal fascia. Contrast medium is then dripped through the catheter under fluoroscopic control, allowing visualization of the conduit and free reflux into the upper urinary tracts (Fig. 17.67). Because it is a freely refluxing system, it is common to see mild dilatation of the upper tracts. If there is no reflux into one or both upper tracts when the loop is filled, this suggests a stricture at the ureteroileal anastomosis, necessitating an antegrade study such as excretory urography or antegrade pyelography to confirm and determine the extent of obstruction (Fig. 17.68). Other complications of ileal conduits

include fibrosis of the loop with significant narrowing of the lumen. Filling defects can represent stones, or, very rarely, tumors. A smooth filling defect in the proximal end of the loop has been reported to occur in up to 20% of cases and represents the inverted tissue of the bowel segment.

Continent Diversions

Continent urinary diversions have gained wide acceptance as suitable alternatives to the ileal conduit. There are basically three types of continent urinary diversions, classified on the basis of the continence mechanism used. The first and oldest method is the diversion of urine into the intact large bowel, where the anal sphincter acts as a continence mechanism. Second, some patients whose bladders have been removed are suitable candidates for orthotopic pouches. These pouches are anastomosed to the remaining urethra in men, and the external sphincter becomes the continence mechanism. Third, for those patients in whom direct bladder replacement is inappropriate, the continent pouch can be situated higher in the abdomen and a continent abdominal wall stoma can be created.

Ureterosigmoidostomy

Ureterosigmoidostomy is the classic example of an anal continence mechanism. This procedure was first reported in 1851 when it was used in a child with exstrophy. However, this procedure has fallen into disrepute because of the 5% incidence of bowel adenocarcinomas developing at the ureterosigmoidostomy sites over a mean period of 25 years (Fig. 17.69). This increased incidence of tumor is believed to be due to urinary nitrates converted by fecal bacteria to active carcinogenic nitrosamines. These carcinogens act preferentially on intestinal cells. During the past decade, several procedures have been devised to form a valve mechanism that will protect the ureteric anastomosis from contact with feces; however, these procedures have not gained wide acceptance.

Orthotopic Pouches

Orthotopic bladder replacement is typically used in men who have had a radical cystoprostatectomy for invasive bladder cancer. In such patients, the external sphincter is intact and in many instances is adequate to provide satisfactory urinary continence. This procedure is not used in women, because cystourethrectomy is the desired procedure for invasive bladder cancer.

Procedures for orthotopic bladder replacement continue to evolve, and currently no consensus regarding an optimal procedure exists. These evolving procedures include the Camey pouch, the ileal neobladder, and the orthotopic Kock pouch. The Camey pouch is composed

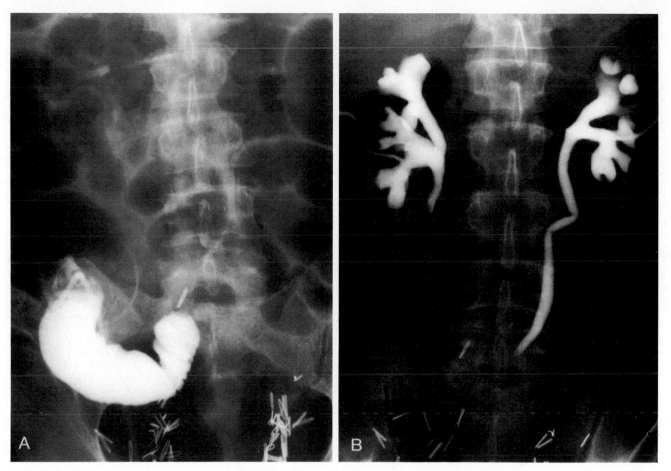

Figure 17.68. Ureteral obstruction. **A,** The absence of reflux on a loopogram implies ureteral obstruction. **B,** Bilateral antegrade pyelograms after percutaneous nephrostomy procedures confirm bilateral ureteral obstruction.

of an isolated U-shaped loop of distal ileum. An opening is created in the most dependent portion of this loop, and this opening is then anastomosed to the urethral stump above the urogenital diaphragm. The ureters are implanted in a mucosal trough at each end of the loop in an effort to prevent reflux. However, reflux does occur in approximately 20% of these patients.

The ileal neobladder and orthotopic Kock pouch are similar in their construction, both using long segments of terminal ileum that are detubularized and reconfigured to form a reservoir. Reflux is prevented by intussuscepting one end of the loop to create a nipple into which both ureters can be reimplanted. Large bowel pouches, which also can be used orthotopically or cutaneously, will be discussed in the next section.

Cutaneous Pouches

The use of this type of continent pouch has been facilitated by the proven safety of clean intermittent catheterization. Self-catheterization with a clean, but not sterile, catheter every 3 to 6 hours is acceptable to patients if continence is maintained during the intervening time. No external collecting device is needed. These are called cutaneous pouches as opposed to the previously described orthotopic pouches.

As with orthotopic pouches, cutaneous pouches are constructed from ileum alone or a combination of terminal ileum and ascending colon. For either type of pouch to function properly, there must be a consistently high capacity with low internal pressure. Low pressure in these reservoirs is obtained by detubularizing the bowel segment used. Detubularization implies interruption of normal bowel continuity, thus preventing organized contractions that cause intermittent high pressures that can compromise continence or result in reflux. Detubularization is especially important in large bowel reservoirs, which are capable of developing very high pressures. The upper urinary tracts should be protected from the effects of reflux or obstruction by special techniques developed for implanting the ureters into the pouch.

The Kock pouch (Fig. 17.70) is constructed entirely

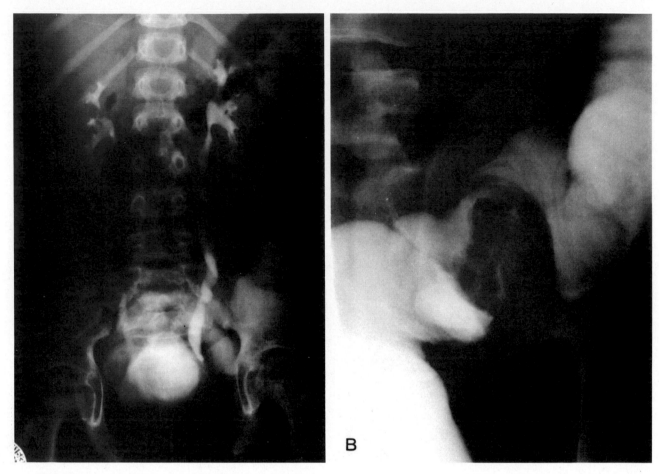

B

Figure 17.69.   Ureterosigmoidostomy. **A,** Diastasis of the symphysis pubis is seen in this patient with bladder exstrophy. A ureterosigmoidostomy was performed and contrast en-hancement can be seen in the sigmoid colon during urogra-phy. **B,** Barium enema demonstrates development of colon cancer.

Figure 17.70.   Kock continent urinary diversion. **A,** A 70- to 80-cm segment of terminal ileum is partially opened on its an-timesenteric border. **B,** The ends of this segment are intussus-cepted. **C,** The pouch itself is constructed from the opened central segment of ileum. **D,** The ureters are anastomosed to the proximal intussuscepted segment, which acts as an antire-flux mechanism. If used orthotopically, the distal intussus-cepted segment is anastomosed to the abdominal wall and be-comes the catheterizing port. **E,** When used orthotopically, only the proximal end of the isolated ileosegment is intussus-cepted. (From Ng C, Amis ES Jr: Radiology of continent uri-nary diversion. *Radiol Clin North Am* 29:557, 1991.)

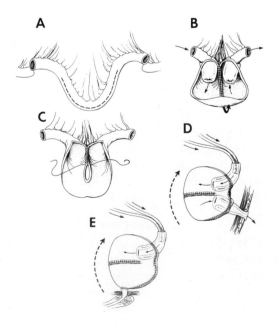

from a long segment of terminal ileum. Both ends of this isolated ileal segment are intussuscepted; the ureters are attached to the proximal segment, the intussusception acting as an antirefluxing mechanism. The intussuscepted distal segment acts as a continent catheterizing port. Pouch capacity can reach 800 to 1000 ml, and reflux and incontinence have been rare.

Large bowel pouches typically are constructed from the cecum and an attached length of terminal ileum. The continent catheterizing stoma may be a plicated segment of terminal ileum (Indiana pouch), an intussuscepted ileocecal valve (King pouch), or a naturally narrow conduit, such as segment of ureter or the appendix may be attached between the skin and a closed cecal pouch (Mitrofanoff technique). The antireflux mechanism in large bowel conduits is created by tunneling of the distal ureters into the taenia of the cecum. Detubularization is typically accomplished by opening the cecum along its antimesenteric border and folding it into a pouch. Cecal pouches have been reported to hold 500 ml or more of urine and to provide satisfactory continence in more than 90% of patients. Reflux has not been a problem.

Postoperative complications and evaluations are similar for both cutaneous and orthotopic pouches. Early problems include leakage of urine, formation of pelvic abscess, obstruction at the point where bowel continuity has been reestablished after segments have been isolated, and pyelonephritis. Late complications include incontinence, stone formation (especially in those patients in whom staples are used for construction of the pouch), difficulty in catheterizing the stoma, and, rarely, rupture of the pouch because of overdistention.

The postoperative radiographic evaluation of continent diversions requires that the radiologist be familiar with the exact procedure performed, as well as the location of any tubes, stents, or drains. For the first few postoperative days, it is not unusual to find ureteral stents and a pouch catheter exiting the stoma of a cutaneous pouch. In an orthotopic pouch, the stents may exit the pouch anteriorly through a separate small incision in the lower abdominal wall. Bilateral stentograms confirm that the upper urinary tracts are not dilated and that contrast medium passes down the ureters around the stents and through the anastomoses without leak. If this study is satisfactory, the stents are usually removed. The pouch itself is studied by dripping contrast medium through the pouch catheter (Figs. 17.71 and 17.72). A relatively small amount of contrast (250 ml), dripped rather than injected into the pouch, is recommended to prevent stressing the fresh suture lines. This should occur under fluoroscopic control, and oblique views can be obtained as necessary to visualize all sides of the pouch for contrast medium extravasation. The presence or absence of reflux should be documented. Follow-up studies after complete healing should document the capacity of the pouch, the postcatheterization residual urine, and whether or not reflux is present.

Many of the initial techniques for constructing continent pouches used metallic staples. However, these can act as nidi for stone formation (Fig. 17.73). More recent techniques have eliminated this potential complication.

Bladder Augmentation

Augmentation cystoplasty is a corollary of the continent orthotopic pouch in which various bowel segments are used to augment an existing small capacity bladder. A typical example would be primary closure of an extrophic bladder. As with continent pouches, large or small bowel segments or a combination of both have proven effective. Radiographically, the bladder in such cases will reflect the specific method and bowel segment used for its augmentation.

NEUROGENIC BLADDER

The spectrum of neurogenic bladder disease is quite complex and often is poorly understood. Evaluation of this condition is typically conducted by urologists in a laboratory specially equipped to perform video urodynamics, a highly sophisticated method for evaluating neurologic function of the bladder. However, the radiologist can play a major role in detecting previously unsuspected neurologic abnormalities, and thus, can facilitate the definitive diagnosis of neurogenic dysfunction at an early stage. When undiagnosed, the effects of neurogenic bladder on the upper urinary tract can be catastrophic, but when properly diagnosed and treated, renal function can almost always be preserved. This section discusses the basic concepts of neurogenic bladder disease.

Anatomy and Physiology

The bladder is the anatomic unit that stores and eliminates urine. Smooth muscle in the bladder wall is the detrusor, which consists of numerous interlacing muscle bundles forming a complex meshwork of smooth muscle without identifiable separate layers. The anatomic arrangement is such that when the detrusor contracts the bladder reduces size equally in all dimensions, resulting in efficient emptying. The muscle fibers of the detrusor continue through the bladder neck and surround the proximal urethra, forming the internal sphincter. The detrusor and internal sphincter are smooth muscles, but unlike other types of smooth muscle, they are under voluntary control.

The external urethral sphincter, composed of striated muscle, surrounds and is integral with the urethra, where it passes through the urogenital diaphragm. This sphincter is composed of both slow- and fast-twitch muscle fibers. The slow-twitch fibers have a special importance

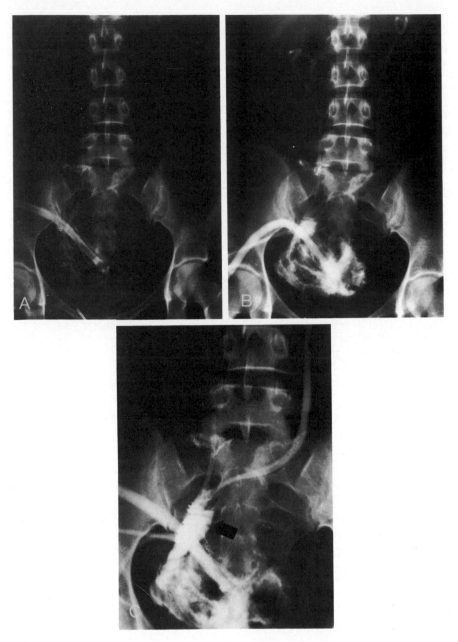

Figure 17.71. Kock pouch. **A,** Preliminary film demonstrates bilateral ureteral stents and a Malecot catheter in the pouch. **B,** No reflux or extravasation is seen after infusion of contrast material into the Malecot catheter. **C,** Injection of contrast into the ureteral stent catheters opacifies the upper urinary tracts and the afferent loop (*arrow*).

in that they allow a more sustained contraction than normal striated muscle. The external sphincter is therefore able not only to close the urethra acutely, but also can serve as a passive continence mechanism for prolonged periods. Because the internal and external sphincters have different nerve supplies, their continence functions are independent of each other. However, the primary continence mechanism in both men and women is the smooth muscle internal sphincter at the bladder neck.

Viscoelastic properties of the normal bladder allow it to enlarge significantly without an attendant increase in

internal pressure. This property is called accommodation and allows the bladder to fill to its maximum capacity (300–1000 ml) with only a slight increase in intravesical pressure. Reflux into the upper urinary tracts is prevented during bladder filling by the course of the distal ureters through the bladder wall to their termination at either end of the trigone. The distal ureters pierce the detrusor at an oblique angle and then course submucosally for a distance of approximately 1.5 cm to their respective orifices. While filling and during voiding, intravesical pressure is exerted evenly at all points

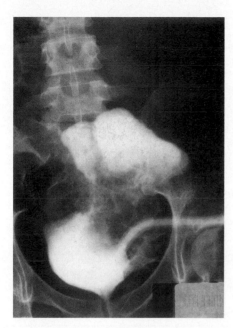

Figure 17.72. Orthotopic continent diversion. Pouch study performed approximately 10 days postoperatively through a catheter left indwelling in the abdominal wall. While there is some spasm of the pouch in its midportion, no extravasation is seen. The anastomosis with the urethral stump is clearly seen inferiorly, and no extravasation is seen in that area either.

on the internal bladder wall. This pressure compresses the submucosal portion of the distal ureter against the muscle behind it, resulting in a functional closure that prevents reflux.

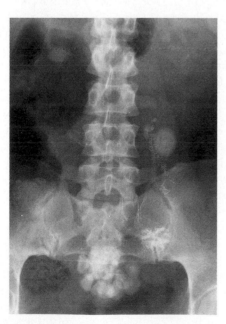

Figure 17.73. Multiple stones have formed in this Kock pouch constructed several years earlier using multiple surgical staples. A surgical staple can be clearly seen as the nidus for each calculus.

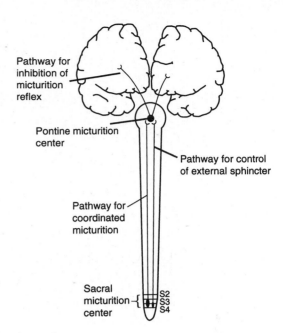

Figure 17.74. Neuroanatomy of voiding, upper urinary tracts. Centers in the cortex consciously inhibit micturition and also provide conscious control of the external sphincter. The pontine micturition center integrates these central control functions. Pathways for control of the bladder and external sphincter travel through the spinal cord from the pontine micturition center to the sacral micturition center.

Voiding is a complicated neurologic event governed by centers in the cerebral cortex that control the detrusor and both sphincters (Fig. 17.74). One cortical center unconsciously inhibits voiding until the bladder nears capacity, then voluntarily controls the detrusor and internal sphincter when voiding is imminent. A second cortical center controls the relaxation and contraction of the external sphincter. The coordination of the detrusor and sphincters occurs in the pontine micturition center in the brain stem. From there, neural tracts travel down the spinal cord to the sacral micturition center and pudendal nucleus, both in the S2-S4 segments of the spinal cord (Fig. 17.75). From the pudendal nucleus, the pudendal nerve extends deep into the pelvis and controls the external sphincter. Efferent and afferent parasympathetic nerves connect the sacral micturition center in the cord with the detrusor and internal sphincter. These nerves form the sacral reflex arc. While detrusor control is parasympathetic, the sympathetic nervous system can block parasympathetic conduction, preventing premature detrusor contractions, and thereby serving to modulate the storage of urine.

The bladder and urethra comprise the lower urinary tract. The urethral sphincters control the storage of urine, and the urethra conveys urine during voiding. During filling, the normal bladder will hold up to 1000 ml of urine at a relatively low pressure because of its viscoelastic

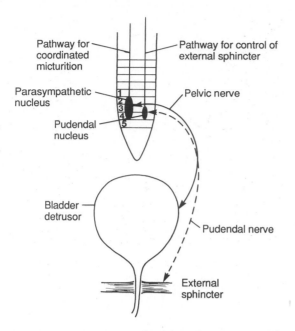

Figure 17.75. Neuroanatomy of voiding, lower tracts. The pelvic nerve connects the parasympathetic nucleus in the sacral micturition center to the bladder detrusor. The pudendal nerve connects the pudendal nucleus in the sacral micturition center to the external sphincter. (From Amis ES Jr, Blaivas JG: Neurogenic bladder simplified. *Radiol Clin North Am* 29:571, 1991.)

Table 17.3.
Classification of Neurogenic Bladder

Uninhibited bladder (essentially normal urinary tract)
   Idiopathic
      Delayed maturation of cortical inhibitory center
      Delayed maturation of detrusor
   Acquired
      Stroke
      Brain tumor
      Normal pressure hydrocephalus
      Parkinson's disease
Detrusor hyperreflexia
   Multiple sclerosis
   Myelodysplasia
   Spinal cord trauma
   Spinal cord tumors
   Spinal arteriovenous malformations
   Herniated intervertebral disc
Detrusor areflexia (large, atonic bladder)
   Herniated intervertebral disc (lower spine)
   Diabetic neuropathy
   Lower spinal cord tumors

properties, because of the modulating action of the sympathetic nerves, and because the normal individual retains voluntary control of the bladder at the level of the cerebral cortex. During normal bladder filling, there is an unconscious inhibition of the micturition reflex in the cerebral cortex. In other words, healthy individuals do not have to consciously think about their bladder to keep it from emptying. However, as the bladder distends toward capacity, the cerebral cortex becomes aware of the need to void. Once a socially acceptable location has been found, micturition is consciously activated.

Coordinated voiding occurs in a well-defined order: relaxation of the external urethral sphincter, detrusor contraction, and, finally, funneling (opening) of the internal sphincter. At the completion of voiding, the external sphincter is voluntarily contracted, resulting in reflex inhibition of detrusor contraction. The internal sphincter then milks any urine remaining in the proximal urethra back into the bladder.

The following sections discuss various types of neurogenic bladder using a simplified classification (Table 17.3).

Uninhibited Bladder

Uninhibited bladder also is known as bladder instability and is a type of detrusor hyperreflexia. However, for the purposes of simplification, uninhibited bladder is considered as a separate entity in this chapter. This condition is caused by failure of the bladder to mature completely or by problems involving the portion of the cerebral cortex that controls voluntary micturition. In patients with uninhibited bladder, coordinated voiding can still occur because the lesion is above the pontine micturition center. Therefore, voiding is physiologic. Uninhibited bladder may be idiopathic in origin, resembling a persistent infantile pattern of voiding. In such cases, there is usually incomplete or delayed maturation of the inhibitory mechanisms controlling the micturition reflex (Fig. 17.76) or of the detrusor itself. While healthy individuals can allow their bladders to fill smoothly to capacity without thinking about it, patients with uninhibited bladder tend to suffer uninhibited (involuntary) bladder contractions. These contractions may occur spontaneously or be provoked by rapid filling of the bladder, change in position of the patient, coughing, or other various triggering mechanisms. In this idiopathic variety, these contractions are sensed by the patient as an urge to void that occasionally progresses to some degree of urge incontinence before the external urethral sphincter can be voluntarily contracted. This condition has been called nonneurogenic neurogenic bladder, or Hinman syndrome. In these patients, a functional bladder outlet obstruction is produced by voluntary contraction of the external sphincter during uninhibited voiding. The resulting pressure increase in the urethra results in dilation of the posterior urethra in male patients (typically young boys) (Fig. 17.77) and of the entire urethra in girls (Fig. 17.78). This has been termed the "spinning top" urethra in both boys and girls. The spinning top urethra in girls has commonly been regarded as a normal

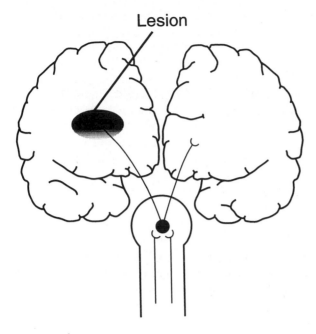

Figure 17.76. Uninhibited bladder. The pontine micturition center and all pathways below it are intact in patients with un-inhibited bladder. This protects the urinary tract and it remains anatomically normal. The lesion in this case usually occurs in the cortex and may be a delayed maturation of the inhibitory mechanism or acquired disease of the cerebral cortex such as stroke, brain tumor, normal pressure hydrocephalus, or Parkin-son's disease.

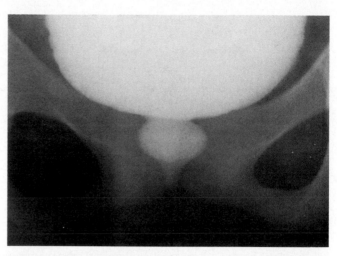

Figure 17.78. Spinning-top urethra in a woman. This is sometimes considered a normal variant. However, this ap-pearance should suggest the possibility of uninhibited bladder.

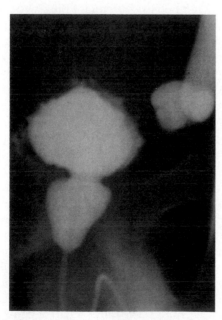

Figure 17.77. Spinning-top urethra in a young boy. Note the dilated posterior urethra which resembles the pattern seen in posterior urethral valves. (From Saxton HM, Borzyskowski M, Robinson LB: Nonobstructive posterior urethral widening (spinning top urethra) in boys with bladder instability. *Radi-ology* 182:81, 1992.)

variant. However, careful study of female patients with this configuration shows that a majority have uninhibited bladder. In boys, the dilated posterior urethra may occa-sionally resemble that seen with posterior urethral valves. In either case, the finding of a spinning top ure-thra in girls or a wide posterior urethra in boys, espe-cially when accompanied by urinary urgency, urge in-continence, daytime wetting, or enuresis, should prompt referral for thorough urologic evaluation.

Uninhibited bladder contractions also can occur as a result of acquired disease in that part of the cerebral cor-tex that exercises voluntary control over micturition. In these patients, there is no ability to initiate or prevent voiding voluntarily, and uninhibited contractions occur that are not sensed and therefore not counteracted. As with the idiopathic or infantile pattern of voiding, the pontine micturition center and all neural pathways be-low it remain intact. This allows physiologically normal voiding, although the patient may not be aware that it is occurring. Conditions that result in this type of inconti-nence include stroke, brain tumor, normal pressure hy-drocephalus, and Parkinson's disease. In most of these patients, because micturition is well-coordinated and complete, the radiographic appearance of the urinary tract remains normal.

Voiding cystourethrography can be standardized to provide a practical urodynamic evaluation of the lower urinary tract in these patients. No special equipment is required. However, interaction with the patient is nec-essary during all phases of the study, because the ex-aminer must know what the patient is trying to do. For example, normal voluntary voiding looks exactly like true incontinence associated with bladder instability when observed during a fluoroscopic examination.

In this standardized technique, the bladder is

catheterized with a small catheter (e.g., 8-French pediatric feeding tube) and diluted contrast medium is dripped into the bladder from a constant height of 30 cm above the level of the pubic symphysis. In a healthy patient, the bladder will fill to its normal capacity without significant slowing or interruption of the drip. This indicates that the intravesical pressure is remaining low and constant. The point of bladder filling at which the patient experiences the first urge to void should be noted; this is typically at a filling level of 100 to 150 ml. A strong urge to void at very small volumes, particularly when associated with cessation or even reversal of flow in the tubing, is typical of an uninhibited detrusor contraction. When observed fluoroscopically, these involuntary contractions may be accompanied by opening of the bladder neck and contrast spilling into the posterior urethra. Conscious tightening of the external sphincter prevents incontinence during these contractions.

Detrusor Hyperreflexia

Detrusor hyperreflexia is caused by lesions of the spinal cord above the sacral segments, but below the pons (Fig. 17.79). These lesions interrupt the neural pathways connecting the pontine micturition center to the sacral micturition center. Such patients have no perception of bladder filling or emptying and voluntary voiding is simply not possible. Voiding, when it does occur, may be associated with simultaneous contractions of

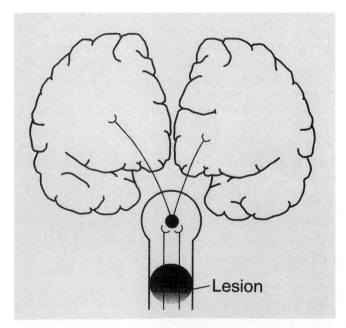

Figure 17.79. Detrusor hyperreflexia. Spinal cord lesion interrupts the neural pathways connecting the pontine micturition center to the sacral micturition center. Coordinated voiding is not possible in these patients. Common lesions include trauma (most common), multiple sclerosis, myelodysplasia, spinal cord tumor, arteriovenous malformation of the spinal cord, and herniated intervertebral disks.

the detrusor and external sphincter muscles. This condition is known as detrusor-external sphincter dyssynergia (DESD). DESD occurs in up to 75% of patients with suprasacral spinal cord lesions. Contraction of the external sphincter can occur involuntarily (without cortical control) at the same time a detrusor contraction occurs, impeding urinary flow and resulting in bladder outlet obstruction. When this type of uncoordinated voiding occurs, intravesical pressure may become very high. This increased pressure ultimately can result in upper urinary tract deterioration. While damage may occasionally be caused by vesicoureteral reflux, it is more common for a functional ureteral obstruction to occur because of the high intravesical pressure that must be overcome in the passage of a urine bolus from the kidney to the bladder.

Common neurologic conditions resulting in DESD include multiple sclerosis, myelodysplasia, spinal cord trauma, spinal cord tumors, arteriovenous malformations of the spinal cord and, occasionally, herniated intervertebral disks. Spinal cord trauma is the most common cause of hyperreflexive bladder, and is typified by a young man suffering spinal injury during a diving or automobile accident.

Radiographically, patients with long-term, untreated DESD have rather characteristic changes of the urinary tract (Fig. 17.80). The bladder often is vertically oriented, with an irregular contour consistent with trabeculation; there are frequently multiple diverticula. Such a bladder often is referred to as a "Christmas tree" or "pine tree" bladder. On voiding cystourethrography, there may or may not be vesicoureteral reflux. When reflux is present, renal parenchymal scarring may occur. When the upper urinary tracts are studied by excretory urography or antegrade pyelography, generalized dilatation and parenchymal thinning is frequently found.

If voiding can be induced during voiding cystourethrography, the posterior urethra is usually seen to be moderately dilated, and there can be massive reflux into the prostatic ducts. When such reflux is present, prostatic calculi on the plain film are a frequent accompaniment. The external sphincter at the level of the membranous urethra remains tightly contracted, and minimal passage of contrast medium into the anterior urethra and poor distention of the anterior urethra are seen. Early in the disease, voiding cystourethrography may demonstrate only persistent urethral narrowing at the level of the external sphincter with mild dilation of the prostatic urethra (Fig. 17.81). Retrograde urethrography in DESD usually also demonstrates external sphincter spasm (Fig. 17.82). The differential diagnosis is a true stricture of the membranous urethra. However, if a 16- or 18-French catheter could be easily passed into the bladder to perform the cystography, significant stricturing in this area can be excluded and the diagnosis of DESD should be made.

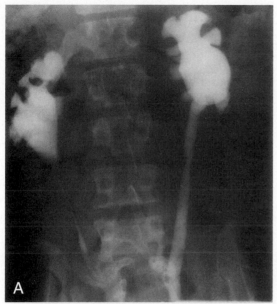

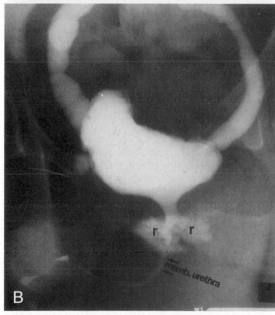

Figure 17.80. Detrusor-external sphincter dyssynergia (DESD). **A,** Voiding cystourethrography shows bilateral reflux with clubbed and dilated calyces. Note the severe sacral dysraphism indicating neurogenic origin of the bladder problem. **B,** On voiding, the bladder is seen to be vertically oriented and trabeculated. Massive reflux (*r*) into the prostatic ducts is also seen. The external sphincter in the region of the membranous urethra (*arrows*) is tightly contracted, and poor distention of the anterior urethra distal to this area is seen. The fact that an 18-French catheter could be passed into the bladder with ease to perform the study rules out a true stricture of the membranous urethra.

In studying patients with suprasacral spinal cord lesions, the radiologist must be aware of autonomic dysreflexia (Fig. 17.83). This is an acute syndrome of massive sympathetic hyperactivity that can be caused by

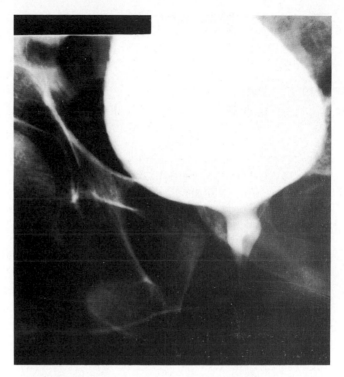

Figure 17.81. Upper motor neuron lesion voiding study after retrograde bladder filling and suprapubic tapping. The bladder neck opens and contrast medium fills the prostatic urethra. The verumontanum is visualized, but detrusor distal sphincter dyssynergia allows only a trickle of contrast medium to pass into the anterior urethra.

stimuli such as urethral catheterization, pressure on the glans penis, bladder distention, manipulation of the renal pelvis (e.g., antegrade pyelography), and ileal conduit loopography. When so stimulated, these patients may exhibit severe paroxysmal hypertension, anxiety, sweating, piloerection, pounding headaches, and bradycardia. Hypertension may be so profound as to result in stroke.

The occurrence and degree of autonomic dysreflexia are largely determined by the level of the suprasacral spinal cord lesion. The major sympathetic splanchnic outflow occurs between T5 and L2. Lesions above T5 isolate this sympathetic outflow from moderating supraspinal influences. Stimuli such as overdistention of the bladder and others mentioned above result in transmission of proprioceptive and pain impulses through the sacral reflex arc to the spinal cord. These impulses travel up to the cord and synapse with sympathetic neurons in the area of splanchnic outflow. If a lesion above the level of T5 prevents normal moderation of this splanchnic response, severe sympathetic hyperactivity occurs. The lower the level of cord compromise, the less severe the autonomic response. Lesions between T6 and T10 usually are associated with only slight blood pressure elevations when the urinary tract is stimulated.

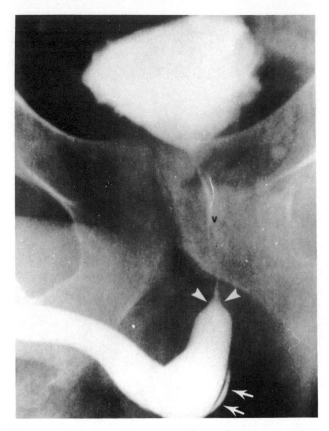

Figure 17.82. Dynamic retrograde urethrogram in upper motor neuron lesion patient with marked distal sphincter dyssynergia. Initially injection of contrast medium did not show contrast enhancement in the posterior urethra. Steady gentle pressure on the barrel of the syringe over a 3-minute period allowed visualization of the posterior urethra, verumontanum (*v*), and bladder neck. Note:unlike the situation in the normal human (convex cone) the cone of the proximal bulbous urethra is symmetric but concave (*arrowheads*). This is commonly seen in the retrograde study in patients with sphincter dyssynergia. Some reflux has occurred into the duct of the gland of Cowper (*arrows*) due to the spasm of the distal sphincters.

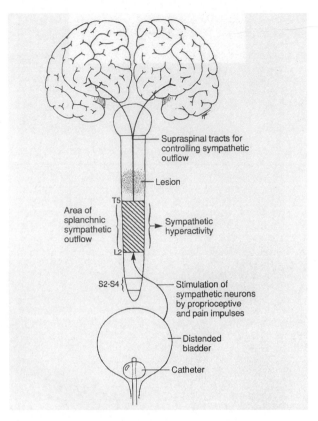

Figure 17.83. Diagram of autonomic dysreflexia. Seen in patients with detrusor hyperreflexia, the cord lesion blocks the moderating influence of supraspinal tracts on sympathetic outflow. A distended bladder or other stimulus therefore results in massive sympathetic hyperactivity.

With lesions below the level of T10, no significant reactions to stimuli are usually seen. The radiologist should be aware of autonomic dysreflexia and should recognize it when it occurs. If the bladder is distended and the patient is noting distress, the bladder should be immediately drained and any indwelling catheter should be removed. The head of the patient's bed should be elevated and the patient's blood pressure should be checked at regular intervals until it returns to normal. Conservative management will result in resolution of the majority of acute episodes of autonomic dysreflexia. When severe hypertension persists, it is advisable to seek assistance from a clinician with expertise in pharmacologic treatment for this condition. It also is extremely important to listen to the patient: many patients with autonomic dysreflexia recognize the onset of symptoms early on and know exactly what should be done to relieve them.

Modern treatment of patients with DESD can prevent deterioration of the kidneys. The external sphincter can be destroyed by sphincterotomy. Alternatively, reasonable results have been reported by disruption of the external sphincter with overdistention of a urethrally placed angioplasty balloon or by transurethral placement of a wire mesh stent to keep the external sphincter widely patent. All of these methods reduce resistance to voiding.

Detrusor Areflexia

Detrusor areflexia is caused by neurologic conditions affecting the sacral micturition center or pathways connecting this center with the bladder or both (Fig. 17.84). Conditions that can result in detrusor areflexia include herniated intervertebral discs in the lower spine, diabetic neuropathy, and lower spinal cord tumors. Pelvic surgery such as radical hysterectomy or abdominoperineal resection of the rectum also has been reported to result in damage of the pelvic and/or pudendal nerves.

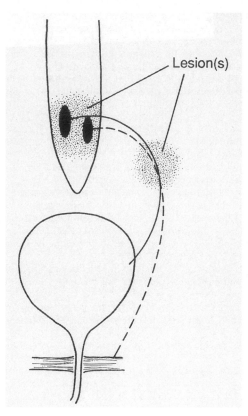

Figure 17.84. Detrusor areflexia. Lesions of the sacral micturition center or sacral reflex arc result in a lack of perception of bladder filling. The bladder therefore continues to fill until its property of accommodation has been overcome. The bladder can easily become grossly distended. Conditions resulting in detrusor areflexia include herniated intervertebral disks in the lower spine, diabetic neuropathy, lower spinal cord tumors, and pelvic surgery with disruption of the pelvic and/or pudendal nerves.

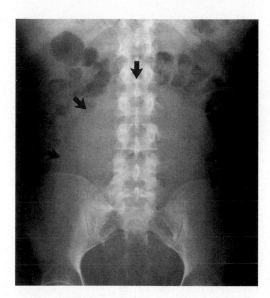

Figure 17.85. Areflexive bladder. Plain-film radiograph of the abdomen reveals a hugely distended bladder (*arrows*) extending to the level of L2.

Because the sacral reflex arc is disrupted, there is no perception of bladder distention. Therefore, the bladder will continue to fill until the viscoelastic accommodating properties of the detrusor are overcome. Intravesical pressure increases rapidly at that point and eventually exceeds that exerted by the intact sphincter mechanisms. Overflow incontinence then occurs until the pressures in the bladder and urethra are equalized, at which point leakage ceases. The clinical pattern is that of a dribbling overflow incontinence that may or may not be constant. The intravesical pressure at which this urine leakage occurs has been called the leak-point pressure. This pressure is not only important in determining when incontinence will occur, it also is an important determinant of upper tract deterioration. Leak-point pressures greater than 40 cm of water result in hydronephrosis with or without vesicoureteral reflux in more than 80% of patients. With lower leak-point pressures, the bladder decompresses by incontinence before upper urinary tract changes occur.

Radiographically, voiding cystourethrography in patients with detrusor areflexia often reveals a smooth, thin-walled bladder with increased capacity, occasionally approaching several liters and extending high into the abdomen. The grossly enlarged bladder also may be easily seen on plain-film radiography (Fig. 17.85). The patient is usually unable to void spontaneously on removal of the filling catheter. Intermittent or total dribbling incontinence of urine may be seen. Even in patients with huge bladders, vesicoureteral reflux is rare because of the persistently low intravesical pressures. If the patient is continent, he or she should be instructed to void by abdominal straining or by the Crede maneuver, and the amount of residual urine should be documented by a postvoid film.

SUGGESTED READING

Benign Bladder Conditions

Allen FJ, De Kock MLS: Pelvic lipomatosis: the nuclear magnetic resonance appearance and associated vesicoureteral reflux. *J Urol* 138:1228, 1987.

Ambos MA, Bosniak MA, Lefleur RS, et al: The pear-shaped bladder. *Radiology* 122:85, 1977.

Amis ES Jr, Cronan JJ, Yoder IC, et al.: Impressions on the floor of the female bladder: "The female prostate." *Urology* 19:441, 1982.

Baath L, Nyman U, Aspelin P, et al.: Computed tomography of pelvic lipomatosis. *Acta Radiol* 3:311, 1986.

Barry KA, Jafri SZH: Eosinophilic cystitis: CT findings. *Abdom Imaging* 19:272, 1994.

Bidwell JK, Dunne MG: Computed tomography of bladder malakoplakia. *J Comput Assist Tomogr* 11:909, 1987.

Blane CE, Zerin JM, Bloom DA: Bladder diverticula in children. *Radiology* 190:695, 1994.

Chen MYM, Zagoria RJ, Dyer RB: Interureteric ridge edema: incidence and etiology. *Abdom Imaging* 20:368, 1995.

Crane DB, Smith MJV: Pelvic lipomatosis: 5-year followup. *J Urol* 118:547, 1977.

Demas BE, Avallon A, Hricak H: Pelvic lipomatosis: diagnosis and characterization by magnetic resonance imaging. *Urol Radiol* 10:198, 1988.

DiSantis DJ, Siegel MJ, Katz ME: Simplified approach to umbilical remnant abnormalities. *RadioGraphics* 11:59, 1991.

Desai SC, Eliot CS, Lawton G: Bladder shape and racial origin. *Clin Radiol* 36:377, 1985.

Farrell B, Martinez R: Urinary schistosomiasis: literature review and case presentations. *Applied Radiology* 24:19, 1995.

Gerber GS, Schoenberg HW: Female urinary tract fistulas. *J Urol* 149:229, 1993.

Goldman IL, Caldamone AA, Gauderer M, et al.: Infected urachal cysts: a review of 10 cases. *J Urol* 140:375, 1988.

Goldman SM, Fishman EK, Gatewood OMB, et al.: CT in the diagnosis of enterovesical fistulae. *AJR* 144:1229, 1985.

Harrison RB, Steir FM, Cochrane JA: Alkaline encrusting cystitis. *AJR* 130:575, 1978.

Izes BA, Larsen CR, Izes JK, et al.: Computerized tomographic appearance of hernias of the bladder. *J Urol* 149:1002, 1993.

Joffe N: Roentgenologic abnormalities of the urinary bladder secondary to Crohn's disease. *AJR* 127:297, 1976.

Jorulf H, Lindstedt E: Urogenital schistosomiasis: CT evaluation. *Radiology* 157:745, 1985.

Klein FA, Smith MJV, Kasenetz I: Pelvic lipomatosis: 35 year experience. *J Urol* 139:998, 1988.

Koziol JA, Clark DC, Gittes RF, et al.: The natural history of interstitial cystitis: a survey of 374 patients. *J Urol* 149:465, 1993.

Martins FE, Bennett CJ, Skinner DG: Options in replacement cystoplasty following radical cystectomy: high hopes or successful reality. *J Urol* 153:1363, 1995.

Moss AA, Clark RE, Goldberg HI, et al.: Pelvic lipomatosis: a roentgenographic diagnosis. *AJR* 115:411, 1972.

Murphy WD, Rovner AJ, Nazinitsky KJ: Condylomata acuminata of the bladder: a rare cause of intraluminal-filling defects. *Urol Radiol* 12:34, 1990.

Pollack HM, Banner MP, Martinez LO, Hodson CJ: Diagnostic considerations in urinary bladder wall calcification. *AJR* 136:791, 1981.

Pope TL, Harrison RB, Clark R, et al.: Bladder base impression in women: "female prostate." *AJR* 136:1105, 1981.

Quint HJ, Drach GW, Rappaport WD, et al.: Emphysematous cystitis: a review of the spectrum of disease. *J Urol* 147:134, 1992.

Rodriguez-de-Velasquez A, Yoder IC, Velasquez PA, et al.: Imaging the effects of diabetes on the genitourinary system. *RadioGraphics* 15:1051, 1995.

Wechsler RJ, Brennan RE: Teardrop bladder: additional considerations. *Radiology* 144:281, 1982.

Zimmermann K, Amis ES Jr, Newhouse JH: Nephrogenic adenoma of the bladder: urographic spectrum. *Urol Radiol* 11;123, 1989.

Bladder Tumors

Amendola MA, Glazer GM, Grossman HB, et al.: Staging of bladder carcinoma: MRI-CT-surgical correlation. *AJR* 146:1179, 1986.

Barentsz JO, Jager G, Mugler JP III, et al.: Staging urinary bladder cancer: value of T1-weighted three-dimensional magnetization prepared-rapid gradient-echo and two-dimensional spin-echo sequences. *AJR* 164:109, 1995.

Barentsz JO, Ruijs SHJ, Strijk SP: The role of MR imaging in carcinoma of the urinary bladder. *AJR* 160:937, 1993.

Brick SH, Friedman AC, Pollack HM, et al.: Urachal carcinoma: CT findings. *Radiology* 169:377, 1988.

Das S, Bulusu NV, Lowe P: Primary vesical pheochromocytoma. *Urology* 21:20, 1983.

Dondalski M, White EM, Ghahremani GG, et al.: Carcinoma arising in urinary bladder diverticula: imaging findings in six patients. *AJR* 161:817, 1993.

Ellis JH, McCullough NB, Francis IR, et al.: Transitional cell carcinoma of the bladder: patterns of recurrence after cystectomy as determined by CT. *AJR* 157:999, 1991.

Filmer RB, Spencer JR: Malignancies in bladder augmentations and intestinal conduits. *J Urol* 143:671, 1990.

Hillman BJ, Silvert M, Cook G, et al.: Recognition of bladder tumors by excretory urography. *Radiology* 138:319, 1981.

Jewett HJ, Strong GH: Infiltrating carcinoma of the bladder: relation of depth of penetration of the bladder wall to the incidence of local extension and metastases. *J Urol* 55:366, 1946.

Kim B, Semelka RC, Ascher SM: Bladder tumor staging: comparison of contrast-enhanced CT, T1- and T2-weighted MR imaging, dynamic gadolinium-enhanced imaging, and late gadolinium-enhanced imaging. *Radiology* 193:239, 1994.

Korobkin M, Cambier L, Drake J: Computed tomography of urachal carcinoma. *J Comput Assist Tomogr* 12:981, 1988.

Lee SH, Kitchens HH, Kim BS: Adenocarcinoma of the urachus: CT features. *J Comput Assist Tomogr* 14:232, 1990.

Miller SW, Pfister R: Calcification in uroepithelial tumors of the bladder. *AJR* 121:827, 1974.

Narumi Y, Kadota T, Inoue E, et al.: Bladder tumors: staging with gadolinium-enhanced oblique MR imaging. *Radiology* 187:145, 1993.

Narumi Y, Sato T, Kuriyama K, et al.: Vesical dome tumors: significance of extravesical extension on CT. *Radiology* 169:383, 1988.

Prout GR: Classification and staging of bladder carcinoma. *Cancer* 45:1932, 1980.

Rozanski TA, Grossman HB: Recent developments in the pathophysiology of bladder cancer. *AJR* 163:789, 1994.

Spataro RF, Davis RS, McLachlan MSF, et al.: Urachal abnormalities in the adult. *Radiology* 149:659, 1983.

Tanimoto A, Yuasa Y, Imai Y, et al.: Bladder tumor staging: comparison of conventional and gadolinium-enhanced dynamic MR imaging and CT. *Radiology* 185:741, 1992.

Tavares NJ, Demas BE, Hricak H: MR imaging of bladder neoplasms: correlation with pathologic staging. *Urol Radiol* 12:27, 1990.

Teefey SA, Baron RL, Schulte SJ, Shuman WP: Abdominal and gastrointestinal radiology. differentiating pelvic veins and enlarged lymph nodes: optimal CT techniques. *Radiology* 175:683, 1990.

Warshawsky R, Bow SN, Waldbaum RS, et al.: Bladder pheochromocytoma with MR correlation. *J Comput Assist Tomogr* 13:714, 1989.

Yu C-C, Huang J-K, Lee Y-H, et al.: Intradiverticular tumors of the bladder: surgical implications-an eleven-year review. *Eur Urol* 24:190, 1993.

Bladder Calculi

Griffith DP, Musher DM, Itin C: Urease: the primary cause of infection-induced stones. *Invest Urol* 13:346, 1976.

McCallum RW, Banner MP: Lower urinary tract calculi and calcifications. In Pollack HM (ed), *Clinical Urography*. Philadelphia, WB Saunders, 1990.

Otnes B: Correlation between causes and composition of urinary stones. *Scand J Urol Nephrol* 17:93, 1983.

Postoperative Bladder Changes

Amis ES Jr, Newhouse JH, Olsson CA: Continent urinary diversions: review of current surgical procedures and radiologic imaging. *Radiology* 168:395, 1988.

Bachor R, Hautmann R: Options in urinary diversion: a review and critical assessment. *Semin Urol* 11:235, 1993.

Banner MP, Pollack HM, Bonavita JA, et al.: The radiology of urinary diversions. *RadioGraphics* 4(6):885, 1984.

Benson MC, Olsson CA: Urinary diversion. *Urol Clin North Am* 19:779, 1992.

Bricker EM: Bladder substitution after pelvic evisceration. *Surg Clin North Am* 30:1511, 1950.

Camey M: Bladder replacement by ileocystoplasty following radical cystectomy. *World J Urol* 3:161, 1985.

Duckett JW, Snyder HMc: The Mitrofanoff principle in continent urinary reservoirs. *Semin Urol* 5:55, 1987.

Filmer RB, Spencer JR: Malignancies in bladder augmentations and intestinal conduits. *J Urol* 143:671, 1990.

Kenney PJ, Hamrick KM, Samuels LJ, et al.: Radiologic evaluation of continent urinary reservoirs. *RadioGraphics* 10:455, 1990.

Middleton AW, Hendren WH: Ileal conduits in children at Massachusetts General Hospital from 1955 to 1970. *J Urol* 115:591, 1976.

Ng C, Amis ES Jr: Radiology of continent urinary diversion. *Radiol Clin North Am* 29:557, 1991.

Ralls PW, Barakos, JA, Skinner DG, et al.: Imaging of the Kock continent ileal urinary reservoir. *Radiology.* 161:477, 1986.

Rowland RG, Mitchell ME, Bihrle R, et al.: Indiana continent urinary reservoir. *J Urol* 137:1136, 1987.

Skinner DG, Lieskovsky G, Boyd SD: Continuing experience with the continent ileal reservoir (Kock pouch) as an alternative to cutaneous urinary diversion: an update after 250 cases. *J Urol* 137:1140, 1987.

Stockle M, Becht E, Voges G, et al.: Ureterosigmoidostomy: an out-dated approach to bladder exstrophy? *J Urol* 143:770, 1990.

Webster GD, Khoury JM: Continent urinary diversions. *Important Adv Oncol* pp 137–154, 1992.

Neurogenic Bladder

Amis ES Jr, Blaivas JG: The role of the radiologist in evaluating voiding dysfunction. *Radiology* 175:317, 1990.

Amis ES Jr, Blaivas JG: Neurogenic bladder simplified. *Radiol Clin North Am* 29:571, 1991.

Chancellor MB, Karasick S, Strup S, et al.: Transurethral balloon dilation of the external urinary sphincter: effectiveness in spinal cord-injured men with detrusor-external urethral sphincter dyssynergia. *Radiology* 187:557, 1993.

Chancellor MB, Karasick S, Erhard MJ, et al.: Placement of a wire mesh prosthesis in the external urinary sphincter of men with spinal cord injuries. *Radiology* 187:551, 1993.

Dangman BC, Lebowitz RL: Urinary tract calculi that form on surgical staples: a characteristic radiologic appearance. *AJR* 157:115, 1991.

Johnson JF III, Hedden RJ, Piccolello ML, et al.: Distention of the posterior urethra: association with nonneurogenic neurogenic bladder (Hinman Syndrome). *Radiology* 185:113, 1992.

Saxton HM, Borzyskowski M, Mundy AR, et al.: Spinning top urethra: not a normal variant. *Radiology* 168:147, 1988.

Saxton HM, Borzyskowski M, Robinson LB: Nonobstructive posterior urethral widening (spinning top urethra) in boys with bladder instability. *Radiology* 182:81, 1992.

Zawin JK, Lebowitz RL: Neurogenic dysfunction of the bladder in infants and children: recent advances and the role of radiology. *Radiology* 182:297, 1992.

18

Prostate and Seminal Vesicles

PROSTATE

Benign Prostatic Hypertrophy

The term prostatic hypertrophy describes hyperplasia of the periurethral glands (transitional zone of McNeal), which are only present above the verumontanum. The benignly enlarged prostate extends above the pubic symphysis, indents the bladder base, and in many cases results in obstructive voiding symptoms, although there is no direct correlation between the degree of prostatic enlargement and the presence or severity of these symptoms.

Etiology

Several factors influence the development of prostatic hypertrophy. Testosterone stimulates prostatic growth, as evidenced by the fact that eunuchs never develop prostatic hypertrophy and that exogenous testosterone causes an increase in the size of the prostate of castrated patients. Estrogen administered to the uncastrated male causes prostatic atrophy; administration of progesterone in patients with obstructive voiding symptoms due to prostate hypertrophy who would be poor surgical risks results in relief of symptoms in 50% of patients. Paradoxically, prostatic hypertrophy occurs in the setting of aging, gonadal involution, and a consequent reduction in the production of testosterone.

Incidence

The prostate in male adults younger than 50 years of age is about the size of a walnut and weighs 15 to 20 g. After 50 years of age, 50% of men have some degree of prostatic hypertrophy. The prostate may double in size before the age of 70 years, and in some elderly men, can weigh several hundred grams. However, only approximately 10% of men require surgical intervention.

Pathology

Prostatic hypertrophy may consist of diffuse enlargement of the stromal and glandular elements in the transitional zone and periurethral glandular tissue, but is more commonly caused by nodular enlargement. Nodules may be stromal without glandular tissue. These nodules may consist of fibrovascular tissue and develop in the transitional zone. Stromal nodules also may consist of fibromuscular tissue; these nodules are prone to infarction and infiltration with plasma cells and histiocytes. Both types of stromal nodules may be incorporated in adenomatous hyperplasia. Fibroadenomas and myoadenomas are the most common and may attain a large size, extending above the pubis and elevating the bladder base. They may interfere with the function of the internal sphincter (Fig. 18.1), creating a large residual volume. Such nodules commonly have areas of hemorrhage, infarction, and calcification.

Clinical Presentation

The clinical presentation of benign prostatic hyperplasia (BPH) depends on the location and size of the nodules, but there is little correlation with the overall size of the prostate. Even small nodules projecting into the prostatic urethra may cause stream reduction and eventual outlet obstruction. Nodules projecting into the bladder neck may interfere with internal sphincter function, resulting in dribbling at the end of micturition. Large nodules may reduce internal sphincter function and may displace the verumontanum and distal sphincters distally so that stress incontinence occurs. Nodules arising laterally generally are asymptomatic until they are so large that the patient experiences difficulty in micturition because of encroachment on the prostatic urethra.

The complex of voiding symptoms due to bladder outlet obstruction from any cause is known as prostatism; while BPH is the most common cause, prostate cancer, bladder neck contracture, or urethral stricture also can be responsible. The initial symptom is most commonly a reduction in force of the urine stream. Nocturia is common and is associated with a feeling of necessity to continue voiding even after voiding has ceased. Difficulty in initiating urination (hesitancy, straining) may have been present for some time before the patient seeks medical advice. Urinary retention may be of

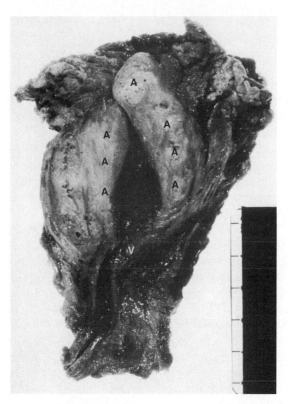

Figure 18.1. Gross specimen showing multiple adenomata (*A*). They project into the bladder neck and interfere with the normal function of the internal sphincter. In addition, the adenomata are all above the verumontanum (*V*), which is pushed inferiorly.

gradual onset or may occur suddenly. Although sudden acute retention often is an indication for prostate surgery, 50% of patients with acute retention are relieved by catheter drainage and may subsequently void relatively well for a period before requiring surgery.

Radiology

The plain-film radiograph is typically normal, although occasionally prostatic adenomata contain calcifications that may be seen behind or extending above the pubic symphysis. Extension above the symphysis is evidence of prostatic enlargement. Excretory urography is a common method of assessing patients with prostatic hypertrophy. The bladder is usually filled with contrast medium toward the end of the study (15-minute films). Anteroposterior or oblique coned films identify the effects of prostatic hypertrophy on the bladder base (Fig. 18.2), and the postvoid film can provide an estimate of residual urine.

As the prostate enlarges, evidence of outlet obstruction may increase. These findings include poor emptying of the bladder, a feathery contour of the bladder suggesting mild trabeculation or a corrugated contour when severe trabeculation is present (Fig. 18.3), the formation of frank diverticula, and a smooth dome-like im-

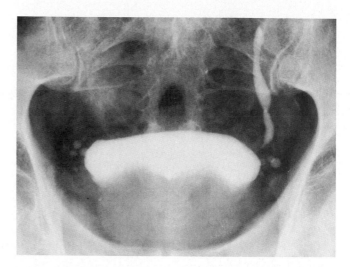

Figure 18.2. Excretory urogram showing bladder base elevation by large bilateral adenomata. The distal left ureter is slightly dilated.

pression on the bladder base representing the enlarged prostate. The enlarged prostate elevates the interureteric ridge, producing a characteristic "J-ing" or "hooking" of the distal ureters (Fig. 18.4). This appearance of the distal ureters is an excellent radiographic indication that the prostate is significantly enlarged.

Other radiographic patterns can be seen with prostate hypertrophy. Zonal anatomy of the prostate has been discussed in an earlier chapter. However, the classic concept of lobar anatomy, including a median lobe at the bladder neck and a vestigial lobe of tissue extending behind the trigone, helps to understand the varied ways in which an enlarged prostate can present. An enlarged median lobe is seen as a transverse ovoid fill-

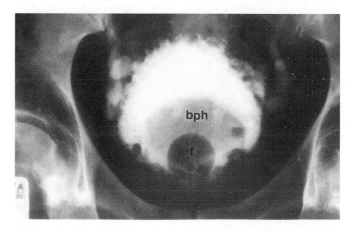

Figure 18.3. Benign prostatic hyperplasia with severe bladder trabeculation and diverticula formation. The urogram reveals a moderately enlarged prostate (*bph*) indenting the bladder base. The bladder is grossly irregular due to trabeculation, and several small diverticula can be seen. A Foley catheter (*f*) is seen at the bladder base.

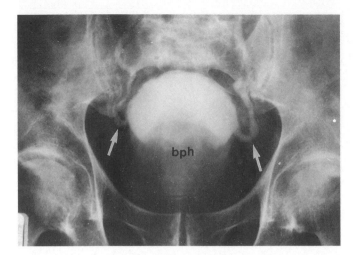

Figure 18.4. "J-ing" of distal ureters. The urogram reveals significant prostate enlargement (*bph*) indenting the bladder base. The distal ureters have a "J" configuration (*arrows*) due to elevation of the trigone and ureteral orifices by the enlarged prostate.

ing defect at the bladder base (Fig. 18.5). The median lobe, by virtue of a narrow attachment to the prostate, can prolapse into the bladder neck and may produce obstruction during voiding. Hypertrophy of tissue behind the trigone indents the bladder posteriorly rather than the far more commonly seen impression on the bladder base. This posterior indentation, when viewed on supine films, looks like a large rounded filling defect in the center of the bladder (Fig. 18.6**A**). This is commonly called the intravesical prostate or the lobe of Albarran. Oblique views confirm the posterior location; computed tomography (CT) or ultrasound clearly show

that the mass is contiguous with more inferior prostatic tissue (Fig. 18.6**B**).

With long-standing severe outlet obstruction, the upper urinary tracts can become dilated because of high intravesical pressure (or occasionally reflux), contrast excretion is delayed, and renal function may be impaired. The rate of contrast medium excretion may be so low that the pelvicalyceal system and ureters do not become visible for 24 hours or more. More typically, there is bilateral symmetric ureteropyelocalyectasis, in which the ureters are dilated to the level of the ureterovesical junctions; in such cases, the bladder is usually poorly opacified because of the presence of a large amount of residual urine (Fig. 18.7). Asymmetric or unilateral upper urinary tract dilation almost never occurs in outlet obstruction and, when present, should lead to the strong suspicion of prostate cancer extend-

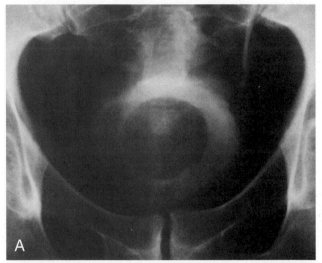

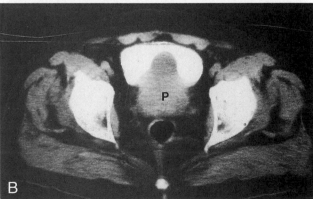

Figure 18.6. Lobe of Albarran. **A,** Excretory urogram reveals a smooth round filling defect in the central portion of the bladder. The patient does not have a Foley catheter indwelling. **B,** Computed tomography scan shows the filling defect in the bladder to directly extend from an enlarged prostate (*P*) immediately behind the bladder. More caudad sections showed this prostatic tissue to be contiguous with the normally situated prostate.

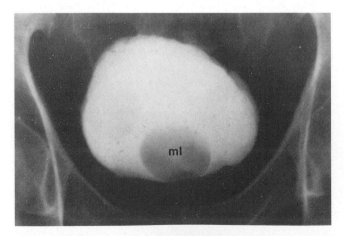

Figure 18.5. Median lobe hypertrophy. The urogram reveals a smooth ovoid filling defect in the bladder base (ml) that remained fixed on various obliquities. This is the classic configuration of an enlarged median lobe. A narrow point of attachment at its base allows this lobe to act as a ball valve at the bladder outlet, causing obstruction during voiding.

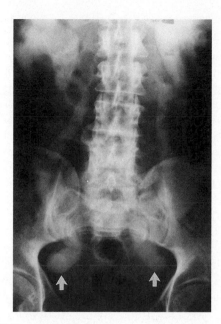

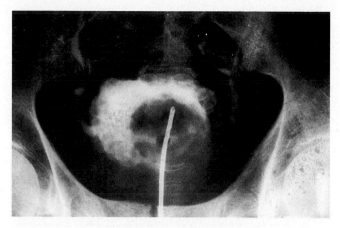

Figure 18.8. Multiple bladder calculi due to outlet obstruction. The bladder is filled with multiple round filling defects representing calculi, and the base is elevated by an enlarged prostate.

Figure 18.7. Bilateral symmetric hydronephrosis due to bladder outlet obstruction. Delayed film from an excretory urogram reveals bilateral symmetric dilatation of the upper tracts to the level of the ureterovesical junctions (*arrows*). Even on this delayed film, no opacification of the bladder is seen. This pattern is consistent with a large residual urine due to bladder outlet obstruction resulting in functional obstruction of the upper urinary tracts.

ing to the level of the trigone or above and involving one or both distal ureters.

Prolonged severe outlet obstruction results in marked trabeculation. When detrusor hypertrophy can no longer compensate for bladder outlet obstruction, the bladder begins to dilate, analogous to the sequence of events occurring when the heart pumps against increased resistance. At this point, urinary retention occurs.

Bladder diverticula result from long-standing outlet obstruction, may be larger than the bladder itself, and may actually deviate the bladder. In such cases, the diverticulum is smooth-walled and the bladder has a thick, irregular (trabeculated) wall.

Excretory urography is commonly requested in patients presenting with symptoms referable to an enlarged prostate. Clinicians say that excretory urography effectively evaluates the upper urinary tracts for dilation and for the presence of unrelated lesions, such as renal cell carcinoma or urothelial tumors. However, it is not clear that urography is justified because the yield of renal lesions is low and the kidneys are well assessed by ultrasound if renal function studies suggest the possibility of obstruction. One benefit of urography may be the identification of unsuspected bladder stones resulting from long-standing outlet obstruction by prostatic hypertrophy (Fig. 18.8), although these stones also may be detected with bladder ultrasound and certainly can be

seen on cystoscopy, which precedes transurethral resection of the prostate.

Transrectal ultrasound (TRUS) can demonstrate significant prostatic enlargement, bladder calculi, and residual urine. TRUS is usually indicated only in those cases in which prostate cancer is suspected (e.g., when a palpable nodule is present or prostate-specific antigen is elevated). However, it is important to be aware of the sonographic appearance of benign hypertrophy. TRUS provides excellent definition of the internal glandular structure, and prostatic adenomata arising in the transitional zone and periurethral glandular tissue are well visualized (Fig. 18.9). The transitional zone and periurethral glandular tissue is normally coarser and slightly less echogenic than the central and peripheral zones. Adenomata arising from the transitional zone vary in echogenicity, but are more commonly hypoechoic or show mixed echogenicity. Large or diffuse calcifications within adenomata produce acoustic shadowing. Digital rectal examination in such cases may reveal a stony hard nodule that suggests the possibility of prostate cancer. Biopsy may be required to distinguish such benign nodules from carcinoma. Benign hypertrophy may cause only a generalized increase in size of the prostate without clearly defined nodules. The echogenicity is, however, coarser, and there may be areas of mixed, hypo-, and hyperechogenicity.

Computed tomography and magnetic resonance imaging (MRI) are both effective methods of assessing the effects of the hypertrophied prostate on the bladder, but are not usually indicated. Generally, CT shows the prostate as a homogeneous organ without internal detail; however, in approximately 25% of contrast-enhanced studies in men with BPH, the posterior peripheral zone can be seen as an area of relatively lower attenuation than the centrally located adenoma. To date, no definite

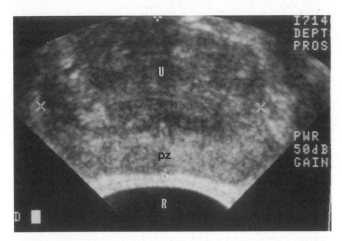

Figure 18.9. Benign prostatic hypertrophy. Transverse section of the prostate from a transrectal ultrasound examination shows the central portion of the prostate (*x markers*) to be enlarged. The mixed echogenicity is consistent with benign prostatic hyperplasia. The centrally placed urethra (*U*) is clearly seen. The peripheral zone (*pz*) can be seen posterior to the adenoma and extending laterally around its margins. The rectum (*R*) is posterior.

value of MRI over ultrasound has been clearly elicited in benign prostatic hypertrophy.

Prostate Cancer

Incidence

The first edition of this book, published in 1991, stated that prostatic carcinoma was the second most common malignancy in men after bronchogenic carcinoma. Since then, the incidence has increased markedly; prostate cancer is now the most common cancer in men other than skin cancer (basal cell and squamous cell cancers). The American Cancer Society estimates that in 1994, 200,000 new cases will be diagnosed, up from 165,000 in 1993. The dramatic increase in incidence is attributed to better reporting of cases plus improved detection with a relatively new screening test known as prostate-specific antigen (PSA).

Prostate cancer is rare in men younger than 50 years of age, but increases dramatically with age thereafter. It accounts for approximately 13% of cancer deaths in men. Significant geographic and racial differences in the incidence of prostate cancer are reported. The incidence of clinical carcinoma is low in China, Japan, Hispanic areas, Israel, Latin and South America, and in American Indians. The incidence is high in North America and Northern Europe. North American blacks have an incidence approximately twice that of white Americans. However, the incidence of occult carcinoma is uniform throughout the world. The geographic incidence may be influenced by the lack of epidemiologic studies in low-incidence countries and by the lack of documentation of prostate cancer.

Etiology

Prostatic carcinoma, like prostatic hypertrophy, has been shown to be androgen dependent. Castrated males do not develop prostatic carcinoma. Marital status, sexual practices, occupation, dietary habits, socioeconomic status, tobacco consumption, and viral and bacterial infection have all been extensively investigated. No definite cause and effect has yet been proven; however, there appears to be a familial tendency for prostate cancer and recent evidence suggests that American men whose diets are rich in fats from red meat face nearly an 80% greater risk of developing prostate cancer than do men with the lowest intake of such foods.

Pathology

More than 95% of prostatic neoplasms are adenocarcinomas, which typically originate in the epithelium of prostatic acini in the outer or peripheral zone of the prostate. Less commonly, adenocarcinoma may arise from ductal epithelium, which also may undergo metaplasia to transitional cells and produce transitional cell carcinoma. Other prostate tumors are rare and include squamous cell carcinomas, endometrioid carcinomas arising from the prostatic utricle, carcinosarcomas, melanomas (Fig. 18.10) and mesenchymal neoplasms such as rhabdomyosarcoma (Fig. 18.11), leiomyosarcoma, or fibrosarcoma. The remainder of this discussion pertains to adenocarcinoma of the prostate.

Grading of prostate cancer involves a histologic evaluation of tissue for glandular pattern, size, and distribution; cells are examined for their degree of differentiation. The margins of the tumor are examined for the degree of definition at the edge of the tumor cell aggregates, and the assessment of stromal invasion is evalu-

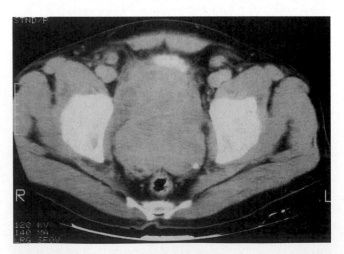

Figure 18.10. Primary malignant melanoma of the prostate. Computed tomography through the prostate shows a large complex mass extending to the right pelvic sidewall. Nothing in this pattern would lead one to suspect melanoma as the most likely diagnosis.

with scores of 8 to 10 almost always have involvement of pelvic lymph nodes.

Staging

The Whitmore-Jewett staging method is the most commonly used system for staging prostate cancer in North America (Fig. 18.12). Stage A carcinoma has no clinical manifestations and is not palpable on digital rectal examination (DRE). It is usually incidentally found in pathology specimens of patients who have had prostatectomy for presumed benign prostatic hypertrophy, but also can be identified by biopsy performed in patients with an elevated PSA. Approximately 10% of all prostatic hypertrophy surgical specimens show histologic carcinoma. Stage A tumors also are found incidentally in autopsy specimens with a frequency that increases with age. The natural history of stage A prostatic carcinoma is not clearly defined. It is generally accepted that a small focus of well-differentiated carcinoma is not likely to progress rapidly to a lethal disease. Most stage A carcinomas fall into this category. Stage A_1 carcinoma is a small focus of tumor entirely within the substance of the prostate. Stage A_2 diffusely involves the prostate, but also is not palpable and does not invade through the capsule.

Stage B is a clinically palpable, firm nodule in the peripheral zone without evidence of capsular transgression or distant extension. Stage B_1 is a palpable nodule less than 1.5 cm in diameter, whereas stage B_2 is a larger nodule usually involving both sides of the prostate.

Stage C carcinomas transgress the capsule. Digital rectal examination reveals a less well-defined firmness, perhaps extending to the seminal vesicles. However, it often is difficult to differentiate stages B and C with DRE, because extension beyond the prostate may be only microscopic, and therefore, is not palpable. At least 50% of patients with stage C carcinoma have metastases to the pelvic lymph nodes.

Patients with stage D carcinoma may present with urinary symptoms, palpable extension of tumor beyond the confines of the prostatic capsule, bone metastases, and hydronephrosis due to ureteral obstruction by carcinoma at the ureterovesical junction. Stage D_1 refers to extraprostatic spread of tumor only to pelvic nodes, whereas stage D_2 pertains to all other types of metastatic spread. Digital rectal examination usually reveals a diffusely hard nodular prostate, but occasionally, only a single hard nodule is felt. Rarely the prostate may feel entirely normal. Presenting symptoms not uncommonly include bone pain due to the skeletal metastases.

The TNM staging method is more descriptively detailed and has been adopted by the American Joint Commission on Cancer, Staging, and End Results Reporting. T refers to tumor stage, N to node involvement, and M to distant metastases. Table 18.1 compares the Whitmore-Jewett and TNM staging systems.

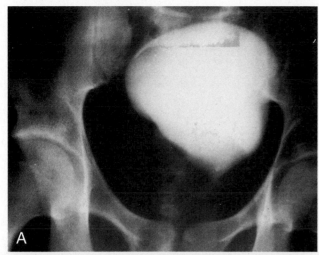
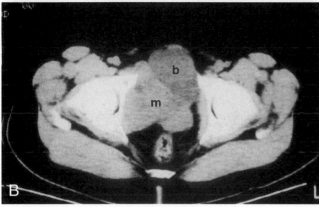

Figure 18.11. Embryonal rhabdomyosarcoma of the prostate in a young man. **A,** Cystogram shows the bladder elevated and displaced to the left by an infravesical mass. **B,** Computed tomography near bladder base shows an irregular soft tissue mass (*m*) displacing bladder (*b*) and extending to right pelvic sidewall. As with the melanoma, nothing indicates the cell type in this case.

ated by tumor glandular cells between stromal planes or destruction of stromal tissue.

The Gleason system for grading prostate cancer is in common use. This system requires that the tumor is studied histologically and that predominant and secondary patterns of tumor are identified. Each of these is assigned a score of 1 through 5. The lower the grade number, the better differentiated is the tumor. The higher the grade, the less differentiation is present. The numbers are then added for the final score, which can range between 2 and 10. For example, a tumor that is predominantly well-differentiated (score of 1), but that has a small focus of moderate dedifferentiation (score of 3) would have a Gleason score of 4 overall. Correlation between tumor grade and degree of spread (stage) is usually good; tumors with a Gleason score of 2 to 4 rarely have metastases to pelvic nodes, whereas tumors

Figure 18.12. Staging of prostate cancer. Diagrammatic comparison of Whitmore-Jewett and TNM staging systems. (Modified from Amis ES Jr: Epidemiology and natural history of carcinoma of the prostate. *American Roentgen Ray Society Categorical Course Syllabus on Uroradiology,* 1989, 87–92. Copyright 1989, American College of Radiology.)

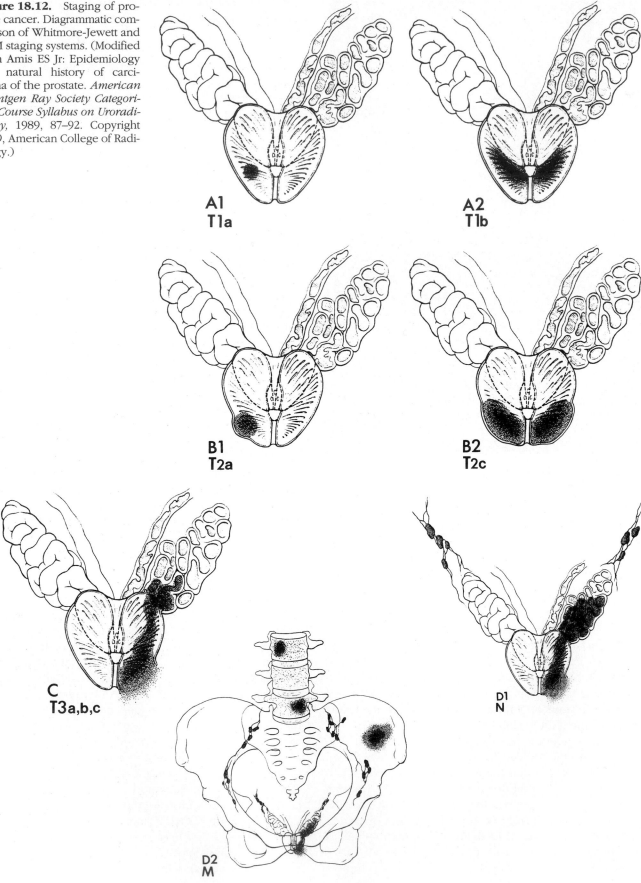

Table 18.1.
Comparison of Staging Systems for Prostate Cancer

Whitmore-Jewett	TNM	Description
—	TO	No evidence of tumor
A_1	T1a	Tumor not palpable; small focus (<5% of gland)
A_2	T1b	Tumor not palpable; diffuse involvement of gland
B_0	T1c	Nonpalpable tumor identified because of an elevated PSA; not visible on TRUS
B_1	T2a	Palpable tumor involving less than half of one lobe
B_1	T2b	Palpable tumor involving more than half of one lobe, but not both lobes
B_2	T2c	Palpable tumor involving both lobes
C	T3a	Unilateral extracapsular extension
C	T3b	Bilateral extracapsular extension
C	T3c	Invasion of one or both seminal vesicles
	T4a	Invasion of bladder neck, external sphincter, or rectum
	T4b	Invasion of levator muscles or fixation to pelvic sidewall
D_1	N	Regional (pelvic) node involvement
D_2	M	Distant metastases

PSA = prostate-specific antigen; TRUS = transrectal ultrasound

Although there is usually a good correlation between tumor grade and stage (Table 18.2), there are exceptions. Stage B_1 lesions have a better prognosis than stage A_2 lesions; this occurs because only 25% of stage A_2 lesions are well differentiated, as opposed to 85% of Stage B_1 lesions. Recent reports indicate that the incidence of diagnosis of stage A carcinomas is increasing. In 1967, the Veterans Administration Cooperative Urological Research Group (VACURG) reported that only 6% of prostatic cancers were diagnosed at stage A. Currently up to 50% of all prostatic carcinomas are stage A when diagnosed.

Table 18.2.
Relation Between Grade and Stage in Prostate Cancer

Grade	Stage (%)			
	A	B	C	D
Well differentiated	61.9	41.0	30.0	18.3
Moderately differentiated	18.5	32.7	31.5	32.1
Poorly differentiated	5.4	13.0	23.0	30.2
Undifferentiated	0.3	1.0	2.5	3.1
Not graded or unknown	13.9	12.3	13.0	16.3

Based on data from the National Survey of Prostate Cancer in the United States by the American College of Surgeons 1982.

Screening for Prostate Cancer

Biochemical studies may be helpful in detecting prostatic cancer and in assessing its spread. The serum acid phosphatase (SAP) level is elevated in 60% of patients with stage C and D carcinoma and in 80% of patients with bone metastases. Estimation of the prostatic fraction of SAP is more precise for prostate cancer, because the SAP may be elevated in other conditions such as multiple myeloma, leukemia, and pancreatic carcinoma.

Far more important in the diagnosis of prostate cancer is the PSA level in the serum. Prostate-specific antigen is a serine protease that was discovered in 1979. It is normally secreted only into the ductal system of the prostate. However, with significant derangement of prostate architecture due to a variety of conditions, PSA can leak from the acini into the stroma of the gland, and from there can enter the circulation through lymphatics and capillaries. There are multiple causes for an elevated PSA level. It can be significantly elevated by cystoscopy (4×), needle core biopsy of the prostate (57×), and by transurethral resection of the prostate (53×). Elevated PSA levels also can be found in association with prostatitis, prostatic infarct, acute urinary retention, and benign hypertrophy of the prostate. Digital rectal examination and TRUS have been shown to have little or no effect on serum PSA levels.

The most common method for determining the serum PSA level is the Hybritech monoclonal antibody assay (Hybritech Inc., San Diego, CA), which has an upper limit of normal of 4.0 ng/ml. Prostate-specific antigen levels between 4 and 10 ng/ml do not distinguish benign from malignant conditions, because BPH is common in older men and is known to elaborate PSA at the rate of 0.3 ng/ml per gram of BPH tissue. The rate of PSA increase over time or the ratio of PSA to prostate volume (PSA density) may be more useful indicators of malignancy. If a serum PSA is drawn annually and a rate of change of 0.75 ng/ml or greater per year or a 20% or more increase in PSA per year occurs, this is far more indicative of prostate cancer than BPH. The PSA density, which requires TRUS for determination of prostate volume, also appears to be a useful way to differentiate malignant from benign disease. The mean PSA density for prostate cancer is 0.581, whereas the mean PSA density for BPH is only 0.044. Typically, BPH has a PSA density of 0.1 or less, whereas almost all patients with a PSA density of greater than 0.1 will have prostate cancer.

Another screening tool, the DRE, is significantly dependent on the skill of the examiner. It detects only approximately 40% of prostate cancers less than 1.5 cm in diameter. Further, more than 50% of prostate cancers are clinically advanced at the time they are detected by DRE. However, there is a significant symbiotic effect of combining DRE with PSA. The PSA level is normal in

21% of patients with biopsy-proven prostate cancer. Therefore, PSA is not capable of finding all cases of this neoplasm. Conversely, DRE can detect some prostate cancers that would be missed if relying on PSA alone. Therefore, if both DRE and PSA are positive, 60% of those patients will have prostate cancer; if both DRE and PSA are normal, only 2% of those patients will have the disease.

Screening for prostate cancer remains a controversial subject, because the natural history of the small tumors detected by elevated PSA levels or by TRUS is unknown. Nonetheless, both the American Cancer Society and the American Urological Association now recommend an annual DRE and PSA beginning at 50 years of age. For high-risk patients such as black men and those with a strong family history of prostate cancer, this screening is recommended to begin at 40 years of age.

Dissemination

Spread of prostatic carcinoma occurs by three methods: direct extension, lymphatic spread, and hematogenous spread. Carcinoma of the prostate typically originates in the peripheral zone closer to the prostatic capsule than to the urethra. Capsular invasion opens a route to perineural lymphatics and to the periprostatic venous plexus of Santorini, allowing distant metastases to the viscera and axial skeleton.

Local spread is to the seminal vesicles, the urethra, the bladder neck, the bladder base, and the interureteric ridge, the latter causing asymmetric or unilateral ureteral obstruction. Less commonly, prostatic cancer spreads posteriorly and superiorly, invades Denonvilliers' fascia, and grows into the rectosigmoid region of the colon, sometimes producing bowel obstruction. Rarely, rectal involvement produces an ulcerating lesion that is extremely difficult to distinguish from rectal carcinoma. Late local spread to the corpus cavernosa, corpus spongiosum, and scrotum has been reported.

Lymphatic spread is initially from lymphatics within the prostate to the pelvic lymph nodes, which are usually dissected for frozen section histologic examination at the time of total prostatectomy (screening lymphadenectomy). There is a high incidence of pelvic lymph node metastases in carcinoma of the prostate. The lymph node groups involved include the obturator, the external iliac, and the internal iliac nodes. The common iliac, paraaortic, mediastinal, and supraclavicular lymph nodes may be involved in advanced disease. Spread from the mediastinal lymph nodes into pulmonary lymphatics resulting in lymphangitic carcinomatosis has been reported. In autopsy cases of patients who died of prostate cancer, up to 20% have pathologic evidence of pulmonary lymphangitic carcinomatosis, but only 5% of these cases were detected radiographically. Suspicion of a prostate primary in such patients is important, because the prognosis can be improved with estrogen therapy.

Hematogenous spread is to the axial skeleton or viscera. Eighty-five percent of patients dying of prostatic carcinoma exhibit bony metastases in the axial skeleton. Sites of skeletal metastases are the lumbar spine, proximal femur, bony pelvis, thoracic spine, ribs, sternum, skull, and proximal humerus in order of decreasing frequency. The route of early hematogenous spread to the spine and pelvis is through the intervertebral venous plexus of Batson, which directly communicates with the periprostatic venous plexus of Santorini. More than 90% of prostatic metastatic lesions to bone are blastic.

Capsular invasion opens the hematogenous route for metastatic disease through the periprostatic venous plexus, which communicates with the pudendal and vesical venous plexuses. Drainage progresses through the veins to the lungs. Metastases to bones below the level of the prostate (i.e., ischia and femora) likely result from malignant shunts with arterial metastases. Brain metastases from carcinoma of the prostate have been reported without lung metastases, which implies arterial embolization. This may occur in the presence of a cardiac right-to-left shunt. When lung metastases are present, microscopic lesions may enter the pulmonary veins returning to the left heart and thus causing arterial embolization, but this is a rare form of tumor embolization.

Clinical Presentation

Prostatic carcinoma often does not produce symptoms until significant local spread has occurred. Up to 25% of patients presenting with urinary retention have prostatic carcinoma, but the urinary retention may be solely the result of prostatic hypertrophy and the carcinoma is a coincidental histologic finding. When the carcinoma has attained sufficient bulk, dysuria, slow urinary stream, dribbling, and some degree of outlet obstruction are the presenting symptoms. Hematuria and rectal or perineal pain are less common symptoms. More commonly, metastases cause bone pain, weight loss, and anemia.

Clinical Diagnosis

Once prostate cancer is suspected based on the DRE, PSA or both, TRUS is usually performed to identify potential abnormal foci within the prostate and to guide biopsy study of these areas. Alternatively, digital guidance of biopsy of a palpable nodule transrectally can be performed. The positive predictive value that a palpable nodule will be cancer is approximately 50%; the remainder prove to be focal areas of prostatitis, old infarcts, or nodular BPH.

The preferred method of diagnosis of a suspicious hypoechoic nodule demonstrated by TRUS is by core needle biopsy. The positive predictive value that such a nodule will be cancer varies between 18 and 60%; by TRUS hypochoic areas also can be prostatitis, infarct, or atypical nodular BPH. A prostatic cyst or a ductal structure such as the ejaculatory duct are anechoic and should be distinguished from hypoechoic lesions. Biopsy can be performed under ultrasound guidance through the transperineal or the transrectal route. Although the incidence of infection is lower with transperineal biopsy, it is more cumbersome and painful. Most prostate biopsy studies are performed through the transrectal route. Mechanical, spring-loaded biopsy devices are used routinely for prostate biopsy procedures because they provide a better core of tissue and are less painful. A biopsy specimen of any suspicious lesion should be obtained. Systematic biopsies of the remainder of the prostate gland are recommended, because since it often contains cancer, despite a benign ultrasound appearance. Antibiotics are recommended before the biopsy to reduce the incidence of septicemia or urinary tract infection.

Radiology

While PSA levels are not routinely used to predict capsular transgression or nodal involvement by prostate cancer, recent studies indicate that it is extremely rare to find bony metastases in patients with a PSA of 10 ng/ml or less. In an era when use of imaging procedures is being closely controlled, obtaining bone scintigraphy for the large majority of patients diagnosed with prostate cancer may not be justified. Radionuclide bone scans should be reserved for those patients with PSA levels greater than 10 ng/ml at the time of diagnosis (Fig. 18.13), or for patients with localized bone pain suggesting the possibility of metastases. When a bone scan is obtained and shows areas of increased activity, plain-film radiographs of the suspicious areas are indicated to

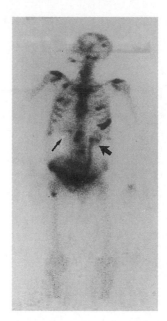

Figure 18.13. Radionuclide bone scan showing multiple metastases. Multiple areas of increased radiopharmaceutical uptake by the osseous metastases are seen. Note the obstructed right kidney (*large arrow*) in this posterior view. The left kidney (*small arrow*) is normal. (From Amis ES Jr, Newhouse JH: *Essentials of Uroradiology.* Boston, Little, Brown and Co, 1991.)

exclude benign lesions such as degenerative change or Paget's disease. Because the radionuclide bone scan can detect metastatic deposits before they become radiographically apparent, negative plain-film radiographs in the light of increased scan activity should lead to the diagnosis of metastases.

Most metastatic bone lesions are seen in the thoracolumbar spine, pelvis, and ribs, and the vast majority are blastic (90%) (Figs. 18.14 and 18.15). The remainder are mixed blastic and lytic. Approximately 1% are bone

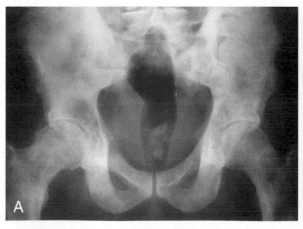
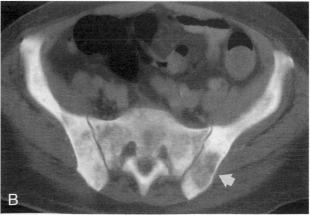

Figure 18.14. Metastatic prostate carcinoma. **A,** Plain-film radiograph of the pelvis showing multiple blastic lesions in the pelvis and femora. **B,** An unenhanced computed tomography scan using "bone windows" in the same patient demonstrates a lytic lesion (*arrow*) in addition to the blastic deposits.

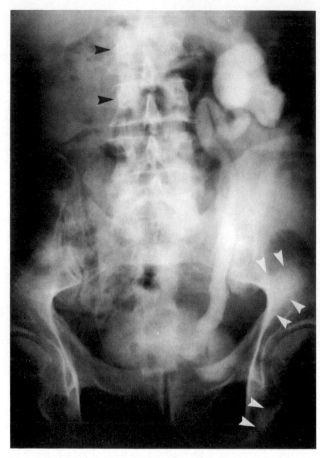

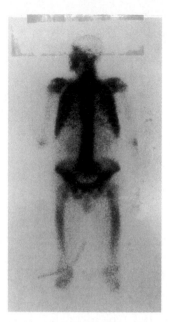

Figure 18.16. Super bone scan in patient with diffuse prostate metastases. Note the absence of renal function indicating diffuse uptake of radiopharmaceutical by metastatic prostate cancer. (From Amis ES Jr, Newhouse JH: *Essentials of Uroradiology.* Boston, Little, Brown and Co, 1991.)

Figure 18.15. Excretory urogram in a patient with carcinoma of the prostate and well demarcated bone metastases (*white arrowheads*). Blastic pedicles are also seen (*black arrowheads*). Carcinoma of the prostate has spread locally to involve the interureteric ridge completely obstructing the right ureter and causing marked pelvicalyceal and ureteric dilatation on the left.

destructive and lytic, but may produce periosteal new bone. Metastatic bone lesions are discrete dense areas varying in size from a few millimeters to several centimeters. Solitary small discrete blastic lesions may represent bone islands, but in the presence of known prostatic carcinoma, follow-up examination is required. Metastatic lesions are commonly adjacent to joint surfaces such as the sacroiliac joints and hip joints, but do not affect the joint space. Difficulty may be experienced when a metastatic lesion abuts a joint affected by degenerative or inflammatory change. Blastic lesions have a well-demarcated edge as opposed to degenerative sclerosis, which is more diffuse. Blastic metastases in pedicles are relatively common, but may be obscured by degenerative arthritic change in the lumbar apophyseal joints, and additional oblique lumbar spine views may be necessary for clarification. Blastic metastatic lesions in the vertebral bodies typically lie adjacent to the vertebral body cortex, but may increase in size to involve the com-

plete vertebral body, resulting in a sclerotic vertebra. Unlike patients with Paget's disease, the sclerotic vertebra is not enlarged in patients with carcinoma of the prostate. Multiple bone islands and osteopoikilosis are small discrete bone densities that never change in size or density, unlike blastic metastases, which are less discrete and increase in size without therapy.

Mixed osteoblastic and lytic lesions may be produced by both carcinoma of the prostate and by Paget's disease. Paget's disease generally produces cortical thickening, coarse trabeculation, and an increase in the size of the affected bone. The lytic lesions in Paget's disease are well demarcated. Areas of repair become blastic, leading to the mixed blastic and lytic appearance. Although the appearance of metastases from carcinoma of the prostate and Paget's disease are similar and can coexist, careful evaluation of the distinguishing features usually allows the correct diagnosis. Difficulty with this differentiation can be clarified by assessing the SAP and serum alkaline phosphatase. Serum alkaline phosphatase is markedly elevated in Paget's disease, whereas the SAP is not. The reverse is true in carcinoma of the prostate with metastases.

Prostate cancer can be so diffusely metastatic that virtually all the bones are involved and dense. A bone scan in such a patient may be difficult to interpret, because it shows no focal areas of involvement. However, the key finding will be the absence of visualization of the kidneys. In normal patients, approximately 15% of the radionuclide is excreted by the kidneys. In patients with diffuse metastases, the radionuclide is completely absorbed by the bones, leaving little or none for the kidneys to excrete. Such a pattern is known as a "super bone scan" (Fig. 18.16). The differential diagnosis of diffusely dense bones includes myelosclerosis, urticaria pigmentosa, and fluorine poisoning in addition to blastic metastases.

The chest radiograph can be a useful study in patients with prostate cancer, and a careful search for small nodular lesions and increased interstitial lung markings is mandatory. Hematogenous nodules in the lungs may vary in size from a few millimeters to several centimeters. Lymphangitic spread may be recognized as hilar lymph node enlargement and increased interstitial lung markings, particularly Kerley A and B lines. Kerley A lines are several centimeters long extending from the hila into the lungs. Kerley B lines are short, extending to the lung periphery in the costophrenic angles. There may be small effusions obliterating the costophrenic angles. Generally, however, chest findings tend to occur late in the disease.

Lymphangiography is no longer indicated in the assessment of prostatic carcinoma, although it is still performed in a few centers. This study has an accuracy of only about 75% for detecting tumor in pelvic nodes; furthermore, the pedal lymphangiogram does not always show the obturator nodes that are most commonly involved in carcinoma of the prostate. The external iliac, common iliac, and paraaortic lymph nodes are visualized in pedal lymphangiography, but involvement of these nodes is less common. When lymphangiography is performed, involved nodes are increased in size, with discrete filling defects.

Computed tomography has no application in the de-

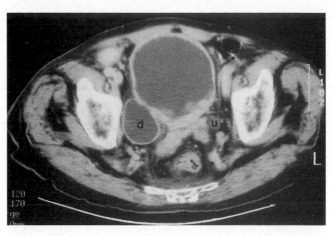

Figure 18.18. Prostate cancer invading posterior bladder wall. Computed tomography at the level of the seminal vesicles shows thickening and irregularity of the posterior bladder wall. On more caudad sections the bladder wall thickening was contiguous with direct extension of tumor through the prostate capsule. Note the right posterolateral wall bladder diverticulum (*d*). The left ureter (*u*) is obstructed by the prostate cancer.

tection of intraprostatic cancer because of the lack of differentiation of the internal anatomy of the gland by this modality. However, CT has been used commonly to stage prostate cancer preoperatively. Gross local spread is typically seen as extension of tumor into the angle between the bladder and seminal vesicle (Fig. 18.17), invasion of one or both seminal vesicles resulting in significant asymmetry, thickening of the posterior bladder wall by direct extension of tumor (Fig. 18.18), an irregular prostatic margin, or rectal invasion (Fig. 18.19). Unfortunately, multiple studies have indicated a poor accuracy for CT in staging this disease. The problem does not lie in showing gross extraprostatic spread, but rather in detecting microscopic transgression of the capsule, a common occurrence.

Computed tomography is of value in the detection of

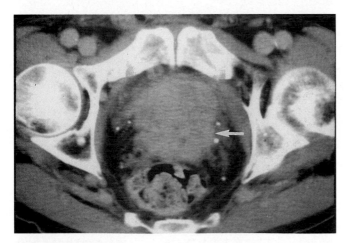

Figure 18.17. Direct extension of prostate cancer through capsule into seminal vesicle angle. Computed tomography through the pelvis shows a soft tissue mass (*arrow*) in the angle between the posterior bladder wall and the seminal vesicles.

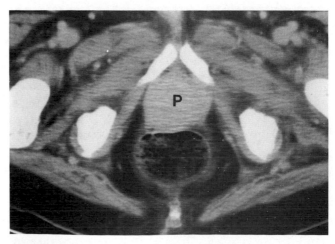

Figure 18.19. Prostate carcinoma. Tumor (*P*) invading the anterior rectal wall is well visualized on pelvic CT.

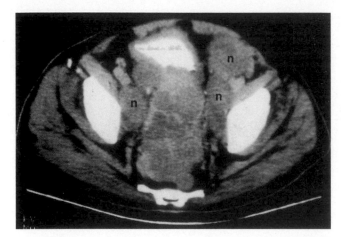

Figure 18.20.   Gleason Grade 8 prostate cancer. Computed tomography through the region of the prostate shows a large complex mass invading the bladder posteriorly and extending to and involving the rectum. Obturator node masses (*n*) are seen bilaterally and a large left external iliac node mass is also present.

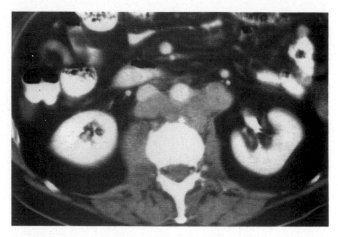

Figure 18.22.   Prostate carcinoma. Paraaortic metastases are clearly distinguished from the opacified aorta and inferior vena cava on this enhanced computed tomography scan.

metastases to the pelvic lymph nodes. Pelvic lymph nodes are usually considered abnormal (and probably involved with metastatic tumor) if they are larger than 1.5 cm in diameter as measured by CT. If the size threshold is reduced, the sensitivity of CT will increase, but at the expense of specificity. One recent study showed that biopsy of lymph nodes 6 mm or larger resulted in a 96.5% accuracy in detecting metastatic prostate cancer. However, aggressive prostate cancers often are associated with bulky pelvic, iliac, and paraaortic node masses (Figs. 18.20–18.22).

Although early reports on TRUS were unimpressive, the development of high-resolution 6- to 7.5-MHz transducers and improved near-field focus have improved results. The aim of this diagnostic procedure is to make

the diagnosis of prostate malignancy while the lesion is still treatable by radical extirpation (i.e., before it has spread beyond the capsule). However, given that many small prostate cancers lie dormant for decades, the clinical effect of early diagnosis is not yet proven.

On TRUS, small carcinomas (stages A and B) are typically hypoechoic relative to the peripheral zone, and the vast majority (80–90%) occur in that zone. Some carcinomas may be well defined without internal echoes (Fig. 18.23) but, unlike cysts, they have no enhanced through-transmission. Others may be irregular and poorly defined. Extension of carcinoma through the capsule is recognized as capsular bulging or actual in-

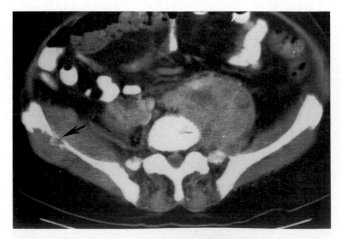

Figure 18.21.   Prostate carcinoma. Bulky metastases to common iliac lymph nodes are seen. Metastatic tumor has also destroyed a portion of the right ilium (*arrow*).

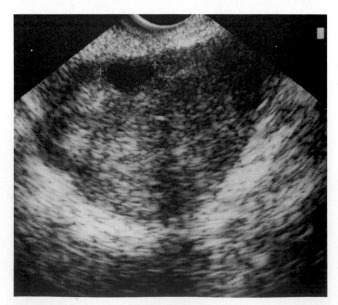

Figure 18.23.   Nonpalpable stage A prostate cancer. Transverse TRUS section shows an anechoic lesion in the peripheral zone (*markers*) without disruption of adjacent hyperechoic capsule.

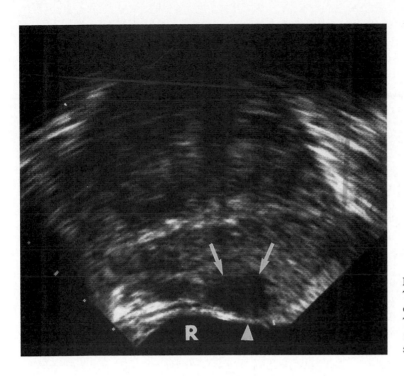

Figure 18.24. Stage C prostate cancer. Transverse TRUS section shows an extensive tumor involving the entire left peripheral zone and extending anteriorly. The tumor can be seen extending directly through (*arrows*) and bulging (*arrowhead*) the hyperechoic capsule. R = rectum.

terruption of the hyperechoic line representing the capsule and pericapsular fat (Fig. 18.24). Such a finding usually indicates stage C carcinoma. However, the experience with TRUS as a staging tool for prostate tumors is variable, with accuracy for detecting capsular transgression ranging from less than 40% to more than 80%. Transrectal ultrasound also has been touted as useful in detection of seminal vesicle involvement by tumor, with a positive examination in more than 90% of histologically proven cases; unfortunately, it also shows sonographic abnormalities in more than 10% of normal seminal vesicles. The normal seminal vesicle is slightly less echogenic than the prostate, and tumor involvement results in a more echogenic appearance.

Hypoechoic foci in the prostate as small as 4 mm in diameter are now detectable with high-resolution equipment. Because the majority of hypoechoic areas in the peripheral zone are not malignant, biopsy is essential for establishing the definitive diagnosis. Ultrasound guidance of transrectal or transperineal biopsy is an accurate and well-tolerated procedure. At least three needle cores are obtained from the lesion, and random biopsy cores are usually obtained from the opposite peripheral zone.

Approximately 25% of prostatic carcinomas are isoechoic or only minimally hypoechoic in relation to the echogenicity of the peripheral zone and are therefore difficult to demonstrate by TRUS. Isoechoic carcinomas can only be suspected when they bulge or invade the capsule. In a minority of cases, prostate cancer can be hyperechoic (Fig. 18.25).

Transurethral prostatectomy for prostatic hypertro-

phy often reveals malignant change on histologic examination of the resected tissue. Ten percent to 20% of prostatic carcinomas develop in the transitional zone around the urethra. Prostatic cancers arising in the tran-

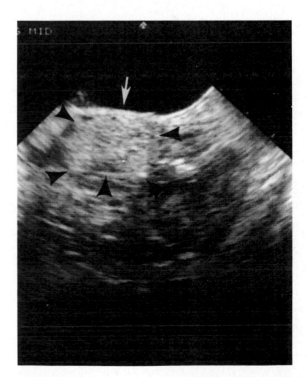

Figure 18.25. Stage C hyperechoic prostate cancer. Transverse TRUS section demonstrates a large hyperechoic mass (*black arrowheads*) which bulges the prostatic capsule (*white arrow*) suggesting the possibility of a Stage C lesion. Biopsy confirmed capsular transgression.

sitional zone are almost impossible to diagnose with transrectal ultrasound since this area is involved by adenomatous hyperplasia (BPH).

Recently color Doppler techniques have been applied to the prostate in an effort to improve diagnostic accuracy. In a series of 132 biopsy proven cancers, 93% had an abnormal flow with a corresponding gray-scale abnormality, typically a hypoechoic nodule, while the remaining 7% showed only a distinctly abnormal flow during color Doppler scanning. The peripheral prostate shows minimal or no flow in normal men. Although the differential diagnosis for abnormal flow is virtually the same as for a palpable nodule on DRE or a hypoechoic nodule on TRUS (e.g., a focus of prostatitis or BPH), the detection of such an area of abnormal flow should prompt biopsy to exclude malignancy.

Ultrasound also shows promise in the treatment of prostate cancer. Excellent results with ultrasound-guided percutaneous cryoablation of prostate tumors have been recently reported. Cryoprobes are selectively used to freeze the area of the tumor, followed by the remainder of the gland. This procedure is performed by a radiologist and urologist working together. Results are preliminary, and longer follow-up will be necessary before this treatment regimen can gain wide acceptance.

Magnetic resonance imaging provides clear visualization of the prostate in transverse, sagittal, and coronal planes. T2-weighted images are necessary for visualiza-

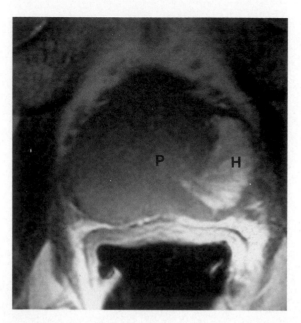

Figure 18.27. Postbiopsy prostatic bleeding. T1-weighted image obtained with an endorectal coil shows a moderate sized high signal intensity hemorrhage (*H*) in the left lateral portion of the prostate (*P*).

tion of the internal architecture of the gland. T1-weighted images show the prostate as a homogeneous gland of medium signal intensity and also clearly demonstrate the neurovascular bundles (Fig. 18.26); these images also can define the extent of postbiopsy bleeding, as hemorrhage is seen as an area of high signal intensity (Fig. 18.27). The central gland is of medium to low signal intensity, whereas the peripheral zone gives a high signal. Inhomogeneous enlargement of the central gland is seen with BPH (Fig. 18.28). Pathologic states within the prostate can be identified by varying areas of signal intensity. Prostate cancer is typically seen as an area of lower signal intensity in the otherwise high-signal peripheral zone (Figs. 18.29–18.31). A recent study showed that MRI was able to detect 62% of proven prostate cancers greater than 5 mm in diameter. The large majority of these cancers were located in the posterior gland; MRI was much less sensitive in demonstrating tumors elsewhere. Therefore, MR is not used for early detection of prostate cancer, because the combination of DRE and PSA is far more accurate and cost-effective for screening.

Magnetic resonance may prove to be a valuable tool for staging prostate cancer. Gross extension of tumor beyond the capsule or into adjacent structures may be seen, especially when an endorectal coil is used. Minor signs of capsular transgression include a smooth or irregular bulge in the contour of the gland in the region of the tumor and asymmetry of the neurovascular bundle secondary to retraction. Smooth capsular bulge is predictive of capsular transgression in approximately

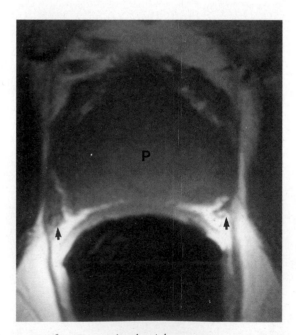

Figure 18.26. T1-weighted axial magnetic resonance image of the prostate obtained with endorectal coil. The prostate (*P*) is seen as a homogeneous medium signal intensity structure. The neurovascular bundles are seen as small, medium signal intensity structures (*arrows*) lying posterolaterally in the rectoprostatic angle where they are contrasted against the higher signal intensity fat.

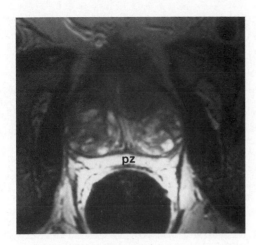

Figure 18.28. Benign prostatic hyperplasia (BPH) without evidence of tumor. Axial T2-weighted magnetic resonance image through the prostate obtained with endorectal coil reveals a large inhomogeneous central gland consistent with BPH. The peripheral zone (*pz*) is somewhat compressed, but of normal high signal intensity without evidence of tumor.

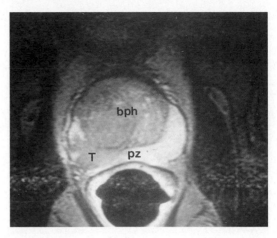

Figure 18.30. Stage B prostate cancer. T2-weighted axial magnetic resonance image of the prostate obtained with endorectal coil shows a slightly irregular medium signal tumor (*T*) in the right posterior zone (*pz*). The capsule is not as clearly seen on this image as it is in Figure 18.29, but there is no bulge and this is consistent with a stage B lesion. The central gland is mildly enlarged consistent with benign prostatic hyperplasia.

25% of cases (Fig. 18.32), while an irregular bulge is indicative of periprostatic spread in 75% (Fig. 18.33). While gross transgression is readily apparent, microscopic involvement can be suggested when asymmetry of the neurovascular bundles is seen in association with other signs of capsular transgression.

The normal seminal vesicles have a high signal intensity on T2-weighted images (Fig. 18.34). Involvement by tumor is seen as an area of lower signal intensity (Fig. 18.35). Unfortunately, lower than normal signal intensity in the seminal vesicles also can be seen after radiation or hormonal therapy, or may be caused by postbiopsy blood.

Currently, the accuracy of MRI in detecting capsular transgression by prostate cancer approaches 80%, although reports indicate there is considerable interobserver variation in interpretation of the images. While MRI is touted by some radiologists as virtually a necessary study for staging prostate cancer, this belief is not universally held. In fact, the lack of diagnostic signs that are uniformly accurate in detecting capsular transgression by tumor, coupled with the high cost of the examination, has precluded widespread use of MRI in staging prostate cancer. With further development and experience in the evaluation of prostate cancer, however, MRI holds promise as a useful staging tool.

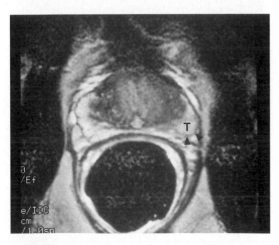

Figure 18.29. Stage B prostate cancer. T2-weighted axial magnetic resonance section through the prostate obtained with endorectal coil shows a small, medium signal tumor (*T*) in the left peripheral zone. The capsule (*arrowheads*) is clearly intact.

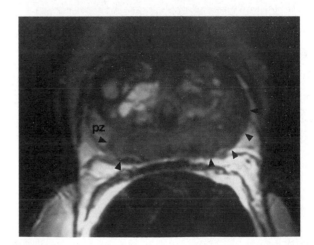

Figure 18.31. Stage B$_2$ prostate cancer. T2-weighted axial magnetic resonance image through the prostate obtained with endorectal coils shows an extensive low signal tumor (*arrowheads*) occupying most of the peripheral zone. A small area of uninvolved peripheral zone (*pz*) is noted on the right side.

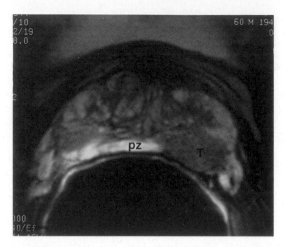

Figure 18.32. Prostate cancer with suggestion of capsular transgression. T2-weighted axial magnetic resonance image through the prostate using endorectal coil shows a moderate size medium signal tumor (*T*) in the left peripheral zone which bulges the capsule posteriorly. This smooth bulge is associated with capsular transgression in about 25% of cases. The uninvolved peripheral zone (*pz*) is seen as a high signal area compressed by BPH involving the central gland.

Prostatitis

Inflammatory conditions of the prostate arise from a variety of causes. The patient with prostatitis presents with frequency, urgency, nocturia, dysuria, fever, perineal pain, urethral discharge, and occasionally sexual dysfunction. In acute prostatitis, DRE reveals an exquisitely tender and swollen prostate that may be firm or "boggy." In patients with chronic prostatitis, the prostate may be normal to the examining finger, stony, asymmetrically hard, or diffusely enlarged and slightly tender.

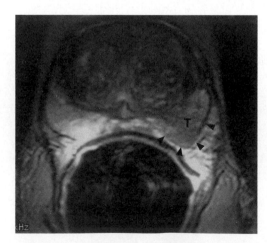

Figure 18.33. Prostate cancer most likely transgressing capsule. T2-weighted axial magnetic resonance image of the prostate using endorectal coil shows a moderate size medium signal tumor in the left peripheral zone (*T*). This tumor produces an angular bulge in the capsule posteriorly (*arrowheads*) suggesting a high possibility of capsular transgression.

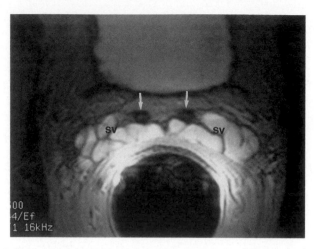

Figure 18.34. Normal seminal vesicles on magnetic resonance imaging. T2-weighted axial section through the seminal vesicles (*sv*) shows them to be convoluted structures of high signal intensity. The convoluted portions of the vasa (*arrows*) are clearly seen as low signal intensity structures.

The etiology of acute prostatitis is bacterial infection. The etiology of chronic prostatitis, which commonly occurs without any acute episode, can be bacterial, inflammatory, or no pathologic lesion may be found (i.e., the patient is symptomatic but all investigations are normal). This last condition is termed prostatosis and may have a psychogenic component. Bacterial prostatitis is more commonly a retrograde infection. *Escherichia coli* infection accounts for more than 80% of bacterial pro-

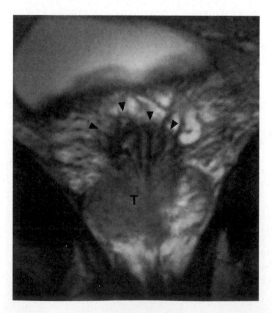

Figure 18.35. Seminal vesicle involvement by prostate cancer. T2-weighted coronal magnetic resonance image through the prostate and seminal vesicles reveals a large medium signal tumor (*T*) arising from the right side of the prostate and extending superiorly into the seminal vesicles. The upper extent of the tumor is defined by arrowheads.

statitis, and an additional 15% are caused by *Klebsiella, Proteus, Pseudomonas,* and *Enterobacter* or *Gonococcus* species. Any of these bacteria may cause acute or chronic prostatitis. Granulomatous prostatitis commonly results from tuberculosis, coccidioidomycosis, histoplasmosis, or blastomycosis.

Clinical diagnosis rests on DRE, culture of prostatic secretions expressed by digital transrectal massage, and biopsy of firm areas in the prostate that remain suspicious for tumor after appropriate antimicrobial therapy. A high index of suspicion for tumor is necessary, because both prostate cancer and prostatitis tend to occur in the peripheral zone.

Radiology

Neither the plain film nor the excretory urogram provides pathognomonic findings for prostatitis. Prostatic calcification and an enlarged prostate indenting the bladder base are more common in prostatic hypertrophy than in prostatitis. Transabdominal ultrasound and CT are nondiagnostic. In chronic prostatitis, TRUS may demonstrate varying areas of altered echogenicity in the bulk of the prostate similar to the findings in prostatic hypertrophy (Fig. 18.36). Areas of low echogenicity may be seen in the peripheral zone that cannot be differentiated from prostatic cancer. Up to 20% of biopsy specimens in such cases reveal chronic prostatitis.

Prostatic abscesses generally demonstrate larger focal areas of decreased echogenicity. Combined with the clinical presentation, a prostatic abscess may be suspected and proven by TRUS-guided aspiration. Computed tomography and MRI, while incapable of diag-

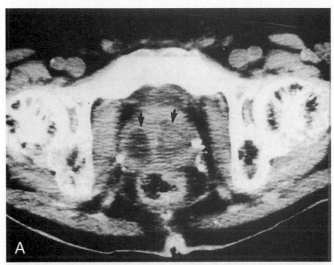

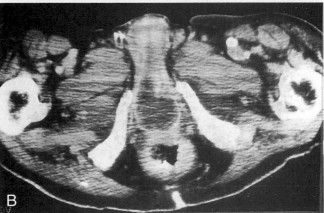

Figure 18.37.   Prostatic abscess. **A,** Computed tomography through the prostate shows two ill-defined areas of low attenuation (*arrows*). (From Putnam CE, Raven CE. *Textbook of Diagnostic Imaging.* Philadelphia, W.B. Saunders, 1988.) **B,** Computed tomography through root of the penis shows that the abscess has extended through the urogenital diaphragm into this region.

nosing acute or chronic prostatitis, are useful in the diagnosis of a prostatic abscess. On CT, the abscess is seen as rounded or irregular areas of fluid attenuation (Fig. 18.37**A**). Care must be taken to carry the examination through the urogenital diaphragm, because prostatic abscesses can extend through that structure into the base of the penis (Fig. 18.37**B**). On MRI, fluid collections within the prostate can be identified on T1- and T2-weighted images. Evidence of an old prostatic abscess that has sloughed into the urethra (Fig. 18.38) may be demonstrated on urethrography as an irregular cavity communicating with the prostatic urethra. Rarely such prostatic cavities are found to contain stones (Fig. 18.39).

Prostatic Calcification

The peripheral zone of the prostate is the seat of the corpora amylacea, where calcifications with no known

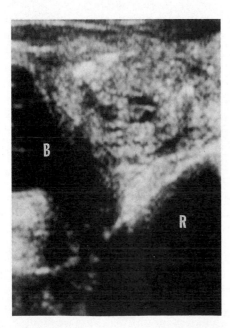

Figure 18.36.   Acute prostatitis. Longitudinal TRUS through the prostate shows ill-defined hypoechoic areas within the gland. B = bladder. R = rectum.

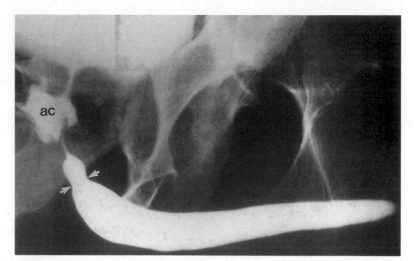

Figure 18.38.   Prostatic abscess drained into prostatic urethra. Retrograde urethrogram reveals opacification of an old abscess cavity (*ac*) adjacent to the prostatic urethra. The abscess was unroofed transurethrally. The mild concentric narrowing of the proximal bulbar urethra (*arrows*) is the musculus compressor nuda.

etiology and without pathologic effects tend to occur. These calcifications are discrete, vary in size from 1 to 5 mm, and are usually multiple. Rarely these calcifications may erode into a prostatic duct and be passed per urethra. Corpora amylaceous calcifications are calcium phosphate (apatite).

Prostatic calcification also occurs in areas of necrosis that may develop in adenomata, carcinoma, granulomatous prostatitis, or after radiation therapy. Calcification occurs in 7 to 10% of patients with prostatic adenomata. In prostatic adenomatous calcification, the only distinguishing feature from corpora amylacea calcification is the position, seen on plain-film radiography. Adenomatous calcification is commonly seen above the symphysis pubis, whereas corpora amylacea calcification is seen in the normal prostate position behind or below the pubic symphysis. Calcification in prostatic carcinoma occurs with about the same frequency as in BPH, and is therefore not a good differentiating factor between benign and malignant disease. Most of the calcifications seen in the prostate in patients with carcinoma are in corpora amylacea. In a small number of carcinomas, necrotic calcification is seen.

Granulomatous prostatitis resulting from tuberculosis may cause significant calcification. Calcifications may be small, or the entire prostate may be calcified. Schistosomal calcification of the prostate is extremely rare, although *Schistosoma hematobium* is a very destructive lesion in the prostate and urethra. Up to 15% of abacterial granulomatous prostatitis shows dystrophic calcification.

Radiology

Plain-film examination is essential in assessing prostatic calcification. These calcifications, usually stippled and lying behind or above the pubic symphysis are seen on 15 to 30% of abdominal radiography in men older than 50 years of age. To this end, the abdominal radiography should be exposed to include the entire pubic symphysis. Prostate calcification may be difficult to see, because corpora amylacea calcification tends to occur in a relatively normal-sized prostate, and therefore, may overlie the pubic symphysis. Dystrophic calcification such as tuberculous granulomatous calcification is usually well visualized on plain-film radiography, because it is more extensive (Fig. 18.40). This is rarely seen in young patients. Excretory urography is useful in assessing bladder indentation by calcified prostatic adenomata (Fig. 18.41). Transabdominal ultrasound shows calcification within the prostate as bright echoes producing

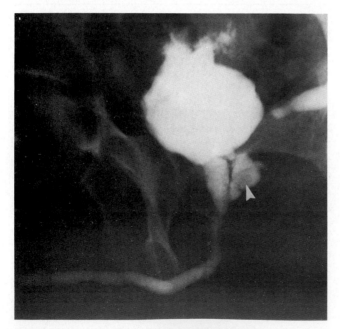

Figure 18.39.   Retrograde urethrocystogram showing a prostatic cavity containing a filling defect (*arrowhead*) which proved to be calcium encrusted debris.

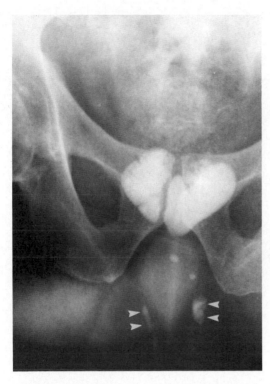

Figure 18.40. Plain film in a patient with known pulmonary and renal tuberculosis. The prostate is almost completely calcified due to tuberculous granulomatous prostatitis. Calcification also is seen in the epdidymides bilaterally (*arrows*) from tuberculous epidydimitis. (From McCallum RW, Colapinto V: *Urological Radiology of the Adult Male Lower Urinary Tract.* Springfield, IL, Charles C Thomas, 1976.)

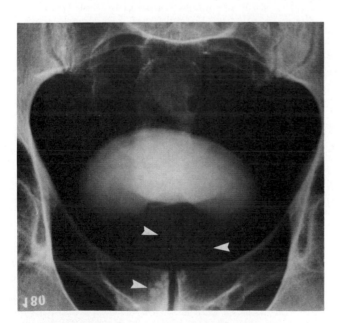

Figure 18.41. Excretory urogram in a patient with a large median lobe adenoma contains dystrophic calcification. (From Pollack HM (ed): *Clinical Urography.* Philadelphia, WB Saunders, 1990.)

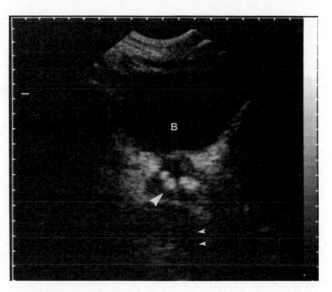

Figure 18.42. Transabdominal ultrasound showing the urine filled bladder (*B*) and the prostate posteriorly, containing several calcifications (*arrowhead*) producing acoustic shadowing (*small arrowheads*). (From Pollack HM (ed): *Clinical Urography.* Philadelphia, WB Saunders, 1990.)

acoustic shadowing if the calcific foci are large enough (Fig. 18.42). Computed tomography is more accurate in showing faint calcification (Figs. 18.43 and 18.44) not apparent on plain-film radiography or transabdominal ultrasound; these calcifications may be seen on CT in up to 60% of men older than 50 years of age.

SEMINAL VESICLES

Symptoms caused by seminal vesicle disease often are difficult to differentiate from those related to prostatic abnormalities. Patients frequently complain of painful ejaculation, bloody semen (hematospermia), perineal or suprapubic pain, and infertility.

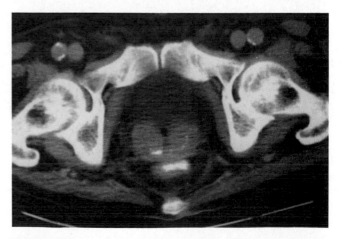

Figure 18.43. Computed tomography of the prostate showing faint calcification within the prostate. This calcification was not visualized on plain film.

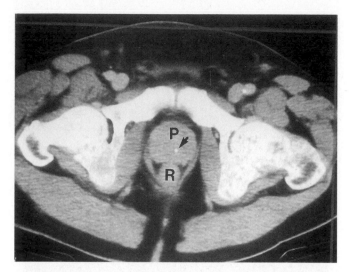

Figure 18.44. Computed tomography through the prostate (*P*) shows a single punctate calcification (*arrow*). R = rectum.

The seminal vesicles are paired structures located immediately posterior to the bladder and just above the prostate. Conditions affecting the seminal vesicles include calculi, cysts, infection, and neoplasms.

Radiology

Until the advent of cross-sectional imaging, the seminal vesicles could only be visualized by seminal vesiculography (Fig. 18.45). This required making a small incision at the neck of the scrotum, and cannulating and injecting contrast proximally into the vas deferens. The contrast medium then opacified the vas deferens, the seminal vesicle, and the ejaculatory duct, and could usually be seen entering the prostatic urethra. The only clin-

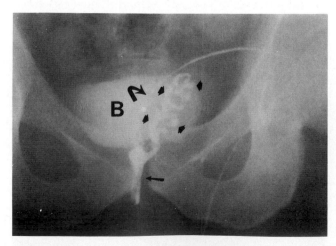

Figure 18.45. Normal seminal vesiculogram. Contrast medium injected into the left vas deferens opacifies the vas, the ampulla of the vas deferens (*curved arrow*), the seminal vesicle (*arrowheads*), and the ejaculatory duct (*arrow*). Contrast medium in the bladder (*B*) indicates patency.

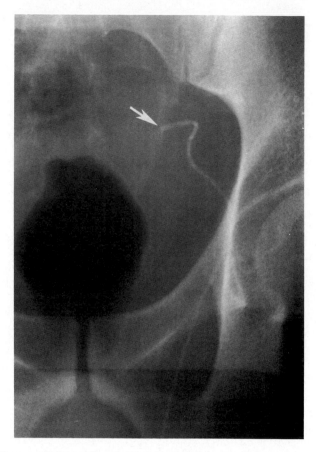

Figure 18.46. Obstructed vas deferens. A left vasogram demonstrates complete obstruction (*arrow*) of the vas deferens.

ical value of direct opacification of the male genital system is to evaluate the vasa for obstruction (Fig. 18.46) in infertile men with no sperm in the ejaculate (azoospermia), but in whom a testis biopsy shows normal spermatogenesis.

The seminal vesicles are now best imaged by TRUS, CT, or MRI. On TRUS, normal seminal vesicles are seen on axial sections as a uniformly echogenic bow-tie-shaped structure just superior to the prostate (Fig. 18.47); on longitudinal images, they are seen as soft tissue cephalad extensions of the posterolateral prostate bilaterally (Fig. 18.48). The soft tissue or somewhat cystic bow-tie configuration also is appreciated on CT in the sections immediately above the prostate (Fig. 18.49). On MR images, the seminal vesicles exhibit medium signal intensity on T1-weighted images and become bright on T2-weighted images.

Seminal vesicle stones, while uncommon, are usually opaque and are related to stone disease elsewhere in the urinary tract or ectopic insertion of a ureter into the ipsilateral seminal vesicle. Stone size may range from tiny to several centimeters in diameter; they may be single or multiple. Ultrasound shows typical acoustic shadowing if the stones are large enough, and on CT the cal-

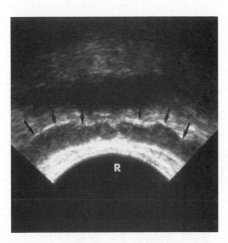

Figure 18.47. Normal seminal vesicles on transrectal ultrasound. Transverse section just above the prostate shows a uniformly echogenic "bowtie" structure extending to both sides of midline (*arrows*). R = rectum. (Case courtesy of Matthew Rifkin, M.D.; From Amis ES Jr, Newhouse JH: *Essentials of Uroradiology*. Boston, Little, Brown & Co, 1991.)

culi are easily identified as such because of their high attenuation (>150 Hounsfield units [HU]). Stone disease should not be confused with wall calcification that can be found in the seminal vesicles in diabetic men. Smaller stones may become impacted in the duct from the seminal vesicle or the ejaculatory duct and may result in pain and hematospermia.

Seminal vesicle cysts are uncommon. In at least two thirds of patients with a congenital seminal vesicle cyst, there is associated ipsilateral renal agenesis. Therefore, when a seminal vesicle cyst is identified, imaging of the kidneys should be mandatory (Fig. 18.50). Acquired cysts can occur in the seminal vesicles secondary to obstruction or inflammation. Congenital or acquired cysts

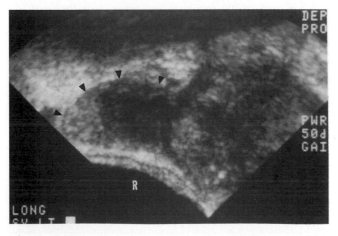

Figure 18.48. Normal seminal vesicle on transrectal ultrasound. Longitudinal views shows the moderately echogenic elliptical structure (*arrowheads*) extending cephalad to the prostate. This section is through the left seminal vesicle. The right seminal vesicle had an identical appearance. R = rectum.

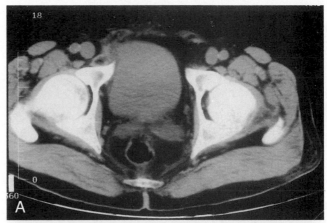

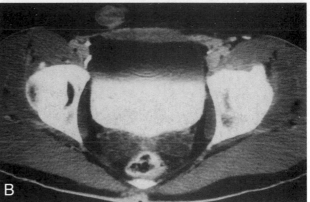

Figure 18.49. Normal seminal vesicles on computed tomography. **A,** In this patient, the seminal vesicles have a normal "bow-tie" configuration behind the bladder and soft tissue attenuation. **B,** The seminal vesicles have a somewhat cystic appearance. This is also considered normal.

may become quite large and may indent the bladder posteriorly. There are no imaging characteristics that differentiate congenital from acquired cysts. Either type of cyst can have water density (Fig. 18.51) or a thick wall. Hemorrhage into the lumen of the cyst may result in a solid appearance on CT (Fig. 18.52). Ultrasound will exhibit specious echoes or dependent debris in hemorrhagic cysts. Magnetic resonance imaging will typically show a high signal intensity of a hemorrhagic cyst on both T1- and T2-weighted images.

Isolated infection of the seminal vesicles is rare. Conversely, seminal vesiculitis in conjunction with prostatitis is common. Imaging findings in such cases are usually nonspecific. Even when frank abscess has formed, the appearance on imaging studies is similar to noninfected cysts. In such cases, fever and leukocytosis favor the diagnosis of abscess. Seminal vesicle tuberculosis can result from primary involvement of the genital tract, or may result from descending infection in the urine after hematogenous spread of the disease to the kidneys. Imaging findings are relatively nonspecific, including

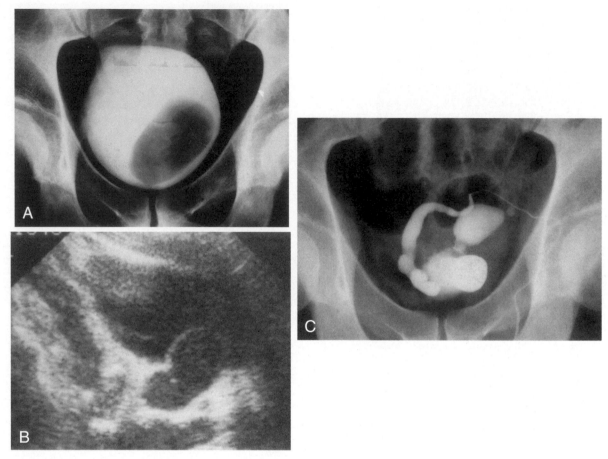

Figure 18.50. Seminal vesicle cyst. **A,** A small mass is seen indenting the bladder on this excretory urogram which also revealed absence of the left kidney. **B,** Ultrasound demonstrates a cystic mass protruding into the bladder lumen. **C,** The seminal vesicle cyst is opacified after injection of the left vas deferens.

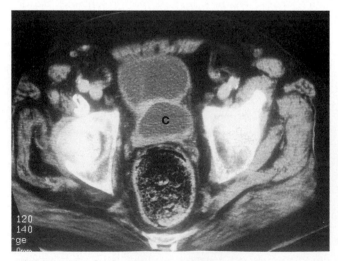

Figure 18.51. Left seminal vesicle cyst. Computed tomography shows a cystic structure (*c*) behind the bladder and just to the left of midline. Computed tomography through the upper abdomen proved left renal agenesis associated with this congenital left seminal vesicle cyst.

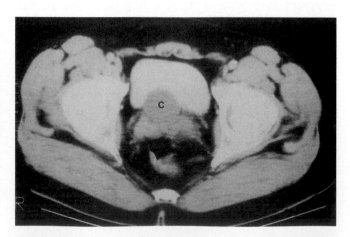

Figure 18.52. Hemorrhagic seminal vesicle cyst. Computed tomography shows a relatively high attenuation seminal vesicle cyst (*c*) in this patient with right renal agenesis. The high attenuation of this cyst is probably due to hemorrhage.

thickening of the walls, cystic dilatation, and irregularity of the seminal vesicles. Calcification may occur with end stage disease.

Primary neoplasms of the seminal vesicles are extremely rare. The most common cause of neoplastic involvement is direct invasion of the seminal vesicles by prostate cancer. Rectal and bladder cancers also can secondarily involve the seminal vesicles.

SUGGESTED READING

Prostatic Hypertrophy

Haylen BT, Parys BT, West CR: Transrectal ultrasound to measure bladder volumes in men. *J Urol* 143:687, 1990.

Doble A: Chronic prostatitis. *Br J Urol* 74:537, 1994.

Mirowitz SA, Hammerman AM: CT depiction of prostatic zonal anatomy. *J Comput Assist Tomogr* 16:439, 1992.

Pope TL Jr, Harrison RB, Clark RL, et al.: Bladder base impressions in women: "female prostate." *AJR* 136:1105, 1981.

Talner LB: Routine urography in men with prostatism. *AJR* 147:960, 1986.

Villers A, Terris MK, McNeal JE, et al.: Ultrasound anatomy of the prostate: the normal gland and anatomical variations. *J Urol* 143:732, 1990.

Wasserman NF, Lapointe S, Eckmann DR, et al.: Assessment of prostatism: role of intravenous urography. *Radiology* 165:831, 1987.

Prostate Cancer

Ajzen SA, Goldenberg SL, Allen GJ, et al.: Palpable prostatic nodules: comparison of US and digital guidance for fine-needle aspiration biopsy. *Radiology* 171:521, 1989.

Amis ES Jr: Role of CT and CT-guided nodal biopsy in staging of prostatic cancer [editorial]. *Radiology* 190:309, 1994.

Andriole GL, Kavoussi LR, Torrence RJ, et al.: Transrectal ultrasonography in the diagnosis and staging of carcinoma of the prostate. *J Urol* 140:758, 1988.

Benson CB, Doubilet PM, Richie JP: Sonography of the male genital tract. *AJR* 153:705, 1989.

Benson MC, Whang IS, Pantuck A, et al.: Prostate specific antigen density: a means of distinguishing benign prostatic hypertrophy and prostate cancer. *J Urol* 147:815, 1992.

Boring CC, Squires TS, Tong T, et al.: Cancer statistics, 1994. *Ca Cancer J Clin* 44:7, 1994.

Carter HB, Pearson JD, Metter J, et al.: Longitudinal evaluation of prostate-specific antigen levels in men with and without prostate disease. *JAMA* 267:2215, 1992.

Catalona WJ, Smith DS, Ratliff TL, et al.: Detection of organ-confined prostate cancer is increased through prostate-specific antigen-based screening. *JAMA* 270:948, 1993.

Chang P, Friedland GW: Hypoechoic lesions of the prostate: clinical relevance of tumor size, digital rectal examination, and prostate specific antigen. *Radiology* 175:581, 1990.

Choyke PL: Imaging of prostate cancer. *Abdom Imaging* 20:505, 1995.

Cooner WH, Mosley BR, Rutherford CL, et al.: Prostate cancer detection in a clinical urological practice by ultrasonography, digital rectal examination and prostate specific antigen. *J Urol* 143:1146, 1990.

Desmond PM, Clark J, Thompson IM, et al.: Morbidity with contemporary prostate biopsy. *J Urol* 150:1425, 1993.

Devonec M, Fendler JP, Monsallier M, et al.: The significance of the prostatic hypoechoic area: results in 226 ultrasonically guided prostatic biopsies. *J Urol* 143:316, 1990.

Donohue RE, Fauver HE, Whitesel JA, et al.: Prostatic carcinoma. Influence of tumor grade on results of pelvic lymphadenectomy. *Urology* 17:435, 1981.

Donohue RE, Fauver HE, Whitesel JA, et al.: Staging prostatic cancer. A different distribution. *J Urol* 122:327, 1979.

Ellis JH, Tempany C, Sarin MS, et al.: MR imaging and sonography of early prostatic cancer: pathologic and imaging features that influence identification and diagnosis. *AJR* 162:865, 1994.

Engeler CE, Wasserman NF, Zhang G: Preoperative assessment of prostatic carcinoma by computerized tomography. *Urology* 40:346, 1992.

Gleason DF: Histologic grading and clinical staging of prostatic carcinoma. In Tannenbaum M (ed): *Urologic Pathology: The Prostate*. Philadelphia, Lea & Febiger, 1977, p 171.

Hricak H, White S, Vigneron D, et al.: Carcinoma of the prostate gland: MR imaging with pelvic phased-array coils versus integrated endorectal-pelvic phased-array coils. *Radiology* 193:703, 1994.

Hodge KK, McNeal JE, Stamey T: Ultrasound guided transrectal core biopsies of the palpably abnormal prostate. *J Urol* 142:66, 1989.

Lee F, Bahn DK, McHugh TA, et al.: US-guided percutaneous cryoablation of prostate cancer. *Radiology* 192:769, 1994.

Lee F, Littrup PJ, Torp-Pedersen ST, et al.: Prostate cancer: comparison of transrectal US and digital rectal examination for screening. *Radiology* 168:389, 1988.

Newman JS, Bree RL, Rubin JM: Prostate cancer: diagnosis with color Doppler sonography with histologic correlation of each biopsy site. *Radiology* 195:86, 1995.

Oesterling JE, Martin SK, Bergstralh EJ, et al.: The use of prostate-specific antigen in staging patients with newly diagnosed prostate cancer. *JAMA* 269:57, 1993.

Olson MC, Posniak HV, Fisher SG, et al.: Directed and random biopsies of the prostate: indications based on combined results of transrectal sonography and prostate-specific antigen density determinations. *AJR* 163:1407, 1994.

Outwater EK, Petersen RO, Siegelman ES, et al.: Prostate carcinoma: assessment of diagnostic criteria for capsular penetration on endorectal coil MR images. *Radiology* 193:333, 1994.

Oyen RH, Van Poppel HP, Ameye FE, et al.: Lymph node staging of localized prostatic carcinoma with CT and CT-guided fine-needle aspiration biopsy: prospective study of 285 patients. *Radiology* 190:315, 1994.

Platt JF, Bree RL, Schwab RE: The accuracy of CT in the staging of carcinoma of the prostate. *AJR* 149:315, 1987.

Pollack HM, Resnick MI: Prostate-specific antigen and screening for prostate cancer: much ado about something? *Radiology* 189:353, 1993.

Presti JC Jr, Hricak H, Narayan PA, et al.: Local staging of prostatic carcinoma: comparison of transrectal sonography and endorectal MR imaging. *AJR* 166:103, 1996.

Renfer LG, Schow D, Thompson IM, Optenberg S: Is ultrasound guidance necessary for transrectal prostate biopsy? *J Urol* 154:1390, 1995.

Rifkin MC, Sudakoff GS, Alexander AA: Prostate: techniques, results, and potential applications of color Doppler US scanning. *Radiology* 186:509, 1993.

Rifkin MD, McGlynn ET, Choi H: Echogenicity of prostate cancer correlated with histologic grade and stromal fibrosis: endorectal US studies. *Radiology* 170:549, 1989.

Rorvik J, Halvorsen OJ, Espeland A, et al.: Inability of refined CT to assess local extent of prostatic cancer. *Acta Radiologica* 34:39, 1993.

Schiebler ML, Schnall MD, Pollack HM, et al.: Current role of MR imaging in the staging of adenocarcinoma of the prostate. *Radiology* 189:339, 1993.

Schiebler ML, Yankaskas BC, Tempany C, et al.: MR imaging in adenocarcinoma of the prostate: interobserver variation and efficacy for determining stage C disease. *AJR* 158:559, 1992.

Schmidt JD: Editorial: Prostate cancer: improvements in detection and diagnosis. *J Urol* 155:243, 1996.

Schnall MD, Imai Y, Tomaszerski J, et al.: Prostate cancer: local staging with endorectal surface coil MR imaging. *Radiology* 178: 797, 1991.

Schroder FH, Hermanek P, Denis L, et al.: The TNM classification of prostate cancer. *Prostate* 4:129, 1992.

Stamey TA: Editorial: The central role of prostate specific antigen in diagnosis and progression of prostate cancer. *J Urol* 154:1418, 1995.

Steele GD, Osteen RT, Winchester DP, et al.: Clinical highlights from the National Cancer Data Base: 1994. *Ca Cancer J Clin* 44:71, 1994.

Tempany CM, Rahmouni AD, Epstein JI, et al.. Invasion of the neurovascular bundle by prostate cancer: evaluation with MR imaging. *Radiology* 181:107, 1991.

Tempany CM, Zhou X, Zerhouni EA, et al.: Staging of prostate cancer: results of Radiology Diagnostic Oncology Group Project comparison of three MR imaging techniques. *Radiology* 192:47, 1994.

Seminal Vesicles

Banner MP, Hassler R: The normal seminal vesiculogram. *Radiology* 128:339, 1978.

Ford K, Carson CC, Dunnick NR, et al.: The role of seminal vesiculography in the evaluation of male infertility. *Fertil Steril* 37(4):552, 1982.

Heaney JA, Pfister RC, Meares EM Jr: Giant cyst of the seminal vesicle with renal agenesis. *AJR* 149:139, 1987.

Kenney PJ, Leeson MD: Congenital anomalies of the seminal vesicles: spectrum of computed tomographic findings. *Radiology* 149:247, 1983.

King BF, Hattery RR, Lieber MM, et al.: Seminal vesicle imaging. *RadioGraphics* 9(4):653, 1989.

Littrup PJ, Lee F, McLeary RD, et al.: Transrectal US of the seminal vesicles and ejaculatory ducts: clinical correlation. *Radiology* 168:625, 1988.

Premkumar A, Newhouse JH: Seminal vesicle tuberculosis: CT appearance. *J Comput Assist Tomogr* 12(4):676, 1988.

Schabsigh R, Lerner S, Fishman IJ, et al.: The role of transrectal ultrasonography in the diagnosis and management of prostatic and seminal vesicle cysts. *J Urol* 141:1206, 1989.

Schwartz JM, Bosniak MA, Hulnick DH, et al.: Computed tomography of midline cysts of the prostate. *J Comput Assist Tomogr* 12(2):215, 1988.

Silverman PM, Dunnick NR, Ford KK: Computed tomography of the normal seminal vesicles. *Comput Radiol* 9(6):379, 1985.

19

··

Urethra and Penis

··········

NORMAL MALE URETHRA

Although the normal anatomy of the male urethra has been described in Chapter 1, a brief review of urethral anatomy as defined by radiographic landmarks is in order before discussing urethral strictures and tumors. During dynamic retrograde urethrography, the entire urethra can be visualized (Fig. 19.1). If properly performed, contrast medium can be seen jetting through the bladder neck into the bladder. The verumontanum is seen as an ovoid filling defect in the posterior (prostatic) urethra. The distal end of the verumontanum marks the proximal boundary of the membranous urethra. The distal boundary of the membranous urethra is the conical tip of the bulbar urethra. The membranous urethra is approximately 1 cm in length and is that portion of the urethra that passes through the urogenital diaphragm. This also is the region of the external sphincter of the urethra. The anterior urethra extends from its junction with the membranous urethra to the urethral meatus. It is divided into the bulbar (most dependent) segment and the penile or pendulous segment. There is usually mild angulation of the urethra where these two segments join at the penoscrotal junction.

On voiding studies, the bladder neck opens widely and becomes funnel-shaped. While the verumontanum can usually still be seen, the proximal bulbar urethra has less of a conical appearance. However, the membranous urethra remains the narrowest segment between these parts of the urethra, although it may dilate up to 6 or 7 mm in diameter during voiding.

The landmarks of the membranous urethra must be recognized, so that it can be accurately located on retrograde or voiding studies. If the membranous urethra can be identified, it will not be confused for a stricture. Narrowing elsewhere in the urethra will be clearly defined as separate from the membranous urethra, and therefore, most likely representative of a pathologic stricture (Fig. 19.2).

ACQUIRED URETHRAL STRICTURES IN MEN

Gonorrhea

Gonorrhea is a sexually transmitted disease more prevalent in underdeveloped countries where low hygienic standards prevail; sexual promiscuity is a major contributing factor. The estimated number of cases of gonorrhea in North America in 1974 reached 2.7 million. Since the early 1980s, sexual promiscuity has decreased because of fear of acquired immunodeficiency syndrome (AIDS), and thus the incidence of gonorrhea also has decreased. The estimated number of cases of gonorrhea in North America in 1985 was 1.8 million. Adequate early antibiotic treatment of gonorrhea eradicates the disease without sequelae. No treatment or inadequate treatment results in a chronic inflammatory reaction that can cause a urethral stricture.

Approximately 40% of all urethral strictures in the United States are caused by gonorrhea, while the remainder are caused by other diseases such as chlamydia or mycoplasma, tuberculosis, schistosomiasis, tumor, trauma, or iatrogenic injury.

Gonococcus ascends the anterior urethra after sexual contact with an infected partner, affecting the columnar epithelial cells, which become congested. The submucosal glands of Littre, which line the anterior urethra and have a lubricating function, become infected and produce a thick, purulent urethral discharge within 48 hours after exposure. Without adequate treatment, the infection extends into the corpus spongiosum surrounding

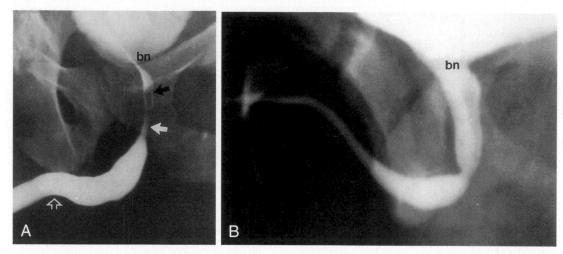

Figure 19.1. Normal male urethra. **A,** Dynamic retrograde urethrogram shows opacification of the entire urethra. Contrast can be seen jetting through the closed bladder neck (*bn*). The verumontanum (*black arrow*) is an ovoid filling defect in the prostatic urethra. The membranous urethra (*white arrow*) lies between the distal end of the verumontanum and the conical tip of the bulbous urethra. The mild angulation in the anterior urethra (*open arrow*) is the penoscrotal junction, dividing the bulbar and penile urethral segments. **B,** Voiding urethrogram in same patient shows funnelling of the bladder neck (*bn*). The verumontanum is still clearly seen as a mound of tissue in the prostatic urethra. The membranous urethra is the narrow junction between the prostatic urethra and the bulbar urethra. Note that the membranous urethra is significantly wider during voiding. (From Amis ES Jr, Newhouse JH: *Essentials of Uroradiology*. Boston, Little, Brown and Company, 1991.)

the anterior urethra, resulting in venous thrombosis and surrounding tissue necrosis. Granulation tissue develops where columnar cells have desquamated and sloughed. The combination of necrosis and granulation develops

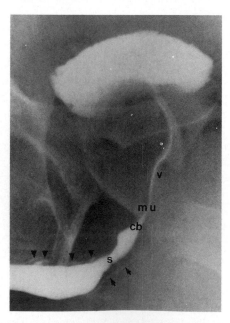

Figure 19.2. Proximal bulbar stricture. Retrograde urethrogram reveals a moderately smooth tapered stricture (*s*) of the proximal bulbar urethra. The glands of Littre are opacified (*arrowheads*) as is one of Cowper's ducts (*arrows*). The membranous urethra (*mu*) can be clearly defined by the distal end of the verumontanum (*v*) and the cone of the bulbar urethra (*cb*).

into fibrous scarring that is more prominent in the bulbar urethra, owing to less effective flushing by urination and the preponderance of glands of Littre in this area. Over a period of months or years, the scarring becomes irregular. Some scarring is hard fibrous tissue that is difficult to dilate, whereas other scarring is softer and more easily dilated. Gonococcal scarring or stricture is typically several centimeters long, and 70% of the hard fibrous scars are present in the most dependent portion of the bulbous urethra. Surgical or radiologic intervention is usually required to alleviate obstructive symptoms secondary to such strictures.

Infection may spread for several centimeters proximal and distal to the hard fibrous scar, producing further scarring that is not as advanced as the initial site and is consequently softer. The proximal spread of the infection may extend as far as the membranous urethra, but the obstructive symptoms, including straining to void, weak stream, and a feeling of incomplete emptying of the bladder, are caused by the hard scarring in the bulbar urethra. This is the primary stricture, and the adjacent softer scars are secondary strictures. The hydrostatic pressure in the urethra during voiding is quite high proximal to hard scarring, resulting in dilation of the urethra proximal to the scar. At least some of this dilation occurs in areas of softer proximal scarring (Fig. 19.3).

Pseudodiverticulum formation results from a gonococcal periurethral abscess that eventually ruptures into the urethra, leaving a cavity. The majority of pseudodiverticula affect the inferior aspect of the urethra, but

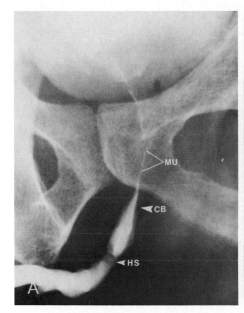
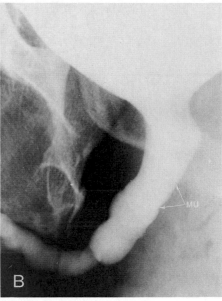

Figure 19.3.   **A,** Dynamic retrograde urethrogram in a patient who had a previous anterior urethroplasty for gonococcal stricture and developed outlet obstruction 2 years after urethroplasty. Note recurrent hard scar (*HS*) in the proximal bulbous urethra. Abnormal irregular narrowed cone to the proximal bulbous urethra (*CB*) indicates scarring which extends into the membranous urethra (*MU*). **B,** Same patient voiding. Note marked dilatation of urethra from bladder neck to hard scar. The soft scarring in the membranous urethra (*MU*) is markedly dilated due to the high hydrostatic back-pressure produced by the hard scar in the proximal bulbous urethra.

they can occur anteriorly in the region of the penoscrotal junction. They vary in size from small (approximately 1 cm) to huge (up to 10 cm) (Fig. 19.4).

Occasionally a periurethral abscess is large enough to extend to the perineum and penetrate both into the urethra and through the perineum, creating a urethrocutaneous fistula. It is not unusual for multiple fistulae to form. Consequently, urination usually occurs through the perineal fistulae, resulting in the so-called "watering can perineum." While this clinical finding can occur as

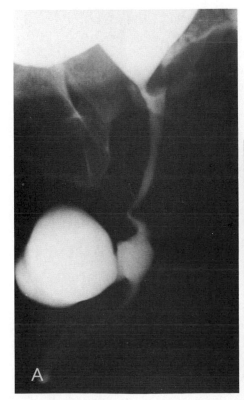
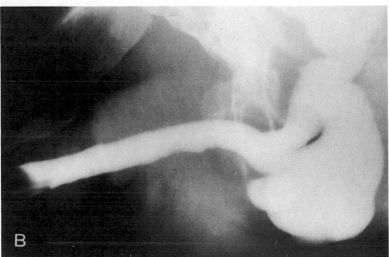

Figure 19.4.   **A,** A voiding cystourethrogram in a patient with bulbous urethra scarring and old sloughed periurethral abscess at the penoscrotal junction producing an anterior diverticulum. **B,** Dynamic retrograde urethrogram in a patient with two diverticula (one large) extending posteroinferiorly from the bulbomembranous urethra.

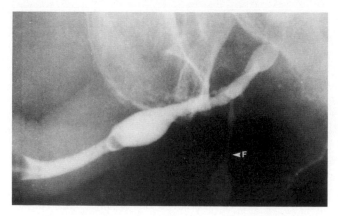

Figure 19.5. Dynamic retrograde urethrogram showing irregular scarring in the bulbous urethra with a fistula extending from the bulbous urethra to the perineum.

a rare complication of gonorrhea, it is more typical of tuberculosis or schistosomiasis. The abscess cavity resulting in the fistula generally contracts by fibrosis leaving only the narrow fistulous tract from the urethra to the perineum (Fig. 19.5).

High intraurethral pressure proximal to a stricture not only results in dilation of the urethra, but also can cause reflux of urine into the prostatic ducts. Ostia for these ducts, 30 to 40 in number, are found in the floor of the prostatic urethra around the verumontanum. This reflux may be massive and may allow infection to enter the prostate, potentially resulting in a prostatic abscess or formation of multiple prostatic calculi (Fig. 19.6). As with other causes of bladder outlet obstruction, the pressure necessary to urinate through a hard stricture may be high enough to result in hypertrophy of the detrusor muscle of the bladder, leading to trabeculation and diverticulum formation. In some cases, vesicoureteral reflux occurs, with eventual dilation of the one or both upper urinary tracts. Residual urine in the bladder can result in recurrent infections and stone formation.

Dynamic retrograde urethrography is the most efficacious way of imaging gonococcal strictures and commonly shows several centimeters of irregular urethral narrowing. The stricture may be smooth or have a beaded appearance (Fig. 19.7). While the bulbar urethra is the most common area of occurrence, gonorrheal strictures may occur anywhere in the anterior urethra or may even involve the entire anterior urethra. If the dis-

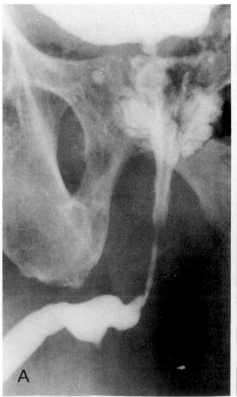
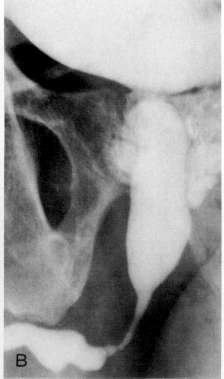

Figure 19.6. **A,** Dynamic retrograde urethrogram showing grossly abnormal cone to proximal bulbous urethra indicating scarring extends into the membranous urethra. Marked reflux of contrast medium into dilated open prostatic ducts indicating previous prostatitis and outlet obstruction. **B,** The same patient voiding. There is marked paradoxical dilatation with increased reflux into the prostatic ducts.

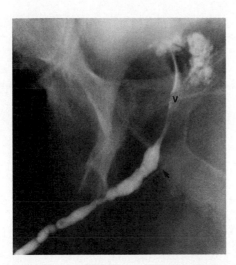

Figure 19.7. Gonococcal stricture. Retrograde urethrogram shows an irregular, beaded stricture involving the pendulous urethra and distal two thirds of the bulbar urethra. The conical tip of the bulbar urethra is preserved and the verumontanum (*v*) can be clearly seen allowing easy identification of the membranous urethra. Cowper's duct is opacified (*arrows*) and reflux can be seen into the prostate.

ease has spread proximally to the membranous urethra, the normal cone shape of the proximal bulbous urethra becomes asymmetric and narrowed, giving an elongated appearance to the membranous urethra (Fig. 19.8). Abnormality of the normal convex cone shape of the proximal bulbous urethra indicates scarring extending into the membranous urethra. This radiologic finding is of prime importance to the urologist, since surgical treatment may involve cutting the scar tissue and consequently the distal sphincter, which can result in iatrogenic incontinence. The verumontanum can almost always be seen on the dynamic retrograde urethrogram. If the cone of the bulbous urethra is distorted, resulting in loss of the distal landmark for identifying the membranous urethra, its location can be inferred to be just below the distal end of the verumontanum.

A voiding cystourethrogram may occasionally be of use in defining the proximal extent of a urethral stricture, assuming a catheter can be passed through the stricture to allow filling of the bladder with contrast medium. An 8-French pediatric feeding tube may be useful in passing some strictures. The presence of a urethral stricture may alter the bladder capacity. In men with urethral stricture, the bladder capacity may increase to 1000 ml before the urge to void is felt. It is usually a mistake to remove the catheter for voiding when the patient first indicates that he is ready to void; he may not void after catheter removal, resulting in lost time and necessitating reinsertion of the catheter. Rather, it is wise to instill a further 50 to 100 ml of contrast medium into the bladder after the patient indicates he is ready to

void. This usually results in an immediate and good voiding study.

In the presence of a gonococcal stricture, the voiding study usually shows dilation of the proximal urethra (Fig. 19.9). The dilation may include the membranous urethra, even when the dynamic retrograde study indicates scarring extending into the membranous urethra. Dilation of a scarred membranous urethra indicates softer scarring in the membranous urethra than the hard scarring in the bulbous urethra.

The dynamic retrograde and voiding examinations also may indicate other complications of gonococcal urethral stricture. Reflux into prostatic ducts, or Cowper's duct, as well as the development of bladder trabeculation and diverticula are common findings. Reflux into the ejaculatory ducts, seminal vesicles, and vasa deferentia is uncommon (Fig. 19.10), as is reflux into the prostatic utricle, which may be somewhat dilated (Fig. 19.11).

Recent literature has emphasized the use of ultrasound in the assessment of urethral disease. While ul-

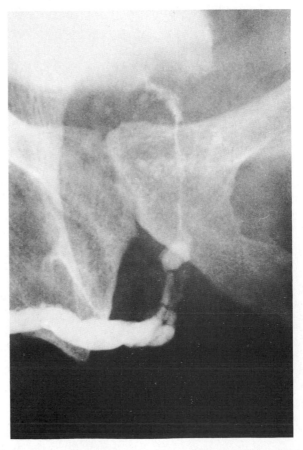

Figure 19.8. Dynamic retrograde urethrogram showing infectious scarring in the bulbous urethra, marked hard scarring in the proximal bulbous urethra, abnormal cone of the proximal bulbous urethra indicating scarring extends into the membranous urethra. By permission. (From Putman CE, Ravin CE: Textbook of Diagnostic Imaging. Philadelphia, WB Saunders, 1989.)

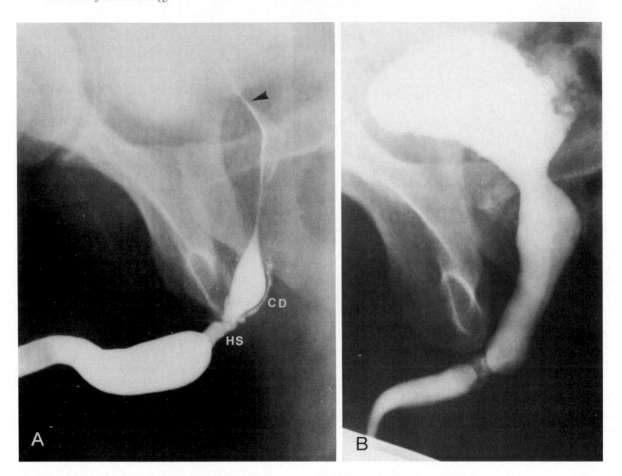

Figure 19.9. **A,** Dynamic retrograde urethrogram showing hard scar in mid-bulbous urethra (*HS*). Contrast medium also outlines Cowper's duct (*CD*). *Black arrow* indicates closed bladder neck. **B,** The same patient voiding. Note that the bladder neck is open. The urethra is dilated down to the hard scar in the mid bulbous urethra.

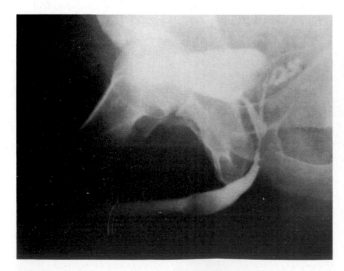

Figure 19.10. Dynamic retrograde urethrogram showing bulbomembranous stricture and reflux into ejaculatory duct, seminal vesicle, and vas deferens.

trasound can give adequate information regarding scarring in the anterior urethra, this procedure is unlikely to indicate bulbous urethral scarring extending into the membranous urethra. The assessment of bulbous urethral scarring extending into the membranous urethra is essential for the urologist in the decision regarding operative procedure. Consequently, it appears that dynamic retrograde urethrography is of more value than ultrasound, because the urologist gains more information on the need for a transsphincter urethroplasty.

Tuberculosis

Tuberculous stricture of the urethra is rare without evidence of tuberculous involvement of the prostate. Usually genital tuberculosis is a descending infection and renal tuberculosis is evident. However, in some patients with genital tuberculosis, the kidneys are normal, indicating the possibility of hematogenous spread directly to the urethra. The prostate is involved in 70% of patients with genital tuberculosis. Prostatic abscesses may rupture into any surrounding structure, resulting in

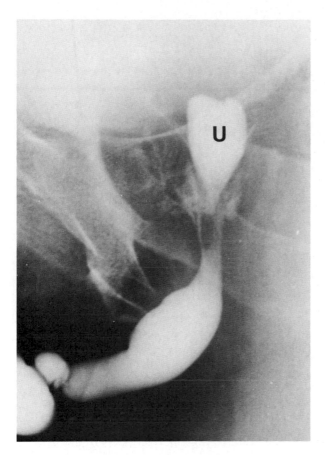

Figure 19.11. Dynamic retrograde urethrogram in a patient with multiple anterior urethral strictures. A dilated prostatic utricle (*U*) is arising from the verumontanum.

prostatorectal and prostatoperineal fistulae and sinus tracts extending from the posterior urethra. Tuberculous epididymitis and scrotal abscess with fistula formation also may be seen with genital tuberculosis, but less than 4% of cases have urethral involvement. When urethral infection occurs, stricturing is followed by periurethral abscesses, producing numerous perineal and scrotal fistulae. The end result is the watering-can perineum.

Dynamic retrograde urethrography and voiding cystourethrography typically show an anterior urethral stricture associated with multiple prostatocutaneous and urethrocutaneous fistulae, as well as blind-ending sinus tracts extending from the urethra. It may not be possible to visualize the entire urethra by standard means if most of the contrast medium exits the urethra through the perineal fistulae. It may then be necessary to insert catheters into the perineal fistulae and to inject the fistulae and urethra at the same time to obtain a satisfactory study (Fig. 19.12).

Schistosomiasis

Schistosomiasis hematobium is the parasite that involves the urinary tract; the life cycle involved is discussed in detail in chapter 18. In this disease, multiple fistulae develop between the urethra and the suprapubic area, the perineum, and the scrotum. Unlike tuberculosis, in which urethral stricture precedes fistula formation, in schistosomiasis urethral strictures result from fistulous tract formation. These strictures are most common in the bulbous urethra. In patients who have had schistosomal fistulae for more than 4 years, virtually all develop urethral strictures. Radiographic study is the same as described for tuberculous urethral disease.

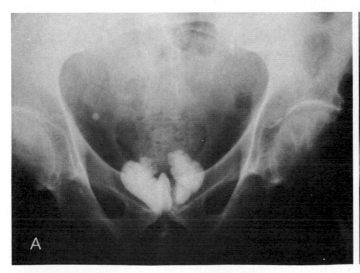

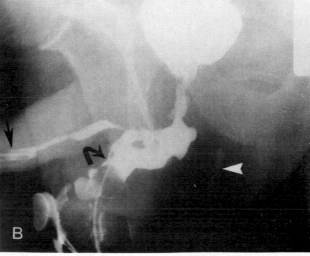

Figure 19.12. **A,** A plain film in a patient with known pulmonary and renal tuberculosis. The prostate gland is almost completely calcified. **B,** Same patient. Dynamic retrograde urethrogram with injection of contrast medium into the catheter (*arrow*) in the fossa navicularis shows a perineal fistula. A second catheter (*curved arrow*) is inserted into the perineal fistula orifice. Injection of both catheters simultaneously outlines a urethro-perineal abscess cavity and scarred urethra. Calcification is seen in the epididymis (*arrowhead*).

Iatrogenic Injury

Instrument Strictures in Men

The initial insult to the urethra in iatrogenic stricturing is pressure necrosis resulting from the passage of a straight metallic instrument along an S-shaped urethra that is fixed at two points. These points of relative fixation are the penoscrotal junction, where angulation is caused by the suspensory ligament of the penis, and the membranous urethra which is fixed by the urogenital diaphragm. When a straight rigid instrument is passed along the urethra, a fulcrum is created at the penoscrotal junction; a second fulcrum is present at the bulbomembranous urethra. If the instrument is of large diameter, is left in the urethra for too long, or is moved in the urethra without appropriate lubrication, pressure necrosis can occur, resulting in tissue necrosis, scar formation, and subsequent stricturing.

The most common instrument to cause such urethral damage is the resectoscope used in transurethral resection for prostatic hypertrophy. The incidence of urethral stricture after transurethral resection of the prostate (TURP) has been reported to be as high as 14%, and urethral contour irregularities or serrations are seen postoperatively in up to 30% of patients. However, meticulous technique results in a much lower complication rate. Urethrography has demonstrated that strictures arising from instrumentation are short and well defined. The majority of instrument-related strictures occur in the

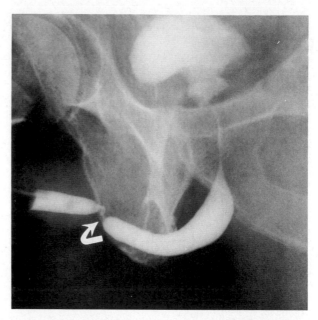

Figure 19.14. Instrument stricture: post-TURP. Dynamic retrograde urethrogram shows a short tight instrument stricture (*arrow*) at the penoscrotal junction. Note resected prostatic bed. The cone of the bulbous urethra is elongated and narrowed suggesting bulbomembranous urethral scarring.

bulbomembranous region (Fig. 19.13), and less than 20% occur at the penoscrotal junction (Fig. 19.14).

Catheter Strictures

Indwelling urethral catheters may cause pressure necrosis at the fixed points of the urethra and almost invariably cause infection if the catheter is left in position for more than a few days. The catheter causes pressure necrosis if it is too large for the urethra or if the catheter is allowed to dangle from the penis, draining into a bag strapped to the lower thigh. Penoscrotal junction pressure necrosis due to catheterization can usually be avoided if the catheter is taped to the anterior abdominal wall, thus removing the bend at the penoscrotal junction.

Occasionally catheter material (rubber, latex, plastic, Teflon, silicone) may evoke an inflammatory response that may lead to a superimposed infection. With long-term indwelling catheters, a diffuse urethritis is almost unavoidable. This superimposed infection spreads along the urethra involving the glands of Littre and extending into the submucosal tissues and corpus spongiosum. Urethrography typically reveals long and irregular strictures, often with visualization of the glands of Littre (Fig. 19.15). Clinical history is necessary to differentiate between previous gonorrhea or catheterization as the etiology of the stricture. Catheter strictures affecting the bulbomembranous urethra cause irregularity and asymmetry of the cone of the proximal bulbous ure-

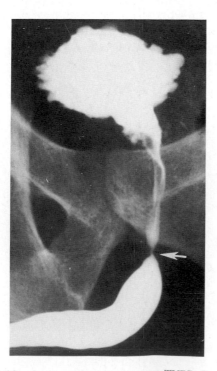

Figure 19.13. Instrument stricture: post-TURP. Dynamic retrograde urethrogram shows a short tight instrument stricture (*arrow*) in the bulbous urethra.

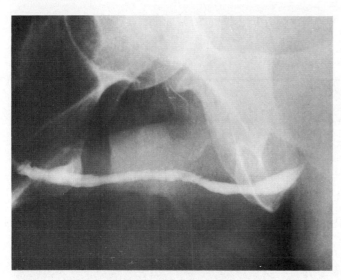

Figure 19.15. Catheter stricture: dynamic retrograde urethrogram 1 year following abdominal operation requiring 7 days of bladder catheterization. The penile and distal bulbous urethra is markedly narrowed and irregular—most marked at the penoscrotal junction. Glands of Littre are visualized.

thra. The glands of Littre are not visualized because they are sparse proximal to the middle, or most dependent portion, of the bulbous urethra. One study reported that 12% of patients who had indwelling urethral catheters during recovery from major surgery subsequently developed urethral strictures.

Treatment of Urethral Stricture

All patients with urethral strictures should be assessed by dynamic retrograde and voiding urethrography and urethroscopy. Anterior urethral strictures 1.5 cm or more below the membranous urethra are far enough from the external sphincter to be managed by internal visual urethrotomy if simple dilation fails. Urethrotomy involves incising the stricture with a urethrotome under direct visualization. Urethroplasty may be necessary when more conservative measures fail. A patch or pedicle penile skin graft is the usual method used for widening an area of urethral stricturing. Transsphincter urethroplasty is necessary to repair a bulbomembranous urethral stricture and should not be taken lightly because it involves compromising the external sphincter at the urogenital diaphragm. A flap of scrotal skin is used to construct a new urethra extending from the verumontanum to healthy urethra distal to the stricture. Follow-up urethrography may be necessary at regular intervals until the urethra has stabilized.

Urethral stricture also may be treated by balloon dilation. This may be accomplished with inflation of the balloon in the strictured area (Fig. 19.16). Strictures that cannot be dilated from below require an antegrade approach through a suprapubic cystostomy tract. A guidewire is passed through the strictured area via the bladder neck and is grasped as it exits the urethral meatus. With the guidewire anchored at both ends, the balloon catheter is passed per urethra over the guidewire to the strictured area and the balloon is inflated (Fig. 19.17). Balloon dilation of urethral strictures requires visualization of the membranous urethra by retrograde urethrography before the balloon is inflated to prevent damage to the external sphincter. The balloon should then be inflated for several minutes until the "waist" of the stricture is effaced. Several inflations may be required.

PERIURETHRAL ABSCESS

Periurethral abscesses arise when a gland of Littre becomes obstructed by inspissated pus or fibrosis. Because the tunica albuginea resists the dorsal spread of infection, the abscess tracks ventrally into the corpus spongiosum, where it is confined by Buck's fascia. The abscess may spread into the anterior abdominal wall, thighs, or buttocks if Buck's fascia is perforated.

Scrotal swelling and fever are the most common presenting complaints. Occasionally the abscess may occlude the urethra, causing urinary retention. Most patients have a history of urethral strictures and many are associated with recent urethral instrumentation or catheterization. The most common infecting organisms are Gram-negative rods, enterococci, and anaerobes.

If the abscess drains into the urethra, it may be demonstrated by urethrography. Edema and fluid collections may be recognized by computed tomography (CT) or ultrasound.

Approximately 10% of periurethral abscesses drain spontaneously. Percutaneous aspiration and catheter drainage may be performed, usually through the perineal route.

URETHRAL TUMORS

Benign Tumors

Benign tumors of the urethra are rare. They may be of epithelial or mesenchymal origin.

Epithelial Origin

Three types of epithelial cells make up the mucosa of the urethra. Transitional cell epithelium lines the prostatic urethra to the membranous urethra, where it changes to pseudostratified tall columnar epithelium. This type continues from the membranous throughout the bulbous and penile urethra to the fossa navicularis where it becomes stratified squamous epithelium. How-

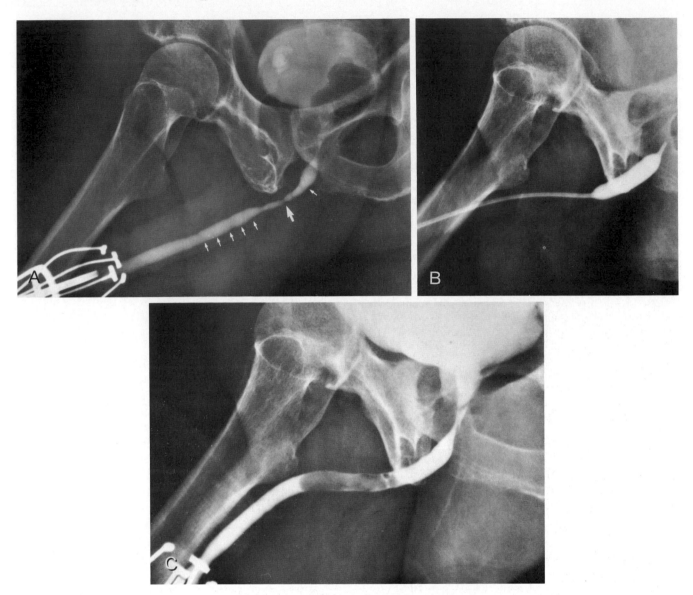

Figure 19.16. **A,** Dynamic retrograde urethrogram done using a Brodny clamp. Severe scarring is seen in the bulbous urethra (*large arrow*). Lesser softer scarring is present both proximal and distal to the hard scar. **B,** A balloon catheter has been inserted into the stricture area, and the balloon inflated with dilute contrast medium. **C,** Postdilatation urethrogram showing stricture is dilated to a normal urethral caliber. (From Russinovich NAE, Lloyd LK, Griggs WP, et al.: Impassable urethral strictures: Percutaneous transvesical catheterization and balloon dilatation. *Urol Radiol* 2:33, 1980.)

ever, there may be rests of squamous or transitional epithelium throughout the bulbous and penile urethra.

Transitional cell papilloma is the most common benign tumor in the prostatic urethra. It arises from the transitional cell epithelium, has a vascular stroma, and is difficult to identify radiographically at the time of presentation. Patients with transitional cell papilloma present with hematuria, nocturia, and stream reduction (in elderly males) and are usually diagnosed by urethroscopy. It is seen as a sessile polyp with multiple papillary outgrowths. The lesion is not associated with multifocal origin or malignant change, and recurrence is unlikely after urethroscopic resection. However, many pathologists consider transitional cell papillomas to be very low grade carcinomas.

Adenomatous tumors in the prostatic urethra develop in the prostatic epithelium and project into the prostatic urethra. They commonly have a sessile base, but may be polypoid or papillary. There is a covering of transitional cell epithelium, but this benign tumor clearly originates from the prostate. This lesion usually presents with hematuria or hematospermia and may be identified on cystourethrography as a filling defect in the prostatic urethra just below the verumontanum. Recurrence is rare after resection. Although considered a benign lesion, adenocarcinoma within an adenomatous polyp has been reported.

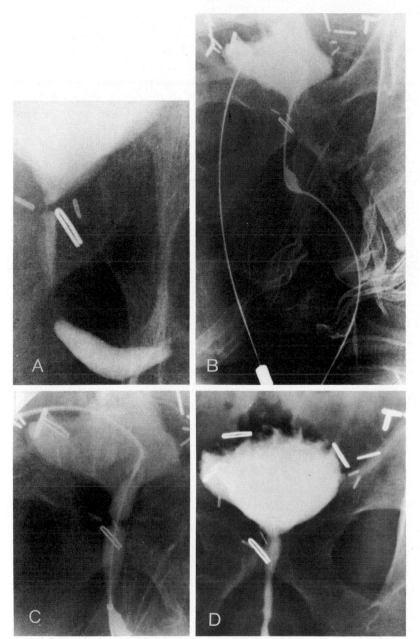

Figure 19.17. **A,** A voiding cystourethrogram in a patient after total suprapubic prostatectomy. A tight stricture has developed at the anastomosis of the cut bladder ends and the membranous urethra. This stricture is impassable from below. **B,** Via a suprapubic cystostomy tube a guidewire is passed through the stricture and extends from the external urethral orifice. **C,** The balloon catheter is then passed over the guidewire to the strictured area, and the balloon is inflated with contrast medium. Note the waist in the balloon at the stricture site. The balloon may require several deflations and inflations until the waist disappears. (From Scales FE, Katzen BT, van Breda A, et al.: Impassable urethral strictures: Percutaneous transvesical catheterization and balloon dilatation. *Radiology* 157:59, 1985.) **D,** Postdilatation voiding cystourethrogram showing marked improvement in the caliber of the urethra at the stricture site.

Nephrogenic adenoma is a rare metaplastic process that is more common in the bladder than in the urethra. However, it may be present only in the prostatic urethra and is found in elderly men who have had a previous history of bladder or urethral trauma or previous bladder, prostatic, or urethral surgery. Histologically, these lesions resemble the nephron. Grossly, they are small (5 mm or less) and may be multiple. They are friable and tend to present with gross hematuria. Diagnosis is made using urethroscopy, although a slightly irregular appearance to the prostatic urethra may be seen on cystourethrography.

Papillary urethritis (polypoid urethritis) in the prostatic urethra is an inflammatory reaction resulting in transitional cell proliferation, ectatic capillaries, and edema, producing multiple small cystic strictures similar to ureteritis cystica. The ectatic capillaries bleed, producing hematuria, which is the most common presentation. There may be a reduction in the urinary stream. Cystoscopically, polypoid urethritis is difficult to differentiate from the lesions discussed in the preceding paragraphs.

Inflammatory polyps in the anterior urethra are the result of previous urethral infection or previous urethral surgery for stricture. They are usually symptomless, but may increase in size to more than 1 cm, when they may produce obstructive voiding symptoms. They may be diagnosed by urethrography (Fig. 19.18) or urethroscopy.

Squamous cell papillomas occur in younger men and

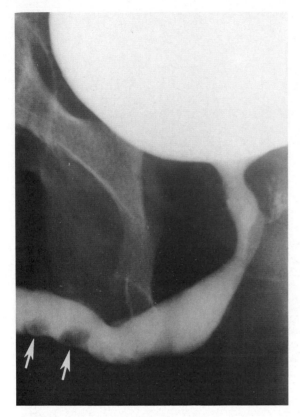

Figure 19.18. Voiding cystourethrogram showing inflammatory polyps (*arrows*) in the anterior urethra following urethroplasty for gonococcal stricture.

present at the urethral meatus. These lesions recur after surgical excision, and malignant change has been reported. Squamous cell papillomas arising elsewhere in the urethra develop in squamous cell rests amid the columnar epithelium.

Mesenchymal Origin

Fibrous polyps are congenital lesions arising in the prostatic urethra. The polyp may protrude into the bladder when resting and may prolapse as far as the membranous or bulbous urethra on voiding (Fig. 19.19). The growth of fibrous polyps commonly initiates intermittent obstructive symptoms and is found in male children; it has not been reported in female patients. Frequency, dysuria, and occasional microhematuria accompany intermittent obstructive symptoms. The lesion is easily demonstrated by dynamic retrograde and voiding cystourethrography. Transurethral resection is the treatment.

Hemangioma and myoblastoma occurring in the urethra are exceedingly rare, but have been reported.

Tumor-Like Lesions

Amyloidosis of the urethra is characterized by penile bleeding and a palpable hard mass along the ventral surface of the penile or bulbous urethra. Fewer than 25

cases have been reported, and most have occurred in men younger than 50 years of age. Amyloidosis should be considered in any young male presenting with penile bleeding and a palpable mass without previous urethral disease or trauma. Urethrography shows an irregular narrowed anterior urethra that may be indistinguishable from infective urethral stricture, but glands of Littre are not visualized in amyloidosis.

Condylomata acuminata (venereal warts) is a viral infection that usually produces sessile squamous papillomas on the glans and shaft of the penis and on the prepuce. Occasionally these warts spread along the urethra (Fig. 19.20) and may even reach the bladder. Urethral involvement is a serious complication and may require numerous treatment sessions with the instillation of podophyllin, thiotepa, or 5-fluorouracil into the urethra. If urethral involvement is suspected clinically, the patient should not have any urethral instrumentation or catheterization because of the possibility of retrograde seeding. Retrograde urethrography should not be performed for the same reason. The diagnostic procedure of choice is voiding cystourethrography at the end of excretory urography (excretory voiding urethrography). The urethrographic study shows characteristic multiple frond-like papillary filling defects in the area of involvement. Occasionally only isolated filling defects are seen in the penile urethra.

Balanitis xerotica obliterans (BXO) is rare and affects the glans penis, prepuce, and urethral meatus. The le-

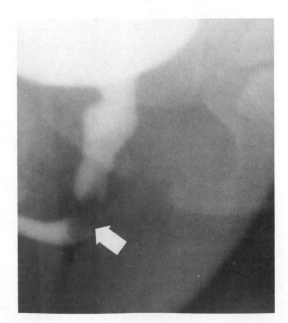

Figure 19.19. Voiding cystourethrogram in a child with difficulty in micturition. The filling defect in the bulbomembranous urethra is a fibrous polyp (*arrow*) on a stalk arising from the verumontanum. (Courtesy of Dr. R. Lebowitz. From Pollack HM ed: *Clinical Urography.* vol 2 Philadelphia, WB Saunders, 1990.)

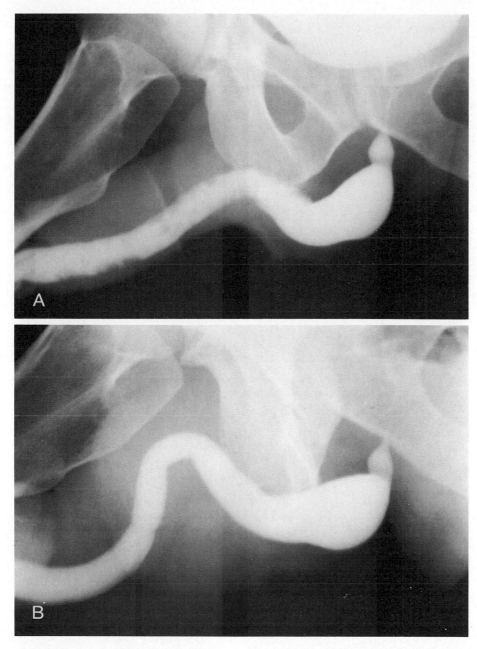

Figure 19.20. Condylomata acuminata. **A,** Multiple filling defects are seen in the anterior urethra. **B,** After treatment with podophyllin, there is complete clearing of the urethra.

sion is seen as white, dry, hyperkeratotic plaques. Rarely BXO extends into the anterior urethra and may cause pain on micturition. It may be premalignant and may be associated with squamous cell carcinoma. The typical radiographic finding is meatal stenosis.

Malignant Tumors

Malignant tumors of the urethra are rare and are almost all of epithelial origin. Leiomyosarcoma, malignant melanoma, and urethral metastases have been reported, but are exceedingly rare. Malignant urethral tumors are twice as common in the female urethra than in the male urethra. The most common urethral carcinomas are squamous cell carcinoma and transitional cell carcinoma (TCC). Adenocarcinoma is rare and develops in Skene's glands in women and in Cowper's gland or duct or the glands of Littre in men. In both men and women, carcinoma of the urethra usually occurs after 50 years of age.

Malignancy of the Male Urethra

Approximately 80% of male urethral carcinomas are squamous cell tumors that occur almost exclusively in

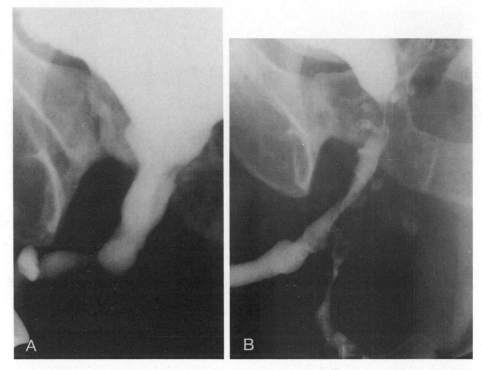

Figure 19.21.   Urethal carcinoma **A,** Voiding cystourethrogram in a patient who had previous urethroplasty for proximal bulbous urethral stricture. The stricture has recurred and proximal dilatation is present. No biopsy was performed at this time. **B,** The same patient 1 year later. The patient had a perineal mass and fistula. The retrograde urethrogram shows the perineal fistula with a fixed mass producing a scalloped appearance in the bulbous urethra at the site of origin of the fistula. (From McCallum RW, Colapinto V: *Urological Radiology of the Adult Lower Urinary Tract.* Springfield, IL, Charles C Thomas, 1976.)

the anterior urethra. Fifteen percent are TCCs and are usually found in the prostatic urethra. The remainder are adenocarcinomas or undifferentiated carcinomas. Fewer than 500 cases of urethral carcinoma in men have been reported.

Squamous cell carcinoma is associated with previous urethral stricture in up to 75% of cases. Chronic irritation producing squamous metaplasia in a preexisting urethral stricture is common, and therefore, the tumor most often is seen in the bulbomembranous region. Approximately 50% are associated with urethral stricture because of previous external or iatrogenic trauma. Consequently, any condition that may result in urethral stricture should be considered a predisposing factor to squamous cell carcinoma. These include gonococcal urethritis, long-term urethral catheterization, and urethral trauma. The diagnosis often is difficult and unsuspected. Excess bleeding after stricture dilatation, or the development of perineal fistula (Fig. 19.21) or a palpable hard mass in the bulbar region are all clues to the development of squamous cell carcinoma (Fig. 19.22). The incidence of squamous cell carcinoma after successful urethroplasty for stricture is low, only a few such cases having been reported. While successful urethro-

plasty appears to reduce the incidence of squamous cell carcinoma of the urethra, failure of urethroplasty should lead to consideration of biopsy of the recurrent strictured area to exclude carcinoma.

Spontaneous squamous cell carcinoma in patients

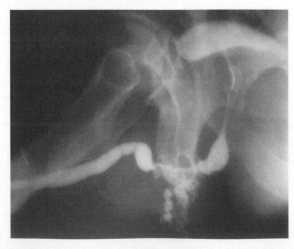

Figure 19.22.   Squamous cell carcinoma. A spontaneous perineal fistula was the presenting complaint in this man with urethral carcinoma.

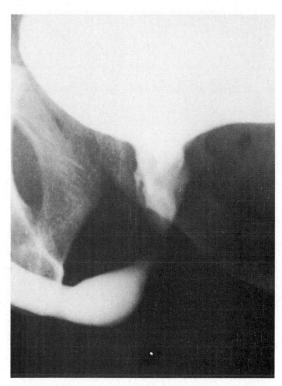

Figure 19.23. Spontaneous transitional cell carcinoma in the prostatic urethra causing gross hematuria in a 55-year-old man. The remainder of the urinary tract was free of transitional cell carcinoma. (From Pollack HM (ed): *Clinical Urography,* Philadelphia, WB Saunders, 1990, Vol 2.)

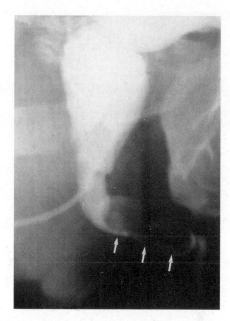

Figure 19.24. Squamous cell carcinoma arising de novo in the bulbar urethra. Voiding study performed via suprapubic tube shows the tumor (*arrows*) as a large filling defect in the bulbar urethra. There is gross dilation of the urethra proximal to the tumor. (From Amis ES Jr, Newhouse JH: *Essentials of Uroradiology.* Boston, Little Brown and Company, 1991.)

without previous history of urethral disease or trauma is thought to arise in rests of squamous cell epithelium within the normal stratified columnar epithelium.

Transitional cell carcinoma tends to occur in the prostatic urethra (Fig. 19.23), but can be found elsewhere in the urethra. The multicentric origin of TCC in the urinary tract may account for some occurrences in the prostatic urethra. In some patients, TCC is found in the posterior urethra as a direct extension of tumor in the bladder base or in the region of the bladder neck. Yet another possibility is seeding of malignant transitional cells from elsewhere in the urinary tract to the prostatic urethra, especially by instrumentation. Transitional cell carcinoma of the anterior urethra has been associated with carcinoma of the bladder and probably represents "drop" metastases.

Adenocarcinoma of the urethra is rare. It may arise from the glands of Littre or Cowper's glands or ducts.

Patients with urethral carcinoma may present with obstructive symptoms, serosanguineous discharge, perineal fistula, periurethral abscess, or palpable mass in the perineum or along the shaft of the urethra. Obstructive symptoms are most common, occurring in approximately 60% of patients.

Radiographically, urethral tumors may have varied presentations. When associated with existing strictures, neoplastic change typically produces more narrowing and grossly irregular margins of the stricture. Such changes should lead to a high suspicion for tumor. In the absence of an existing stricture, urethral neoplasms may present as a de novo stricture or as a filling defect in the urethra (Fig. 19.24); in either case, obstructive changes consisting of dilation and possibly extravasation into prostatic ducts may be seen proximal to the tumor. Early tumors may be detected as small mucosal nodules without proximal urethral dilation.

Secondary tumors of the male urethra are uncommon. Bladder TCC may be spread to the anterior urethra by seeding during urethral instrumentation or at the time of cystectomy; these are usually seen as multiple small mucosal nodules during urethrography (Fig. 19.25). Contiguous spread of carcinoma of the prostate (Fig. 19.26), rectum, spermatic cord, and testis may involve the corpus spongiosum, causing extensive urethral narrowing and irregularity. Erosion into the urethra from metastases to the corpus spongiosum (Fig. 19.27) may produce urethral irregularities (Fig. 19.27), although hematogenous metastases to the corpora cavernosa and corpus spongiosum are exceedingly rare.

Malignancy of Female Urethra

Although twice as common as male urethral carcinoma, carcinoma of the female urethra is still a rare con-

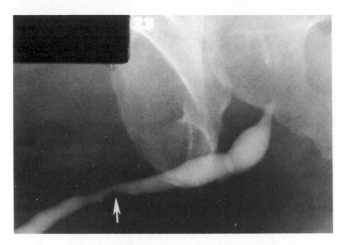

Figure 19.25. Transitional cell carcinoma of the anterior urethra producing irregular narrowing (*arrow*). This patient had cystectomy 1 year previously for transitional cell carcinoma of the bladder. (From Pollack HM (ed): *Clinical Urography*. Philadelphia, WB Saunders, 1990, Vol 2.)

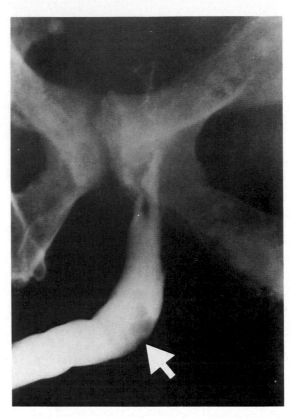

Figure 19.27. Carcinoma of the prostate metastasizing to bones and corpus spongiosum producing an irregular filling defect (*arrow*) in the bulbous urethra.

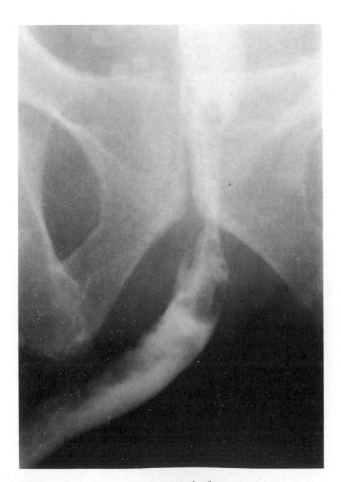

Figure 19.26. Contiguous spread of carcinoma of prostate into urethra. Multiple filling defects are appreciated in the bulbous and membranous portions of the urethra.

dition and accounts for less than 1% of genitourinary malignancies. Ninety-two percent of female malignant urethral tumors are carcinomas, of which 74% are squamous cell carcinomas and 16% are adenocarcinomas. The remainder are TCCs, undifferentiated carcinomas, or an extremely rare mucinous adenocarcinoma. Other malignancies reported in the female urethra include sarcomas and malignant melanomas. Carcinoma of the female urethra has been recorded in patients between 30 and 90 years of age, but 75% of patients are older than 50 years of age.

The etiology of female urethral carcinomas remains controversial, but previous urethral infection, urethral trauma, and urethral caruncle may be predisposing factors. Approximately 2.5% of patients with urethral caruncle have an associated carcinoma. Female urethral diverticula may contain carcinomas as well as stones. The female urethral mucosa consists of transitional cells in the proximal one third of the urethra; squamous epithelium is present in the distal two thirds of the urethra. Carcinomas presenting in the distal one third of the urethra are classified as "anterior" urethral tumors and are usually low-grade tumors with early presentation and good prognosis. Tumors involving the proximal two thirds of the urethra are classified as "entire" urethral tu-

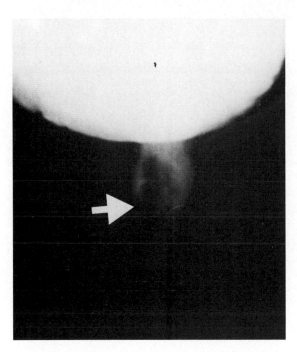

Figure 19.28.   A voiding cystourethrogram in a female complaining of dysuria and poor urinary stream. The filling defect in the proximal urethra (*arrow*) represents transitional cell carcinoma. (From Pollack HM (ed): *Clinical Urography.* Philadelphia, WB Saunders, 1990, Vol 2.)

mors and are of more advanced grade, become apparent later, and have a less favorable prognosis (Fig. 19.28). Clinically, "anterior" urethral tumors present with a mass projecting from the urethral orifice, urethral bleeding, dysuria, and frequency. Entire urethral tumors may have a similar presentation early in the course of the disease, but may not present until urinary retention, urethral abscess, or urethrovaginal fistula have developed. Urethral and pelvic pain are late and uncommon presentations. The diagnosis of urethral tumor in a woman is usually clinical. Imaging has little to offer beyond staging evaluation once the diagnosis has been established.

FEMALE URETHRAL DIVERTICULUM

Urethral diverticulum in women may be more common than has been suspected and should be excluded in patients with chronic irritative voiding symptoms (female urethral syndrome). Nonspecific chronic infection of the urethra may result in periurethral inflammation and edema as well as polyps near the bladder neck. In addition, patients with urethral diverticulum often complain of postvoid dribbling and dyspareunia. These diverticula are currently thought to be acquired. Infection of one of the periurethral Skene's glands is believed to

be the initial event, followed by obstruction of the ostium of the gland and abscess formation. Subsequently, the abscess ruptures into the urethra, resulting in a cavity communicating with the urethra.

A diverticulum causes irritative symptoms by harboring infected debris, postvoid dribbling because it fills during voiding and then empties afterward, and dyspareunia because of its frequent location in the urethrovaginal septum where it can be easily traumatized during intercourse. While most diverticula lie posterior to the urethra, they also can be located laterally or anteriorly, or even surround the urethra ("saddle" diverticulum). When a diverticulum originates from the proximal urethra, there may be mass effect on the bladder base similar to that seen in elderly men with enlarged prostates. This is termed the "female prostate," which is discussed in more detail in chapter 18.

An unobstructed diverticulum often can be demonstrated on the postvoid film during excretory urography. However, the denser contrast medium used for voiding cystourethrography allows an even greater likelihood of opacifying the cavity (Fig. 19.29). When suspicion remains after these studies, a double-balloon retrograde urethrogram (Fig. 19.30) may be diagnostic. The catheter is passed through the urethra and the balloon nearest the catheter tip is inflated in the bladder and snugged against the bladder neck. The second balloon, located outside the urethra, is then inflated, isolating the urethra. The Davis double-balloon catheter has an outside balloon that can be moved on the catheter shaft, and therefore provides even better isolation of the urethra. Contrast medium injected through the catheter exits through an opening between the balloons and opacifies the diverticulum, if present (Fig. 19.31). A filling defect in a diverticulum is a rare finding but, when pres-

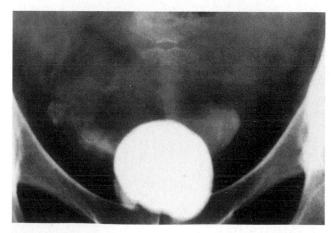

Figure 19.29.   Female urethral diverticulum. Postvoid film from a voiding cystourethrogram reveals a large collection of contrast in the suprapubic area. This is superimposed upon the minimal amount of contrast remaining in the bladder.

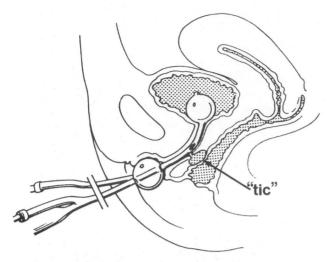

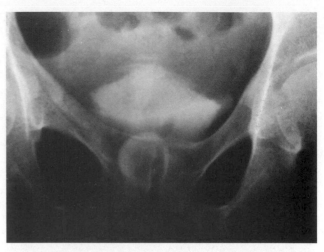

Figure 19.30. Double balloon retrograde urethrography technique. The more distal balloon on the catheter tip is inflated and snugged against the bladder neck. The second balloon is inflated at the urethral meatus, effectively isolating the urethra. Contrast injected through the catheter exits from the opening between the two balloons, distends the urethra, and opacifies a urethral diverticulum, if present. (From Amis ES Jr, Newhouse JH. *Essentials of Uroradiology.* Boston, Little, Brown and Company, 1991.)

Figure 19.32. Tumor in female urethral diverticulum. Postvoid film from an excretory urogram reveals a collection of contrast below the bladder base. This is typical for a urethral diverticulum. The filling defect in the diverticulum proved to be adenocarcinoma. (From Amis ES Jr, Newhouse JH: *Essentials of Uroradiology.* Boston, Little, Brown and Company, 1991.)

ent, may be caused by stone, debris, or tumor (Fig. 19.32). Although squamous cell carcinoma is the most common neoplasm in the female urethra, adenocarcinoma is the most frequently diagnosed tumor in a diverticulum.

More recently, transvaginal sonography and magnetic resonance imaging (MRI) have been reported as useful in detecting urethral diverticula. Ultrasound shows a relatively echo-free cavity adjacent to the urethra (Fig. 19.33); it also may demonstrate inflammatory debris and/or surrounding inflammatory edema. The high cost of MRI should preclude its use for detecting a diverticulum.

URETHRAL CALCULI

Calculi from the upper urinary tract or bladder that are small enough to pass through the bladder neck into the urethra are usually small enough to be passed through the urethra during voiding. Occasionally, however, a stone may be large enough to become lodged at a point of urethral narrowing such as the membranous urethra (Fig. 19.34) or a urethral stricture (Fig. 19.35). Primary formation of a stone in the urethra is usually only seen within a congenital or acquired diverticulum (Fig. 19.36). Symptoms of urethral stone include weak stream, dysuria, and hematuria. Retrograde urethrography will usually identify a rounded filling defect in the urethra. If one is careful to obtain a low abdominal radiograph, the stone may be identified before contrast medium is injected.

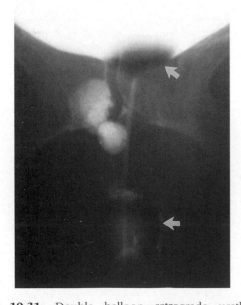

Figure 19.31. Double balloon retrograde urethrogram demonstrating urethral diverticulum. Both balloons have been inflated with air (*arrows*) to make them more readily visualized on radiography. After contrast has been injected a bilobed diverticulum is noted. With this technique contrast invariably leaks around the inner balloon into the bladder resulting in its opacification as seen here.

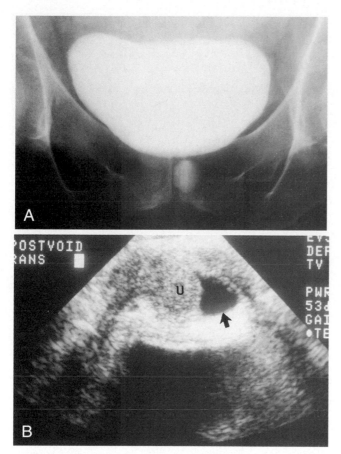

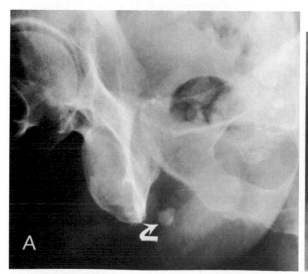

Figure 19.33. Female urethral diverticulum. **A,** Postvoid film from a voiding cystourethrogram reveals a collection of contrast below the bladder base and slightly to the left of midline. **B,** Transvaginal sonography reveals a cystic mass (*arrow*) adjacent to the urethra (*U*).

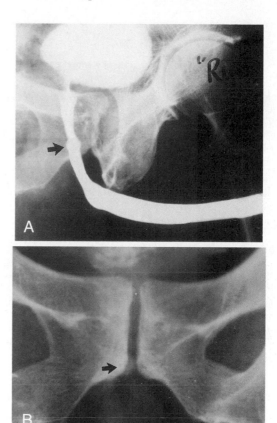

Figure 19.34. Urethral calculus. **A,** Retrograde urethrogram shows widening rather than narrowing in the membranous urethra (*arrow*). There is a question of a filling defect in this area. **B,** Careful evaluation of the scout film reveals a calculus (*arrow*) lodged in the membranous urethra. (From Amis ES Jr, Newhouse JH: *Essentials of Uroradiology.* Boston, Little, Brown and Company, 1991.)

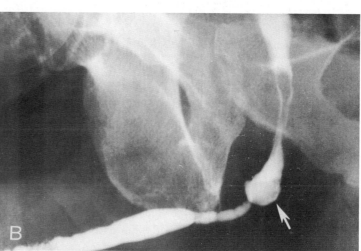

Figure 19.35. **A,** Plain film showing a stone (*curved arrow*) in the expected position of the urethra. **B,** Dynamic retrograde urethrogram showing severe scarring in the bulbous urethra. The filling defect (*arrow*) in the dilated urethra proximal to the scarring is a urethral stone.

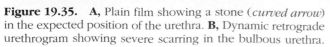

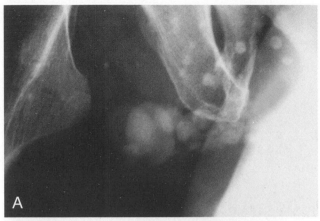

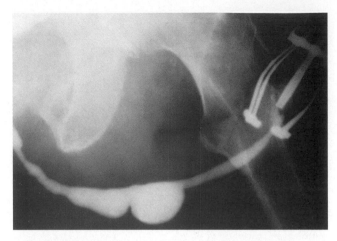

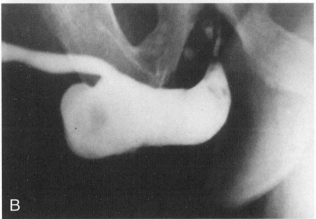

Figure 19.36. Calculi in acquired anterior urethral diverticulum. **A,** Multiple calculi are appreciated on the scout radiograph. **B,** Their location in an acquired urethral diverticulum is apparent on the retrograde urethrogram.

Figure 19.37. Post urethroplasty sacculations. Retrograde urethrogram using Brodny clamp shows two saccular dilations of the mid anterior urethra in a patient who has undergone urethroplasty for urethral stricture. (From Taveras JM and Ferrucci JT: *Radiology: Diagnosis-Imaging-Intervention.* Philadelphia, J.B. Lippincott Company, 1986.)

POSTOPERATIVE URETHRAL CHANGES

Urethroplasty

Urethroplasty, particularly two-stage procedures performed as definitive therapy for anterior urethral strictures, may sometimes result in fusiform dilations of the urethra, particularly near the proximal and distal ends of the repair (Fig. 19.37). These dilations are called sacculations and may be so large as to resemble urethral diverticula. Because of their size they may collect urine during voiding and cause significant postvoid dribbling. Retrograde urethrography easily demonstrates sacculations or acquired diverticula.

Prostatectomy

Transurethral resection of the prostate (TURP) is a commonly performed operation for relieving obstructive voiding symptoms in men with benign enlargement of the prostate. As part of the procedure, the internal sphincter at the bladder neck is widely resected as is prostatic tissue surrounding the posterior urethra. While

urography in patients who have not had prostate surgery shows a smooth bladder base with no contrast enhancement in the posterior urethra, after TURP the urogram will demonstrate a collection of contrast medium below the bladder base in the region of prostate resection (Fig. 19.38); this occurs since the internal sphincter has been resected and continence is being provided by the slow-twitch muscle fibers in the external sphincter at the urogenital diaphragm. This so-called "TURP defect" also can

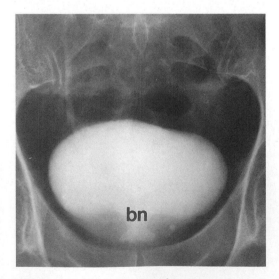

Figure 19.38. Urethral changes after transurethral resection of the prostate (TURP). The bladder phase of an excretory urogram shows mild elevation of the bladder base by an enlarged prostate. Since the internal sphincter has been resected, contrast flows through the bladder neck (*bn*) and fills the resected area of the prostate. (From Amis ES Jr, Newhouse JH: *Essentials of Uroradiology.* Boston, Little, Brown and Company, 1991.)

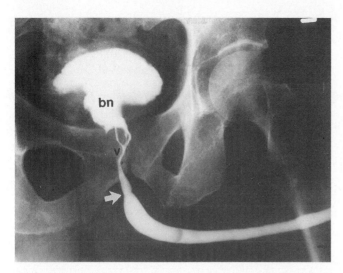

Figure 19.39.   Recurrent nodule of BPH after TURP. Retrograde urethrogram shows a widely resected prostatic urethra and bladder neck (*bn*). Immediately above the verumontanum (*v*) there is a nodule protruding into the urethral lumen. This proved to be regrowth of BPH. The narrowing of the proximal bulbar urethra (*arrow*) is the musculus compressor nuda.

be seen on cross-sectional studies such as transrectal sonography, CT, and MRI. In rare instances, nodules of benign prostatic hyperplasia can reform in the resected urethra; these are most commonly found near the distal end of the resection, because the urologist may be less vigorous in resecting this area in an effort not to compromise the external sphincter. These nodules are typically smooth and round or ovoid, and are best demonstrated by retrograde urethrography (Fig. 19.39). Inflammatory polyps also can result in urethral nodules after TURP. Another, although fortunately rare, complication of TURP or other interventions in the region of the bladder neck is bladder neck contracture (Fig. 19.40). After open prostatectomy for benign disease, the proximal prostatic urethra may appear patulous and irregular when imaged by urethrography, CT, MRI, or transrectal ultrasound.

Radical prostatectomy for cancer can be performed through the retropubic or transperineal route. In either case, the entire prostate and both seminal vesicles are removed en bloc. Continuity of the lower urinary tract must then be reestablished by anastomosing the bladder neck to a stump of membranous urethra extending from the urogenital diaphragm. The end result is a funnel shape of the bladder base that extends well below the top of the pubic symphysis (Fig. 19.41). This finding is virtually pathognomonic of a radical prostatectomy, and, if it was accomplished using the retropubic approach, there will be multiple surgical clips along the paths of the pelvic node chains as evidence of a staging lymphadenectomy.

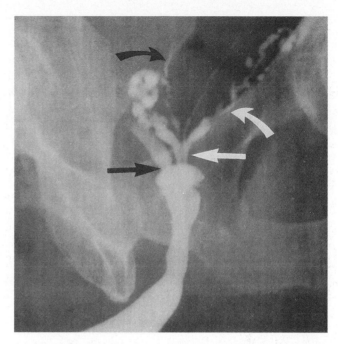

Figure 19.40.   Bladder neck contracture after TURP. Retrograde urethrogram shows a very narrow bladder neck (*straight black arrow*). Normally, following TURP the bladder neck is widely open. In this case, contrast can be seen taking the path of least resistance and opacifying the ejaculatory ducts (*straight white arrow*) and subsequently the convoluted portion of the vasa (*curved black arrow*) and the seminal vesicles (*curved white arrow*). (From Amis ES Jr, Newhouse JH, Cronan JJ: Radiology of male periurethral structures. *AJR* 151:321, 1988.)

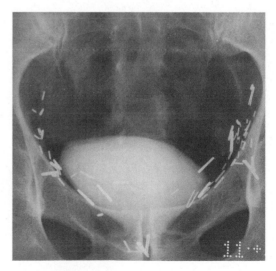

Figure 19.41.   Postoperative radical prostatectomy changes. An excretory urogram reveals funnelling of the bladder base behind the pubic symphysis. The entire prostate and prostatic urethra have been removed. The free edges of the bladder have been pulled down and anastomosed to the remaining stump of membranous urethra just above the urogenital diaphragm. This results in the funnelled appearance of the bladder base. The multiple surgical clips are evidence of a pelvic lymph node dissection. (From Taveras JM and Ferrucci JT: *Radiology. Diagnosis-Imaging-Intervention.* Philadelphia, J.B. Lippincott, 1988.)

PENIS

Benign and malignant lesions of the penis are readily visible and may be diagnosed clinically. These include condylomata acuminata, chancres, melanomas, basal cell carcinomas, and squamous cell carcinomas. Radiologic examination makes little or no contribution to the diagnosis of these lesions. However, radiology procedures are useful in the investigation of organic impotence, penile prostheses, and Peyronie's disease.

Organic Impotence

In men older than 50 years of age, erectile impotence has an organic cause in 90% of patients; in younger men, psychogenic impotence is more common. In either case, the impact is devastating to the 10 million or more impotent men in the United States. Fortunately, with better knowledge of the physiologic changes that

result in erection, methods for diagnosing the abnormalities that prevent this essential element of sexual function have been devised. Radiology can play a significant role in the evaluation of impotence.

Parasympathetic neural control of erection is mediated through the pelvic nerves that course between the prostate and rectum, which explains the high incidence of impotence after radical surgery involving these structures. In the penis, the result of pelvic nerve stimulation is smooth muscle relaxation in the walls of the cavernosal arteries and in the walls of sinusoids that fill both corpora cavernosa (Fig. 19.42). As the sinusoids and cavernosal arteries relax, there is a resultant decreased resistance to arterial flow into the cavernosa. Eventually, the pressure in the cavernosa is the same as systolic blood pressure. As the sinusoids distend with blood, they compress and block small emissary veins that extend from lacunar spaces around the peripheral sinu-

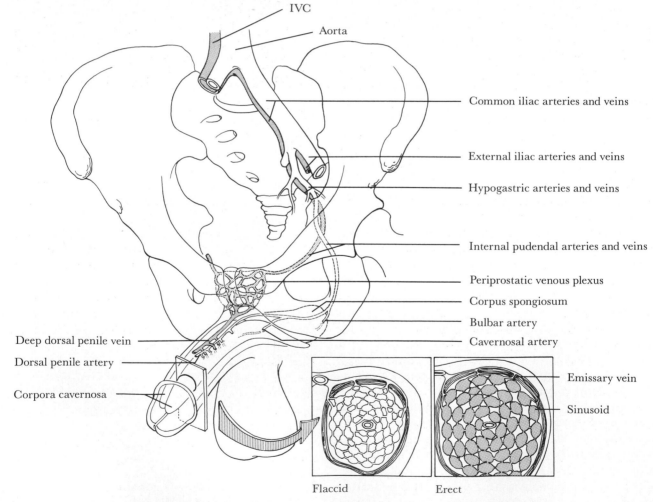

Figure 19.42. Simplified diagram of erectile function. Note that during erection the sinusoids in the corpora cavernosa distend and compress the emissary veins against the rigid tunica albuginea, thus occluding venous outflow. Leakage via these veins is the cause of venogenic impotence. Obstruction of the arterial supply to the penis (e.g., atherosclerotic plaques) is the cause of arteriogenic impotence. (IVC = inferior vena cava) (From Amis ES Jr, Newhouse JH: *Essentials of Uroradiology.* Boston, Little, Brown and Company, 1991.)

soids through the relatively rigid tunica albuginea surrounding the cavernosa to enter the deep dorsal vein of the penis. Thus, increased inflow of blood into the corpora directly inhibits the venous outflow of blood and results in an erection. Arteriogenic impotence implies an inability to increase the flow of blood into the cavernosa, such as can occur with posttraumatic or atheromatous occlusion of the internal pudendal or common penile arteries. In fact, atherosclerotic disease of the penile arteries is the primary cause in more than half of impotent men older than 50 years of age. Venogenic impotence results from the failure to occlude venous outflow, allowing continuous venous leakage from the emissary veins. While vascular problems are the most common cause of impotence, other etiologies include endocrine disorders, neurologic conditions, various systemic diseases, psychological factors, medications, and the abuse of tobacco and/or alcohol.

Arteriogenic impotence can be evaluated by selective pudendal arteriography with vasodilation and magnification. Intrapenile arterial anatomy is best shown by penile magnification pharmacoarteriography. This method has shown a high degree of variability of penile arteries, often differing from the classic arterial descriptions found in anatomy textbooks. The method consists of the use of a low-osmolar, high-concentration contrast medium, the intrapudendal arterial injection of nitroglycerin and papaverine, or the intracavernosal injection of papaverine alone to achieve vasodilation and to obviate arterial small vessel spasm. In experienced hands, internal pudendal artery catheterization can be achieved in 95% of patients. Direct magnification is necessary to visualize intrapenile arteries.

Originating as a branch from the internal pudendal artery, each penile artery gives rise to a dorsal penile artery, a cavernous artery, an artery to the corpus spongiosum, and a urethral artery. The corpus spongiosum artery forms small anastomoses with the urethral arteries. However, penile magnification pharmacoangiography demonstrates variable branching patterns to the dorsal penile and cavernosal arteries. Numerous intrapenile arterial communications are demonstrated that may act as collateral pathways in patients with intrapenile arterial obstructive disease.

Doppler ultrasound has recently been reported as a noninvasive way to access the deep penile arteries. Recent reports also indicate that sequential contrast-enhanced MRI may be able to provide additional morphologic information that will aid in the evaluation of erectile dysfunction. Currently, however, initial evaluation may simply be the injection of prostaglandin E1 or papaverine (with or without phentolamine) directly into one corpus cavernosum; these vasodilators facilitate maximal arterial flow into the penis and an arteriogenic cause of impotence can be excluded if an erection re-

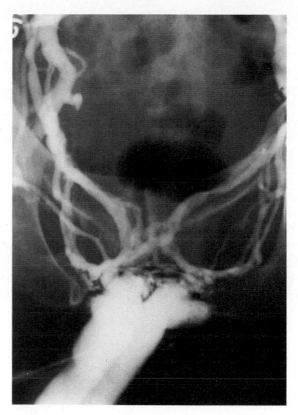

Figure 19.43. Venous leak. Both corpora cavernosa are filled, but the erection is not maintained. Rapid filling of large veins indicates a venous leak.

sults. In patients with severe vascular disease, however, blood flow may not be increased enough to cause an erection.

Cavernosography and cavernosometry (*see* Chapter 3) have been shown to be of value in the evaluation of venogenic impotence. This method involves the continuous injection of contrast medium directly into one corpus cavernosum (cavernosogram) at a rate necessary to achieve an intracavernosal pressure near that of systolic blood pressure. Only one side is injected, because the septum between the corpora is fenestrated and both corpora will fill (Fig. 19.43). A needle for measuring pressure (cavernosometry) is inserted in the opposite corpus cavernosum. Significant venous leakage into the deep dorsal vein of the penis seen with a flow rate necessary to maintain intracavernosal pressure in the 90 to 100 mmHg range is considered evidence of venogenic impotence.

Penile Prostheses

Better understanding of the etiologies of impotence has allowed more physiologic treatment to minimize the problem of erectile dysfunction. Failure to initiate an erection can be treated with intracorporeal injections as described above. Selected patients with arteriogenic impotence may be treated with large vessel angioplasty or microvascular bypass techniques. Patients who are unable to maintain erection may suffer from a venous leak that can be treated with ligation or transvascular occlusion of the draining veins of the penis. However, many patients have an organic cause of impotence that is not amenable to these treatment options. Implantable penile prostheses have become an attractive alternative treatment, and in many cases, are the preferred option.

The first successful penile prostheses were semirigid or malleable rods designed for placement into each corpus cavernosum. The Small-Carion semirigid prosthesis (Heyer-Schulte Corp., Minneapolis, MN) consists of a silicone sponge interior surrounded by a medical-grade silicone exterior. This prosthesis is only faintly radioopaque (Fig. 19.44). Malleable prostheses consist of braided stainless steel or silver wire cores surrounded by Teflon (Fig. 19.45). Although less rigid than the solid silicone prostheses, they are more malleable and concealable. These prostheses come in many sizes and widths or can be tailored to an individual patient. However, rigidity, length, and width cannot be altered once a particular device has been inserted. Patient satisfaction has been high, greater than 80%. Complications including pain, infection, perforation, and erosion have been observed in 7 to 16% of patients.

The development of an inflatable penile prosthesis provided significant improvement as both erect and flaccid states could be achieved. Concealment was no

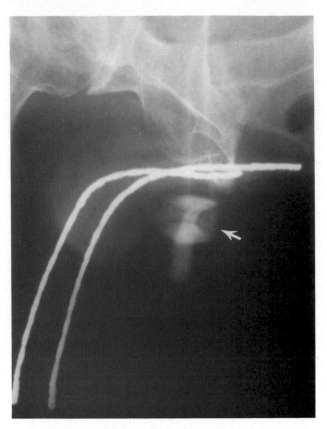

Figure 19.45. Malleable prosthesis. The braided wire cores are readily visualized but the silicone shell can only barely be appreciated. An artificial urethral sphincter (*arrow*) is also present. (From Cohan RH: Radiology of penile prostheses: Normal appearance and evaluation of malfunctions. In *Uroradiology Syllabus—American Roentgen Ray Society:* 1989.)

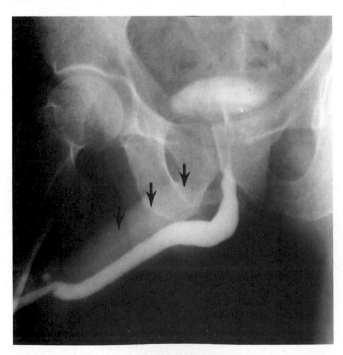

Figure 19.44. Semirigid prosthesis. The faint opacification of a Small-Carion prosthesis (*arrows*) is appreciated during retrograde urethrography. (From Cohan RH: Radiology of penile prostheses: Normal appearance and evaluation of malfunctions. In *Uroradiology Syllabus—American Roentgen Ray Society:* 1989.)

longer a problem and the quality of the erection was superior to that obtained with the noninflatable devices. Early versions suffered from a high mechanical failure rate because of the increased number of components. However, revised versions have significantly reduced the incidence of malfunction.

Two of the newer multicomponent inflatable prostheses have a 97% likelihood of remaining functional 3 to 4 years after implantation. The AMS 700 (American Medical Systems) and Mentor IPP (Mentor Corp. Goleta, CA) consist of four components interconnected by kink-resistant plastic tubing (Fig. 19.46). A spherical reservoir comprising a single piece of silicone rubber is implanted immediately beneath the rectus abdominus muscle in the pelvis. It is filled with isoosmolar contrast media so that the status of the fluid can be followed with plain-film radiographs. Two inflatable penile cylinders are made of expansile silicone rubber that widens and stiffens when inflated. These are inserted into the corpora cavernosa. The pump mechanism is placed in the scrotum, where it is easily accessible for activation. Recent modifications (Mentor Mark II, Mentor Corp., Goleta, CA

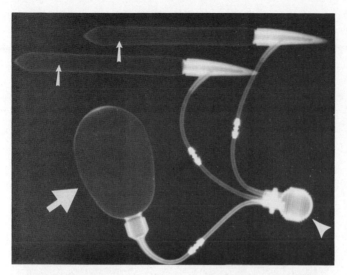

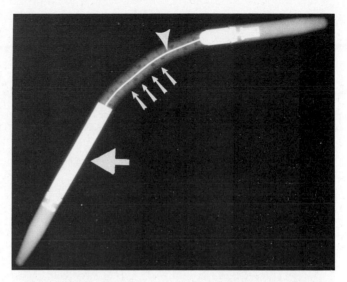

Figure 19.46. Multicomponent inflatable penile prosthesis (IPP). This specimen radiograph of a Mentor IPP demonstrates the reservoir (*large arrow*), valve mechanism (*arrowhead*), and penile cylinders (*small arrows*). (From Cohan RH: Radiology of penile prostheses: Normal appearance and evaluation of malfunctions. In *Uroradiology Syllabus—American Roentgen Ray Society:* 1989.)

Figure 19.48. Omni Phase prosthesis. The spring action cable (*arrowhead*) and interconnecting plastic segments (*small arrows*) are well seen. The spring action assembly is housed in the radioopaque metallic segment (*large arrow*). (From Cohan RH: Radiology of penile prostheses: Normal appearance and evaluation of malfunctions. In *Uroradiology Syllabus— American Roentgen Ray Society:* 1989.)

and Uni-Flate 1000, Surgitek, Racine, WI) have eliminated the reservoir by using a larger, more capacious pump, so the reservoir is not needed (Fig. 19.47). Patient satisfaction of greater than 90% is reported.

Self-contained cylindrical units for implantation in each corpora have also been developed. The DuraPhase and OmniPhase prostheses (Dacomed Corp., Minneapolis, MN) employ articulating plastic segments and a tensioning wire for positioning in a flaccid or erect state (Fig. 19.48). Another self-contained unit is the Flexi-Flate II

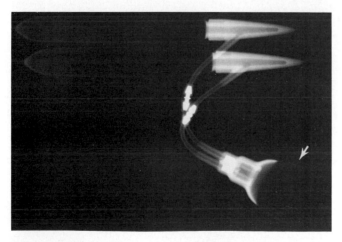

Figure 19.47. Multicomponent inflatable penile prosthesis. This newer version has the reservoir (*arrow*) contained in the valve mechanism. (From Cohan RH: Radiology of penile prostheses: Normal appearance and evaluation of malfunctions. In *Uroradiology Syllabus—American Roentgen Ray Society:* 1989.)

(Surgitek, Racine, WI), in which both the reservoir and inflatable chamber are contained in the cylinder implanted in each corpora.

These devices are constantly undergoing modification, and new prostheses are under development. It is therefore wise for radiologists practicing in a community where urologists treat impotence by implantation of prosthetic devices to keep abreast of developments in this field if they are to continue to provide expert radiologic evaluation of these patients.

Plain-film radiographs are usually sufficient for radiographic evaluation of the malfunctioning prosthesis. Fracture or erosion may be seen with semirigid or malleable prostheses. These are usually obvious on physical examination and radiographic confirmation is not necessary. The silver braided core of the older Jonas malleable prosthesis may break or fray. Patients may complain of loss of rigidity or audible crackling on movement. Although these breaks may be detected radiographically, their severity often is underestimated because of breaks or fraying of individual wire braids that comprise the core.

Radiography plays a much more important role in identifying the cause of mechanical malfunction of inflatable penile prostheses. A single anteroposterior or oblique pelvic radiograph with the prosthesis inflated often is diagnostic.

Fluid may leak from an inflatable prosthesis due to erosion of the tubing against the cylinders or kinks in the tubing leading to breakage. This complication has been seen in as many as 50% of patients with older

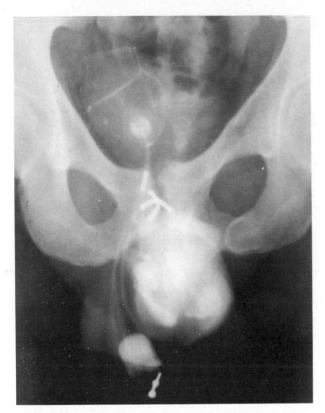

Figure 19.49. Fluid leak from an inflatable penile prosthesis. Only a minimal amount of fluid remains within the reservoir and penile cylinders, indicating fluid leak.

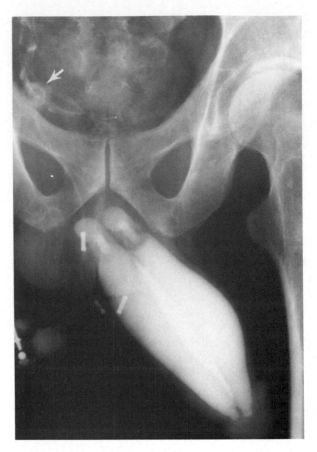

Figure 19.50. Aneurysmal ballooning of inflatable penile cylinders. The reservoir (*arrow*) is empty. (From Cohan RH, Dunnick NR, Carson CC: Radiology of penile prostheses. *AJR* 152:925, 1989.)

models, but is less commonly encountered with newer devices. Cohan and colleagues reported that 20% of 179 patients with a variety of inflatable penile prostheses had leaks from the cylinders, connectors, or tubing.

If there has been a leak of fluid, the prosthesis will not inflate adequately, and the patient will be unable to achieve erection. A pelvic radiograph reveals a decrease or complete absence of fluid in the reservoir and the penile cylinders will not completely inflate (Fig. 19.49).

Structural weakness may develop in the cylinders themselves after multiple inflations and deflations. These weaknesses may be apparent as buckling of the cylinders or even aneurysmal dilatation (Fig. 19.50). Weakness of the tunica albuginea may predispose to the development of these problems. Such structural weaknesses tend to occur in approximately 2% of patients. These problems can frequently be detected on physical examination and can be confirmed with a pelvic radiograph. The defective cylinders must be replaced, and because the surrounding tunica albuginea has been expanded, it must be reinforced.

Kinks in the tubing connecting the reservoir and pump were reported in approximately 5% of patients. They usually develop within the first few months of surgery. Kinks cannot be detected on physical exami-

nation, but may be identified on abdominal radiography (Fig. 19.51). This problem is seen less frequently with the introduction of "kinkproof" tubing. Separation of the tubing from the reservoir, pump, or cylinder is rare, but can easily be detected on a plain radiograph.

Erosions of a pelvic reservoir, usually into the bladder, can be encountered in 1 to 3% of patients, probably a result of local tissue ischemia. Cylinder and pump erosions are detected on physical examination. A reservoir erosion can be suggested on the plain radiograph by identifying an unusual position of the reservoir or change in position since the previous film. Confirmation may require cystoscopy or surgery.

Any prosthetic device can incite a surrounding infection. While this is usually clinically apparent, Gallium-67 scanning has been reported to show increased activity along the infected corporal implant in questionable cases.

Peyronie's Disease

Peyronie's disease is the development of fibrous plaques in the corpora cavernosa, resulting in painful deformity of the penis when erect. Plain-film radiography

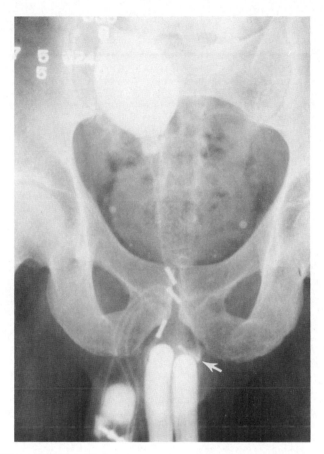

Figure 19.51.   Kink in connecting tubing. The abrupt angulation (*arrow*) indicates a kink in the connecting tubing. (From Cohan RH: Radiology of penile prostheses: Normal appearance and evaluation of malfunctions. In *Uroradiology Syllabus—American Roentgen Ray Society:* 1989.)

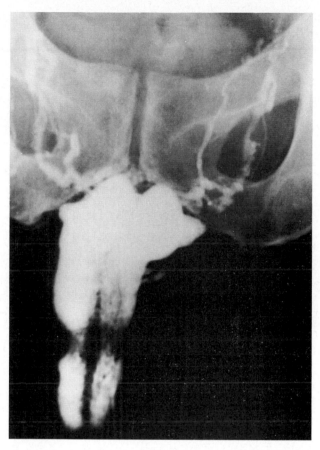

Figure 19.53.   Cavernosogram in a patient with Peyronie's disease. Filling defects are present in both corpora cavernosa due to fibrous plaques. Excess venous drainage is also present contributing to the patient's impotence. (From Gray R, Grosman H, St. Louis EL, et al.: The use of corpus cavernosography· a review. *J Can Assoc Radiol* 35:338, 1984.)

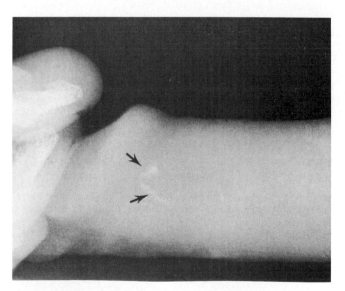

Figure 19.52.   A plain film of the penis showing several calcified plaques (*arrows*) in the distal penis. (From Gray R, Grosman H, St. Louis EL, et al.: The use of corpus cavernosography: a review. *J Can Assoc Radiol* 35:338, 1984.)

may show calcification (Fig. 19.52) in these plaques, but this is uncommon. Computed tomography of the penis has been reported to show faint calcifications in penile plaques that cannot be demonstrated on plain-film radiography. Cavernosography shows contour defects in the contrast media–filled corpora (Fig. 19.53). The septum between the corpora may be involved and significantly thickened. In patients with severe Peyronie's disease, cavernosography may show areas of fibrous obliteration of the corpora.

SUGGESTED READING

Urethra

Al-Ghorab NM: Radiological manifestations of genitourinary bilharziasis. *Clin Radiol* 10:100, 1968.

Amis ES Jr, Newhouse JH, Cronan JJ: Radiology of male periurethral structures. *AJR* 151:321, 1988.

Bolduan JP, Farah RN: Primary urethral neoplasms: review of 30 cases. *J Urol* 125:198, 1981.

Campbell JE, Sniderman KW: Urethral diverticula in the adult female. *J Can Assoc Radiol* 27:232, 1976.

Colodny AH, Lebowitz RL: Lesions of Cowper's ducts and glands in infants and children. *Urology* 9:321, 1978.

Cranston D, Davies AH, Smith JC: Cobb's collar—a forgotten entity. *Brit J Urol* 66:294, 1990.

de Gonzalez EL, Cosgrove DO, Joseph AE, et al.: The appearances on ultrasound of the female urethral sphincter. *Brit J Radiol* 61:687, 1988.

DiSantis DJ: Urethral inflammation. In Pollack HM (ed): *Clin Urography,* Philadelphia, WB Saunders, 1990.

Donald JJ, Rickards D, Milroy EJG: Stricture disease: radiology of urethral stents. *Radiology* 180:447, 1991.

Gluck CD, Bundy AL, Fine C, et al.: Sonographic urethrogram: comparison to roentgenographic techniques in 22 patients. *J Urol* 140:1404, 1988.

Greenberg M, Stone D, Cochran ST, et al.: Female urethral diverticula: double-balloon catheter study. *AJR* 136:259, 1981.

Hricak H, Secaf F, Buckley DW, et al.: Female urethra: MR imaging. *Radiology* 178:527, 1991.

Keefe B, Warshauer DM, Tucker MS, et al.: Diverticula of the female urethra: diagnosis by endovaginal and transperineal sonography. *AJR* 156:1195, 1991.

Kim B, Hricak H, Tanagho EA: Diagnosis of urethral diverticula in women: value of MR imaging. *AJR* 161:809, 1993.

Levine RL: Urethral cancer. *Cancer* (Phila) 45(8):1965, 1980.

McCallum RW: Urethral disease and interventional cystourethrography. *Radiol Clin North Am* 24:651, 1986.

McCallum RW: Urethral neoplasms. In Pollack HM (ed): *Clinical Urography,* Philadelphia, WB Saunders, 1990.

McCallum RW, Colapinto V: *Urological Radiology of the Adult Male Lower Urinary Tract.* Springfield, IL, Charles C Thomas, 1976.

McCallum RW, Rogers JM, Alexander MW: The radiologic assessment of iatrogenic urethral injury. *J Can Assoc Radiol* 36:122, 1985.

Morikawa K, Togashi K, Minami S, et al.: MR and CT appearance of urethral clear cell adenocarcinoma in a woman. *J Comput Assist Tomogr* 19(6):1001, 1995.

Palmer PES, Reeder MM: Parasitic disease of the urinary tract. In Pollack HM (ed): *Clinical Urography,* Philadelphia, WB Saunders, 1990.

Paulk SC, Khan AU, Malek RS, et al.: Urethral calculi. *J Urol* 116:436, 1976.

Pollack HM, DeBenedictis TJ, Marmar JL, et al.: Urethrographic manifestations of venereal warts (condyloma acuminata). *Radiology* 126:643, 1978.

Russinovich NAE, Lloyd LK, Griggs WP, et al.: Balloon dilatation of urethral strictures. *Urol Radiol* 2:33, 1980.

Scales FE, Katzen BT, van Breda A, et al.: Impassable urethral strictures: percutaneous transvesical catheterization and balloon dilatation. *Radiology* 157:59, 1985.

Shaver WA, Richter PH, Orandi A: Changes in the male urethra produced by instrumentation for transurethral resection of the prostate. *Radiology* 116:623, 1975.

Stern AJ, Patel SK: Diverticulum of the female urethra. *Radiology* 121:222, 1976.

Symes JM, Blandy JP: Tuberculosis of the male urethra. *Br J Urol* 5:432, 1973.

Tines SC, Bigongiari LR, Weigel JW: Carcinoma in diverticulum of the female urethra. *AJR* 138:582, 1982.

Wasserman NF, Reddy PK, Zhang G, et al.: Transurethral balloon dilatation of the prostatic urethra: effectiveness in highly selected patients with prostatism. *AJR* 157:509, 1991.

Yoder IC, Papanicolaou N: Imaging the urethra in men and women. *Urol Radiol* 14:24, 1992.

Penis

Better N, Ahn C-S, Drum DE, et al.: Identification of penile prosthetic infection on 67-gallium scan. *J Urol* 152:475, 1994.

Bookstein JJ, Lang EV: Penile magnification pharmacoarteriography: details of intrapenile arterial anatomy. *AJR* 148:883, 1987.

Cohan RH, Dunnick NR, Carson CC: Radiology of penile prostheses. *AJR* 152:925, 1989.

Delcour C, Wespes E, Vandenbosch G, et al.: Impotence: evaluation with cavernosography. *Radiology* 161:803, 1986.

Frank RG, Gerard PS, Wise GJ: Human penile ossification: a case report and review of the literature. *Urol Radiol* 11:179, 1989.

Fuchs AM, Mehringer CM, Rajfer J: Anatomy of penile venous drainage in potent and impotent men during cavernosography. *J Urol* 141:1353, 1989.

Goldstein I, Krane RM, Greenfield AJ, et al.: Vascular disease of the penis: impotence and priapism. In Pollack HM (ed): *Clinical Urography,* Philadelphia, WB Saunders, 1990.

Gomella LG: Impotence—defining the role of minimally invasive therapy. *J Urol* 155:147, 1996.

Gray R, Grosman H, St. Louis EL, et al.: The uses of corpus cavernosography: a review. *J Can Assoc Radiol* 35:338, 1984.

Hattery RE, King BF Jr, Lewis RW, et al.: Vasculogenic impotence: duplex and color Doppler imaging. *Radiol Clin North Am* 29:629, 1991.

Hovsepian DM, Amis ES: Penile prosthetic implants: a radiographic atlas. *RadioGraphics* 9(4):707, 1989.

Hricak H, Marotti M, Gilbert TJ, et al.: Normal penile anatomy and abnormal penile conditions: evaluation with MR imaging. *Radiology* 169:683, 1988.

Kaneko K, De Mouy EH, Lee BE: Sequential contrast-enhanced MR imaging of the penis. *Radiology* 191:75, 1994.

Krysiewicz S, Mellinger BC: The role of imaging in the diagnostic evaluation of impotence. *AJR* 153:1133, 1989.

Lerner SE, Melman A, Christ GJ: A review of erectile dysfunction: new insights and more questions. *J Urol* 149:1246, 1993.

Malhotra CM, Balko A, Wincze JP, et al.: Cavernosography in conjunction with artificial erection for evaluation of venous leakage in impotent men. *Radiology* 161:799, 1986.

Morgentaler A: Current diagnosis and management of impotence. *Comprehensive Therapy* 17:25, 1991.

Morley JE: Management of impotence. *Postgrad Med* 93:65, 1993.

Mulcahy JJ, Krane RJ, Lloyd LK, et al.: DuraPhase penile prosthesis: results of clinical trials in 63 patients. *J Urol* 143:518, 1990.

Paushter DM: Role of duplex sonography in the evaluation of sexual impotence. *AJR* 153:1161, 1989.

Porst H, van Ahlen H, Vahlensieck W: Relevance of dynamic cavernosography to the diagnosis of venous incompetence in erectile dysfunction. *J Urol* 137:1163, 1987.

Quam JP, King BJ, James EM, et al.: Duplex and color Doppler sonographic evaluation of vasculogenic impotence. *AJR* 153:1141, 1989.

Rajfer J, Canan V, Dorey FJ, Mehringer CM: Correlation between penile angiography and duplex scanning of cavernous arteries in impotent men. *J Urol* 143:1128, 1990.

Rajfer J, Mehringer M: Cavernosography following clinical failure of penile vein ligation for erectile dysfunction. *J Urol* 143:514, 1990.

Rajfer J, Rosciszewski A, Mehringer M: Prevalence of corporeal venous leakage in impotent men. *J Urol* 140:69, 1988.

Schwartz AN, Lowe MA, Ireton R, et al.: A comparison of penile brachial index and angiography: evaluation of corpora cavernosa arterial flow. *J Urol* 143:510, 1990.

St. Louis EL, Gray RR, Grosman H: Simplified technique of internal pudendal angiography in the investigation of impotence. *Cardiovasc Intervent Radiol* 9:22, 1986.

Velcek D, Evans JA: Cavernosography. *Radiology* 144:781, 1982.

Vickers MA, Benson CB, Richie JP: High resolution ultrasonography and pulsed wave Doppler for detection of corporovenous incompetence in erectile dysfunction. *J Urol* 143:125, 1990.

Wespes E, Schulman CC: Venous leakage: surgical treatment of a curable cause of impotence. *J Urol* 133:796, 1985.

Wespes E, Schulman C: Venous impotence: pathophysiology, diagnosis and treatment. *J Urol* 149:1238, 1993.

20

Scrotum and Contents

The most commonly used examination to detect and characterize scrotal and intrascrotal pathology is ultrasound, which is usually performed with color Doppler imaging (Figs. 20.1–20.3). Using surface coils, magnetic resonance imaging (MRI) can produce high-quality images of the scrotum and its contents, but MRI seldom provides important clinical information not obtainable by ultrasound. Computed tomography (CT) is not used to examine the scrotum and its contents, although CT of the lower abdomen may display hernias that extend into the scrotum, and CT is probably the most useful modality to detect abdominal metastases arising from intrascrotal malignancies. Computed tomography also is useful to detect and characterize mediastinal and pulmonary metastatic disease. Radiography of the scrotum is very rarely used as a first-line imaging technique, but it may be used to demonstrate calcifications from old hematomas; high-resolution radiography has occasionally been used to confirm a diagnosis of testicular microlithiasis.

INTRATESTICULAR LESIONS

Testicular Tumors

Testicular cancer accounts for approximately 1% of all cancers in male patients. Testicular tumors may be classified as germ cell tumors, tumors arising from the gonadal stroma, metastases (including lymphoma), and adrenal rest tumors. Germ cell tumors include seminoma, embryonal cell carcinoma, choriocarcinoma, teratoma, and yolk-sac tumors. They may be of single or mixed cell type and constitute approximately 95% of testicular tumors and 5% of male genitourinary tumors. Germ cell tumors are the most common solid tumors of men between 20 to 34 years of age. In adults, 40 to 45% of germ cell tumors are seminomas; in order of decreasing frequency are embryonal carcinoma, choriocarcinoma, teratoma, teratocarcinoma, and other rare tumors. In children, approximately 70% of testis tumors are of germ-cell origin, and, of these, yolk-sac tumors and teratomas comprise about 85%.

There is a strong association between testis tumors and cryptorchidism. Approximately 10% of testis tumors occur in cryptorchid testes, and the risk of a tumor appearing in a cryptorchid testis is more than 30 times greater than for a normal descended testis.

The clinical presentation of testis tumors may involve the detection of an enlarged or mass-containing testis by the patient or his physician. The enlargement often is painless; acute scrotal pain may indicate hemorrhage. In patients with advanced disease, the initial symptoms such as supraclavicular lymphadenopathy, dyspnea, and back pain may be caused by metastases.

Occasionally, testicular tumors may present with metastases, but without a palpable primary tumor in the scrotum; in these cases, ultrasound is particularly important in searching for the primary tumor. Sometimes the primary tumor is "burned out" and is seen as little more than a hyperechoic area or a linear calcification.

Ultrasound of a testis tumor usually reveals the primary lesion to be an intratesticular mass; indeed, deciding whether the mass is in the testis or not is an important step toward determining whether it is a malignancy, because so few extratesticular scrotal lesions are neoplasms. Most testis tumors are shown to be hypervascular by Doppler examination, except cystic and very small tumors. The abnormal vessels are commonly disorganized, but may be relatively regular in configuration with infiltrative tumors such as lymphomas and focal leukemic deposits.

Modalities that directly display testicular parenchymal tissue (ultrasound and MRI) usually reveal a region of

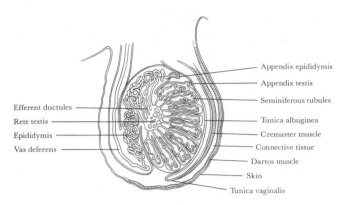

Figure 20.1. Diagram of scrotal and testicular anatomy. (From Amis ES Jr, Newhouse JH: *Essentials of Uroradiology.* Boston, Little, Brown and Co, 1991.)

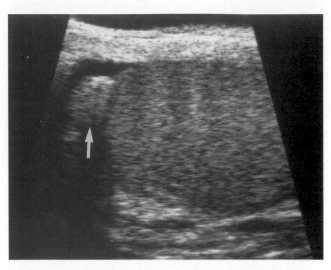

Figure 20.3. Longitudinal sonogram of normal testis, including head of epididymis (*arrow*). Note the homogeneous echo texture. (From Amis ES Jr, Newhouse JH: *Essentials of Uroradiology.* Boston, Little, Brown and Co, 1991.)

normal parenchyma in the involved testis; even if the tumor is quite large, a displaced rim of normal parenchyma can usually be found at some portion of the tumor's periphery. Ultrasound will show this parenchyma to be similar to the contralateral testis in echogenic pattern; MRI will almost always reveal solid tumor tissue to be less intense than the normal parenchyma, which in turn will almost always be identical in intensity to the contralateral testicular tissue. Acute or missed torsion, however, will cause the entire parenchyma of the involved testis to be abnormal. Orchitis may involve the entire testis or may be focal, but when focal, orchitis can usually be distinguished from a tumor by its acute history and tenderness, and by its tendency to appear adjacent to an inflamed epididymis.

Tumors confined to the scrotum are defined as stage I lesions; stage II disease involves lymph nodes inferior to the diaphragm; and stage III disease has metastasized to sites other than retroperitoneal lymph nodes. Staging is usually performed by CT of the abdomen and chest.

Serologic tumor markers, including α-fetoprotein (AFP) and human chorionic gonadotropin (HCG) also are valuable in assessing initial stage and recurrence.

Testis tumors may spread by direct invasion of the epididymis or spermatic cord, by involvement of retroperitoneal nodes, and by hematogenous spread, which usually appears in the lungs. Retroperitoneal nodal involvement often appears first at the approximate level of the renal hila on the left and slightly lower on the right. Inguinal and inferior iliac nodes are usually spared unless the primary tumor has invaded the skin of the scrotum or has recurred in the scrotum after orchiectomy.

Inguinal orchiectomy involves minimal morbidity and functional impairment, and provides excellent local con-

Figure 20.2. Mediastinum testis. **A,** Sagittal section. **B,** Transverse section. The bright linear echo represents the mediastinum testis.

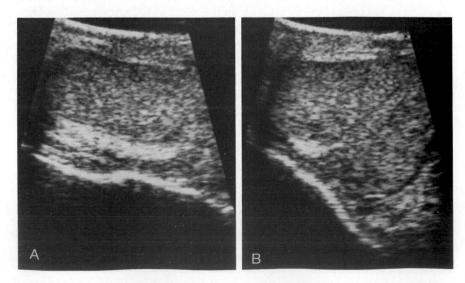

trol of testicular neoplasms. Subsequent treatment depends on the stage and histologic nature of the tumor, and usually involves combinations of external-beam radiation, chemotherapy, and retroperitoneal lymphadenectomy. Seminomas are quite sensitive to radiation therapy and have a cure rate of more than 95% when diagnosis is made before metastases have occurred; lymphadenectomy often is not needed. But nonseminomatous germ-cell tumors are less sensitive to radiation and usually require a combined therapeutic approach. The 5-year survival rate for patients with stage I disease is 90 to 95%.

Seminoma

Seminomas are the most common testicular neoplasm. They account for approximately 40% of all germ cell tumors. Seminomas occur in slightly older men than do other types of testicular tumors; patients often are 30 to 45 years of age.

Ultrasound usually reveals testicular seminomas as intratesticular masses that are less echogenic than the adjacent normal testicular tissue (Figs. 20.4–20.7). They may be discrete and small, or may involve most of the testis. They rarely involve the tunica albuginea, or become necrotic, cystic or hemorrhagic. T2-weighted MR images usually reveal the lesions to be of lower intensity than the normal testes. The lesions often are uniform in appearance, but may be heterogeneous. Lymph node metastases in the retroperitoneum or mediastinum are manifested as nodal enlargement by CT or MRI, which are roughly equivalent in sensitivity. Malignancy in normal-size nodes is extremely difficult to detect. Before CT, bipedal lymphangiography was widely used for staging testicular tumors, but is less frequently employed currently. Some practitioners have suggested that patients who have negative or equivocal CT exam-

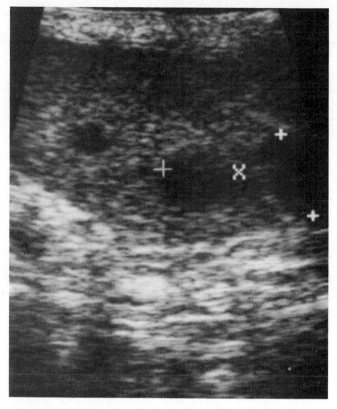

Figure 20.5. Seminoma. Several small hypoechoic foci are appreciated in this 32-year-old man with a testicular seminoma.

inations undergo lymphangiography to attempt to find small tumor deposits.

Other Germ Cell Tumors

Embryonal cell carcinomas account for approximately 30% of germ cell neoplasms and usually occur in

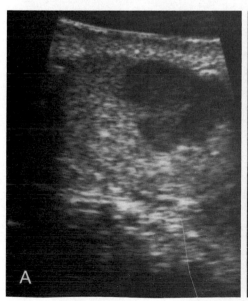

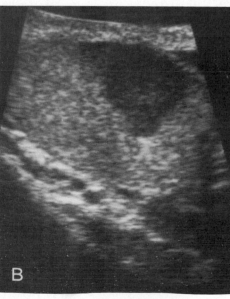

Figure 20.4. Seminoma. **A,** Sagittal and **B,** transverse scans demonstrate well-defined hypoechoic areas corresponding to a 1.5-cm seminoma.

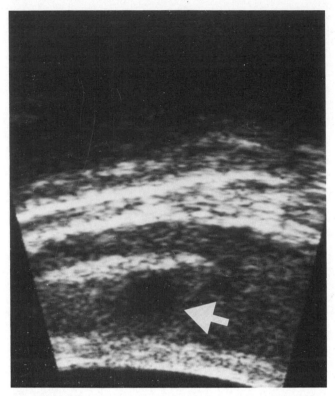

Figure 20.6.   Seminoma. A large seminoma with bleeding was found in this 45-year-old man presenting with a swollen right testicle.

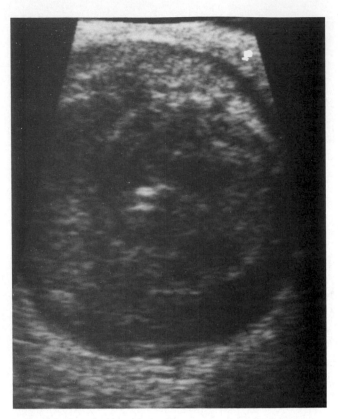

Figure 20.7.   Recurrent seminoma. Five years after orchiectomy for left seminoma, this recurrent seminoma was found in the right testis.

men younger than patients with seminomas. These aggressive tumors may invade the tunica albuginea and may alter the testicular shape. Sonographically, the lesions are poorly circumscribed, hypoechoic, and more likely to be of nonuniform echogenicity than seminomas (Fig. 20.8). They often contain focal areas of increased echogenicity that represent regions of necrosis and hemorrhage, and may demonstrate dense echogenic foci. They are easily detected by MRI, but no specific MRI patterns permit reliable differentiation of different types of testicular tumors.

Choriocarcinoma is less common and accounts for only 2% of testicular tumors. The tumor is aggressive, metastasizes early, and is more likely to present with symptoms from the metastases. The primary lesion may be small; sonography reveals it to be primarily hypoechoic with mixed areas of increased echogenicity due to necrosis, hemorrhage, and calcification.

Most of the remaining germ cell tumors are of mixed histologic pattern and show more than one germ layer. These include teratoma, teratocarcinoma, seminoteratoma, and seminoembryonal cell carcinoma. The most common of these tumors are teratoma and teratocarcinoma.

Teratomas account for 10 to 20% of testicular tumors. They commonly form well-differentiated squamous cystic

lesions containing keratinaceous fatty material, muscle, cartilage, bone, and mucous glandular tissue. These tumors are only rarely poorly differentiated. Although many of these tumors are considered benign, nearly one third of patients may develop metastases within 5 to 10 years of

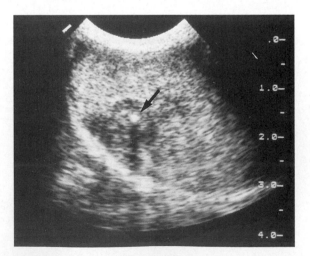

Figure 20.8.   Embryonal cell carcinoma. Longitudinal sonography of testis shows an irregular, hypoechoic tumor nodule with a small, bright echogenic focus (*arrow*) and faint acoustic shadowing. (From Amis ES Jr, Newhouse JH: *Essentials of Uroradiology*. Boston, Little, Brown and Co, 1991.)

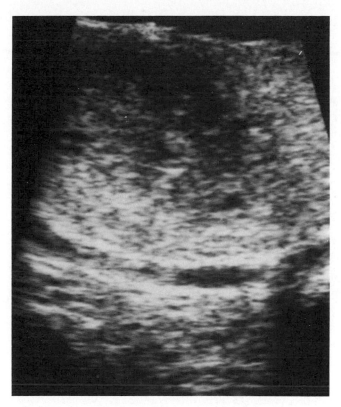

Figure 20.9. Teratocarcinoma. Cystic areas in hyperechoic lesions are seen in this 32-year-old man with teratocarcinoma.

These tumors are usually benign and are rare. On ultrasound, Sertoli cell tumors cause spotty hypoechoic areas, with several associated cysts.

Other rare primary testicular tumors do not arise from germ cells. These include gonadoblastoma, adenocarcinoma of the rete testes, and mesenchymal neoplasms such as fibromas and leiomyomas. Adenomatoid tumors, which are small and benign, may occur in the testis, but are usually found in the epididymis.

Metastatic disease to the testes is more common than germ cell tumors in men older than 50 years of age. Metastases have been reported from primary tumors in the prostate, kidney, lung, gastrointestinal tract, skin, and other sites. Testicular metastases are usually bilateral, multiple, and hypoechoic, although hyperechoic metastases have been observed.

Testicular lymphoma may be primary in the testis without nodal or systemic involvement, or it may be a complication of systemic disease. Lymphoma accounts for 25% of testicular tumors in men older than 50 years of age. Poorly differentiated lymphoma is more likely to be bilateral. Lymphoma may appear as one or more focal hypoechoic regions (Fig. 20.10) or as a diffusely enlarged hypoechoic testis. Patients with leukemia may develop leukemic deposits in the testes, which look similar to the abnormalities seen with lymphoma (Fig. 20.11). In patients with leukemia, the testes may be the

diagnosis. Ultrasonography shows cystic hypoechoic areas with other areas of marked hypoechogenicity.

Teratocarcinoma is a mixture of teratoma and embryonal cell carcinoma, and is slightly less common than seminoma. This tumor is very aggressive, metastasizes early, and may break through the tunica albuginea. It is subject to necrosis and hemorrhage. Ultrasound shows a hypoechoic cystic lesion that is poorly demarcated and may contain areas of increased echogenicity (Fig. 20.9).

Intratesticular papillary adenocarcinoma is a rare cystic malignancy; fewer than 25 cases have been reported. The sonographic findings as reported in one case are that of a well-defined echo-free, multicystic, septated intratesticular lesion. Within the cysts are solid echogenic nodules, some of which develop in the septations.

Nongerminal Testis Tumors

Primary tumors that arise from the gonadal stroma are Leydig cell or Sertoli cell tumors. Leydig cell tumors develop in the interstitial cells of the fibrovascular stroma; they may produce testosterone and therefore may result in increased muscle mass. Leydig cell hyperplasia has been described in the presence of seminoma. Sertoli cell tumors develop from the basement membranes of seminiferous tubules and produce estrogen.

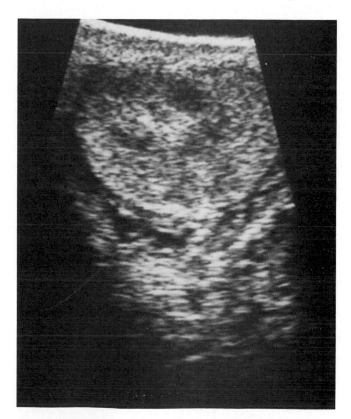

Figure 20.10. Lymphoma. Focal hypoechoic areas are seen within an enlarged testis.

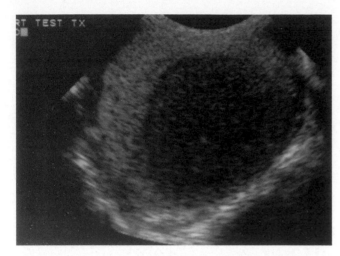

Figure 20.11. Leukemic nodule in testis. Longitudinal ultrasound shows large, hypoechoic nodule almost replacing testis in patient with chronic myelogenous leukemia. (From Amis ES Jr, Newhouse JH: *Essentials of Uroradiology.* Boston, Little, Brown and Co, 1991.)

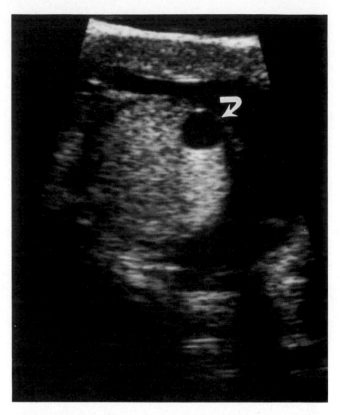

Figure 20.12. Cysts. A well-defined anechoic mass with increased through-transmission in the testis indicates a cyst (*arrow*). A hydrocele also is present.

first site of extramedullary disease and may appear before hematologic relapse.

Rarely, in patients with increased levels of corticotropin (ACTH), adrenal rest tumors of the testes may develop. These may occur in patients with congenital adrenal hyperplasia or primary adrenal insufficiency. They probably represent hypertrophy of ectopic adrenal rests that migrated with the testes during fetal development. The tumors are usually multiple and produce testicular enlargement. On ultrasound, the lesions are eccentrically placed intratesticular hypoechoic nodules, some of which may produce acoustic shadowing. In one case associated with Addison's disease, hyperechoic nodules that also produced acoustic shadowing were seen.

Benign Testicular Conditions

Cysts

Testicular cysts are rare. They are usually idiopathic, but may be postinflammatory or posttraumatic. They arise from efferent ductules of the rete testes and are located peripherally within or adjacent to the mediastinum testis. Their average size is 5 to 7 mm. Histologic examination demonstrates that the cysts are lined by cuboidal or low columnar epithelium and, in some cases, demonstrate cilia. Testicular cysts are not palpable. Ultrasound examination reveals peripheral, well-defined anechoic lesions with normal surrounding testicular echogenicity (Fig. 20.12). Cysts of the rete testis often are accompanied by cysts or other abnormalities of the epididymis.

Ten to twenty percent of benign testicular cysts de-

velop in the tunica albuginea. These cysts are palpable as small (2 to 5 mm) masses at the periphery of the testes. Palpation does not permit distinction of cyst from tumor, but ultrasound examination reveals the typical findings of cysts elsewhere in the testes. When they are adjacent to the epididymis, acoustic enhancement may not be apparent.

Epidermoid cysts of the testes are rare. These cysts usually present as palpable masses and, on ultrasound, are seen as solitary cystic structures with echogenic rims.

Microlithiasis

Testicular microlithiasis is a rare benign condition diagnosed in vivo by ultrasound or by pathologic examination of testicular tissue. It consists of multiple small calcifications, 1 or 2 mm in diameter. They are usually uniformly scattered throughout both testes, but may be predominately in the peripheral portions or even unilateral. Testicular microlithiases are different from the calcifications that occasionally appear within focal testicular lesions. Although often isolated abnormalities, they are frequently found in conjunction with other testicular abnormalities, notably neoplasms. Some authors believe that testicular microlithiases cannot be considered entirely benign. However, it is unclear whether their asso-

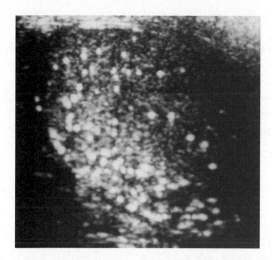

Figure 20.13. Testicular microlithiasis. Multiple small echogenic foci scattered throughout the testis.

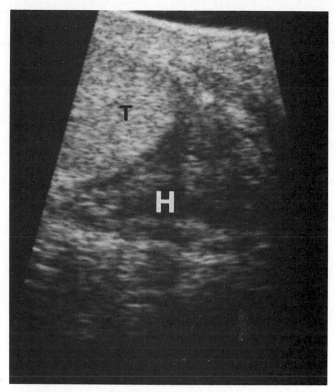

Figure 20.14. Hematoma. A hematoma (*H*) is identified adjacent to the testis (*T*).

ciation with testicular pathology is real, or merely apparent because most patients who have the ultrasound examinations necessary to detect testicular microlithiasis have been referred because they already have known signs or symptoms of the other testicular diseases.

Ultrasound demonstrates multiple small echogenic foci, usually diffusely scattered throughout the testicular parenchyma. (Fig. 20.13) Rarely are they large enough to shadow. There is great variability from patient to patient in the number of foci.

SCROTAL TRAUMA

Testicular trauma is unusual. Testicular rupture results most commonly from athletic injuries, vehicular accidents, and assaults. It often results from compression of the testes between the pubic or ischial bones and an external object. The tunica albuginea ruptures, and hemorrhage occurs into the scrotum. Gross injury to the testicle is an indication for emergency surgery. If surgical intervention occurs within 72 hours, the testis can be saved in approximately 90% of cases, whereas later surgery is associated with a salvage rate of only 55%. Therefore, testicular trauma is an indication for emergency ultrasound examination, which is extremely accurate in diagnosing or excluding testicular hematomas and lacerations.

Testicular rupture or intratesticular hematoma produces focal alterations of the normal testicular echogenicity; the lesions may be hypo- or hyperechoic (Figs. 20.14 and 20.15). A focal region of testicular injury may not be distinguishable from a focal tumor on ultrasonographic grounds alone; the history is necessary. It may be useful to perform serial examinations, because injured regions tend to evolve in appearance, whereas tumors change very slowly.

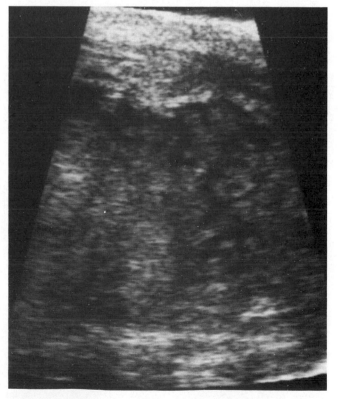

Figure 20.15. Testicular rupture. The testis cannot be visualized, but a large hematoma of mixed echogenicity is seen.

With severe lacerations, it may be impossible to distinguish even a portion of the normal testicular outline or tissue, and only a large mass comprising hematoma and portions of remaining testis and producing an appearance of heterogeneous echogenicity, may be seen. A hydrocele or hematocele may accompany testicular injury; hematoceles may sometimes demonstrate low-level echoes. Traumatic hematomas also may appear in the epididymis and in the scrotal wall. Focal testicular infarction also may accompany trauma and may produce alterations in echogenicity.

TESTICULAR TORSION

Testicular torsion produces acute severe ischemia of the testis, and can present with scrotal pain at any age; most patients are boys or young men. The onset of symptoms is usually spontaneous, but may follow trauma. Normally, the leaves of the tunica vaginalis converge posteriorly, fix the testis, and prevent it from twisting on the spermatic cord. But an anatomic anomaly, known as the "bell-clapper" deformity, may occur in which this fixation is absent. If the testis twists on the spermatic cord, the testicular artery may become occluded. The clinical conditions to be considered in patients with acute painful scrotal swelling include epididymitis, orchitis, acute hydrocele, strangulated inguinal hernia, hemorrhage into a testicle, or fat necrosis of the spermatic cord.

Acute severe testicular ischemia from torsion requires immediate surgery. The testicular salvage rate in the first few hours of symptoms approaches 100%, but decreases rapidly to approximately 20% by 12 to 24 hours. Complete testicular ischemia lasting longer than 24 hours virtually always causes irreversible infarction, which is known as a "missed torsion." When the testis can be salvaged, surgical orchiopexy fixes it to the scrotum. Because the bell-clapper deformity tends to be bilateral,

orchiopexy often is performed bilaterally and may be indicated even for the normal testes in patients who have had missed torsions.

Severe testicular ischemia may be revealed by radionuclide scanning or Doppler ultrasound (Fig. 20.16). If the torsion has been transient and brief, and has been reversed before the examination, radionuclide scan or Doppler ultrasound may be normal. Later, dynamic scintigraphy demonstrates diminished perfusion of the torsed testis, and static images reveal a low-activity "cold" region in the scrotum that reflects the nonperfused testis. Scintigraphy is relatively accurate in making the diagnosis, but a "cold spot" in the scrotum may be produced by a hematoma, tumor or hydrocele, and differential diagnosis may require other examinations. Static ultrasound images may reveal an acutely torsed testis as inhomogeneous and hypoechoic, but it also may appear normal during the first few hours of torsion. Markedly diminished or absent intratesticular flow is demonstrated by Doppler studies, as may be diminished or absent flow in the ipsilateral testicular artery. Rarely, spontaneous reversal of the torsion may produce return of blood flow. Extratesticular findings of torsion include enlargement of the epididymis, thickening of the scrotal skin, and hydrocele; occasionally, a torsed testis may be accompanied by an extratesticular hematoma.

Magnetic resonance imaging may reveal an enlarged spermatic cord in patients with testicular torsion, and the cord may produce a pattern revealing a knot or twisted "whirlpool" pattern.

A missed torsion, while still evolving, may produce scintigraphic findings of a peripheral rim of increased activity surrounding the cold spot of the infarcted testis. However, this finding is nonspecific, because it has been reported with tumor, trauma, and inflammation. Ultrasound usually reveals a chronic torsed testis to be small and echopenic.

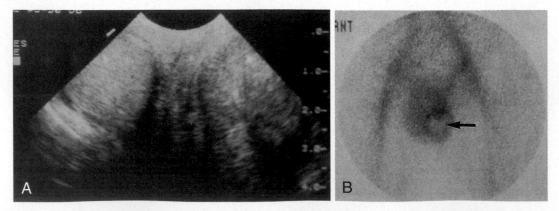

Figure 20.16. Acute testicular torsion. **A,** Transverse scrotal sonography shows the left testis to be slightly inhomogeneous and hypoechoic as compared with the normal right testis. **B,** Static scintigraphy demonstrates a "cold" defect in the region of the left testis (*arrow*). (From Amis ES Jr, Newhouse JH: *Essentials of Uroradiology*. Boston, Little, Brown and Co, 1991.)

UNDESCENDED TESTES

The embryonal gonad descends to the internal inguinal ring. Descent through the inguinal ring is guided by the gubernaculum, which leads the testicle into the scrotum. This process occurs between the 34th and 36th week of fetal life. Premature infants, therefore, have a high incidence (approximately 30%) of undescended testicle at birth; the incidence is about 3.5% in full-term babies, and spontaneous descent after birth reduces the prevalence to only about 1% at the age of 1 year. Approximately 10% of cases of undescended testes are bilateral. Although 75% of undescended testes are found in the inguinal canal, the descent may be arrested at any level, and the testicle may be found within the abdominal cavity from the level of the kidneys to the pelvis.

Normal testicular development occurs only if the testicle is in the scrotum. Undescended testes are sterile and have high incidences of malignant change, especially when they are within the abdomen. Consequently, orchiopexy is usually performed at about 1 year of age. In patients who are beyond the age of puberty, an undescended testis is usually resected to avoid malignancy.

In many cases, the undescended testis lies high in the scrotum, is palpable, and does not require imaging. Undescended testes that lie within the inguinal canal can be detected by ultrasound or CT. Intraabdominal testes may be imaged by CT, MRI, arteriography, or venography, but not infrequently elude imaging detection altogether.

Ultrasound accurately localizes undescended testes in more than 90% of cases when the organ is in or near the inguinal canal. The examination should begin with the scrotum in order to identify the normal descended testis. On the abnormal side, the empty scrotum is examined, and the inguinal canal, where the undescended testis is commonly found, should be scrutinized. The undescended testis is usually smaller and more elongated than the normal testis, but has similar echogenicity. The mediastinum testis in the undescended testis must be identified, because the bulbous end of the gubernaculum (pars infravaginalis gubernaculi) may be of similar size and echogenicity as the testis; only the identification of the mediastinum testis reliably identifies a structure as a testicle.

The reported sensitivity of CT in the detection of undescended testes in or near the inguinal canal is excellent. An ovoid mass of soft tissue density is seen along the line of testicular descent (Fig. 20.17); the mass usually enhances very little with intravenous contrast medium. Intraabdominal testes may be missed by this modality and, for that matter, by all others.

Magnetic resonance imaging also may be used to localize undescended testes. Cryptorchid testes have similar tissue signal intensities (medium to low on T1-weighted spin-echo examinations; bright on T2-weighted spin-echo examinations) as normal testes.

Gonadal venography was used for many years to localize undescended testes. Identification of the pampiniform plexus permits identification of the testicular site, and a blind-ending internal spermatic vein suggests that the testis is absent. These criteria are not completely accurate, however, and valves in the gonadal vein may prevent contrast medium from reaching the most terminal portion of the vein. Gonadal venography is currently only infrequently used for localization of undescended testes.

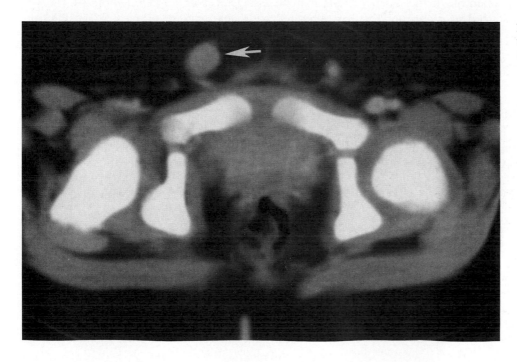

Figure 20.17. Undescended testis. The right testis is seen (*arrow*) in the inguinal canal.

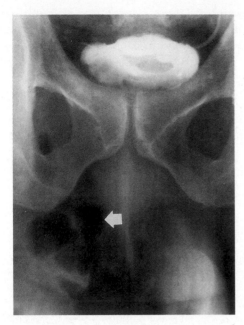

Figure 20.18. Inguinal hernia. Multiple loops of small bowel (*arrow*) are noted within the scrotum on a postvoid radiograph from an excretory urogram.

EXTRATESTICULAR SCROTAL PATHOLOGY

Hernia

Hernias containing structures normally found within the abdomen frequently extend through the inguinal canal into the scrotum. If bowel loops are in the hernia, air or contrast medium may be seen within them on plain-film radiography (Fig. 20.18) or CT. Ultrasound examination usually reveals the intrascrotal portion of gut to undergo peristalsis, and to contain air. If the hernia contains fat, it can usually be detected by ultrasound or CT; however, the hernia may be difficult to distinguish from a spermatic cord lipoma.

If the bladder extends into the scrotum, it may be diagnosed if the intrascrotal portion is opacified on urography, or if it can be seen to be continuous with the main portion of the bladder at CT. Ultrasound of portions of the bladder that extend into the scrotum may be confusing, however, because the urine within the bladder may be difficult to distinguish from a hydrocele.

Hydrocele

A hydrocele is an abnormal collection of fluid between the visceral and parietal layers of the tunica vaginalis. It may be congenital or acquired. A congenital hydrocele is usually caused by a patent communication between the peritoneum and the processus vaginalis. A hydrocele is not uncommon in premature infants, and may be demonstrated in the male fetus after 30 weeks gestation. Normally, the communication closes and the hydrocele resolves late in gestation. A persistent hydro-

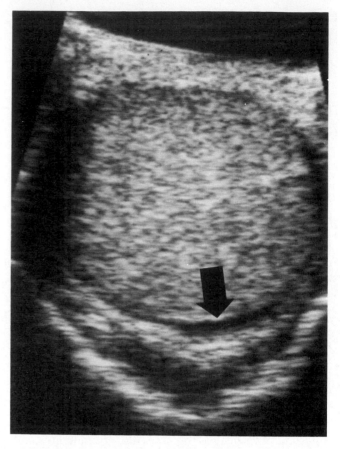

Figure 20.19. Hydrocele. Small hydroceles (*arrow*) are found in as many as 60% of normal males.

cele often indicates persistence of the communication, and may be associated with an inguinal hernia.

Acquired hydrocele may be primary (idiopathic), in which case it is usually insidious in onset. Small hydroceles may be present in more than 60% of otherwise normal men. Hydroceles are less frequently secondary to inflammatory disease, tumor, or trauma. Hydroceles secondary to trauma also may contain blood and may be termed a hematocele; hydroceles due to inflammation may contain pus.

The common type of small idiopathic hydrocele (Fig. 20.19) usually involves only a fraction of the testicular circumference. A large hydrocele (Fig. 20.20) may surround the entire testis, but usually can be seen posterolaterally, where the tunica vaginalis invests the testis and epididymis. Occasionally, thin septae can be demonstrated within a hydrocele. Low-level echoes may indicate blood, pus, or necrotic debris.

Epididymal Cysts

Epididymal cysts are caused by dilatation of the tubules in the epididymis. They may be small and multiple, but also may range up to several centimeters in di-

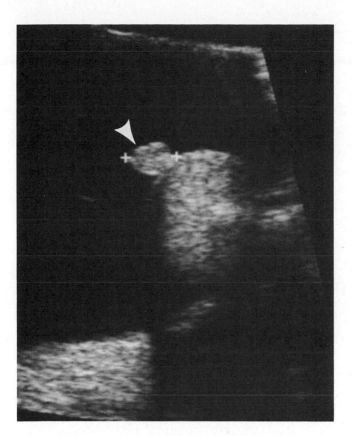

Figure 20.20.   Hydrocele. A large hydrocele almost completely surrounds the testis. The appendix testis is seen (*arrowhead*) projecting off the testis.

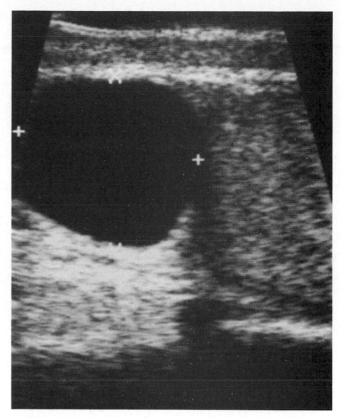

Figure 20.21.   Spermatocele. A large cystic mass in the region of the epididymis is consistent with a spermatocele, but cannot be distinguished from an epididymal cyst.

ameter. Epididymal cysts contain serous fluid and may occur anywhere within the epididymis.

Spermatoceles usually represent retention cysts of the small tubules in the epididymal head and may be loculated. They contain thicker sperm-filled fluid than that found in serous epididymal cysts. Both epididymal cysts and spermatoceles (Fig. 20.21) may be unilateral or bilateral, and are usually palpated as extratesticular masses posterior to the testes. Cystic replacement of the epididymis is rare, but has been reported after vasectomy.

Ultrasound examinations show these lesions to be well-defined anechoic structures with enhanced through-transmission. They can usually be distinguished from hydrocele by their position. A hydrocele surrounds the testis, usually anteriorly, whereas epididymal cysts and spermatoceles lie in the epididymis superior or posterior to the testis. Spermatoceles and epididymal cysts usually cannot be distinguished, but occasionally a spermatocele may have a few internal echoes.

Varicocele

Varicoceles consist of dilated veins draining the testis. The dilation usually involves the pampiniform plexus, which is the main venous drainage of the testis, and also

has been reported to occur in the cremasteric plexus, which drains the epididymis and the scrotal wall. Primary varicoceles are idiopathic, whereas secondary varicoceles usually result from incompetent valves in the left spermatic (gonadal) vein. Rarely, they indicate left spermatic vein occlusion, such as may occur with extension of a renal tumor into the left renal vein. Ten to twenty percent of healthy men have a varicocele, and up to 50% of men evaluated for infertility have varicoceles. Bilateral varicoceles are common in infertile men. The causal relationships between varicoceles in male infertility are not certain. Increased scrotal temperature, preferential drainage of renal or adrenal metabolites to the testis, testicular hypoxemia, and inefficient testicular hormone production all have been postulated. Because many varicoceles in infertile men cannot be palpated, they should be sought with imaging. Doppler ultrasound, spermatic venography, and radionuclide scanning have been proposed. Surgical varicocelectomy often is followed by an improvement in sperm quality and increased fertility.

High-resolution real-time Doppler ultrasound is an excellent method for demonstrating varicocele. Small varicoceles may be made more visible by examining the pa-

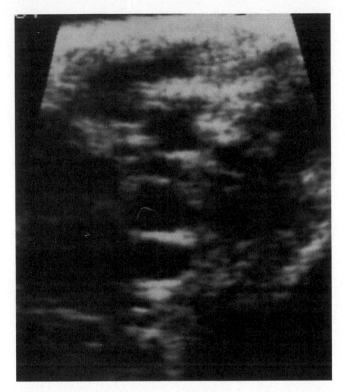

Figure 20.22. Varicocele. A serpiginous, fluid-containing structure is consistent with varicocele.

tient in the upright position or by using the Valsalva maneuver in the supine position. Small varicoceles may be demonstrated as serpentine, tubular, elongated anechoic fluid collections in the spermatic cord adjacent to the testis (Fig. 20.22). These veins usually measure more than 3 mm in diameter and should increase in caliber with a Valsalva maneuver. Doppler ultrasound may reveal antegrade flow, stasis, or retrograde flow. The lesions and their component veins may be large. On occasion, varicoceles may mimic other multicystic extratesticular masses, such as spermatoceles, but demonstration of flow should remove nonvascular lesions from consideration.

Spermatic venography is reserved for men who require surgical intervention for varicocele-associated infertility or other symptoms. Because of the frequency of bilateral varicoceles, both sides should be studied; either a transfemoral or transjugular approach can be used to catheterize the internal spermatic vein. The left vein drains into the left renal vein, whereas the right vein usually empties directly into the inferior vena cava slightly inferior to the renal veins. When the valves are incompetent, a hand injection of contrast medium usually demonstrates retrograde flow down the spermatic vein into the pampiniform plexus and varicocele. Anomalies in course and number are common. There may be collaterals through which contrast medium passes into the cremasteric vein, the vein of the vas def-

erens, or both, finally emptying into a common iliac vein and the inferior vena cava.

Angiographic techniques permit occlusion of the internal spermatic vein as an alternative to surgical ligation. Agents used have included sclerosing solutions, stainless steel coils, compressed Ivalon (Ivalon Inc., San Diego, CA) plugs, and detachable balloons. The demonstration of multiple collaterals occasionally makes angiographic techniques impractical, but, if they are performed, the recurrence rate of varicocele (which is approximately 10%) is comparable to the rate that follows surgical ligation of the internal spermatic vein.

Radioisotope examination with technetium-99m–pertechnetate demonstrates many clinically palpable varicoceles. The dynamic study provides an isotope angiogram demonstrating increased uptake in the varicocele. Stasis may be demonstrated by increased uptake in the late static images. There are sources of error with these techniques: there may be no blood pooling in small subclinical varicoceles, and the asymmetry that constitutes an abnormal sign in scintigraphy may not be detectable in patients with bilateral varicoceles.

INFLAMMATORY LESIONS

Epididymitis and Orchitis

Epididymitis is the most common inflammatory process in the scrotum. Adolescents and middle-aged men, especially those who have undergone prostatectomy, are most commonly affected. The condition is rare in children. Epididymitis is accompanied by orchitis in a minority of cases. Orchitis alone may be caused by the mumps virus or syphilis.

The most common pathogens causing epididymitis are *Escherichia coli, Pseudomonas sp.,* and *Aerobacter sp.;* gonococcal urethritis also may progress to epididymitis. The epididymis also may be infected by schistosomiasis and tuberculosis.

Acute epididymitis presents as acute pain and tenderness in the scrotum. The patient may present with fever, dysuria, and pyuria with urethral discharge. It may be difficult to distinguish epididymitis from acute torsion, and, rarely, testicular tumor may have a similar initial presentation.

Ultrasound examination reveals that the head and body of the epididymis are enlarged and of altered echogenicity (Fig. 20.23). The echogenicity is usually decreased, but epididymitis also may present with hyperechoic regions in the epididymal head. The entire epididymis or only a part may be affected. A reactive hydrocele often is associated. A focal region of very low or absent echoes suggests an epididymal abscess. Doppler evidence of increased flow may be seen in the epididymis.

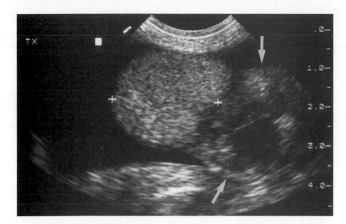

Figure 20.23. Epididymitis. Transverse sonography shows the testis (*defined by markers*) to be normal. The epididymis (*arrow*) is grossly enlarged and inhomogeneous. (From Amis ES Jr, Newhouse JH: *Essentials of Uroradiology.* Boston, Little, Brown and Co, 1991.)

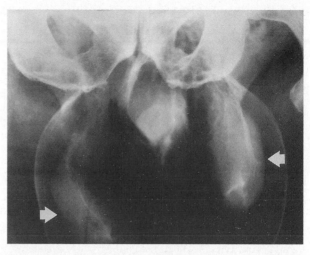

Figure 20.25. Fournier's gangrene. A plain radiograph of the pelvis demonstrates an air-filled scrotum outlining the testicles (*arrows*).

When orchitis coexists with epididymitis, the testicle is enlarged and of reduced echogenicity (Fig. 20.24). Focal orchitis is less common than involvement of the entire testis, but it may occur immediately adjacent to the inflamed epididymis. The inflamed regions may display increased flow on Doppler examination. Focal areas of markedly reduced echogenicity within the testis indicate abscesses. Chronic epididymitis, which may present clinically as a painless nodular mass on palpation, may appear relatively hypoechoic on ultrasound examination.

On radionuclide studies, increased perfusion through the spermatic cord vessels is visualized as linear or curved areas of increased activity in the region of the epididymis.

A complication of severe acute epididymitis is ischemia of the testis, sometimes followed by infarction, which is caused by compression of the testicular vessels from epididymal swelling.

Superficial Inflammation

Occasionally, infection of the skin and superficial layers of the scrotum may be a complication of epididymoorchitis, or may result from infection or trauma to the scrotum that extends deep to the skin. Ultrasound may help diagnose or exclude inflammation of the testis or epididymis in these cases.

Fournier's Gangrene

A rare but fulminant necrotizing fasciitis of the penis, scrotum and perineum was described by Fournier in 1883. Predisposing conditions include diabetes mellitus, paraplegia, and alcohol abuse. Most patients have had an underlying urinary tract infection, recent urologic instrumentation, or perirectal or colonic disease. The condition may progress rapidly to extensive gangrene and may require vigorous antibiotic therapy and surgical debridement. The diagnosis usually does not require imaging, but subcutaneous emphysema may be seen on plain film radiographs (Fig. 20.25) or CT.

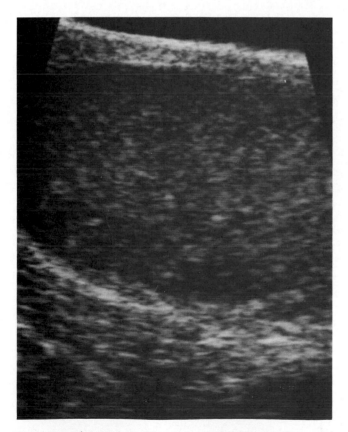

Figure 20.24. Orchitis. The testis is enlarged with decreased echogenicity.

SUGGESTED READINGS

Amendola MA, Casillas J, Joseph R, et al.: Fournier's gangrene: CT findings. *Abdom Imaging* 19:471, 1994.

Atkinson GO Jr., Patrick EL, Ball TI, Jr., et al.: The normal and abnormal scrotum in children: evaluation with color Doppler sonography. *AJR* 158:613, 1992.

Backus ML, Mack LA, Middleton WD, et al.: Testicular microlithiasis: Imaging appearance and pathologic correlation. *Radiology* 192:781, 1994.

Baker LI, Hajek PC, Burkhard TK, et al.: MR imaging of the scrotum: normal anatomy. *Radiology* 163:89, 1987.

Baker LI, Hajek PC, Burkhard TK, et al.: MR imaging of the scrotum: pathologic conditions. *Radiology* 163:93, 1987.

Benson CB, Doubilet PM, Richie JP: Sonography of the male genital tract. *AJR* 153:705, 1989.

Brown DL, Benson CB, Doherty FJ, et al.: Cystic testicular mass caused by dilated rete testis: sonographic findings in 31 cases. *AJR* 158:1257, 1992.

Brown JM, Hammers LW, Rosenfield AT: Scrotal ultrasound 1995: part 1, anatomy and acute disease. *Applied Radiology* 24(7):28, 1995.

Brown JM, Hammers LW, Rosenfield AT: Scrotal ultrasound 1995: part 2, imaging of the nonacute scrotum. *Applied Radiology* 24(8):23, 1995.

Burks DD, Markey BJ, Burkhard TK, et al.: Suspected testicular torsion and ischemia: evaluation with color Doppler sonography. *Radiology* 175:815, 1990.

Comiter CV, Benson CJ, Capelouto CC, et al.: Nonpalpable intratesticular masses detected sonographically. *J Urol* 154:1367, 1995.

Cramer BM, Schlegel EA, Thueroff JW: MR imaging in the differential diagnosis of scrotal and testicular disease. *RadioGraphics* 11:9, 1991.

Dewire DM, Begun FP, Lawson RK, et al.: Color Doppler ultrasonography in the evaluation of the acute scrotum. *J Urol* 147:89, 1992.

Dunn EK, Macchia RJ, Solomon NA: Scintigraphic pattern in missed testicular torsion. *Radiology* 139:175, 1981.

Fan CM, Whitman GJ, Chew FS: Necrotizing fasciitis of the scrotum (Fournier's Gangrene). *AJR* 166:1164, 1996.

Friedland GW, Chang P: The role of imaging in the management of the impalpable undescended testis. *AJR* 151:1107, 1988.

Fritzsche PJ, Hricak H, Kogan BA, et al.: Undescended testis: value of MR imaging. *Radiology* 164:169, 1987.

Gooding GAW: Sonography of the spermatic cord. *AJR* 151:721, 1988.

Gooding GAW, Leonhardt W, Stein R: Testicular cysts: US findings. *Radiology* 163:537, 1987.

Hamm B, Fobbe F, Loy V: Testicular cysts: Differentiation with US and clinical findings. *Radiology* 168:19, 1988.

Horstman WG, Middleton WD, Melson GL: Color Doppler US of the scrotum. *RadioGraphics* 11:941, 1991.

Horstman WG, Middleton WD, Melson GL: Scrotal inflammatory disease: color Doppler US findings. *Radiology* 179:55, 1991.

Janzen DL, Mathieson JR, Marsh JI, et al.: Testicular microlithiasis: sonographic and clinical features. *AJR* 158:1057, 1992.

Jarvis JL, Dubbins PA: Changes in the epididymis after vasectomy: sonographic findings. *AJR* 152:531, 1989.

Joyce JM, Grossman ST: Scrotal scintigraphy in testicular torsion. *Focus on Radiology* Part II 10(1), 1992.

Kim SH, Pollack HM, Cho KS, et al.: Tuberculous epididymitis and epididymo-orchitis: sonographic findings. *J Urol* 150:81, 1993.

Leibovitch I, Foster RS, Kopecky KK, et al.: Improved accuracy of computerized tomography based clinical staging in low stage nonseminomatous germ cell cancer using size criteria of retroperitoneal lymph nodes. *J Urol* 154:1759, 1995.

Lupetin AR, King W, Rich P, Lederman RB: Ultrasound diagnosis of testicular leukemia. *Radiology* 146:171, 1983.

Middleton WD, Siegel BA, Melson GL, et al.: Acute scrotal disorders: Prospective comparison of color Doppler US and testicular scintigraphy. *Radiology* 177:177, 1990.

Middleton WD, Melson GL: Testicular ischemia: color Doppler sonographic findings in five patients. *AJR* 152:1237, 1989.

Mueller DL, Amundson GM, Rubin SZ, Wesenberg RL: Acute scrotal abnormalities in children: diagnosis by combined sonography and scintigraphy. *AJR* 150:643, 1988.

Petros JA, Andriole GL, Middleton WD: Correlation of testicular color Doppler ultrasonography, physical examination and venography in the detection of left varicoceles in men with infertility. *Urology* 145:785, 1991.

Ralls PW, Jensen MC, Lee KP: Color Doppler sonography in acute epididymitis and orchitis. *J Clin Ultrasound* 18:383, 1990.

Rozanski TA, Bloom DA: The undescended testis: theory and management. *Urol Clin North Am* 22:107, 1995.

Rholl KS, Lee JKT, Heiken JP, et al.: MR imaging of the scrotum with a high resolution surface coil. *Radiology* 163:99, 1987.

Rifkin MD: Inflammation of the lower urinary tract: the prostate, seminal vesicles and scrotum. In Pollack HM (ed): *Clinical Urography*. Philadelphia, WB Saunders, 1990.

Rifkin MD: Scrotal ultrasound. *Urol Radiol* 9:119, 1987.

Seidenwurm D, Smathers RL, Kan P, et al.: Intratesticular adrenal rests diagnosed by ultrasound. *Radiology* 155:479, 1985.

Seidenwurm D, Smathers RL, Lo RK, et al.: Testes and scrotum: MR imaging at 1.5 T. *Radiology* 164:393, 1987.

Sheinfeld J: Nonseminomatous germ cell tumors of the testis: current concepts and controversies. *Urology* 44:2, 1994.

Smith SJ, Vogelzang RL, Smith WM, et al.: Papillary adenocarcinoma of the rete testis: sonographic findings. *AJR* 148:1147, 1987.

Spirnak JP, Resnick MI, Hampel N, et al.: Fournier's gangrene: report of 20 patients. *J Urol* 131:289, 1984.

Steinfeld AD: Testicular germ cell tumors: review of contemporary evaluation and management. *Radiology* 175:603, 1990.

Sussman EB, Hadju SI, Lieberman PH, et al.: Malignant lymphoma of the testis: a clinicopathologic study of 37 cases. *J Urol* 118:1004, 1977.

Thurnher S, et al.: Imaging the testis: comparison between MR imaging and US. *Radiology* 167:631, 1988.

Trambert MA, Mattrey RF, Levine D, et al.: Subacute scrotal pain: evaluation of torsion versus epididymitis with MR imaging. *Radiology* 175:53, 1990.

Tumeh SS, Benson CB, Richie JP: Acute diseases of the scrotum. *Semin Ultrasound CT MR* 12(2):115, 1991.

Wilbert DM, Schaerfe CW, Stern WD, et al.: Evaluation of the acute scrotum by color-coded Doppler ultrasonography. *J Urol* 149:1475, 1993.

Winter TC III, Zunkel DE, Mack LA: Testicular carcinoma in a patient with previously demonstrated testicular microlithiasis. *J Urol* 155:648, 1996.

Index

Note: Page numbers in *italics* indicate figures; page numbers followed by t indicate tables.